Imaging in
SPINE
SURGERY

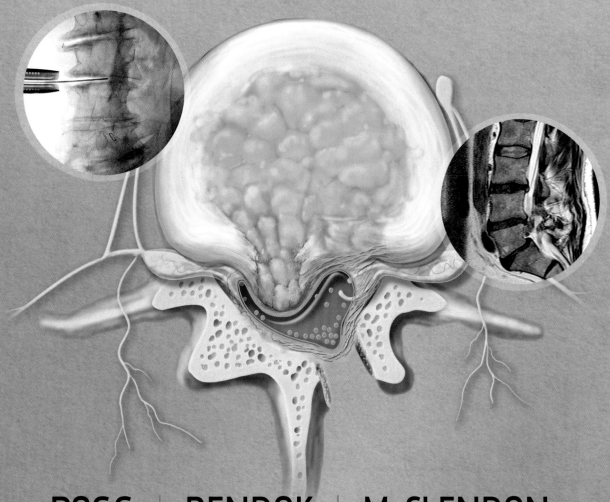

ROSS | BENDOK | McCLENDON

ELSEVIER

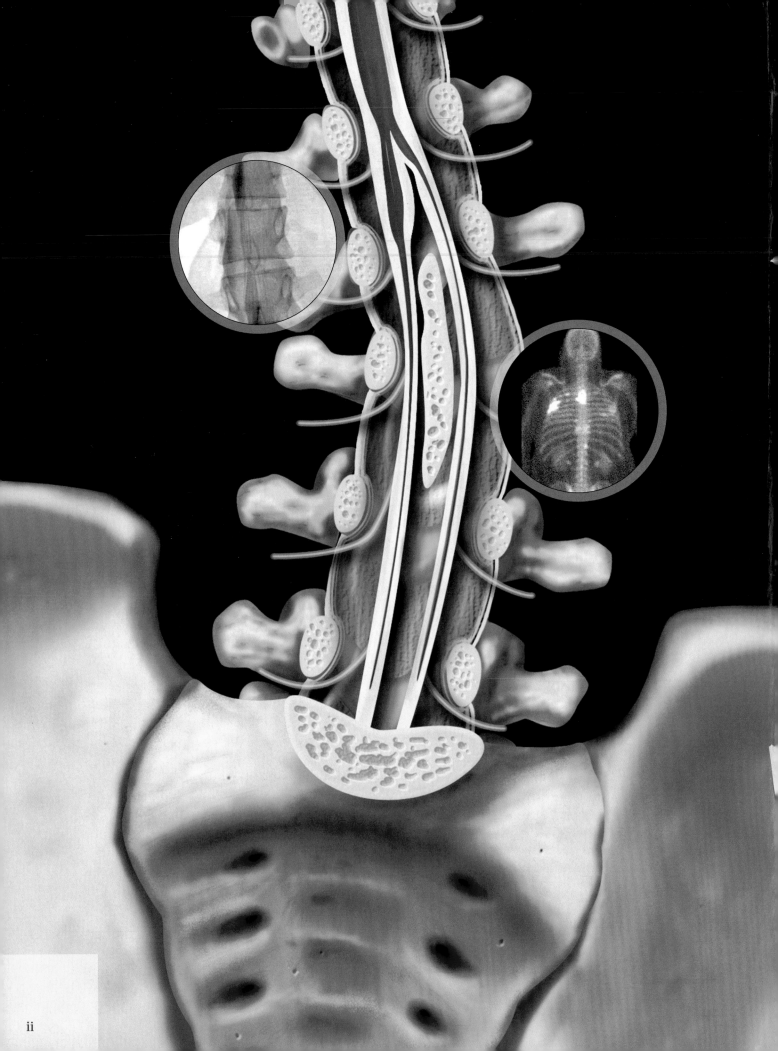

Imaging in
SPINE
SURGERY

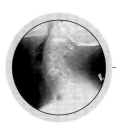

Jeffrey S. Ross, MD

Senior Associate Consultant
Neuroradiology Division
Department of Radiology
Mayo Clinic Arizona
Professor of Radiology
Mayo Clinic College of Medicine
Phoenix, Arizona

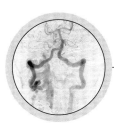

Bernard R. Bendok, MD, FAANS

Chair, Neurologic Surgery
William J. and Charles H. Mayo Professor
Professor of Neurosurgery, Radiology, and Otolaryngology
Mayo Clinic Arizona
Phoenix, Arizona

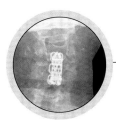

Jamal McClendon, Jr., MD

Senior Associate Consultant
Neurological Surgery
Mayo Clinic Arizona
Phoenix, Arizona

ELSEVIER

1600 John F. Kennedy Blvd.
Ste 1800
Philadelphia, PA 19103-2899

IMAGING IN SPINE SURGERY

ISBN: 978-0-323-48554-8

Notices

Knowledge and best practice in this field are constantly changing. As new research and experience broaden our understanding, changes in research methods, professional practices, or medical treatment may become necessary.

Practitioners and researchers must always rely on their own experience and knowledge in evaluating and using any information, methods, compounds, or experiments described herein. In using such information or methods they should be mindful of their own safety and the safety of others, including parties for whom they have a professional responsibility.

With respect to any drug or pharmaceutical products identified, readers are advised to check the most current information provided (i) on procedures featured or (ii) by the manufacturer of each product to be administered, to verify the recommended dose or formula, the method and duration of administration, and contraindications. It is the responsibility of practitioners, relying on their own experience and knowledge of their patients, to make diagnoses, to determine dosages and the best treatment for each individual patient, and to take all appropriate safety precautions.

To the fullest extent of the law, neither the Publisher nor the authors, contributors, or editors, assume any liability for any injury and/or damage to persons or property as a matter of products liability, negligence or otherwise, or from any use or operation of any methods, products, instructions, or ideas contained in the material herein.

Publisher Cataloging-in-Publication Data

Names: Ross, Jeffrey S. (Jeffrey Stuart) | Bendok, Bernard R. | McClendon, Jamal, Jr.
Title: Imaging in spine surgery / [edited by] Jeffrey S. Ross, Bernard R. Bendok, and Jamal McClendon, Jr.
Description: First edition. | Salt Lake City, UT : Elsevier, Inc., [2017] | Includes bibliographical references and index.
Identifiers: ISBN 978-0-323-48554-8
Subjects: LCSH: Spine--Surgery--Handbooks, manuals, etc. | Spine--Imaging--Handbooks, manuals, etc. | MESH: Spine--surgery--Atlases. | Spine--anatomy & histology--Atlases. | Spine--radiography--Atlases. | Spinal Diseases--diagnosis--Atlases.
Classification: LCC RD768.I43 2017 | NLM WE 725 | DDC 617.3'7507548--dc23

International Standard Book Number: 978-0-323-48554-8

Cover Designer: Tom M. Olson, BA

Printed in Canada by Friesens, Altona, Manitoba, Canada

Last digit is the print number: 9 8 7 6 5 4 3 2 1

Dedications

Wise words bring many benefits,
And hard work brings rewards.
                    ~ Proverbs 12:14
JR

To my parents, wife, and children.
BB

To my family.
JM

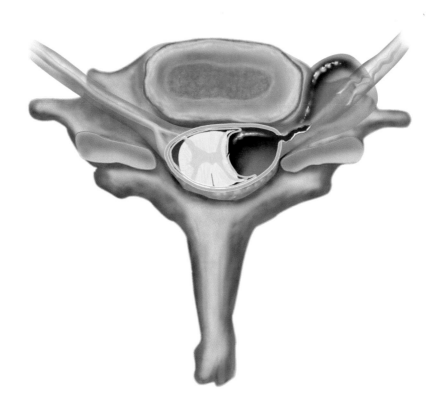

Contributing Authors

Bryson Borg, MD
Chief of Neuroradiology
David Grant Medical Center
Travis Air Force Base, California

Michael P. Federle, MD, FACR
Professor and Associate Chair for Education
Department of Radiology
Stanford University School of Medicine
Stanford, California

Bronwyn E. Hamilton, MD
Professor of Radiology
Director of Head & Neck Radiology
Oregon Health & Science University
Portland, Oregon

R. Brooke Jeffrey, MD
Professor and Vice Chairman
Department of Radiology
Stanford University School of Medicine
Stanford, California

Donald V. La Barge, III, MD
Adjunct Assistant Professor of Radiology
Diagnostic and Interventional Neuroradiology
University of Utah School of Medicine
Salt Lake City, Utah
Assistant Professor of Radiology
Uniformed Services University of the Health Sciences
Bethesda, Maryland

Kevin R. Moore, MD
Pediatric Neuroradiology
Intermountain Pediatric Imaging
Primary Children's Hospital
Salt Lake City, Utah

Anne G. Osborn, MD, FACR

University Distinguished Professor
William H. and Patricia W. Child Presidential Endowed Chair
University of Utah School of Medicine
Salt Lake City, Utah

C. Douglas Phillips, MD, FACR

Professor of Radiology
Director of Head and Neck Imaging
Weill Cornell Medical College
NewYork-Presbyterian Hospital
New York, New York

Lubdha M. Shah, MD

Associate Professor of Radiology
Division of Neuroradiology
University of Utah School of Medicine
Salt Lake City, Utah

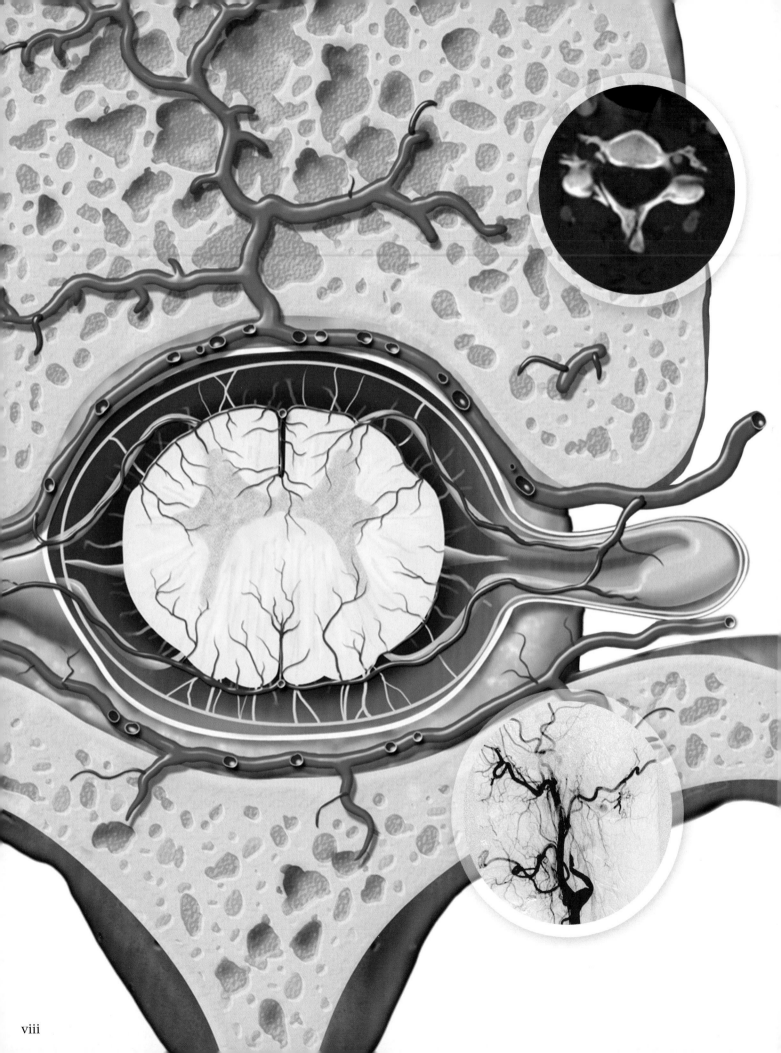

Preface

The spine is complicated, the variety of pathologies legion, and you are busy. Where can you go for up-to-date, easily accessible information regarding spine imaging? Look no further!

This book's purpose is to provide key imaging findings for the most common and important spine surgical disorders in an easy-to-understand format, using typical imaging examples, pathologic examples when appropriate, and spectacular illustrations that demonstrate key findings.

This book covers a wide variety of pathologic conditions with sections on congenital and genetic disorders, disorders of alignment, trauma, degenerative arthritides, infection and inflammation, neoplasms, vascular disorders, and peripheral nerve and plexus diseases. There are overview chapters to problematic subjects like scoliosis, fracture classifications, degenerative disc disease nomenclature, surgical complications, and instrumentation. There are anatomic overviews of the cervical, thoracic, lumbar, and sacral spine as well as craniovertebral junction, vascular anatomy, and brachial and lumbar plexus. The wide variety of common image-guided procedures are also covered, including epidural, nerve root, and facet injections, as well as more complicated procedures such as kyphoplasty/vertebroplasty and percutaneous discectomy.

Each chapter is written to point out the main imaging findings for each disorder or anatomic area. Then, the key clinical features are addressed. The organization of each chapter makes it easy for a surgeon to quickly know the key terminology, imaging findings, pathologic underpinnings, and important clinical details. The images were specifically chosen to be classic examples with the liberal use of arrows describing the key findings.

We see this book being of value to every practicing surgeon or physician who sees patients with spine pathology. Additionally, we see residents using this book to study for board and in-service examinations.

We hope you find this resource of value in providing ongoing care to your patients.

Jeffrey S. Ross, MD
Senior Associate Consultant
Neuroradiology Division
Department of Radiology
Mayo Clinic Arizona
Professor of Radiology
Mayo Clinic College of Medicine
Phoenix, Arizona

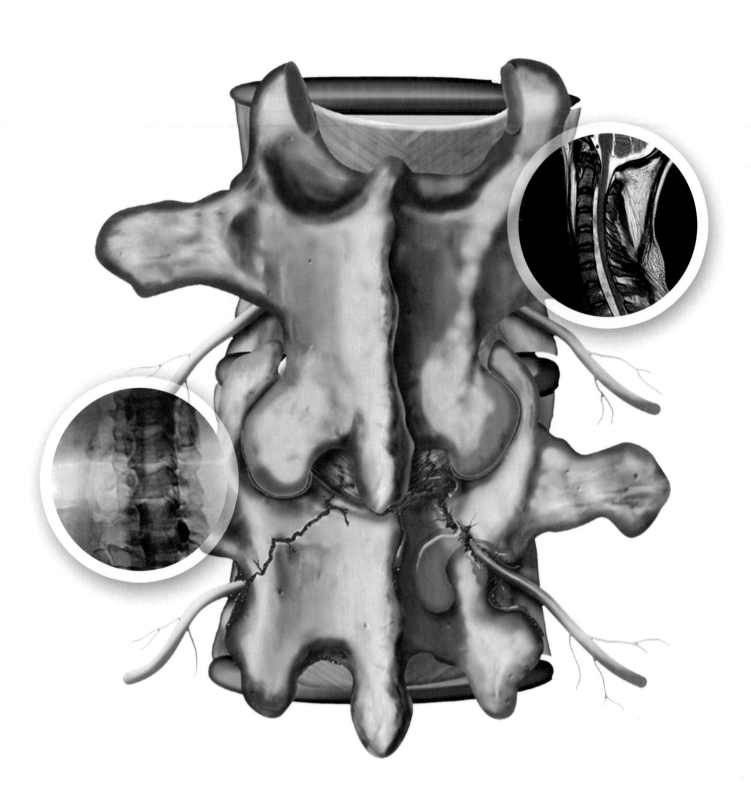

Acknowledgments

Text Editors

Arthur G. Gelsinger, MA
Terry W. Ferrell, MS
Lisa A. Gervais, BS
Karen E. Concannon, MA, PhD
Matt W. Hoecherl, BS
Megg Morin, BA

Image Editors

Jeffrey J. Marmorstone, BS
Lisa A. M. Steadman, BS

Illustrations

Lane R. Bennion, MS
Richard Coombs, MS
Laura C. Sesto, MA

Art Direction and Design

Tom M. Olson, BA
Laura C. Sesto, MA

Lead Editor

Nina I. Bennett, BA

Production Coordinators

Angela M.G. Terry, BA
Rebecca L. Hutchinson, BA
Emily C. Fassett, BA

ELSEVIER

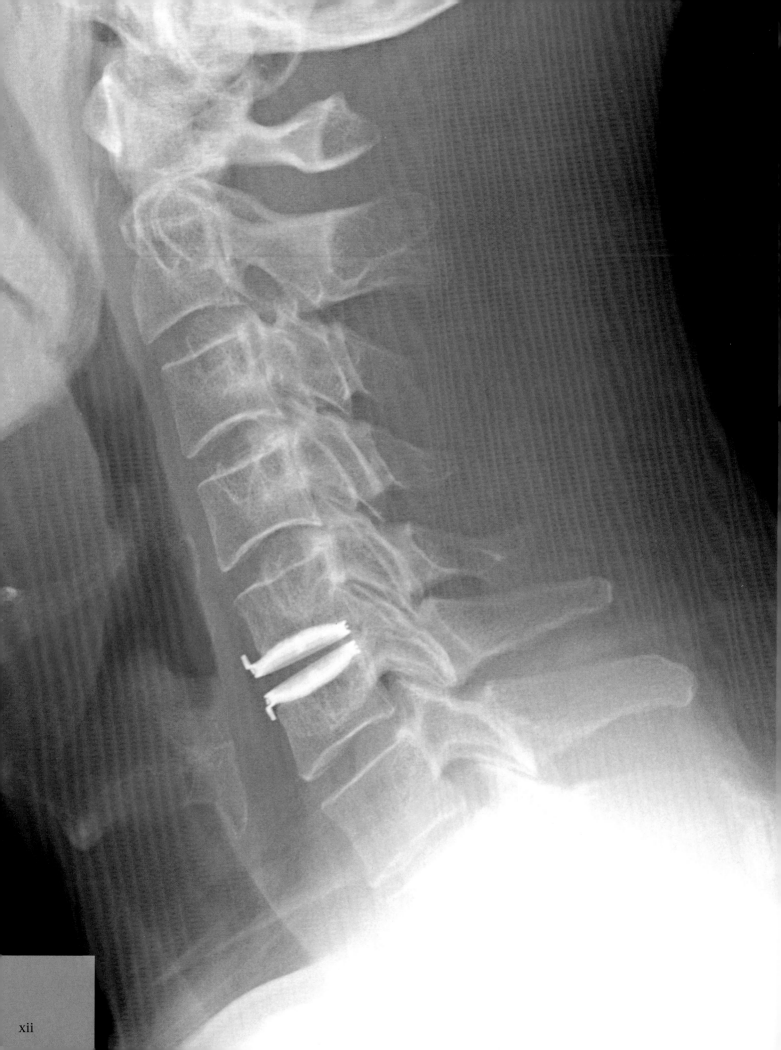

Sections

TABLE OF CONTENTS

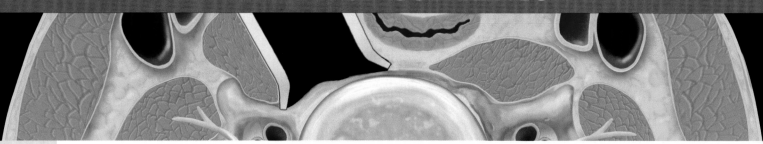

TABLE OF CONTENTS

TABLE OF CONTENTS

TABLE OF CONTENTS

TABLE OF CONTENTS

TABLE OF CONTENTS

Imaging in
SPINE
SURGERY

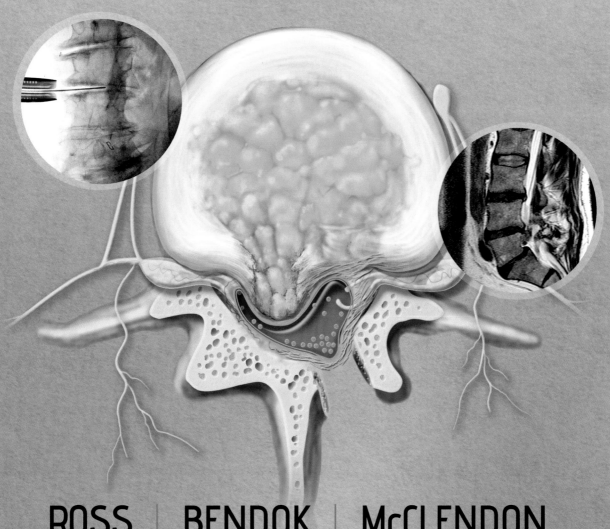

ROSS | BENDOK | McCLENDON

ELSEVIER

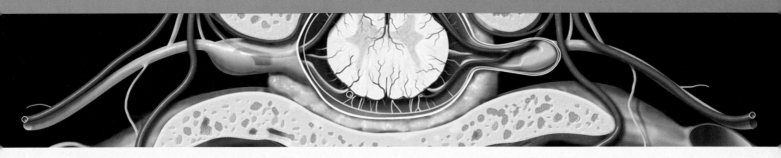

SECTION 1
Normal Anatomy and Techniques

Imaging Anatomy

There are **33** spinal vertebrae, which are composed of 2 components: A cylindrical ventral bone mass, which is the vertebral **body**, and the dorsal **arch**.

7 cervical, 12 thoracic, 5 lumbar bodies
- 5 fused elements form sacrum
- 4-5 irregular ossicles form coccyx

Arch
- 2 pedicles, 2 laminae, 7 processes (1 spinous, 4 articular, 2 transverse)
- Pedicles attach to dorsolateral aspect of body
- Pedicles unite with pair of arched flat laminae
- Lamina capped by dorsal projection called spinous process
- Transverse processes arise from sides of arches
- 2 articular processes (zygapophyses) are diarthrodial joints: Superior process bearing facet with surface directed dorsally and inferior process bearing facet with surface directed ventrally

Pars interarticulars is the part of the arch that lies between the superior and inferior articular facets of all subatlantal movable elements. The pars are positioned to receive biomechanical stresses of translational forces displacing superior facets ventrally, while inferior facets remain attached to dorsal arch (spondylolysis). C2 exhibits a unique anterior relation between the superior facet and the posteriorly placed inferior facet. This relationship leads to an elongated C2 pars interarticularis, which is the site of the hangman fracture.

Cervical
- Cervical bodies are small and thin relative to size of arch and foramen with transverse > AP diameter; lateral edges of superior surface of body are turned upward into uncinate processes; transverse foramen perforates transverse processes
- C1 has no body and forms circular bony mass; superior facets of C1 are large ovals that face upward, and inferior facets are circular in shape; large transverse processes are present on C1 with fused anterior and posterior tubercles
- C2 complex consists of axis body with dens/odontoid process; odontoid embryologically arises from centrum of 1st cervical vertebrae
- C7 shows transitional morphology with prominent spinous process

Thoracic
- Bodies are heart-shaped and increase in size from superior to inferior
- Facets are present for rib articulation, and laminae are broad and thick; spinous processes are long, directed obliquely caudally; superior facets are thin and directed posteriorly
- T1 shows complete facet for capitulum of 1st rib and inferior demifacet for capitulum of 2nd rib
- T12 resembles upper lumbar bodies with inferior facet directed more laterally

Lumbar
- Lumbar vertebral bodies are large, wide, and thick and lack transverse foramen or costal articular facets; pedicles are strong and directed posteriorly; superior articular processes are directed dorsomedially and

almost face each other; inferior articular processes are directed anteriorly and laterally

Joints
- **Synarthrosis** is immovable joint of cartilage and occurs during development and in 1st decade of life; neurocentral joint occurs at union point of 2 centers of ossification for 2 halves of vertebral arch and centrum
- **Diarthrosis** is true synovial joint that occurs in articular processes, costovertebral joints, and atlantoaxial and sacroiliac articulations; pivot type joint occurs at median atlantoaxial articulation; all others are gliding joints
- **Amphiarthroses** are nonsynovial, movable connective tissue joints; **symphysis** is fibrocartilage fusion between 2 bones, as in intervertebral disc; **syndesmosis** is ligamentous connection common in spine, such as paired ligamenta flava, intertransverse ligaments, and interspinous ligaments; unpaired syndesmosis is present in supraspinous ligament
- Atlantooccipital articulation is composed of diarthrosis between lateral mass of atlas and occipital condyles and syndesmoses of atlantooccipital membranes; anterior atlantooccipital membrane is extension of anterior longitudinal ligament (ALL); posterior atlantooccipital membrane is homologous to ligamenta flava
- Atlantoaxial articulation is pivot joint; transverse ligament maintains relationship of odontoid to anterior arch of atlas; synovial cavities are present between transverse ligament/odontoid and atlas/odontoid junctions

Disc
- Intervertebral disc is composed of 3 parts: Cartilaginous endplate, annulus fibrosis, and nucleus pulposus
- Height of lumbar disc space generally increases as one progresses caudally; annulus consists of concentrically oriented collagenous fibers, which serve to contain the central nucleus pulposus (these fibers insert into vertebral cortex via Sharpey fibers and also attach to anterior and posterior longitudinal ligaments)
- Type I collagen predominates at periphery of annulus, while type II predominates in inner annulus; normal contour of posterior aspect of annulus is dependent upon contour of its adjacent endplate (typically this is slightly concave in axial plane, although commonly at L4-5 and L5-S1 these posterior margins will be flat or even convex; convex shape on axial images alone should not be interpreted as degenerative bulging)
- Nucleus pulposus is remnant of embryonal notochord and consists of well-hydrated noncompressible proteoglycan matrix with scattered chondrocytes; proteoglycans form major macromolecular component, including chondroitin 6-sulfate, keratan sulfate, and hyaluronic acid
- Proteoglycans consist of protein core with multiple attached glycosaminoglycan chains; nucleus occupies eccentric position within confines of annulus and is more dorsal with respect to center of vertebral body
- At birth, ~ 85-90% of nucleus is water; this water content gradually decreases with advancing age; within nucleus pulposus on T2-weighted sagittal images, there is often linear hypointensity coursing in anteroposterior direction, intranuclear cleft (this region of more prominent fibrous tissue should not be interpreted as intradiscal air or calcification)

Anterior Longitudinal Ligament
- Runs along ventral surface of spine from skull to sacrum; ALL is narrowest in cervical spine and is firmly attached at ends of each vertebral body; it is loosely attached at midsection of disc

Posterior Longitudinal Ligament (PLL)
- Runs on dorsal surface of bodies from skull to sacrum; PLL has segmental denticulate configuration and is wider at disc space but narrows and becomes thicker at vertebral body level

Craniocervical Ligaments
- Located anteriorly to spinal cord and occur in 3 layers: Anterior, middle, and posterior
- Anterior ligaments consist of odontoid ligaments (apical and alar); apical ligament is small fibrous band extending from dens tip to basion; alar ligaments are thick, horizontally directed ligaments extending from lateral surface of dens tip to anteromedial occipital condyles; middle layer consists of cruciate ligament
- Transverse ligament is strong horizontal component of cruciate ligament extending from behind dens to medial aspect of C1 lateral masses; craniocaudal component consists of fibrous band running from transverse ligament superiorly to foramen magnum and inferiorly to C2; posteriorly, tectorial membrane is continuation of PLL and attaches to anterior rim of foramen magnum

Vertebral Artery
- Vertebral artery arises as 1st branch of subclavian artery on both sides; vertebral artery travels cephalad within foramen transversarium within transverse processes
- 1st segment of vertebral artery extends from its origin to entrance into foramen of transverse process of cervical vertebrae, usually 6th; most common variation is origin of left vertebral from arch, between left common carotid and left subclavian arteries (2-6%) (vertebral artery in these cases almost always enters foramen of the transverse process of C5)
- 2nd segment runs within transverse foramen to C2 level; nerve roots pass posterior to vertebral artery
- 3rd segment starts at C2 level where artery loops and turns lateral to ascend in C1 transverse foramen; it then turns medial crossing on top of C1 in groove 4
- 4th segment starts where artery perforates dura and arachnoid at lateral edge of posterior occipitoatlantal membrane, coursing ventrally on medulla to join with other vertebral artery to make basilar artery

Vertebral Column Blood Supply
- Paired segmental arteries (intercostals, lumbar arteries) arise from aorta and extend dorsolaterally around middle of vertebral body; near transverse process, segmental artery divides into lateral and dorsal branches
- Lateral branch supplies dorsal musculature, and dorsal branch passes lateral to foramen giving off branch(es) providing major vascular supply to bone and vertebral canal contents; posterior central branch supplies disc and vertebral body, while prelaminal branch supplies inner surface of arch and ligamenta flava, regional epidural tissue
- Neural branch entering neural foramen supplies pia, arachnoid, and cord; postlaminar branch supplies musculature overlying lamina and branches to bone

Nerves
- Spinal nerves are arranged in 31 pairs and grouped regionally: 8 cervical, 12 thoracic, 5 lumbar, 5 sacral, 1 coccygeal
- Ascensus spinalis is apparent developmental rising of cord related to differential spinal growth
- Course of nerve roots becomes longer and more oblique at lower segments
- C1 nerve from C1 segment and exits above C1
- C8 nerve from C7 segment and exits at C7-T1
- T6 nerve from T5 segment and exits at T6-T7
- T12 nerve from T8 segment and exits at T12-L1
- L2 nerve from T10 segment and exits at L2-3
- S3 nerve from T12 segment and exits at the S3 foramen

Meninges are divided into dura, arachnoid, and pia.
- **Dura** is dense, tough covering corresponding to meningeal layer of cranial dura; epidural space is filled with fat, loose connective tissue, and veins; dura continues with spinal nerves through foramen to fuse with epineurium; cephalic attachment of dura is at foramen magnum and caudal attachment at back of coccyx
- **Arachnoid** is middle covering, which is thin, delicate, and continuous with cranial arachnoid; arachnoid is separated from dura by potential subdural space
- **Pia** is inner covering of delicate connective tissue closely applied to cord; longitudinal fibers are laterally concentrated as denticulate ligaments lying between posterior and anterior roots and attach at 21 points to dura; longitudinal fibers are concentrated dorsally as septum posticum attaching dorsal cord to dorsal midline dura

Selected References
1. Modic MT et al: Lumbar degenerative disk disease. Radiology. 245(1):43-61, 2007
2. Battie MC et al: Lumbar disc degeneration: epidemiology and genetics. J Bone Joint Surg Am. 88 Suppl 2:3-9, 2006
3. Grunhagen T et al: Nutrient supply and intervertebral disc metabolism. J Bone Joint Surg Am. 88 Suppl 2:30-5, 2006
4. Haughton V: Imaging intervertebral disc degeneration. J Bone Joint Surg Am. 88 Suppl 2:15-20, 2006
5. Roh JS et al: Degenerative disorders of the lumbar and cervical spine. Orthop Clin North Am. 36(3):255-62, 2005
6. Fardon DF et al: Nomenclature and classification of lumbar disc pathology. Recommendations of the Combined Task Forces of the North American Spine Society, American Society of Spine Radiology, and American Society of Neuroradiology. Spine (Phila Pa 1976). 26(5):E93-E113, 2001

SPINE ANATOMY GENERAL OVERVIEW

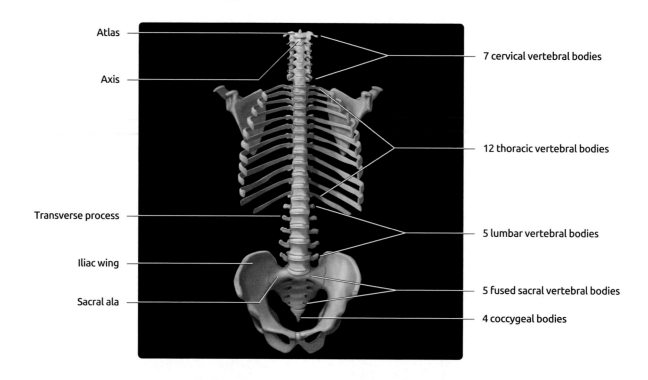

Atlas

Axis

7 cervical vertebral bodies

12 thoracic vertebral bodies

Transverse process

5 lumbar vertebral bodies

Iliac wing

Sacral ala

5 fused sacral vertebral bodies

4 coccygeal bodies

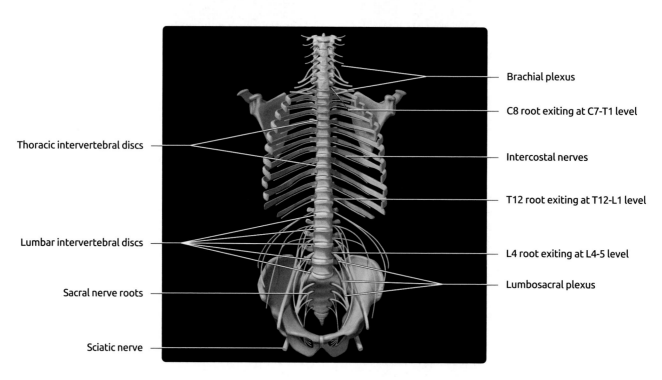

Brachial plexus

C8 root exiting at C7-T1 level

Thoracic intervertebral discs

Intercostal nerves

T12 root exiting at T12-L1 level

Lumbar intervertebral discs

L4 root exiting at L4-5 level

Lumbosacral plexus

Sacral nerve roots

Sciatic nerve

(Top) *Coronal graphic of the spinal column shows the relationship of 7 cervical, 12 thoracic, 5 lumbar, 5 fused sacral, and 4 coccygeal bodies. Note the cervical bodies are smaller with the neural foramina oriented at 45° and capped by the unique C1 and C2 morphology. Thoracic bodies are heart-shaped, have thinner intervertebral discs, and are stabilized by the rib cage. Lumbar bodies are more massive with prominent transverse processes and thick intervertebral discs. (Bottom) Coronal graphic demonstrates exiting spinal nerve roots. C1 exits between the occiput and C1, while the C8 root exits at the C7-T1 level. Thoracic and lumbar roots exit below their respective pedicles.*

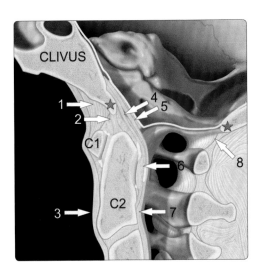

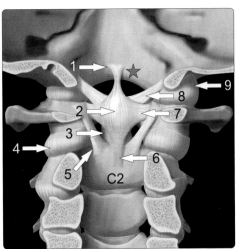

(Left) Sagittal CVJ graphic shows 1) ant. atlantooccipital membrane, 2) apical ligament, 3) ALL, 4) cruciate ligament, 5) tectorial membrane, 6) transverse ligament, 7) post. longitudinal ligament, 8) post. atlantooccipital membrane: Red star = basion, blue star = opisthion. (Right) Posterior CVJ graphic shows 1) sup. cruciate ligament, 2) cruciate lig., 3) odontoid ant. to cruciate lig., 4) atlantoaxial jt., 5) accessory atlantoaxial lig., 6) inf. cruciate lig., 7) transverse lig., 8) alar lig., and 9) atlantooccipital jt. (Red star = basion).

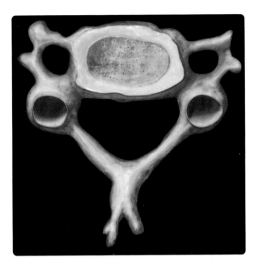

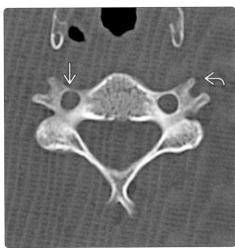

(Left) Graphic shows the cervical vertebra from above. The vertebral body is broad transversely; the central canal is large & triangular in shape; the pedicles are directed posterolaterally; the laminae are delicate. Lateral masses contain the vertebral foramen for passage of vertebral artery & veins. (Right) Mid C5 body at the pedicle level shows transverse foramina are prominent ➡, encompassing the vertical course of the vertebral artery. The anterior and posterior tubercles ➡ give rise to muscle attachments in the neck.

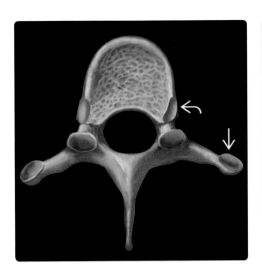

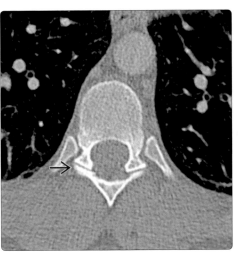

(Left) Graphic shows thoracic vertebral body from above. Thoracic bodies are characterized by long spinous processes and transverse processes. Complex rib articulation includes both costotransverse joints ➡ & costovertebral joints ➡. Facet joints are oriented in the coronal plane. (Right) Image through the pedicle level of the thoracic spine shows the coronal orientation of the facet joints is well identified ➡ in this section. The pedicles are thin & gracile with adjacent rib articulations.

(Left) *Graphic shows the lumbar body from above. Large, sturdy lumbar bodies connect to thick pedicles and transversely directed transverse processes. Facets maintain oblique orientation favoring flexion/extension.* **(Right)** *Lateral 3D scan of the lumbar spine shows large bodies joined by thick posterior elements with superior and inferior articular processes angled in the lateral plane. Transverse processes jut out laterally for muscle attachments. Pars interarticularis form junction between articular processes.*

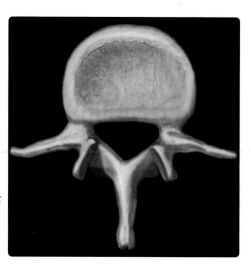
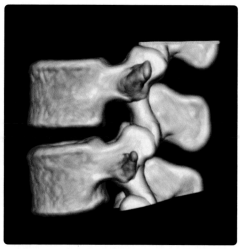

(Left) *Oblique view of the lumbar spine shows the typical Scotty dog appearance of the posterior elements. The neck of the dog is the pars interarticularis ➡. * **(Right)** *Oblique 3D exam of the lumbar spine shows the surface anatomy of the "Scotty dog": Transverse process (nose) ➡, superior articular process (ear) ➡, inferior articular process (front leg) ➡, and intervening pars interarticularis (neck) ➡. The pedicle that forms the "eye" on CT reconstructions is obscured.*

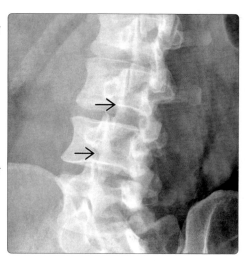
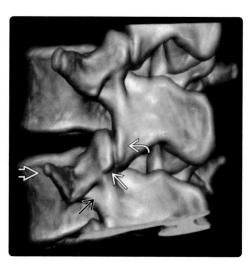

(Left) *Graphic shows lumbar vertebral bodies joined by disc & ant. & post. longitudinal ligaments. Posteriorly are paired pedicles, transverse processes, articular facets, lamina, & spinous process. Paired ligamentum flavum & interspinous ligaments join posterior elements with midline supraspinous ligaments.* **(Right)** *Graphic shows spinal cord & coverings: 1) dura mater, 2) subdural space, 3) arachnoid mater, 4) subarachnoid space, 5) pia mater, 6) ant. spinal artery, 7) epidural space, & 8) root sleeve.*

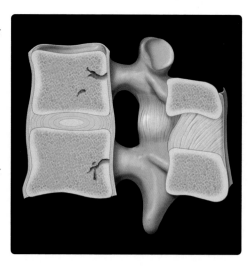
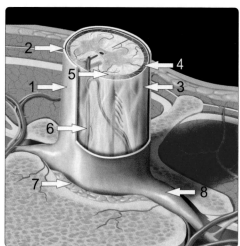

VASCULAR ANATOMY

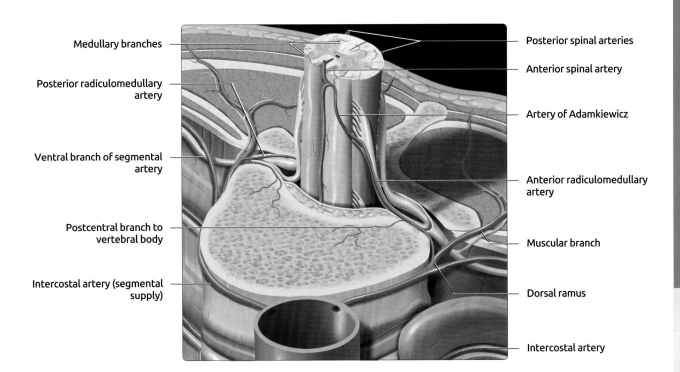

Medullary branches

Posterior radiculomedullary artery

Ventral branch of segmental artery

Postcentral branch to vertebral body

Intercostal artery (segmental supply)

Posterior spinal arteries

Anterior spinal artery

Artery of Adamkiewicz

Anterior radiculomedullary artery

Muscular branch

Dorsal ramus

Intercostal artery

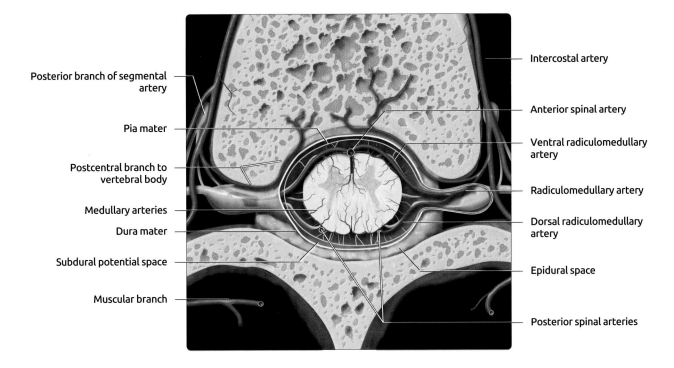

Posterior branch of segmental artery

Pia mater

Postcentral branch to vertebral body

Medullary arteries

Dura mater

Subdural potential space

Muscular branch

Intercostal artery

Anterior spinal artery

Ventral radiculomedullary artery

Radiculomedullary artery

Dorsal radiculomedullary artery

Epidural space

Posterior spinal arteries

(Top) *Axial oblique graphic of the thoracic spinal cord and arterial supply at T10 shows segmental intercostal arteries arising from the lower thoracic aorta. The artery of Adamkiewicz is the dominant segmental feeding vessel to the thoracic cord, supplying the anterior aspect of the cord via the anterior spinal artery. Adamkiewicz has a characteristic hairpin turn on the cord surface as it first courses superiorly, then turns inferiorly.* **(Bottom)** *Axial graphic shows the anterior and posterior radiculomedullary arteries anastomosing with the anterior and posterior spinal arteries. Penetrating medullary arteries in the cord are largely end-arteries with few collaterals. The cord "watershed" zone is at the central gray matter.*

TERMINOLOGY

Definitions

- Craniocervical junction (CCJ) = C1, C2, and articulation with skull base

GROSS ANATOMY

Overview

- Craniocervical junction comprises occiput, atlas, axis, their articulations, ligaments

Components of Craniocervical Junction

- Bones
  - **Occipital bone**
    - Occipital condyles are paired, oval-shaped, inferior prominences of lateral exoccipital portion of occipital bone
    - Articular facet projects laterally
  - **C1 (atlas)**
    - Composed of anterior and posterior arches, no body
    - Paired lateral masses with their superior and inferior articular facets
    - Large transverse processes with transverse foramen
  - **C2 (axis)**
    - Large body and superiorly projecting odontoid process
    - Superior articulating facet surface is convex & directed laterally
    - Inferior articular process + facet surface is typical of lower cervical vertebrae
    - Superior facet is positioned relatively anteriorly; inferior facet is posterior with elongated pars interarticularis
- Joints
  - **Atlantooccipital joints**
    - Inferior articular facet of occipital condyle: Oval, convex surface, projects laterally
    - Superior articular facet of C1: Oval, concave anteroposteriorly, projects medially
  - **Median atlantoaxial joints**
    - Pivot-type joint between dens + ring formed by anterior arch + transverse ligament of C1
    - Synovial cavities between transverse ligament/odontoid & atlas/odontoid articulations
  - **Lateral atlantoaxial joints**
    - Inferior articular facet of C1: Concave mediolaterally, projects medially in coronal plane
    - Superior articular facet of C2: Convex surface, projects laterally
- Ligaments (from anterior to posterior)
  - **Anterior atlantooccipital membrane**: Connects anterior arch C1 with anterior margin foramen magnum
  - **Odontoid ligaments**
    - Apical ligament: Small fibrous band extending from dens tip to basion
    - Alar ligaments: Thick, horizontally directed ligaments extending from lateral surface of dens tip to anteromedial occipital condyles
  - **Cruciate ligament**
    - Transverse ligament: Strong horizontal component between lateral masses of C1, passes behind dens
    - Craniocaudal component: Fibrous band running from transverse ligament superiorly to foramen magnum and inferiorly to C2
  - **Tectorial membrane**: Continuation of posterior longitudinal ligament; attaches to anterior rim foramen magnum (posterior clivus)
  - **Posterior atlantooccipital membrane**
    - Posterior arch C1 to margin of foramen magnum
    - Deficit laterally where vertebral artery enters on superior surface of C1
- Biomechanics
  - Atlantooccipital joint: 50% cervical flexion/extension and limited lateral motion
  - Atlantoaxial joint: 50% cervical rotation

IMAGING ANATOMY

Overview

- Lateral assessment of CCJ
  - **C1-C2 interspinous space**: ≤ 10 mm
  - **Atlantodental interval (ADI)**
    - Adults < 3 mm, children < 5 mm in flexion
  - **Pseudosubluxation**
    - Physiologic anterior displacement seen in 40% at C2-C3 level and 14% at C3-C4 level to age 8
    - Anterior displacement of C2 on C3 up to 4 mm
  - **Posterior cervical line**: Line is drawn from anterior aspect of C1-C3 spinous processes → anterior C2 spinous process should be within 2 mm of this line
  - **Wackenheim line**
    - Posterior surface of clivus → posterior odontoid tip should lie immediately inferior
    - Relationship does not change in flexion/extension
  - **Welcher basal angle**
    - Angle between lines drawn along plane of sphenoid bone and posterior clivus
    - Normal < 140°, average 132°
  - **Chamberlain line**
    - Between hard palate and opisthion
    - Odontoid tip ≥ 5 mm above line abnormal
  - **McGregor line**
    - Between hard palate to base of occipital bone
    - Odontoid tip ≥ 7 mm above line abnormal
  - **Clivus canal angle**
    - Junction of Wackenheim line and posterior vertebral body line
    - 180° extension, 150° flexion, < 150° abnormal
  - **McRae line**
    - Drawn between basion and opisthion
    - Normal 35-mm diameter
- Frontal assessment of CCJ
  - Lateral masses of C1 and C2 should align
    - Overlapping lateral masses can be normal variant in children
  - **Atlantooccipital joint angle**
    - Angle formed at junction of lines traversing joints
    - 125-130° normal, < 124° may reflect condyle hypoplasia

LIGAMENT ANATOMY

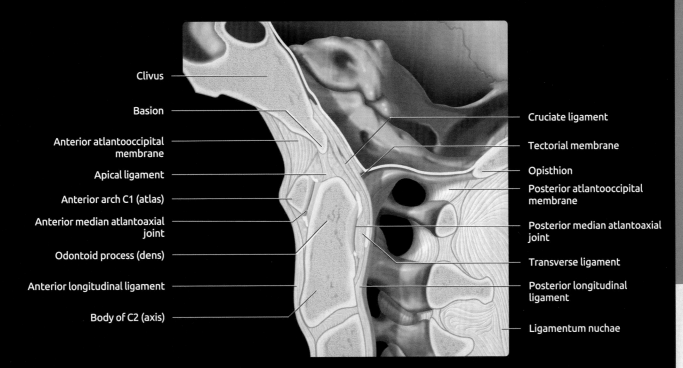

Clivus

Basion

Anterior atlantooccipital membrane

Apical ligament

Anterior arch C1 (atlas)

Anterior median atlantoaxial joint

Odontoid process (dens)

Anterior longitudinal ligament

Body of C2 (axis)

Cruciate ligament

Tectorial membrane

Opisthion

Posterior atlantooccipital membrane

Posterior median atlantoaxial joint

Transverse ligament

Posterior longitudinal ligament

Ligamentum nuchae

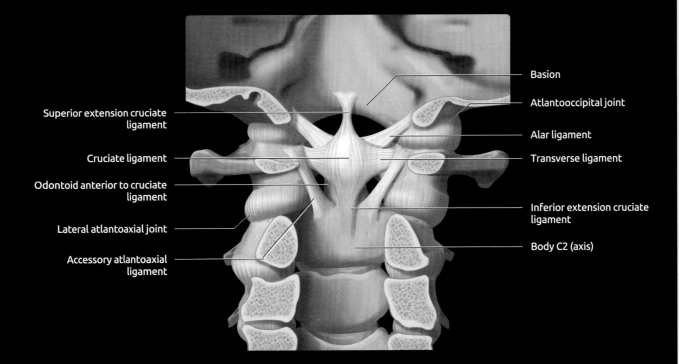

Superior extension cruciate ligament

Cruciate ligament

Odontoid anterior to cruciate ligament

Lateral atlantoaxial joint

Accessory atlantoaxial ligament

Basion

Atlantooccipital joint

Alar ligament

Transverse ligament

Inferior extension cruciate ligament

Body C2 (axis)

(Top) Sagittal midline graphic shows the craniocervical junction. The complex articulations and ligamentous attachments are highlighted. The midline atlantoaxial articulations consist of anterior and posterior median atlantoaxial joints. The anterior joint is between the posterior aspect of the anterior C1 arch and the ventral aspect of odontoid process. The posterior joint is between the dorsal aspect of the odontoid process and the cruciate ligament. The midline view shows a series of ligamentous connections to the skull base including the anterior atlantooccipital membrane, apical ligament, superior component of cruciate ligament, tectorial membrane, and posterior atlantooccipital membrane. (Bottom) Posterior view of the craniocervical junction with posterior elements cut away to define the components of the cruciate ligament and alar ligaments is shown.

C1 GRAPHICS

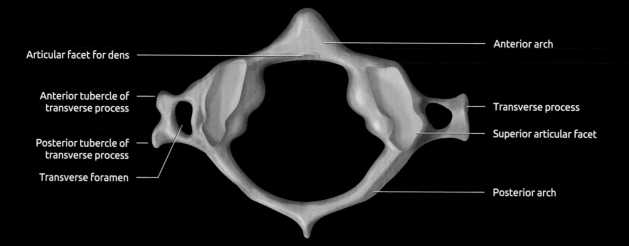

Articular facet for dens

Anterior tubercle of transverse process

Posterior tubercle of transverse process

Transverse foramen

Anterior arch

Transverse process

Superior articular facet

Posterior arch

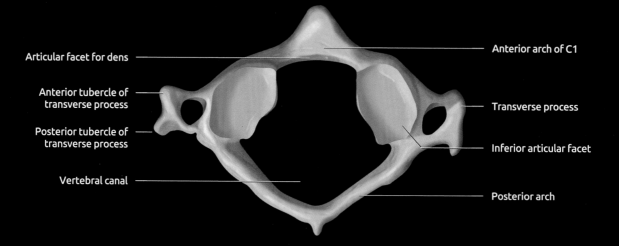

Articular facet for dens

Anterior tubercle of transverse process

Posterior tubercle of transverse process

Vertebral canal

Anterior arch of C1

Transverse process

Inferior articular facet

Posterior arch

(Top) *Axial graphic shows the atlas viewed from above. The characteristic ring shape is shown, composed of anterior and posterior arches and paired large lateral masses. The superior articular facet is concave anteroposteriorly and projects medially for articulation with the convex surface of the occipital condyle at the atlantooccipital joint. The anterior arch articulates with the odontoid process at the anterior median atlantoaxial joint.* **(Bottom)** *In this atlas viewed from below, the large inferior facet surface is concave mediolaterally and projects medially for articulation with the convex surface of the superior articular facet of C2. The canal of the atlas is ± 3 cm in AP diameter: The spinal cord, odontoid process, and free space for the cord are each about 1 cm in diameter. The size of the anterior midline tubercle of the anterior arch and spinous process of posterior arch are quite variable.*

C2 GRAPHICS

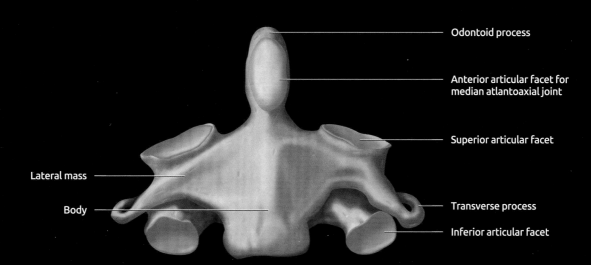

Odontoid process

Anterior articular facet for median atlantoaxial joint

Superior articular facet

Lateral mass

Body

Transverse process

Inferior articular facet

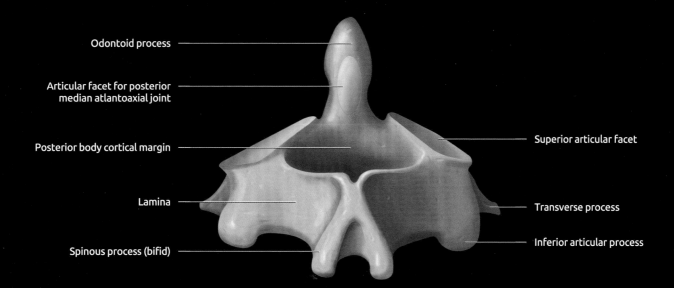

Odontoid process

Articular facet for posterior median atlantoaxial joint

Posterior body cortical margin

Lamina

Spinous process (bifid)

Superior articular facet

Transverse process

Inferior articular process

(Top) *In this atlas viewed from the anterior perspective, the odontoid process is the "purloined" embryologic centrum of C1, which is incorporated into C2, giving C2 its unique morphology. The C2 body laterally is defined by large lateral masses for articulation with the inferior facet of C1. The elongated pars interarticularis of C2 ends with the inferior articular process for articulation with the superior articular facet of C3.* (Bottom) *The atlas viewed from the posterior perspective shows that the odontoid process has anterior and posterior joints for articulation with C1. The anterior median joint articulates with the C1 arch, while the posterior median joint (shown*

RADIOGRAPHY

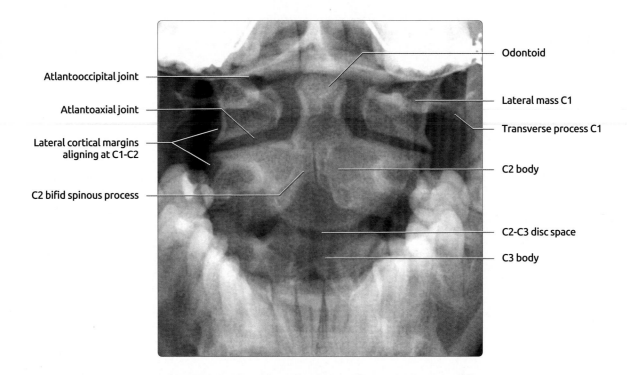

Atlantooccipital joint

Atlantoaxial joint

Lateral cortical margins aligning at C1-C2

C2 bifid spinous process

Odontoid

Lateral mass C1

Transverse process C1

C2 body

C2-C3 disc space

C3 body

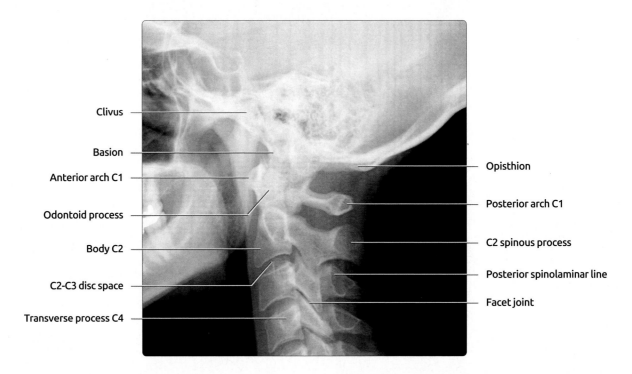

Clivus

Basion

Anterior arch C1

Odontoid process

Body C2

C2-C3 disc space

Transverse process C4

Opisthion

Posterior arch C1

C2 spinous process

Posterior spinolaminar line

Facet joint

(Top) *AP open-mouth view shows the odontoid process. With proper positioning, the odontoid process is visualized in the midline with symmetrically placed lateral C1 masses on either side. The medial space between the odontoid and C1 lateral masses should be symmetric as well. The lateral cortical margins of the C1 and C2 lateral masses should align. The atlantooccipital and atlantoaxial joints are visible bilaterally with smooth cortical margins. The bifid C2 process should not be confused for fracture.* (Bottom) *In this lateral radiograph of craniocervical junction, there is smooth anatomic alignment of the posterior vertebral body margins and the posterior spinolaminar line of the posterior elements. The anterior arch of C1 should assume a well-defined oval appearance with sharp margination between the anterior C1 arch and the odontoid process.*

CORONAL BONE CT

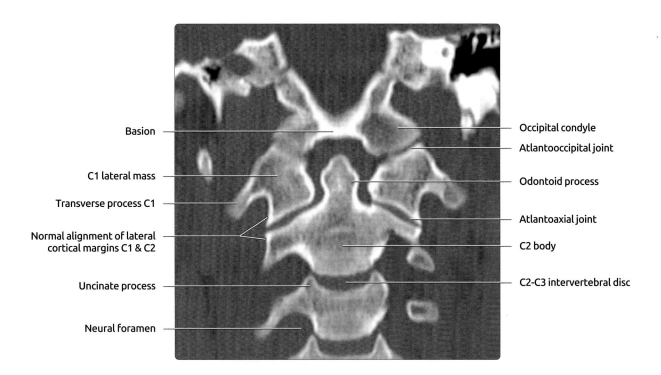

Basion — | — Occipital condyle
| — Atlantooccipital joint
C1 lateral mass — | — Odontoid process
Transverse process C1 — |
| — Atlantoaxial joint
Normal alignment of lateral cortical margins C1 & C2 — | — C2 body
Uncinate process — | — C2-C3 intervertebral disc
Neural foramen — |

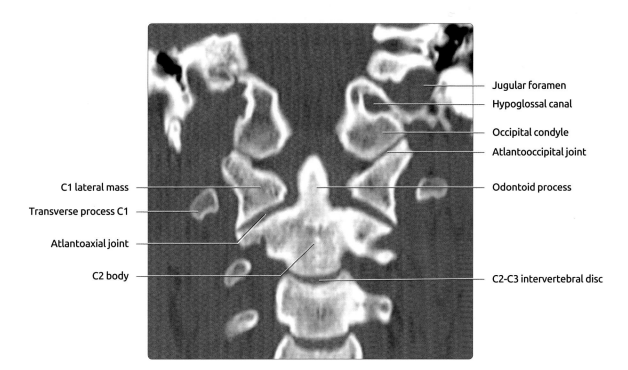

| — Jugular foramen
| — Hypoglossal canal
| — Occipital condyle
| — Atlantooccipital joint
C1 lateral mass — | — Odontoid process
Transverse process C1 — |
Atlantoaxial joint — |
C2 body — | — C2-C3 intervertebral disc

(Top) *The 1st of 2 coronal bone CT reconstructions of the craniocervical junction presented from anterior to posterior is shown. The odontoid process is visualized in the midline as a sharply corticated bony peg with symmetrically placed lateral C1 masses on either side. The lateral cortical margins of the C1 lateral masses and the C2 lateral masses should align. The atlantooccipital and atlantoaxial joints are visible bilaterally with even joint margins and sharp cortical margins.* (Bottom) *The more posterior view of the craniocervical junction shows that both the atlantooccipital joints are now well defined with smooth cortical margins, sloping superolateral to inferomedial. The atlantoaxial joints are smoothly sloping inferolateral to superomedial.*

AXIAL BONE CT

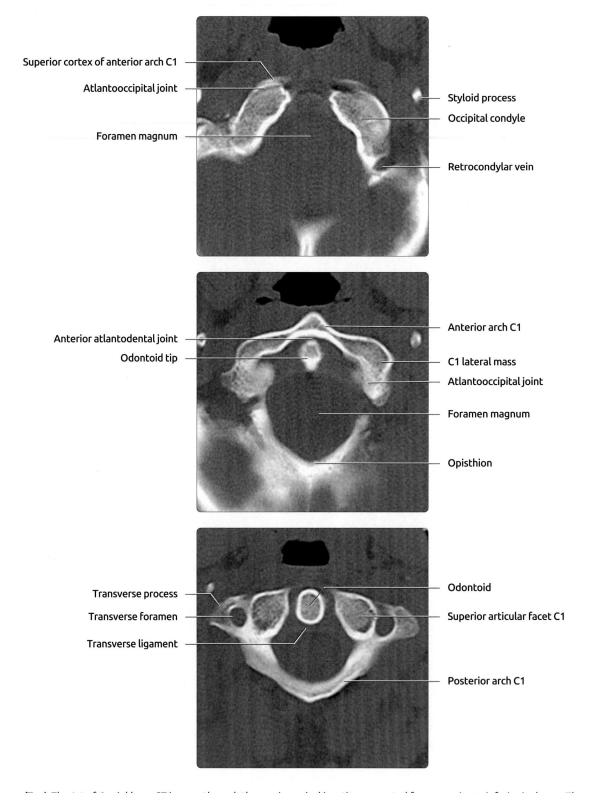

Superior cortex of anterior arch C1

Atlantooccipital joint

Foramen magnum

Styloid process

Occipital condyle

Retrocondylar vein

Anterior atlantodental joint

Odontoid tip

Anterior arch C1

C1 lateral mass

Atlantooccipital joint

Foramen magnum

Opisthion

Transverse process

Transverse foramen

Transverse ligament

Odontoid

Superior articular facet C1

Posterior arch C1

(Top) *The 1st of 6 axial bone CT images through the craniocervical junction presented from superior to inferior is shown. The anterolateral margin of the foramen magnum is formed by the prominent occipital condyles, which articulate with the superior articular facets of the C1 lateral masses.* (Middle) *This more inferior image of the craniocervical junction shows that the anterior arch of C1 is now well defined with the odontoid process of C2 coming into plane. The atlantooccipital joint is seen in oblique section and therefore has poorly defined margins. The odontoid is tightly applied to the posterior margin of the C1 arch, held in place by the strong transverse component of the cruciate ligament.* (Bottom) *Image at the level of the atlas shows the unique morphology of the C1 body, defined with its large transverse process, with a transverse foramen and ring shape.*

AXIAL BONE CT

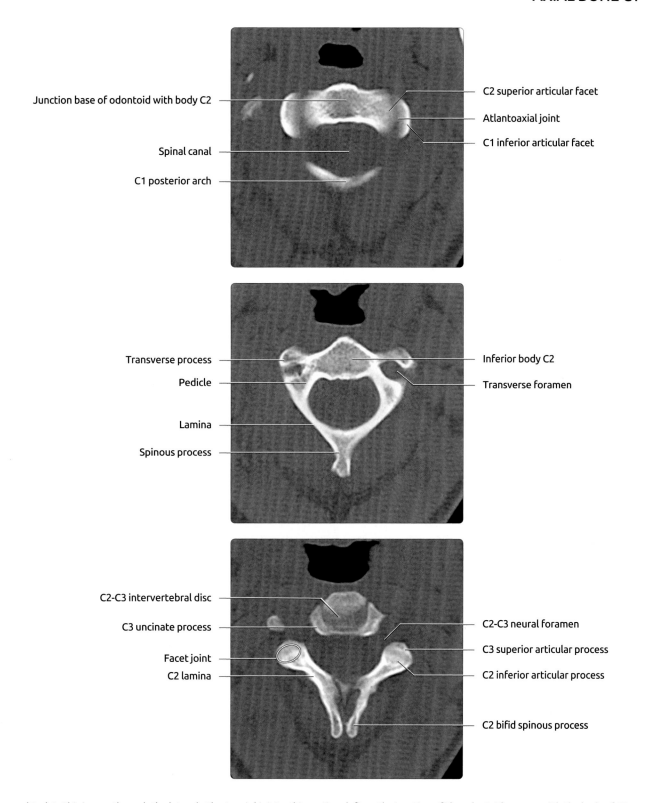

Junction base of odontoid with body C2

C2 superior articular facet

Atlantoaxial joint

Spinal canal

C1 inferior articular facet

C1 posterior arch

Transverse process

Inferior body C2

Pedicle

Transverse foramen

Lamina

Spinous process

C2-C3 intervertebral disc

C3 uncinate process

C2-C3 neural foramen

Facet joint

C3 superior articular process

C2 lamina

C2 inferior articular process

C2 bifid spinous process

(Top) *In this image through the lateral atlantoaxial joints, this section defines the junction of the odontoid process with the body of C2. The obliquely oriented atlantoaxial joints are partially seen with the C1 component lateral to the joint space and the C2 component medial.* (Middle) *This image through the inferior C2 body level shows a large C2 vertebral body and vertebral arch formed by gracile pedicles and laminae.* (Bottom) *This image through the C2-C3 intervertebral disc level shows the C2-C3 neural foramen well defined with the posterior margin formed by the superior articular process of C3. The spinous process of C2 is large and typically bifid. The C2-C3 disc assumes the characteristic cervical cup-shaped morphology bound by uncinate processes.*

SAGITTAL CT & MR

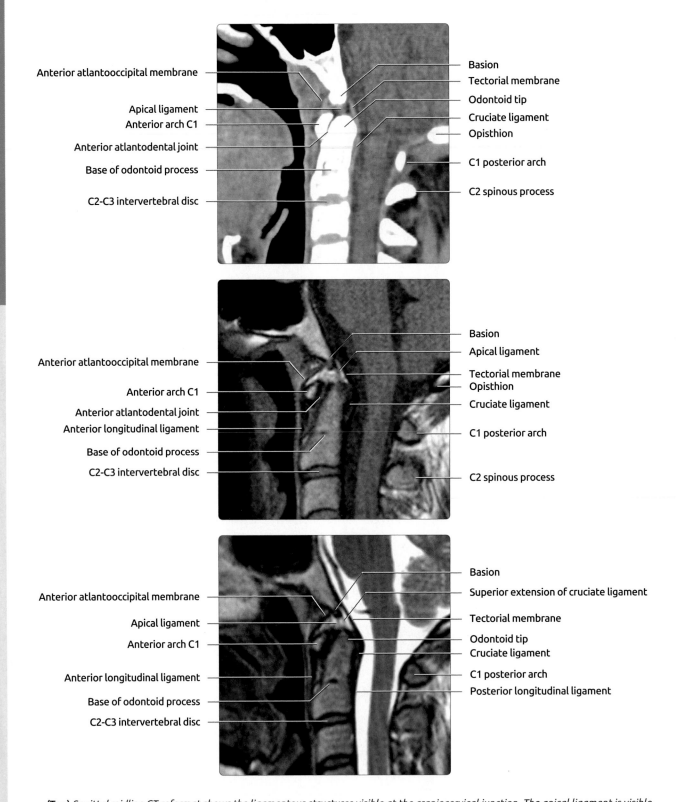

Anterior atlantooccipital membrane

Apical ligament
Anterior arch C1
Anterior atlantodental joint
Base of odontoid process
C2-C3 intervertebral disc

Basion
Tectorial membrane
Odontoid tip
Cruciate ligament
Opisthion
C1 posterior arch
C2 spinous process

Anterior atlantooccipital membrane
Anterior arch C1
Anterior atlantodental joint
Anterior longitudinal ligament
Base of odontoid process
C2-C3 intervertebral disc

Basion
Apical ligament
Tectorial membrane
Opisthion
Cruciate ligament
C1 posterior arch
C2 spinous process

Anterior atlantooccipital membrane
Apical ligament
Anterior arch C1
Anterior longitudinal ligament
Base of odontoid process
C2-C3 intervertebral disc

Basion
Superior extension of cruciate ligament
Tectorial membrane
Odontoid tip
Cruciate ligament
C1 posterior arch
Posterior longitudinal ligament

(Top) Sagittal midline CT reformat shows the ligamentous structures visible at the craniocervical junction. The apical ligament is visible as a linear band between the odontoid tip and clivus. The tectorial membrane is the superior extension of the posterior longitudinal ligament. The anterior atlantooccipital membrane is the extension of the anterior longitudinal ligament. (Middle) Sagittal T1 MR midline image shows the craniocervical junction. The atlantodental interval is well defined by the adjacent low signal cortical margins of the C1 anterior arch and the odontoid process. The cruciate ligament is a low signal band dorsal to the odontoid. (Bottom) Sagittal T2 MR shows the craniocervical junction. The tectorial membrane, superior extension of the cruciate ligament, apical ligament, and anterior atlantooccipital membranes are evident.

SAGITTAL T1 MR

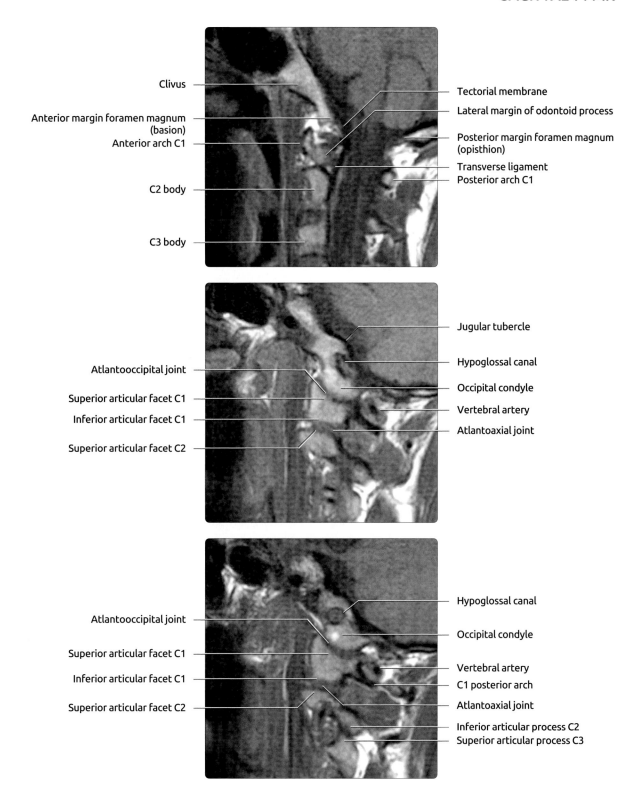

Clivus

Anterior margin foramen magnum (basion)

Anterior arch C1

C2 body

C3 body

Tectorial membrane

Lateral margin of odontoid process

Posterior margin foramen magnum (opisthion)

Transverse ligament

Posterior arch C1

Atlantooccipital joint

Superior articular facet C1

Inferior articular facet C1

Superior articular facet C2

Jugular tubercle

Hypoglossal canal

Occipital condyle

Vertebral artery

Atlantoaxial joint

Atlantooccipital joint

Superior articular facet C1

Inferior articular facet C1

Superior articular facet C2

Hypoglossal canal

Occipital condyle

Vertebral artery

C1 posterior arch

Atlantoaxial joint

Inferior articular process C2

Superior articular process C3

(Top) *The 1st of 3 parasagittal T1 MR images shown from medial to lateral through the atlantooccipital joint is shown. This image extends through the lateral cortical margin of the odontoid, which is incompletely visualized. The anterior arch of C1 is obliquely visualized as it curves posterolaterally. The lateral extension of the cruciate ligament and the transverse ligament is prominent.* (Middle) *The relationship of the occipital condyle, C1 lateral mass + the atlantoaxial joint is highlighted in this image. The articular surface of occipital condyle is convex, and the superior facet of C1 is concave allowing for flexion/extension.* (Bottom) *More lateral image of the craniocervical junction shows the atlantooccipital joint and atlantoaxial joints with sharp, smooth cortical margins.*

TERMINOLOGY

Synonyms

- Uncovertebral joint (joint of Luschka)
- C1 (atlas), C2 (axis)

Definitions

- Subaxial cervical spine = C3-C7

GROSS ANATOMY

Overview

- Consists of 7 vertebrae (C1-C7)
  o **Craniocervical junction (CCJ)**: C1, C2, & articulation with skull base constitute craniocervical junction
  o **Subaxial spine**: C3-C7
    - C3-C6 typical cervical vertebrae
    - C7 has features that differ slightly from C3-C6

Components of Subaxial Cervical Spine

- **Bones C3-C7**
  o **Body**
    - Small, broader transversely than in AP dimension
    - Posterolateral edges of superior surface are turned upward = uncinate process
  o **Vertebral arches**
    - Pedicle: Delicate, project posterolaterally
    - Lamina: Thin and narrow
    - Vertebral foramen: Large, triangle-shaped
  o **Transverse processes**
    - Project laterally and contain foramen for vertebral artery
    - Anterior and posterior tubercles are separated by superior groove for exiting spinal nerve
  o **Articular processes**
    - Superior and inferior articular processes with articular facets oriented ~ 45° superiorly from transverse plane
    - Form paired osseous shafts posterolateral to vertebral bodies = articular pillars
  o Spinous process: Short and bifid
  o **C7 unique features**
    - Spinous process: Long, prominent
    - Transverse process: Short and project inferolaterally compared with T1 spinous processes, which are long & project superolaterally
- **Intervertebral foramen**
  o Oriented anterolaterally below pedicles at ~ 45° to sagittal plane
- **Joints**
  o Intervertebral disc
    - Narrowest in cervical region
    - Thinner posteriorly than anteriorly
    - Do not extend to lateral margins of vertebral bodies in cervical spine → joints of Luschka
  o **Uncovertebral joint** (joints of Luschka)
    - Oblique, cleft-like cavities between superior surfaces of uncinate processes & lateral lips of inferior articular surface of next superior vertebra
    - Lined by cartilaginous endplate of vertebral body
    - No true synovial lining present; contains serum, simulating synovial fluid

- Uncinate process develops during childhood with uncovertebral joint forming by fibrillation and fissuring in fibers of annulus fibrosus
  o **Facet (zygapophyseal) joints**
    - Facet joints oriented ~ 45° superiorly from transverse plane in upper cervical spine; assume more vertical orientation toward C7
    - Formed by articulation between superior & inferior articular processes = articular pillars
    - Form 2 sides of flexible tripod of bone (vertebral bodies, right and left articular pillars) for support of cranium
- **Ligaments**
  o Anterior & posterior longitudinal, ligamentum flavum, interspinous & supraspinous ligaments
  o Additional ligaments of CCJ include apical, alar, and cruciate ligaments
- **Biomechanics**
  o Subaxial cervical spine shows free motion range relative to remainder of presacral spine
    - Cervical extension checked by anterior longitudinal ligament & musculature
    - Cervical flexion checked by articular pillars & intertransverse ligaments

IMAGING ANATOMY

Lateral Assessment of Subaxial Spine

- Principles apply equally to radiography, CT, or MR
- **Prevertebral soft tissues**: Distance between air column and anterior aspect of vertebral body
  o Adults: < 7 mm at C2 & < 22 mm at C6
  o Child: < 14 mm at C6
- Bony alignment
  o **Anterior vertebral line**: Smooth curve paralleling anterior vertebral cortex
    - Less important than posterior cortical line
  o **Posterior vertebral line**: Smooth curve paralleling posterior vertebral cortex
    - Translation > 3.5 mm is abnormal
    - Flexion and extension allow physiological offset < 3 mm of posterior cortical margin of successive vertebral bodies
  o **Spinolaminar line**: Smooth curve from opisthion to C7 formed by junction of laminae with spinous processes
  o **Spinous process angulation**: Cervical spinous processes should converge toward common point posteriorly
    - Widening is present when distance is > 1.5x interspinous distance of adjacent spinal segments

Frontal Assessment of Subaxial Spine

- Lateral masses: Bilateral smooth undulating margins
- Spinous processes: Midline
  o Lateral rotation of 1 spinous process with respect to others is abnormal
- Interspinous distance: Symmetric throughout
  o Interspinous distance 1.5x distance of level above or below is abnormal

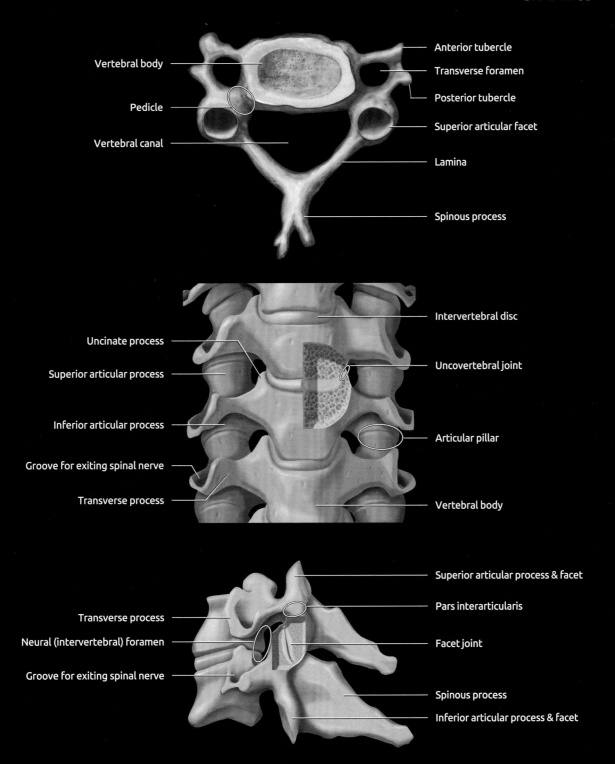

(Top) *Graphic of a typical cervical vertebra viewed from above demonstrates important morphology. The vertebral body is broader transversely than in the AP dimension, the central vertebral canal is large and triangular in shape, the pedicles are directed posterolaterally, and the laminae are delicate and give rise to a spinous process with a bifid tip. Lateral masses contain the vertebral foramen for passage of vertebral artery and veins.* **(Middle)** *Frontal graphic of subaxial cervical spine with cutout shows the intervertebral disc and uncovertebral joints. Paired lateral articular pillars are formed by articulation between the superior and inferior articular processes.* **(Bottom)** *Lateral graphic of 2 consecutive typical cervical vertebrae with cutout shows facet (zygapophyseal) joint detail. Note also the prominent groove on the superior surface of the transverse process for exiting spinal nerves.*

GRAPHIC & 3D VRT NECT

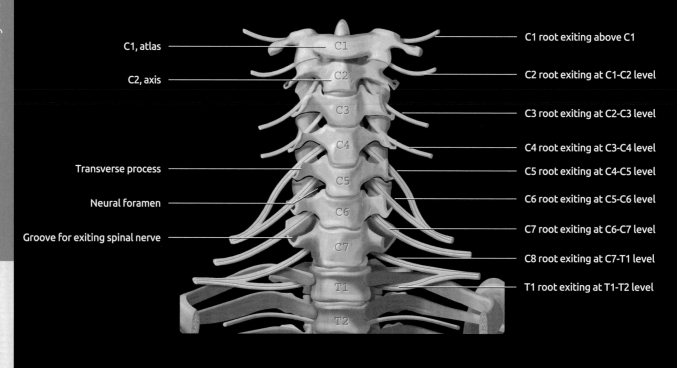

C1, atlas — C1 root exiting above C1

C2, axis — C2 root exiting at C1-C2 level

C3 root exiting at C2-C3 level

C4 root exiting at C3-C4 level

Transverse process — C5 root exiting at C4-C5 level

Neural foramen — C6 root exiting at C5-C6 level

Groove for exiting spinal nerve — C7 root exiting at C6-C7 level

C8 root exiting at C7-T1 level

T1 root exiting at T1-T2 level

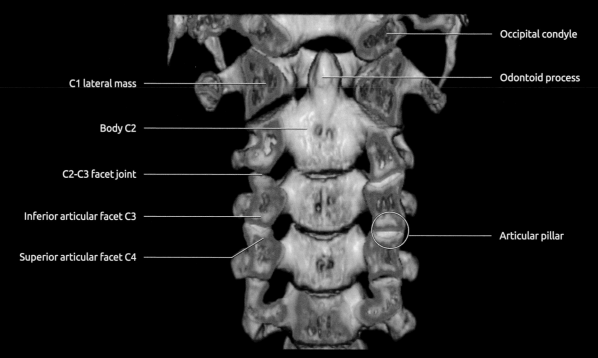

Occipital condyle

C1 lateral mass — Odontoid process

Body C2

C2-C3 facet joint

Inferior articular facet C3 — Articular pillar

Superior articular facet C4

(Top) *Coronal graphic of the cervical spine shows vertebrae and corresponding cervical nerves. The vertebrae are numbered and are shown with their exiting nerves. There are 8 cervical nerves, with the C1 nerve exiting above the C1 body and the C2 nerve exiting at the C1-C2 level. The C8 nerve exits at C7-T1. Below this level, the thoracic roots exit below their respective numbered vertebrae. The roots exit inferiorly within the neural foramen along the bony groove in the transverse process.* (Bottom) *Coronal 3D-VRT examination shows the cervical spine, viewed posteriorly with the dorsal elements partially removed to show the dorsal vertebral body surface. The concept of the cervical articular pillars is well shown in this view with the facets forming paired columns of bone with superior and*

RADIOGRAPHY

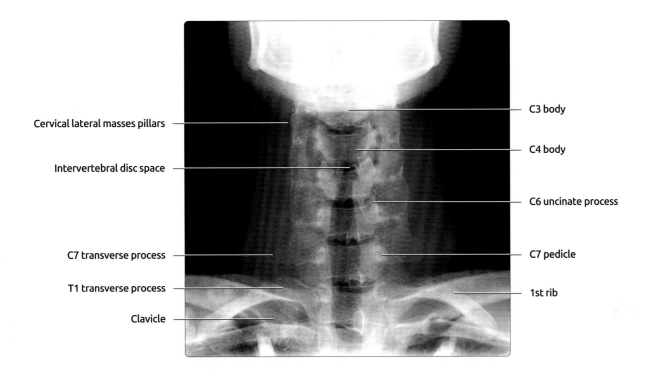

Cervical lateral masses pillars

Intervertebral disc space

C7 transverse process

T1 transverse process

Clavicle

C3 body

C4 body

C6 uncinate process

C7 pedicle

1st rib

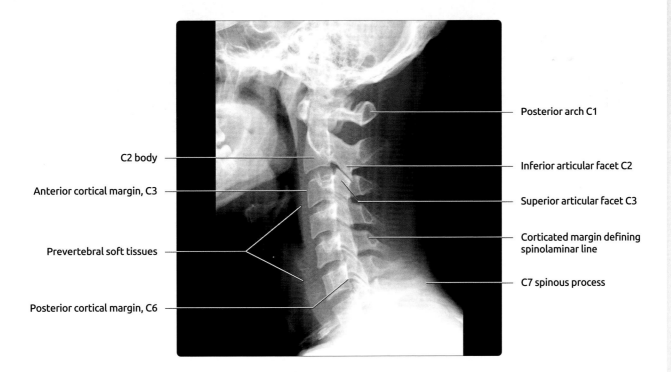

C2 body

Anterior cortical margin, C3

Prevertebral soft tissues

Posterior cortical margin, C6

Posterior arch C1

Inferior articular facet C2

Superior articular facet C3

Corticated margin defining spinolaminar line

C7 spinous process

(Top) *AP plain film view shows the cervical spine. The articular facets are viewed obliquely in this projection and therefore not defined, giving the appearance of smoothly undulating lateral columns of bone. The superior and inferior vertebral endplate margins are sharp, with regular spacing of the intervertebral discs. The spinous processes are midline. The C7 transverse process is directed inferolaterally compared with T1, which is directed superolaterally.* (Bottom) *Lateral radiograph shows the cervical spine. The prevertebral soft tissues should form a defined, abrupt "shelf" at approximately C4/5 where the hypopharynx/esophagus begins, hence thickening the prevertebral soft tissues. The bony cervical spine is aligned, from anterior to posterior, with the anterior vertebral body margins, the posterior vertebral body margins, and the ventral margins of the spinous processes (spinolaminar line).*

Normal Anatomy and Techniques

RADIOGRAPHY & 3D VRT NECT

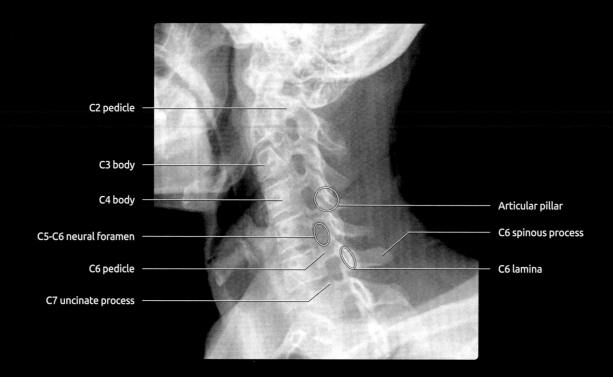

C2 pedicle

C3 body

C4 body

C5-C6 neural foramen

C6 pedicle

C7 uncinate process

Articular pillar

C6 spinous process

C6 lamina

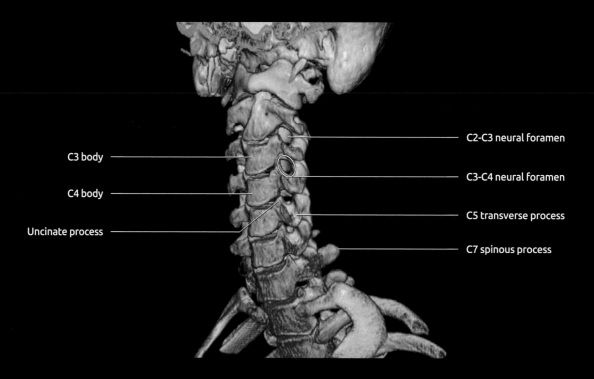

C3 body

C4 body

Uncinate process

C2-C3 neural foramen

C3-C4 neural foramen

C5 transverse process

C7 spinous process

(Top) *Oblique radiograph of the cervical spine best demonstrates the neural foramina, as these are oriented obliquely at ~ 45° from the sagittal plane. With the patient rotated to the left, the radiograph demonstrates the right-sided foramina. The anterior boundary of the neural foramina includes the uncinate process, intervertebral disc, and vertebral body. The posterior boundary is the facet joint complex. The articular pillar facet joints are viewed obliquely and therefore are not well defined. The lamina is seen end-on and hence is sharply corticated.* (Bottom) *Oblique 3D-VRT examination of the cervical spine shows the neural foramina end-on. The groove on the superior surface of the transverse processes fo the exiting spinal nerves is well shown.*

AXIAL BONE CT

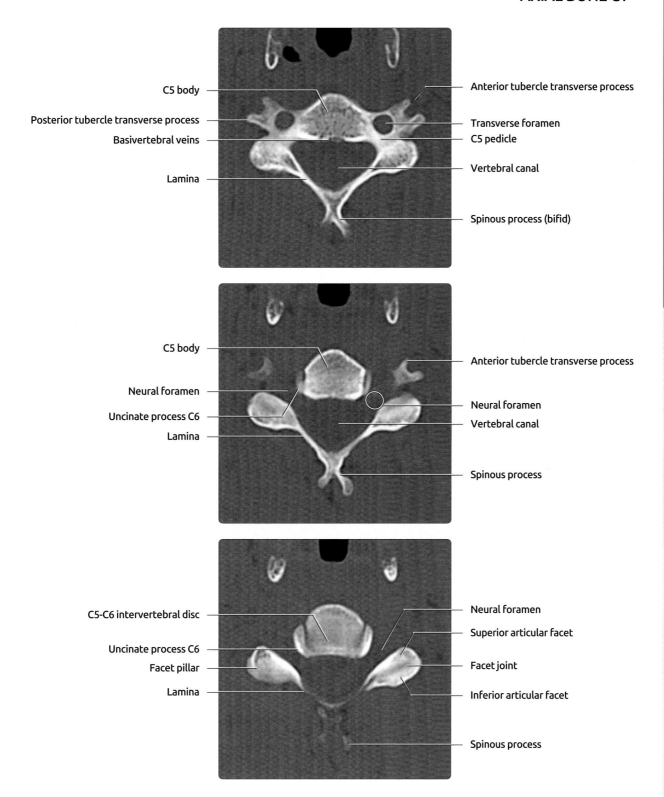

C5 body — Anterior tubercle transverse process

Posterior tubercle transverse process — Transverse foramen

Basivertebral veins — C5 pedicle

Lamina — Vertebral canal

Spinous process (bifid)

C5 body — Anterior tubercle transverse process

Neural foramen — Neural foramen

Uncinate process C6 — Vertebral canal

Lamina — Spinous process

C5-C6 intervertebral disc — Neural foramen

Uncinate process C6 — Superior articular facet

Facet pillar — Facet joint

Lamina — Inferior articular facet

Spinous process

(Top) *Image through mid C5 body at the pedicle level is shown. The transverse foramina are prominent at this level, with the round, sharply marginated transverse foramen encompassing the vertical course of the vertebral artery. The anterior and posterior tubercles give rise to muscle attachments in the neck. The vertebral body is interrupted along the posterior cortical margin for the passage of the basivertebral venous complex.* **(Middle)** *In this image at the inferior C5 body level, the uncinate process arising off of the next inferior vertebral body is coming into view. The inferior margins of the transverse processes are incompletely visualized. The spinous process is well seen joining with the thin lamina.* **(Bottom)** *View at C5-C6 level shows the next neural foraminal level bound by uncovertebral joint anteriorly and facet posteriorly.*

AXIAL BONE CT

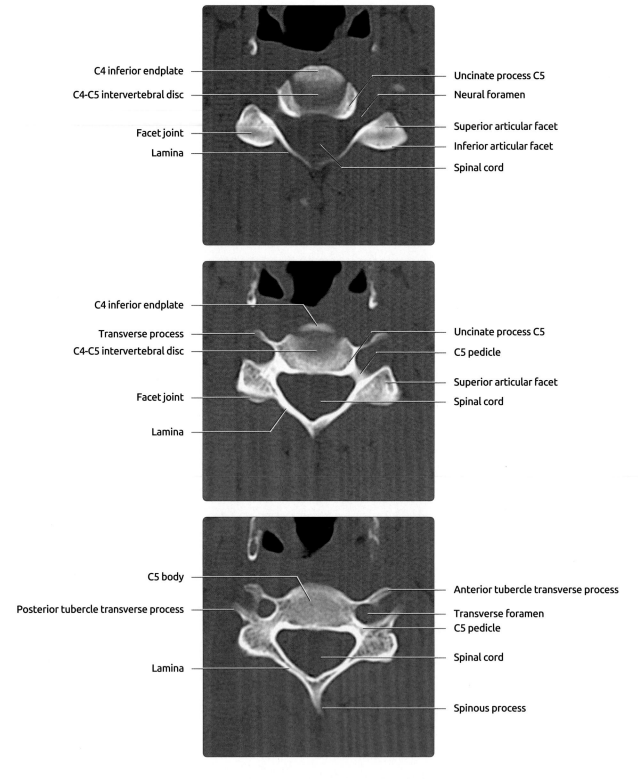

Top image labels:
- C4 inferior endplate
- C4-C5 intervertebral disc
- Facet joint
- Lamina
- Uncinate process C5
- Neural foramen
- Superior articular facet
- Inferior articular facet
- Spinal cord

Middle image labels:
- C4 inferior endplate
- Transverse process
- C4-C5 intervertebral disc
- Facet joint
- Lamina
- Uncinate process C5
- C5 pedicle
- Superior articular facet
- Spinal cord

Bottom image labels:
- C5 body
- Posterior tubercle transverse process
- Lamina
- Anterior tubercle transverse process
- Transverse foramen
- C5 pedicle
- Spinal cord
- Spinous process

(Top) *This is the 1st of 6 axial bone CT images presented from superior to inferior through the cervical spine starting at the C4-C5 level. The cup-shaped intervertebral disc of the cervical region is seen centrally, bound along the posterolateral margin by the uncinate processes. The uncinate process defines the joint of Luschka between adjacent vertebral segments. The neural foramina exit at around 45° in an anterolateral direction, bound posteriorly by the superior articular process.* **(Middle)** *In this image through the inferior margin of the intervertebral disc, the gracile pedicles arise obliquely from the posterolateral margins of the vertebral bodies. The bony canal is large relative to the posterior elements and assumes a triangular configuration.* **(Bottom)** *In this image through the C5 body level, the transverse process contains the transverse foramen for the vertebral artery.*

SAGITTAL T2 MR

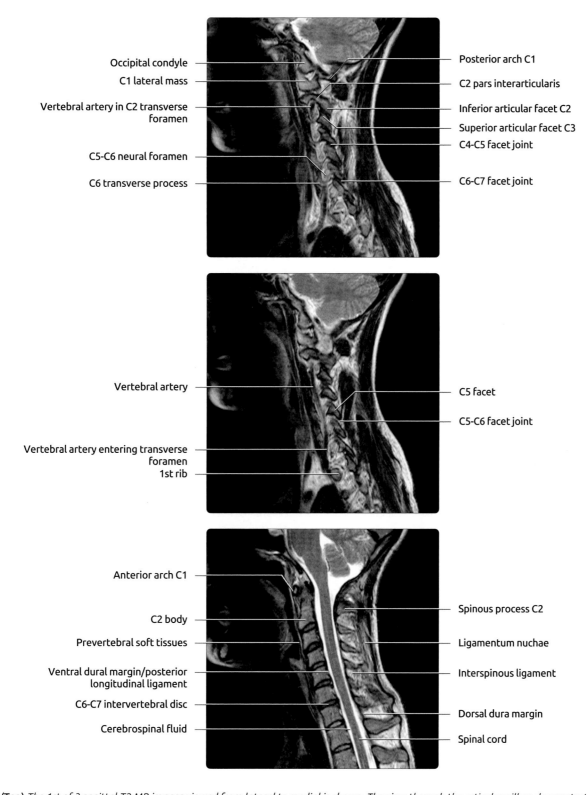

Occipital condyle

C1 lateral mass

Vertebral artery in C2 transverse foramen

C5-C6 neural foramen

C6 transverse process

Posterior arch C1

C2 pars interarticularis

Inferior articular facet C2

Superior articular facet C3

C4-C5 facet joint

C6-C7 facet joint

Vertebral artery

Vertebral artery entering transverse foramen
1st rib

C5 facet

C5-C6 facet joint

Anterior arch C1

C2 body

Prevertebral soft tissues

Ventral dural margin/posterior longitudinal ligament

C6-C7 intervertebral disc

Cerebrospinal fluid

Spinous process C2

Ligamentum nuchae

Interspinous ligament

Dorsal dura margin

Spinal cord

(Top) *The 1st of 3 sagittal T2 MR images viewed from lateral to medial is shown. The view through the articular pillars demonstrates normal alignment of the facet joints. The rhomboidal configuration of the cervical facets is noted, with their complementary superior and inferior articular facets. The exiting spinal nerves run in the groove along the superior aspect of transverse processes.* (Middle) *More medial section shows the overlapping facets at each level and the flow void of the vertebral artery within the transverse foramen.* (Bottom) *Midline image shows the relationship of the cervical cord, vertebral bodies, and spinous processes with smooth, straight margins and alignment. The posterior dural margin merges with the ligamentum flavum and the low signal of the spinous process cortex. The anterior dural margin merges with the posterior body cortex and posterior longitudinal ligament.*

Normal Anatomy and Techniques

AXIAL T2 MR

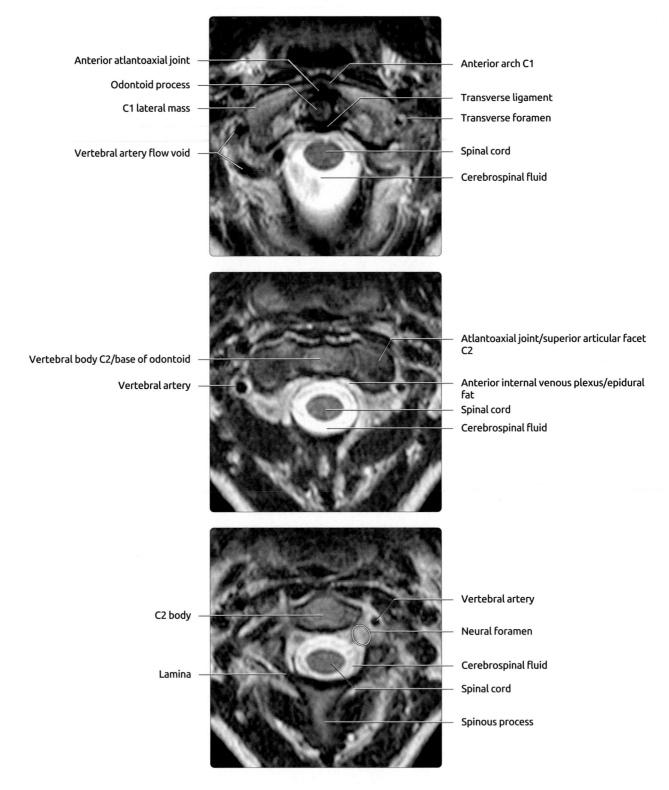

Anterior atlantoaxial joint

Odontoid process

C1 lateral mass

Vertebral artery flow void

Anterior arch C1

Transverse ligament

Transverse foramen

Spinal cord

Cerebrospinal fluid

Vertebral body C2/base of odontoid

Vertebral artery

Atlantoaxial joint/superior articular facet C2

Anterior internal venous plexus/epidural fat

Spinal cord

Cerebrospinal fluid

C2 body

Lamina

Vertebral artery

Neural foramen

Cerebrospinal fluid

Spinal cord

Spinous process

(Top) *The 1st of 6 axial T2 MR images from superior to inferior beginning at the level of the anterior arch of C1 is shown. The anterior atlantodental joint is well identified, bound by the low signal cortical margins of the anterior odontoid and anterior arch of C1. Posterior to the odontoid is the low signal transverse ligament complex.* (Middle) *In this image at odontoid/C2 body level, the base of the odontoid is at the level of the lateral atlantoaxial articulation. This joint is sloped, being more superior at the medial margin. The vertebral arteries are identified by their flow voids located just lateral to the lateral masses and passing superiorly toward the C1 transverse foramen.* (Bottom) *In this image at the C2 body level, the relationship of the vertically oriented vertebral artery to the neural foramen is highlighted.*

AXIAL T2

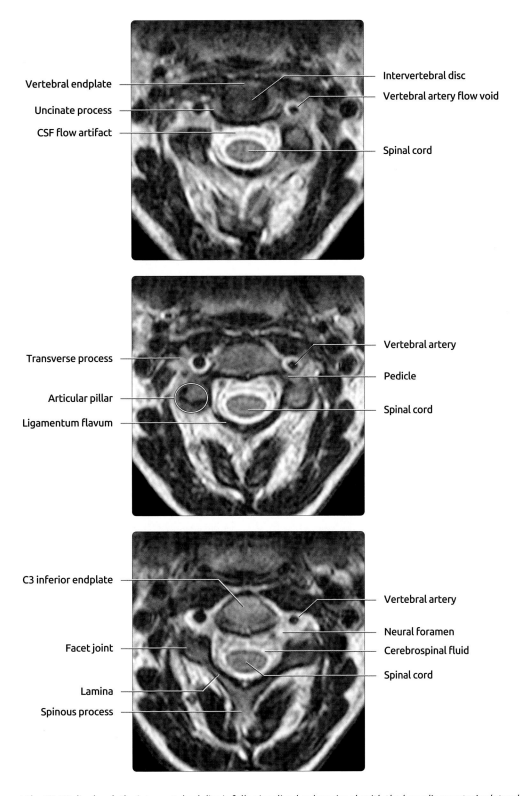

(Top) Vertebral endplate · Uncinate process · CSF flow artifact — Intervertebral disc · Vertebral artery flow void · Spinal cord

(Middle) Transverse process · Articular pillar · Ligamentum flavum — Vertebral artery · Pedicle · Spinal cord

(Bottom) C3 inferior endplate · Facet joint · Lamina · Spinous process — Vertebral artery · Neural foramen · Cerebrospinal fluid · Spinal cord

(Top) *In this image at the C2-C3 disc level, the intervertebral disc is fully visualized as low signal, with the bounding posterior lateral uncovertebral joints.* **(Middle)** *Image through the pedicles of C3 is shown. Pedicles are delicate and are directed posterolaterally from the vertebral body. The superior and inferior articular processes and intervening facet joints form the articular pillars. Prominent vertebral artery flow voids are seen within the transverse foramina of the transverse processes.* **(Bottom)** *Image through the neural foramina of C3 is shown, which are oriented ~ 45° anterolaterally. The posterior margin of the neural foramen is the facet joint; the ventral margin is the disc and uncinate process.*

TERMINOLOGY

Abbreviations

- Costovertebral (CV)

Synonyms

- Costal facet = demifacet

GROSS ANATOMY

Overview

- Consists of 12 vertebrae (T1-12)
- **Thoracic kyphosis**
  - 1 of 2 primary spinal curves (thoracic & sacral) present at birth, maintained throughout life
  - Cervical & lumbar lordoses are secondary curves, more flexible than thoracic, & result of development
    - Considerable variability in amount of kyphosis (20-45°)
    - Each body contributes 3.8° of kyphosis via wedge-shaped angulation
    - Apex at T7
    - Increases with age
    - M < F
- **Thoracolumbar junction**
  - Transition from rigid thoracic spine to more mobile lumbar spine
  - T11, T12 ribs provide less rigidity compared to rest of thoracic spine
  - No connection to sternum (free floating)
  - Only single rib articulation on vertebral bodies
- **Unique features of thoracic spine**
  - Articulation with rib cage
  - Coronal facet orientation
  - Small spinal canal relative to posterior element size

Components

- **Bones**
  - Thoracic vertebrae increase in size from T1 → T12
  - **Body**
    - Typical body contains 2 costal demifacets laterally
    - T1 has complete facet superiorly and demifacet inferiorly; T10 has superior demifacet only; T11 and 12 have complete facet
  - **Arch**
    - Pedicle: Projects directly posterior
    - Transverse process: T1 transverse process projects superolaterally; T1-10 transverse process costal facet articulates with costal tubercle
    - Articular processes: Superior & inferior articular process with coronally oriented facet joint
    - Lamina
    - Spinous process: T1-T9 project inferiorly; T10-T12 project more horizontally
- **Intervertebral foramen**
  - Oriented laterally below pedicle
- **Joints**
  - Intervertebral disc
  - Facet (zygapophyseal) joints
    - Facets oriented near vertical in coronal plane
    - Limit flexion & extension
  - **Rib articulations**

- Costovertebral joint: Rib head articulates with 2 costal demifacets; superior costal facet of same number vertebra as rib & inferior costal facet of next vertebral body
    - **Costotransverse joint**: Transverse process of vertebral body T1-T10
- **Muscles**
  - Superficial muscles include trapezius, rhomboid, latissimus dorsi, & serratus inferior & superior
  - Deep muscles include erector spinae (sacrospinalis), iliocostalis, longissimus, spinalis & semispinalis thoracis, multifidus, rotatores, & interspinalis
- **Ligaments**
  - Anterior & posterior longitudinal, interspinous, supraspinous ligaments & ligamentum flavum
  - Costovertebral ligaments
    - Radiate ligament connects head of rib & adjacent vertebral bodies
    - Costotransverse ligaments (lateral & superior) connect neck of rib with transverse process
- **Biomechanics**
  - Intact rib cage increases axial load resistance 4x
  - Rib cage & facets limit rotation

IMAGING ANATOMY

Radiography

- Short C7 transverse process projects inferolaterally; long T1 transverse process projects superolaterally

MR

- Body: Signal intensity of marrow varies with age
  - Hemopoietic ("red") marrow is hypointense on T1WI, becomes hyperintense with conversion from red → yellow (age 8-12 years)
  - Endplate, reactive marrow changes normally with aging (can be fibrovascular, fatty, or sclerotic)
- Intervertebral disc: Signal intensity varies with age
  - Hyperintense on T2WI in children, young adults; progressive ↓ water → hypointense on T2WI
  - Disc degeneration, desiccation, shape change (bulge) normal after 2nd decade
- Ligaments: Hypointense on both T1 & T2WI

ANATOMY IMAGING ISSUES

Questions

- Thoracic spinal cord is protected & shielded from injury by paraspinal muscles & rib cage
- Narrow spinal canal of thoracic spine allows for easy cord compression with malalignment or trauma
- Normal kyphotic posture increases risk of fracture
- Thoracolumbar junction at more traumatic risk due to lack of rib cage stabilization

Imaging Pitfalls

- **Cervicothoracic junction**
  - Cervical ribs arising from C7 found in 0.5% population
  - Short C7 transverse process projects inferolaterally
  - Long T1 transverse process projects superolaterally

3D VRT NECT

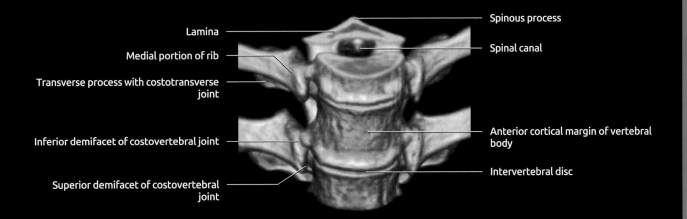

Lamina — Spinous process

Medial portion of rib — Spinal canal

Transverse process with costotransverse joint

Inferior demifacet of costovertebral joint — Anterior cortical margin of vertebral body

Intervertebral disc

Superior demifacet of costovertebral joint

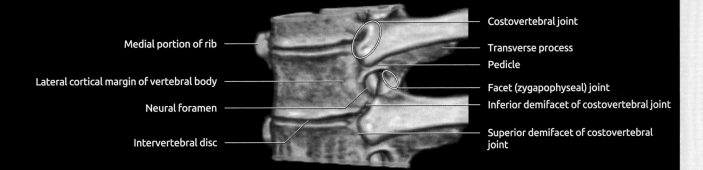

Medial portion of rib — Costovertebral joint

Transverse process

Pedicle

Lateral cortical margin of vertebral body — Facet (zygapophyseal) joint

Neural foramen — Inferior demifacet of costovertebral joint

Intervertebral disc — Superior demifacet of costovertebral joint

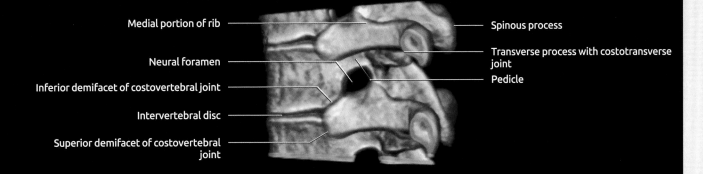

Medial portion of rib — Spinous process

Transverse process with costotransverse joint

Neural foramen — Pedicle

Inferior demifacet of costovertebral joint

Intervertebral disc

Superior demifacet of costovertebral joint

(**Top**) *Oblique anterior 3D VRT examination shows the thoracic spine. The complex costovertebral and costotransverse joints are highlighted in the projection. The superior and inferior demifacets are identified with the joint proper crossing the intervertebral disc space.* (**Middle**) *Lateral oblique 3D VRT examination shows the thoracic spine. The relationship of the neural foramen and the posterior elements and costal joints is visualized in this projection. The foramen is bounded posteriorly by the facet joint, superiorly by the pedicle, and ventrally by the posterior margin of the vertebral body.* (**Bottom**) *Lateral 3D VRT examination shows the thoracic spine. The neural foramina are oriented laterally, therefore viewed en face in this projection and bound by the vertebral body anteriorly, pedicle superiorly, and facet joint posteriorly.*

Normal Anatomy and Techniques

3D VRT NECT

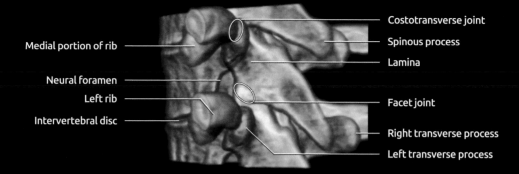

Medial portion of rib

Neural foramen

Left rib

Intervertebral disc

Costotransverse joint

Spinous process

Lamina

Facet joint

Right transverse process

Left transverse process

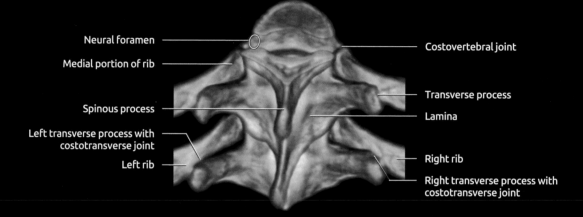

Neural foramen

Medial portion of rib

Spinous process

Left transverse process with costotransverse joint

Left rib

Costovertebral joint

Transverse process

Lamina

Right rib

Right transverse process with costotransverse joint

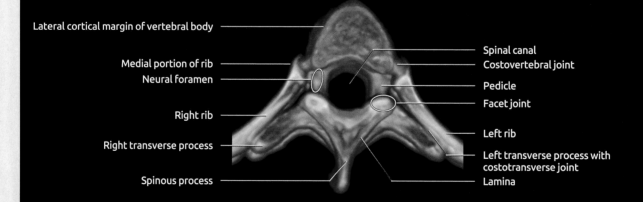

Lateral cortical margin of vertebral body

Medial portion of rib

Neural foramen

Right rib

Right transverse process

Spinous process

Spinal canal

Costovertebral joint

Pedicle

Facet joint

Left rib

Left transverse process with costotransverse joint

Lamina

(Top) Oblique anterior 3D VRT examination shows the thoracic spine. The facet joints are partially seen in this projection, primarily obscured by the posterior surface of the inferior articular facet, which overlaps the dorsal surface of the superior articular facet from the next caudal vertebra. The thoracic spinous processes are long and directed inferiorly, overlapping the next vertebral body level. (Middle) Posterior 3D VRT examination shows the thoracic spine. The posterior bony projections of the thoracic spine are highlighted in this projection, including the spinous processes, transverse processes, and the costotransverse articulations. (Bottom) Axial 3D VRT examination shows the thoracic spine. The 2 costal articulations are viewed in this projection. The neural foramen is immediately adjacent to the costovertebral articulations.

AXIAL BONE CT

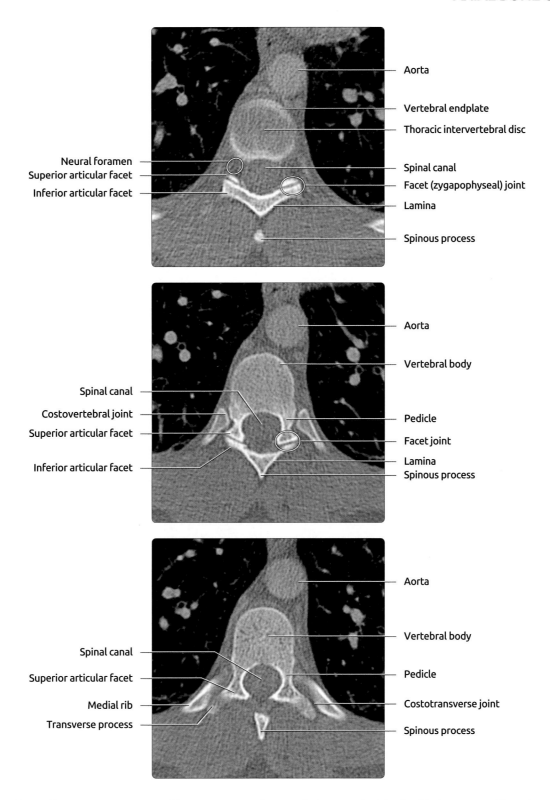

Aorta

Vertebral endplate

Thoracic intervertebral disc

Neural foramen
Superior articular facet
Inferior articular facet

Spinal canal

Facet (zygapophyseal) joint

Lamina

Spinous process

Aorta

Vertebral body

Spinal canal
Costovertebral joint
Superior articular facet

Inferior articular facet

Pedicle

Facet joint

Lamina
Spinous process

Aorta

Vertebral body

Spinal canal

Superior articular facet

Medial rib

Transverse process

Pedicle

Costotransverse joint

Spinous process

(Top) *The 1st of 6 axial bone CT images presented from superior to inferior at the intervertebral disc level is shown. Neural foramina are directed laterally and bound anteriorly by the posterior vertebral body margin and dorsally by the facet joint (superior articular facet). The facet joints are oriented in a coronal plane and strongly resist rotation combined with the costovertebral joints.* (Middle) *In this image through the pedicle level of the thoracic spine, the coronal orientation of the facet joints is well identified. The pedicles are relatively thin and gracile with the adjacent rib articulations.* (Bottom) *In this image through vertebral body level, the posterior bony projections are highlighted, including the spinous process, transverse processes, and medial ribs.*

SAGITTAL T2 MR

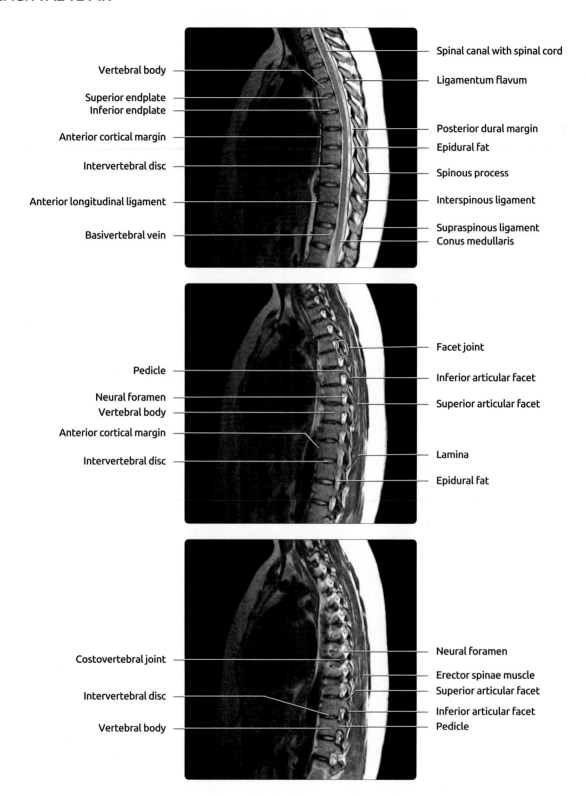

Vertebral body

Superior endplate
Inferior endplate

Anterior cortical margin

Intervertebral disc

Anterior longitudinal ligament

Basivertebral vein

Spinal canal with spinal cord

Ligamentum flavum

Posterior dural margin

Epidural fat

Spinous process

Interspinous ligament

Supraspinous ligament
Conus medullaris

Pedicle

Neural foramen
Vertebral body

Anterior cortical margin

Intervertebral disc

Facet joint

Inferior articular facet

Superior articular facet

Lamina

Epidural fat

Costovertebral joint

Intervertebral disc

Vertebral body

Neural foramen

Erector spinae muscle
Superior articular facet

Inferior articular facet

Pedicle

(Top) The 1st of 3 sagittal T2 MR images of the thoracic spine presented from medial to lateral is shown. The square thoracic vertebral bodies with the small intervening intervertebral discs are identified in this midline view. The spinous processes are large and dominate the dorsal soft tissues. The thoracic cord is seen in its entirety with its smoothly tapering conus medullaris. (Middle) The facet joints are identified on this sagittal image with the coronally oriented joints seen in lateral view. The superior and inferior articular processes and neural foramen are easily viewed in this plane. (Bottom) The more lateral margin of the neural foramen is identified on this section as well as the costovertebral joints at the disc levels.

AXIAL T2 MR

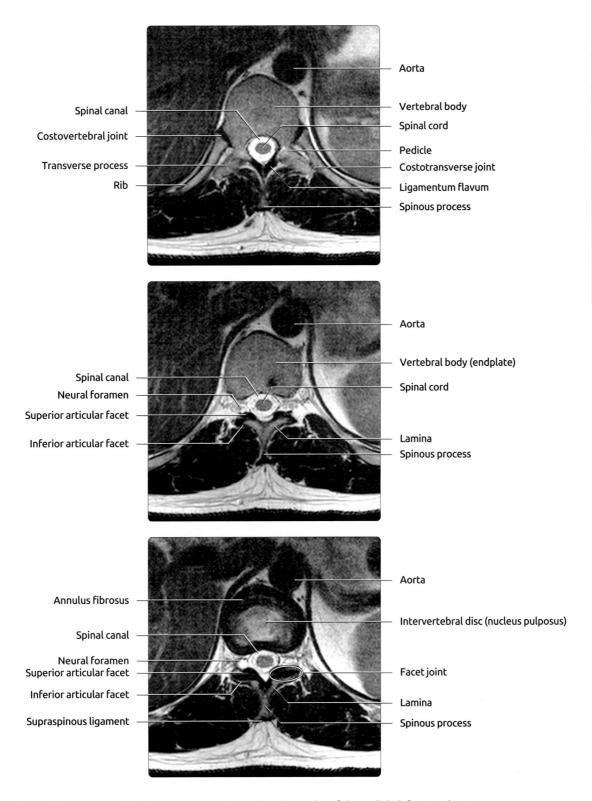

Aorta

Spinal canal

Costovertebral joint

Transverse process

Rib

Vertebral body

Spinal cord

Pedicle

Costotransverse joint

Ligamentum flavum

Spinous process

Aorta

Spinal canal

Neural foramen

Superior articular facet

Inferior articular facet

Vertebral body (endplate)

Spinal cord

Lamina

Spinous process

Annulus fibrosus

Spinal canal

Neural foramen

Superior articular facet

Inferior articular facet

Supraspinous ligament

Aorta

Intervertebral disc (nucleus pulposus)

Facet joint

Lamina

Spinous process

(Top) *The 1st of 3 axial T2 MR images of the thoracic spine is shown. The relationship of the medial rib forming the strong costotransverse and costovertebral joints is highlighted. The transverse processes extend dorsally and laterally to articulate with the medial ribs. The spinous process is large and directed caudally.* **(Middle)** *In this image through the foraminal level of the thoracic spine, the neural foramina are directed laterally with their posterior margin formed by the facet joints and anterior margin by the vertebral body and disc.* **(Bottom)** *In this image through the disc level, the coronal orientation of the facet joints is identified, forming the posterior boundary of the neural foramen. The components of the intervertebral disc are also shown in this section with well-defined nucleus pulposus and annulus fibrosus.*

TERMINOLOGY

Abbreviations

- Anterior longitudinal ligament (ALL)
- Posterior longitudinal ligament (PLL)

Synonyms

- Articular processes = facets = zygapophyses

GROSS ANATOMY

Overview

- 5 discovertebral units (L1-L5)

Components

- **Bones**
  - **Body**
    - Large oval cancellous ventral mass
    - Larger in transverse width than AP diameter
  - **Endplates**
    - Formed by superior & inferior surfaces of vertebral bodies
    - Consist of concave surfaces of 1-mm-thick cortical bone & hyaline cartilage plates
    - Endplates are transitional between fibrocartilage disc & vertebral body
    - Nutrients to disc diffuse via endplates
  - **Arch**
    - Pedicle: Project directly posteriorly
    - Transverse process: Extend out laterally, long and flat on L1-L4, small at L5
    - Articular process: Superior and inferior articular processes with pars interarticularis between; facet joints oriented obliquely
    - Lamina: Broad, thick, overlap minimally
    - Spinous process
- **Intervertebral foramen**
  - Aperture giving exit to segmental spinal nerves and entrance to vessels
  - Oriented laterally below pedicle
  - Boundaries
    - Superior & inferior pedicles of adjacent vertebrae
    - Ventral boundary is dorsal aspect vertebral body above and intervertebral disc below
    - Dorsal boundary is joint capsule of facets and ligamentum flavum
  - Vertical elliptical shape in lumbar region
    - Vertical diameter 12-19 mm
    - Transverse diameter from disc to ligamentum flavum ~ 7 mm; thus, little room for pathologic narrowing
- **Joints**
  - **Intervertebral disc**
    - Outer annulus fibrosus (alternating layers of collagen fibers)
    - Inner annulus fibrosus (fibrocartilaginous component)
    - Transitional region
    - Central nucleus pulposus (elastic mucoprotein gel with high water content)
  - **Facet (zygapophyseal) joints**
    - Facet joints oriented obliquely
    - Superior facet: Concave, faces dorsomedially to meet inferior facet from above
    - Inferior facet: Faces ventrolaterally to meet superior facet from body below
- **Ligaments**
  - ALL and PLL, interspinous and supraspinous ligaments
  - **Ligamentum flavum**
    - Thick in lumbar region
    - Connects adjacent lamina
    - Extends from capsule of facet joint to junction of lamina with spinous process, discontinuous in midline
- **Muscles**
  - Erector spinae: Poorly differentiated muscle mass composed of iliocostalis, longissimus, spinalis
  - Multifidi (best developed in lumbar spine)
  - Deep muscles: Interspinalis, intertransversarius
  - Quadratus lumborum & psoas muscles
- **Biomechanics**
  - Lumbar articulations permit ventral flexion, lateral flexion, extension
  - Facets prevent rotation
  - Lumbosacral junction motion checked by strong iliolumbar ligaments

IMAGING ANATOMY

Radiography

- **"Scotty dog"** demonstrated on oblique view
  - Nose = transverse process, eye = pedicle, ear = superior articular process, neck = pars interarticularis, front leg = inferior articular process

Cross-Sectional Imaging

- **Facet joint orientation**
  - Facet joint angle is measured relative to coronal plane
  - Normal facet joint angle ~ 40°
  - More sagittally oriented facet joints (> 45°) at L4 & L5 levels ↑ incidence of disc herniation & degenerative spondylolisthesis

ANATOMY IMAGING ISSUES

Imaging Pitfalls

- **Lumbosacral junction**
  - Transitional lumbosacral vertebrae
    - Congenital malformation of vertebrae, usually last lumbar or 1st sacral vertebra
    - Bony characteristics of both lumbar vertebrae and sacrum
  - Vertebral facet asymmetry (**tropism**)
    - Asymmetry between left & right vertebral facet (zygapophyseal) joint angles
    - Tropism defined as mild (6-10°), moderate (10-16°), or severe (> 16°)
    - Variable relationship between facet joint tropism & disc herniation at L4 and L5 level

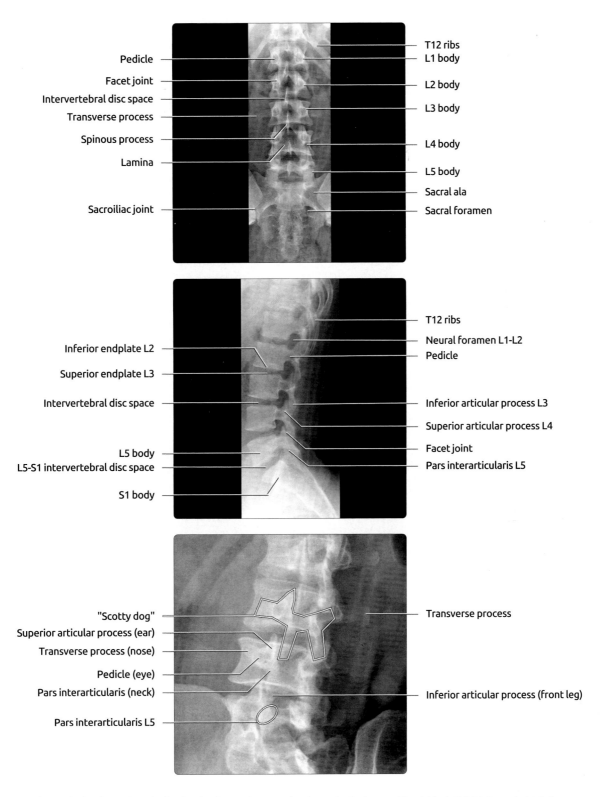

Pedicle — T12 ribs
Facet joint — L1 body
Intervertebral disc space — L2 body
Transverse process — L3 body
Spinous process — L4 body
Lamina — L5 body
— Sacral ala
Sacroiliac joint — Sacral foramen

Inferior endplate L2 — T12 ribs
Superior endplate L3 — Neural foramen L1-L2
— Pedicle
Intervertebral disc space — Inferior articular process L3
— Superior articular process L4
L5 body — Facet joint
L5-S1 intervertebral disc space — Pars interarticularis L5
S1 body

"Scotty dog" — Transverse process
Superior articular process (ear)
Transverse process (nose)
Pedicle (eye)
Pars interarticularis (neck) — Inferior articular process (front leg)
Pars interarticularis L5

(Top) *AP view shows the lumbar spine. The lumbar bodies are large and rectangular in shape with relatively thick intervertebral disc spaces. The pedicles are viewed en face with the adjacent facet joints incompletely visualized due to their obliquity. The large horizontal transverse processes are easily identified at the pedicle levels.* (Middle) *Lateral view shows the lumbar spine. The large, strong lumbar bodies join with the stout lumbar pedicles and posterior elements. The neural foramina are large and directed laterally. The boundary of the neural foramen includes the posterior vertebral body, inferior and superior pedicle cortex, and superior articular process.* (Bottom) *Oblique view shows the lumbar spine. The typical Scotty dog appearance of the posterior elements is visible. The neck of the dog is the pars interarticularis.*

3D VRT NECT

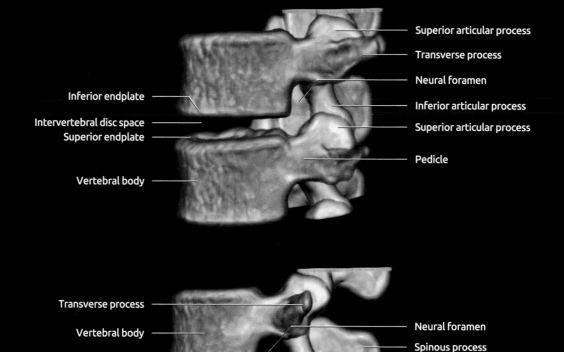

Superior articular process

Transverse process

Neural foramen

Inferior endplate

Inferior articular process

Intervertebral disc space

Superior articular process

Superior endplate

Pedicle

Vertebral body

Transverse process

Vertebral body

Neural foramen

Spinous process

Inferior endplate

Inferior articular process

Intervertebral disc space

Superior articular process

Superior endplate

Pedicle

Pars interarticularis

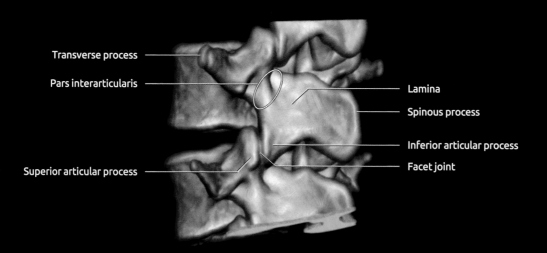

Transverse process

Pars interarticularis

Lamina

Spinous process

Inferior articular process

Facet joint

Superior articular process

(Top) *Left anterior oblique 3D VRT NECT examination shows the lumbar spine. The broad, stout pedicle/vertebral body junction is highlighted in this projection with the superior facet arising as the dorsal extension.* **(Middle)** *Left lateral 3D VRT NECT examination of the lumbar spine shows the neural foramen seen en face as it projects laterally.* **(Bottom)** *Left posterior oblique 3D VRT NECT examination shows the lumbar spine. This view shows the surface anatomy inherent in the "Scotty dog." The transverse process (nose), superior articular process (ear), inferior articular process (front leg), and intervening pars interarticularis (neck) are well defined. The pedicle that forms the "eye" on oblique radiographs is obscured. The oblique sagittal orientation of the facet joints is evident in this view, restricting lumbar rotation and allowing flexion/extension.*

AXIAL BONE CT

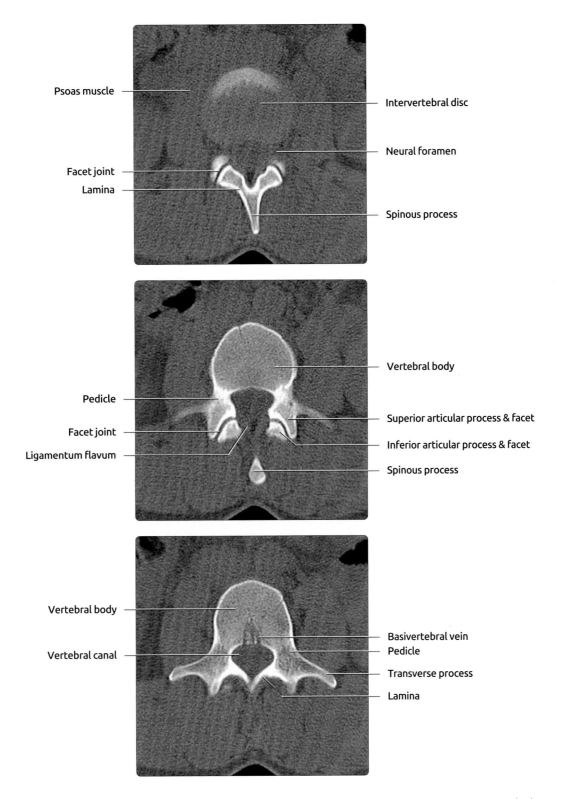

(Top) *The 1st of 6 axial bone CT images through the lumbar spine is presented from superior to inferior. This image is at intervertebral disc and lower neural foraminal level. The posterior intervertebral disc forms the lower anterior border of the neural foramen, which contains primarily fat. Exiting nerves are in the upper neural foramen.* **(Middle)** *This image through the facet joint demonstrates the typical lumbar morphology with the superior facet showing a concave posterior surface and inferior facet showing the complementary convex anterior surface. Facet joints are oriented ~ 40° from the coronal plane. An angle of > 45° from the coronal plane increases incidence of disc herniation and degenerative spondylolisthesis at L4 and L5 levels.* **(Bottom)** *This image shows the triangular central vertebral canal and posteriorly oriented pedicles. Basivertebral veins enter the vertebral body through the posterior cortex.*

AXIAL BONE CT

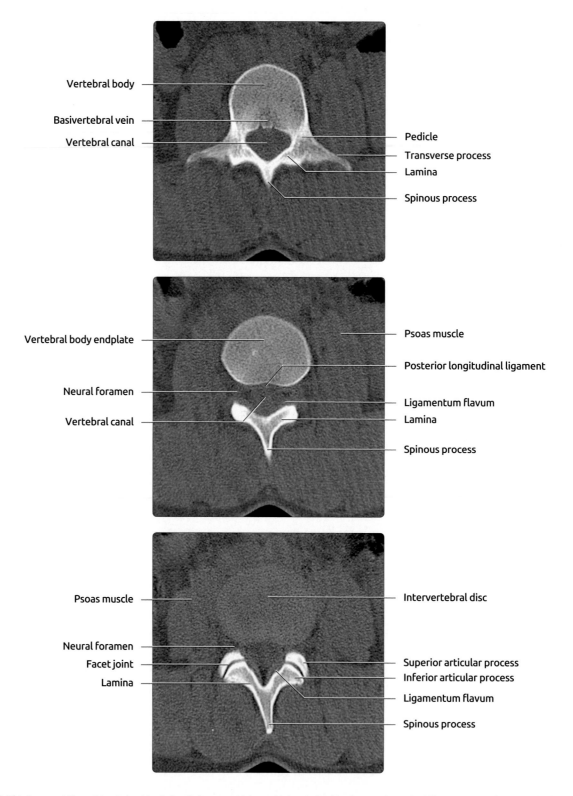

Vertebral body

Basivertebral vein

Vertebral canal

Pedicle

Transverse process

Lamina

Spinous process

Vertebral body endplate

Psoas muscle

Posterior longitudinal ligament

Neural foramen

Vertebral canal

Ligamentum flavum

Lamina

Spinous process

Psoas muscle

Intervertebral disc

Neural foramen

Facet joint

Lamina

Superior articular process

Inferior articular process

Ligamentum flavum

Spinous process

(Top) *This image at the midvertebral body level shows a thick cortical vertebral body margin and midline posterior basivertebral veins. The pedicles are strong, thick, and directed posteriorly. Large transverse processes project from the lateral margins.* **(Middle)** *In this image at the endplate level, the neural foramen is identified, opening laterally. The posterior elements have a T pattern with the large posteriorly directed spinous process.* **(Bottom)** *This image through the intervertebral disc level again demonstrates the lower neural foramen bound anteriorly by intervertebral disc and posteriorly by the superior articular process and facet joint. Oblique coronal orientation of the facet joints is again appreciated. Asymmetry between the left and right vertebral facet joint angles with 1 joint having a more sagittal orientation than the other is termed tropism.*

SAGITTAL T1 MR

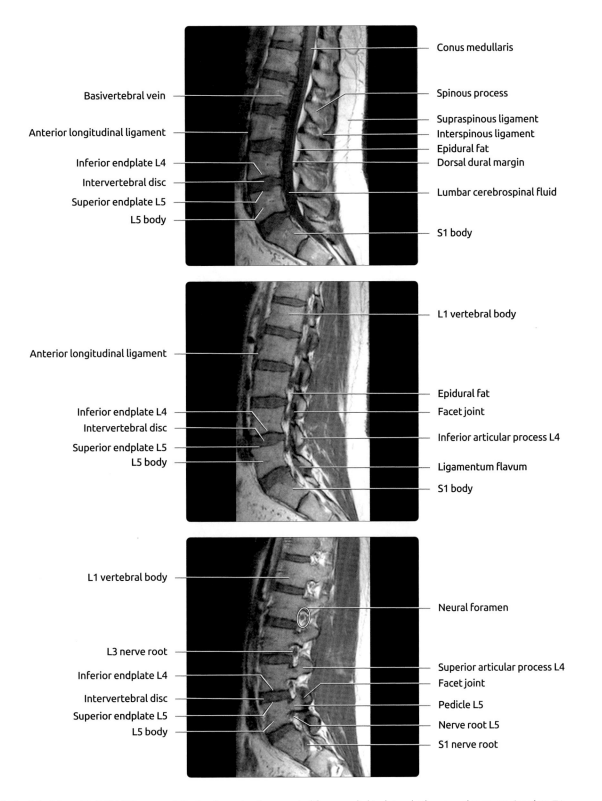

Top image labels:
- Basivertebral vein
- Anterior longitudinal ligament
- Inferior endplate L4
- Intervertebral disc
- Superior endplate L5
- L5 body
- Conus medullaris
- Spinous process
- Supraspinous ligament
- Interspinous ligament
- Epidural fat
- Dorsal dural margin
- Lumbar cerebrospinal fluid
- S1 body

Middle image labels:
- Anterior longitudinal ligament
- Inferior endplate L4
- Intervertebral disc
- Superior endplate L5
- L5 body
- L1 vertebral body
- Epidural fat
- Facet joint
- Inferior articular process L4
- Ligamentum flavum
- S1 body

Bottom image labels:
- L1 vertebral body
- L3 nerve root
- Inferior endplate L4
- Intervertebral disc
- Superior endplate L5
- L5 body
- Neural foramen
- Superior articular process L4
- Facet joint
- Pedicle L5
- Nerve root L5
- S1 nerve root

(Top) *The 1st of 3 sagittal T1 MR images of the lumbar spine is presented from medial to lateral. The normal marrow signal on T1 images is of increased signal compared to the adjacent intervertebral discs in the adult due to fatty marrow content. The basivertebral veins are seen as signal voids in the midline of the posterior vertebral bodies, often with surrounding high signal fatty marrow. The intervertebral disc morphology is poorly identified on this sequence with little differentiation of annulus or nucleus.* **(Middle)** *In this image, the lateral vertebral bodies are evident with the pronounced oblong-shaped inferior articular facets dominating the posterior aspect.* **(Bottom)** *In this image, the anterior boundaries of the neural foramina are evident, as is the relationship of the disc to the exiting nerve.*

AXIAL T2 MR

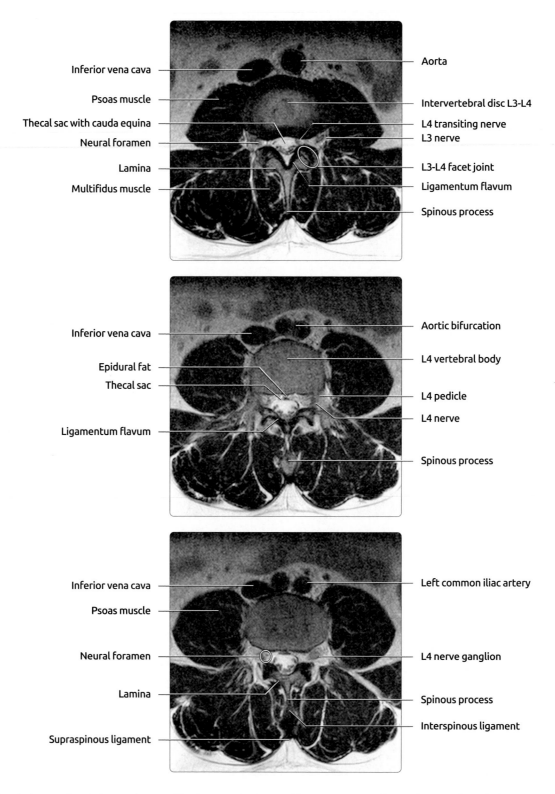

Inferior vena cava — Aorta

Psoas muscle — Intervertebral disc L3-L4

Thecal sac with cauda equina — L4 transiting nerve

Neural foramen — L3 nerve

Lamina — L3-L4 facet joint

Multifidus muscle — Ligamentum flavum

Spinous process

Inferior vena cava — Aortic bifurcation

L4 vertebral body

Epidural fat — L4 pedicle

Thecal sac — L4 nerve

Ligamentum flavum — Spinous process

Inferior vena cava — Left common iliac artery

Psoas muscle

Neural foramen — L4 nerve ganglion

Lamina — Spinous process

Interspinous ligament

Supraspinous ligament

(Top) *The 1st of 6 axial T2 MR images of lumbar spine is presented from superior to inferior. This view through the intervertebral disc shows increased disc signal within the central nucleus pulposus due to its high water content and low signal within the peripheral annulus fibrosus. The margin with the thecal sac is sharp with the cauda equina seen as punctate nerves within the high signal cerebrospinal fluid. The L3 nerve is extraforaminal in location; the L4 nerve is transiting in lateral recess.* (Middle) *This image just below the L4 pedicle shows the exiting L4 nerve passing just below the pedicle within the upper neural foramen.* (Bottom) *This image shows the L4 nerve ganglion and surrounding fat within the midneural foramen. The posterior margin of the neural foramen at this level is the facet joint complex, and the anterior margin is the posterior vertebral body.*

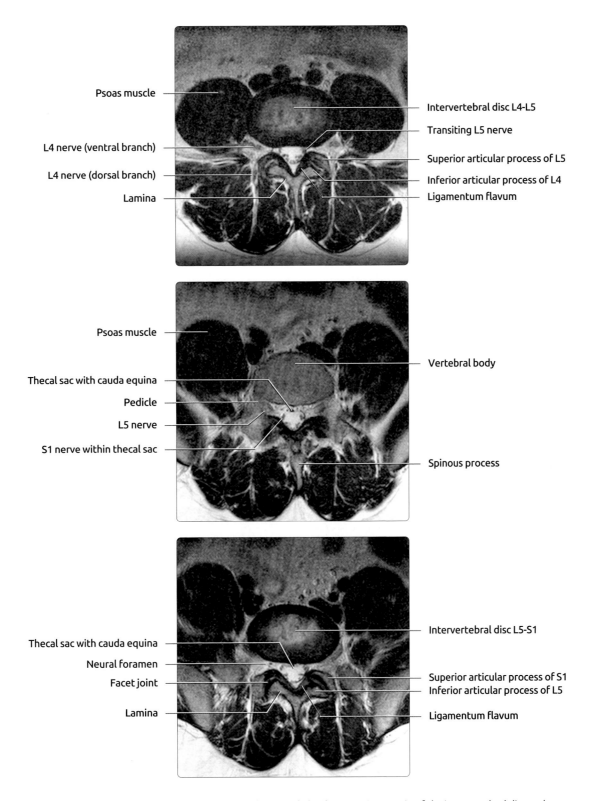

Psoas muscle — **Intervertebral disc L4-L5**

Transiting L5 nerve

L4 nerve (ventral branch) — **Superior articular process of L5**

L4 nerve (dorsal branch) — **Inferior articular process of L4**

Lamina — **Ligamentum flavum**

Psoas muscle

Thecal sac with cauda equina — **Vertebral body**

Pedicle

L5 nerve

S1 nerve within thecal sac

Spinous process

Thecal sac with cauda equina — **Intervertebral disc L5-S1**

Neural foramen

Facet joint — **Superior articular process of S1**
Inferior articular process of L5

Lamina — **Ligamentum flavum**

(Top) *This image through the lower neural foramen is bordered anteriorly by the posterior margin of the intervertebral disc and posteriorly by the facet joint. The L4 nerve has divided into anterior and posterior branches.* **(Middle)** *This image through the upper L5 neural foramina shows the exiting L5 nerves just below the pedicles.* **(Bottom)** *In this image through the L5-S1 intervertebral disc, the typical facet morphology is again identified. The superior articular facet is seen as a convex anterior bony mass with low signal cortical margin. The joint space is seen as a linear focus of high signal due to joint fluid and cartilage. The inferior articular facet is typically convex anteriorly, although it can be seen as a more straight margin or even slightly concave (as is seen on the left). The facet joints are oriented ~ 40° from the coronal plane.*

Terminology

Radiographic measurement techniques, skull base craniometry, skull base lines

Pathology-based Imaging Issues

This chapter provides a broad summary of the varied measurement techniques used to evaluate the spine. The main focus for the reader should be the tables and the multiple schematics that define the variously named lines and angles. These summarize the classic measurement techniques for the skull base and rheumatoid disease as well as some of the most commonly used measurements for trauma assessment. The rest of the measurements defined below are a mixture of miscellaneous measurements and those that do not translate well into a table (i.e., equations).

Torg-Pavlov Ratio

- Diameter of canal to width of vertebral body (initially defined on plain radiographs of subaxial spine)
- Utility is controversial; < 0.80 as seen on lateral view considered to be cervical stenosis, such small canal potentially increases risk for cord injury

Maximum Canal Compromise (%)

- $= 1 - (Di/[(Da+Db)/2]) \times 100\%$
- AP canal diameter at normal levels (immediately above and below level of injury) and at level of maximum compromise are defined; measurement of normal levels is taken at the midvertebral body level: Di is anteroposterior canal diameter at level of maximum injury, Da is AP canal diameter at nearest normal level above level of injury, and Db is AP canal diameter at nearest normal level below level of injury
- In spinal cord injury patients, midline T1 and T2 images provide objective, quantifiable, and reliable assessment of cord compression that cannot be defined by CT alone

Maximum Cord Compression (%)

- $= 1 - (di/[(da+db)/2]) \times 100\%$
- AP cord diameter at normal levels immediately above and below level of injury and at level of maximum cord compression are defined: di is anteroposterior cord diameter at level of maximum injury, da is AP cord diameter at nearest normal level above level of injury, and db is AP cord diameter at nearest normal level below level of injury (if cord edema is present, then measurements are made at midvertebral body level just above or below extent of edema where cord appears normal)

Cobb Measurement of Kyphosis

- Lines are drawn to mark superior endplate of superior next unaffected vertebral body and inferior endplate of inferior next unaffected vertebral body, which are then extended anterior to bony canal; perpendicular lines are then extended, and angle between 2 perpendicular lines is measured

Tangent Method for Kyphosis

- Lines are drawn along posterior vertebral body margin on lateral view of affected body and next most superior body that is unaffected; angle between these 2 vertically oriented lines is measured

Centroid, or the geometric center of the vertebral body, is defined by drawing diagonal lines between opposite corners of the body, with the centroid at the intersection.

Apical Vertebral Translation (AVT)

- Lateral displacement of apex of coronal curve is relative to center sacral vertical line (CSVL) on AP plain film; AVT is horizontal distance between centroid of apical body and CSVL

Sagittal Balance

- Sagittal alignment is defined on lateral view using C7 plumb line; distal reference point is posterior superior aspect of sacrum (positive number if C7 plumb line falls anterior to reference point, negative number if it falls posterior to reference)

Selected References

1. Radcliff KE et al: Comprehensive computed tomography assessment of the upper cervical anatomy: what is normal? Spine J. 10(3):219-29, 2010
2. Rojas CA et al: Evaluation of the C1-C2 articulation on MDCT in healthy children and young adults. AJR Am J Roentgenol. 193(5):1388-92, 2009
3. Angevine PD et al: Radiographic measurement techniques. Neurosurgery. 63(3 Suppl):40-5, 2008
4. Bono CM et al: Measurement techniques for upper cervical spine injuries: consensus statement of the Spine Trauma Study Group. Spine (Phila Pa 1976). 32(5):593-600, 2007
5. Furlan JC et al: A quantitative and reproducible method to assess cord compression and canal stenosis after cervical spine trauma: a study of interrater and intrarater reliability. Spine (Phila Pa 1976). 32(19):2083-91, 2007
6. Pang D et al: Atlanto-occipital dislocation–part 2: The clinical use of (occipital) condyle-C1 interval, comparison with other diagnostic methods, and the manifestation, management, and outcome of atlanto-occipital dislocation in children. Neurosurgery. 61(5):995-1015; discussion 1015, 2007
7. Pang D et al: Atlanto-occipital dislocation: part 1–normal occipital condyle-C1 interval in 89 children. Neurosurgery. 61(3):514-21; discussion 521, 2007
8. Bono CM et al: Measurement techniques for lower cervical spine injuries: consensus statement of the Spine Trauma Study Group. Spine (Phila Pa 1976). 31(5):603-9, 2006
9. Fehlings MG et al: The optimal radiologic method for assessing spinal canal compromise and cord compression in patients with cervical spinal cord injury. Part II: results of a multicenter study. Spine (Phila Pa 1976). 24(6):605-13, 1999
10. Rao SC et al: The optimal radiologic method for assessing spinal canal compromise and cord compression in patients with cervical spinal cord injury. Part I: an evidence-based analysis of the published literature. Spine (Phila Pa 1976). 24(6):598-604, 1999
11. Harris JH Jr et al: Radiologic diagnosis of traumatic occipitovertebral dissociation: 1. Normal occipitovertebral relationships on lateral radiographs of supine subjects. AJR Am J Roentgenol. 162(4):881-6, 1994
12. Harris JH Jr et al: Radiologic diagnosis of traumatic occipitovertebral dissociation: 2. Comparison of three methods of detecting occipitovertebral relationships on lateral radiographs of supine subjects. AJR Am J Roentgenol. 162(4):887-92, 1994
13. Powers B et al: Traumatic anterior atlanto-occipital dislocation. Neurosurgery. 4(1):12-7, 1979

Common CV Junction Measurements

Measurement	Definition	Normal	Abnormal
Chamberlain (palatooccipital) line	Posterior hard palate to opisthion	< 2.5 mm of dens above line	Dens > 2.5 mm above line
McGregor (basal) line	Posterior hard palate to lowest point of occipital bone	Tip of dens < 4.5 mm above line	Tip of dens > 4.5 mm above line
McRae line	Basion to opisthion	Entire dens below line	< 19 mm
Wackenheim clival line	Dorsum sellae to tip of clivus	Entire dens ventral to line	Dens bisects line
Fischgold digastric line	Connects 2 digastric fossae	Entire dens below line	Dens bisects line
Fischgold bimastoid line	Connects tips of mastoid processes	Tip of dens 3 mm below to 10 mm above line	Tip of dens > 10 mm above line
Anterior atlantodental interval	Posterior aspect of anterior C1 arch to anterior margin odontoid process	Plain films in children: < 4-5 mm; plain film in adults: Men < 3.0 mm, women < 2.5 mm; sagittal CT reformats in children: < 2.6 mm; sagittal CT in adults: Both men and women < 2.0 mm	Plain films in children: > 4-5 mm; plain film in adults: Men > 3.0 mm, women > 2.5 mm; sagittal CT reformats in children: > 2.6 mm; sagittal CT in adults: Both men and women > 2.0 mm
Atlantooccipital joint space	Line from midpoint of occipital condyle to C1 condylar fossa	Plain films in children: < 5 mm; CT in children: < 2.5 mm	Plain films in children: > 5 mm; CT in children: > 2.5 mm
Summed condylar distance	Sum of bilateral distances between midpoint of occipital condyle and C1 condylar fossa	CT in adults: < 4.2 mm	
Atlantoaxial joint space	Line defining midpoint of C1-C2 joint on coronal view	CT in adults: < 3.4 mm; CT in children: < 3.9 mm	CT in adults: > 3.4 mm; CT in children: > 3.9 mm

Rheumatoid Arthritis Measurements

Measurement	Definition	Normal	Abnormal
Ranawat	Distance between center of C2 pedicle and transverse axis of atlas measured along axis of odontoid process	< 15 mm in men, < 13 mm in women	≥ 15 mm in men, ≥ 13 mm in women
Redlund-Johnell line	Distance between McGregor line and midpoint of caudal margin C2	< 34 mm in men, < 29 mm in women	≥ 34 mm in men, ≥ 29 mm in women
Clark stations	Dividing odontoid process into 3 parts in sagittal plane	Anterior ring of atlas is level with 1st station	Anterior ring of atlas is level with middle 1/3 (2nd station) or caudal 1/3 (3rd station)
Posterior atlantodental interval	Horizontal distance from posterior dens to anterior aspect of C1 lamina or ring		Smaller is worse and relates to potential neurologic deficit
Space available for cord (SAC)	AP diameter on sagittal MR study between dorsal and ventral dura	> 13 mm	SAC < 13 mm then decompression in RA patients considered
Spinal canal diameter	Horizontal measurement from posterior vertebral body to spinolaminar line		On plain films < 14 mm, canal stenosis warrants MR for further evaluation

CV Junction Trauma Measurements

Measurement	Definition	Normal	Abnormal
Basion dental interval	Basion to superior aspect of odontoid process	< 12-12.5 mm in children on plain films, < 10.5 mm in children by sagittal CT, < 8.5 mm in adults	> 12 mm (Harris measurement)
Basion axial interval	Distance between basion and line drawn along posterior cortical margin of C2	0-12 mm on plain films	Highly variable and not recommended as primary diagnostic method
Powers ratio	Ratio of distance between basion and C1 posterior arch divided by distance between opisthion and midpoint of posterior aspect of anterior C1 arch (BC/OA)	< 1.0	> 1.0 (anterior dislocation only) posterior dissociation or vertical distraction could be missed with normal value

(Left) *Sagittal graphic of the craniocervical junction shows a Wackenheim clival line (red) extending tangent to the normal odontoid position. The line is drawn from the dorsum sellae to the tip of the clivus.*
(Right) *Sagittal graphic of the craniocervical junction shows a Chamberlain line (red), drawn from the posterior hard palate to the opisthion, and McGregor line (yellow), drawn from the posterior hard palate to the lowest point of the occipital bone.*

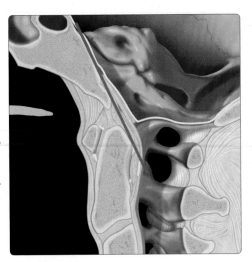
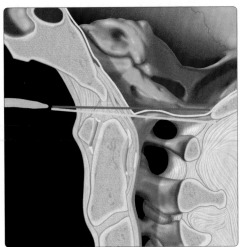

(Left) *Sagittal graphic of the craniocervical junction shows lines comprising the Powers ratio (BC/OA), where normal is < 1: BC = basion to C1 posterior arch; OA = opisthion & midpoint of the posterior aspect of the anterior C1 arch.*
(Right) *Sagittal graphic of the craniocervical junction shows lines comprising the Lee method. BC2SL & C2O should just intersect tangentially with the posterosuperior aspect of the dens and the highest point on the atlas spinolaminar line, respectively, in a normal state.*

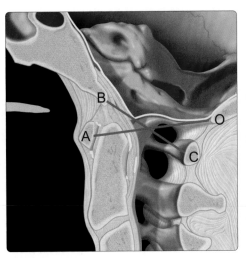
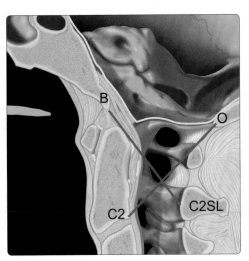

(Left) *Sagittal graphic shows the basion dental interval (BDI) in red, which should be < 12.0-12.5 mm in children on plain films and < 8.5 mm in adults on CT. Black lines define the basion axial interval (BAI) ➡ extending from the basion to the line extended along the posterior margin of C2, which should be < 12 mm on plain films. The C1-C2 spinolaminar line is shown in purple (< 8 mm in adults).*
(Right) *Sagittal graphic shows the atlantodental interval (green) and spinal canal diameter (red).*

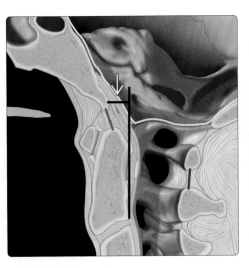
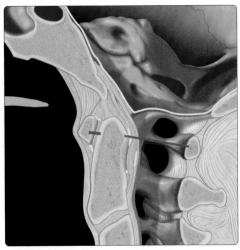

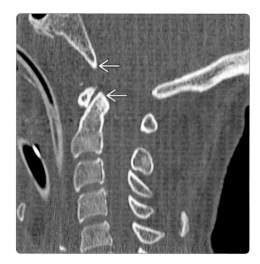

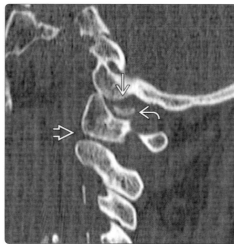

(Left) *Sagittal CT reconstruction in atlantooccipital dislocation (AOD) shows widening ➡ of the BDI > 8.5 mm in this adult. Note the normal Wackenheim line relationship.* (Right) *Sagittal CT reconstruction in AOD shows widening of the C0-C1 junction ➡ with anterior subluxation of the condyle. A condylar fragment is present in the joint space ➡. Note the normal C1-C2 relationship ➡.*

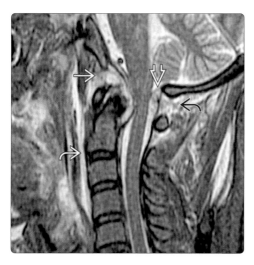

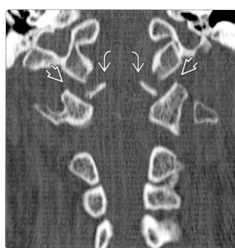

(Left) *Sagittal STIR MR in AOD shows widening of the BDI with ↑ T2 signal ➡ from alar and apical ligament rupture. Note also prevertebral edema ➡ & posterior interspinous ligament disruption ➡. Posterior epidural hemorrhage ➡ contributes to subarachnoid space narrowing.* (Right) *Coronal CT reconstruction in AOD shows marked widening of the C0-C1 joint space ➡, which should be ~ 2 mm. Bilateral symmetric avulsion fractures off of the condyles are present ➡.*

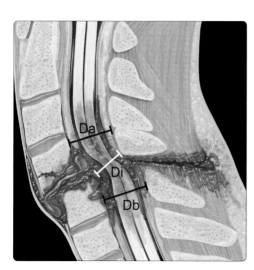

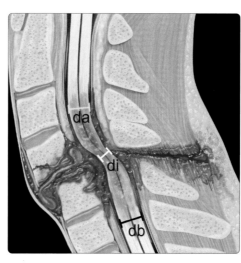

(Left) *Sagittal graphic shows maximum canal compromise. The Di is anteroposterior canal diameter at the level of maximum injury; Da is the AP canal diameter at the nearest normal level above the level of injury. The Db is AP canal diameter at the nearest normal level below the level of injury.* (Right) *Sagittal graphic shows maximum cord compression. The di is AP cord diameter at the level of maximum injury. The da is the AP cord diameter at nearest normal level above injury. db is AP cord diameter at nearest normal level below injury.*

(Left) *Sagittal graphic shows a Redlund-Johnell line (red), which is defined as distance between the McGregor line (yellow) and midpoint of caudal margin of C2 body.*
(Right) *Sagittal graphic shows a Ranawat measurement as the distance between the center of the C2 pedicle (purple) and transverse axis (yellow) of the atlas measured along axis of the odontoid process.*

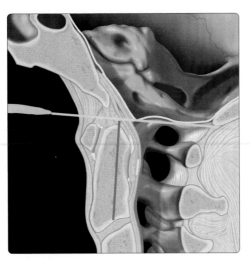
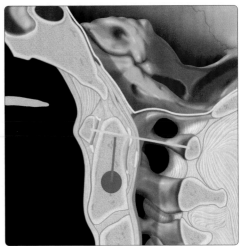

(Left) *Sagittal graphic shows the 3 Clark stations. If the anterior ring of C1 is level with the 2nd or 3rd station, then basilar invagination is present.*
(Right) *Sagittal graphic shows 2 different measurements: McRae line (yellow) is defined from the basion to opisthion, and the dens should be below this line. Length of McRae should be > 19 mm. Lower measurement shows components of Torg-Pavlov ratio, which is diameter of canal (red) to width of vertebral body (black). Normal is > 0.8.*

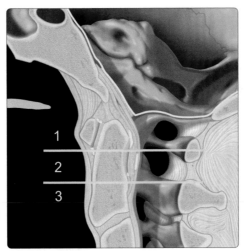
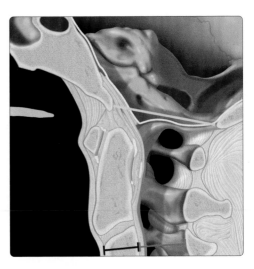

(Left) *Coronal CT shows a Fischgold digastric line (yellow) connecting the 2 digastric fossae (normal when dens below the line) and Fischgold bimastoid line (red) connecting the mastoid processes (abnormal if tip of dens > 10 mm above line).*
(Right) *Sagittal CT study shows upward translocation of odontoid with a Wackenheim clival line & Chamberlain line grossly abnormal. The odontoid is eroded with a thinned pencil tip appearance. Note the markedly increased atlantodental interval.*

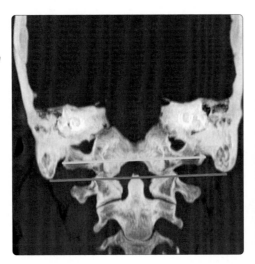
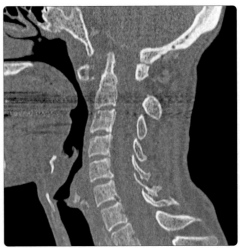

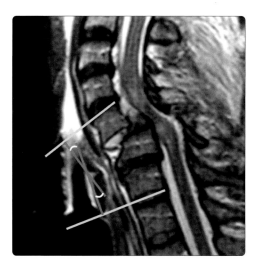

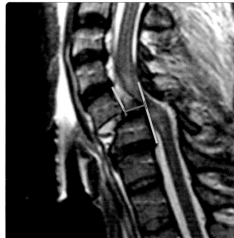

(Left) *Sagittal view shows a Cobb angle method for assessing the cervical kyphosis. Lines are drawn along the superior endplate of the cephalad unaffected body and inferior endplate of caudal unaffected body (yellow). The angle of the perpendiculars (red) from these lines is considered Cobb angle (white).* (Right) *Sagittal view shows posterior vertebral body tangent method. Lines extend from posterior body at fractured level and superior unaffected level. Distance can be measured (red) or angle of lines determined.*

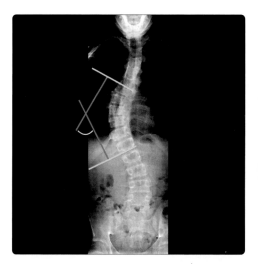

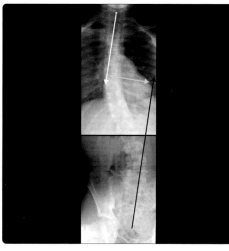

(Left) *AP view shows a Cobb measurement. Lines are drawn (yellow) along end vertebrae, which are upper & lower limits of curve tilting most severely toward concavity. Perpendiculars are drawn from the endplate lines (red), with angle measurement (white).* (Right) *Anteroposterior radiograph shows a measurement of the overall coronal plane balance by the distance (yellow) from the C7 plumb line (white) to the central sacral vertical line (CSVL) (black). Positive displacement is to the right, negative to the left.*

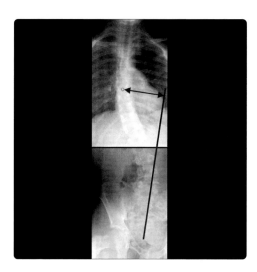

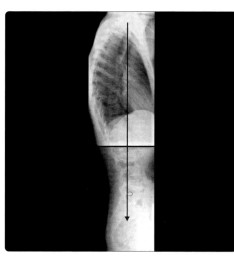

(Left) *AP radiograph shows a measurement of apical vertebral translation (AVT). The distance (line with arrows) from the centroid of the apex of the curve (yellow) is measured relative to the center sacral vertical line (CSVL) (black).* (Right) *Lateral radiograph shows measurement of the sagittal balance in which horizontal displacement is measured from the plumb line extended from the centroid of C7 (black) to posterior superior margin of the sacrum (yellow). Positive balance is identified when line is anterior to reference point.*

TERMINOLOGY

- Substantial imaging overlap in routine early postoperative findings vs. surgical complications
  - Early postoperative imaging not routinely obtained
  - Edema, granulation tissue at operative site may simulate residual/recurrent disc herniation
  - Marrow changes and fluid associated with intervertebral fusion may simulate appearance of spondylodiscitis

IMAGING

- CT: Evaluation of graft position, hardware, bony integrity, and fractures
  - Graft fusion with bony bridging best evaluated by thin-section CT
- MR: Evaluation of endplates, paraspinal soft tissues, epidural space, and intrathecal structures

- Postoperative disc signal dependent on preoperative degree of degeneration, specific surgery and type of implant, and presence or absence of biologic modifiers (i.e., rhBMP-2)
- May see transient increase in disc height and T2 signal immediately after discectomy (not related to infection)
- Discectomy accelerates degenerative appearance of disc with loss of T2 signal and loss of disc height
- Solid fusion typically shown by fatty marrow infiltration/ossification of disc with T1 hyperintensity
- Typical postoperative discectomy enhancement consists of smooth linear enhancement of disc paralleling endplates, with enhancement of dorsal annulus at curettage site

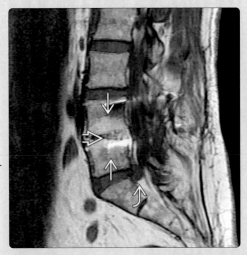
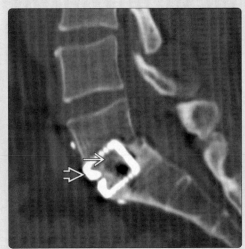

(Left) Sagittal unenhanced T1W MR shows prior laminectomy and fusion with pedicle screws of the L4-L5 level. Fusion appears solid, with high signal fatty marrow conversion of the disc space ⮞ and adjacent fatty type II endplate changes ➡. There is a disc extrusion at the L5-S1 level ⮞. (Right) Sagittal reformatted NECT shows intervertebral fusion of the L5-S1 using fusion cages ⮞. Mature bone bridges the intervertebral space ➡, demonstrating a good bony union.

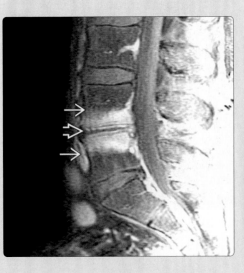
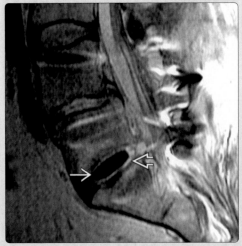

(Left) Sagittal T1 C+ FS MR shows marked endplate ➡ and fine linear enhancement ⮞ of the intervertebral disc due to degeneration. There is no endplate irregularity or paravertebral mass to suggest disc space infection. Fine horizontal linear enhancement is pronounced but not necessarily indicative of disc space infection. (Right) Sagittal T2WI MR shows early look of L5-S1 posterior lumbar invertebral fusion (PLIF) with low signal graft material within the disc space ⮞ and surrounding hyperintense fluid ⮞.

TERMINOLOGY

Definitions

- Discectomy or partial discectomy
  - Surgical removal of herniated portion of intervertebral disc
- Interbody fusion
  - Disc removal by posterior (posterior lumbar intervertebral fusion) or anterior (anterior lumbar intervertebral fusion) approach
  - Insertion of bone graft &/or fusion hardware
  - Goal is arthrodesis (fusion) across disc space
- Disc replacement
  - Variety of intervertebral hardware
  - Preserves motion across segment: Arthroplasty rather than arthrodesis
- Pseudoarthrosis
  - Failure to obtain bony union after fusion
  - Ideally, fused segment will show
    - Mature bridging bone on radiographs, CT
    - Cold on bone scan 6-12 months postop
    - Resolution of type I endplate marrow or conversion to type II
    - No motion on flexion-extension radiographs
  - However
    - Geometry of pseudoarthrosis may be complex and difficult to appreciate on radiographs, CT
    - Bone scan performs poorly, with significant false-negative and false-positive findings
      - Somewhat better performance at 12 months relative to 6 months postop
    - Stability provided by instrumentation may prevent motion on flexion-extension films, despite pseudoarthrosis
      - 2-3° motion may be present with fusion due to compliance of normal bone
    - Pedicle screw fracture can be seen with pseudoarthrosis
      - Instrumentation is temporizing mechanism until bony union can occur
- Peridural fibrosis
  - Some degree of peridural fibrosis along margin of thecal sac is typical finding following discectomy
    - Edema and tissue disruption at discectomy site particularly conspicuous in first 6 weeks postoperatively
- Nerve root clumping, enhancement
  - Transient nerve root clumping can be identified in early postoperative period, often resolves spontaneously
  - Solitary nerve root enhancement may be seen perioperatively; inflammation related to compression, manipulation

IMAGING

Imaging Recommendations

- Best imaging tool
  - CT: Evaluation of graft position, hardware, bony integrity, and fractures
    - Graft fusion with bony bridging best evaluated by thin-section CT
  - MR: Evaluation of endplates, paraspinal soft tissues, epidural space, and intrathecal structures
    - Postoperative disc signal dependent on preoperative degree of degeneration, specific surgery and type of implant, and presence or absence of biologic modifiers (i.e., rhBMP-2)
    - May see transient increase in disc height and T2 signal immediately after discectomy (not related to infection)
    - Discectomy accelerates degenerative appearance of disc with loss of T2 signal and loss of disc height
    - Disc space surrounding implants may initially show T2 hyperintensity (1st few weeks) but should disappear over time
    - Solid fusion typically shown by fatty marrow infiltration/ossification of disc with T1 hyperintensity
    - Typical postoperative discectomy enhancement consists of smooth linear enhancement of disc paralleling endplates, with enhancement of dorsal annulus at curettage site
      - No edema or enhancement of paraspinal soft tissues (this would indicate infection)

SELECTED REFERENCES

1. Yang H et al: MRI manifestations and differentiated diagnosis of postoperative spinal complications. J Huazhong Univ Sci Technolog Med Sci. 29(4):522-6, 2009
2. Tokuhashi Y et al: Clinical course and significance of the clear zone around the pedicle screws in the lumbar degenerative disease. Spine (Phila Pa 1976). 33(8):903-8, 2008
3. Rutherford EE et al: Lumbar spine fusion and stabilization: hardware, techniques, and imaging appearances. Radiographics. 27(6):1737-49, 2007
4. Williams AL et al: CT evaluation of lumbar interbody fusion: current concepts. AJNR Am J Neuroradiol. 26(8):2057-66, 2005
5. Carmouche JJ et al: Epidural abscess and discitis complicating instrumented posterior lumbar interbody fusion: a case report. Spine (Phila Pa 1976). 29(23):E542-6, 2004
6. Ross JS: Magnetic resonance imaging of the postoperative spine. Semin Musculoskelet Radiol. 4(3):281-91, 2000
7. Lonstein JE et al: Complications associated with pedicle screws. J Bone Joint Surg Am. 81(11):1519-28, 1999
8. Fritsch EW et al: The failed back surgery syndrome: reasons, intraoperative findings, and long-term results: a report of 182 operative treatments. Spine (Phila Pa 1976). 21(5):626-33, 1996
9. Larsen JM et al: Assessment of pseudarthrosis in pedicle screw fusion: a prospective study comparing plain radiographs, flexion/extension radiographs, CT scanning, and bone scintigraphy with operative findings. J Spinal Disord. 9(2):117-20, 1996
10. Ross JS: Magnetic resonance assessment of the postoperative spine. Degenerative disc disease. Radiol Clin North Am. 29(4):793-808, 1991
11. Ross JS et al: Lumbar spine: postoperative assessment with surface-coil MR imaging. Radiology. 164(3):851-60, 1987
12. Ross JS et al: Postoperative cervical spine: MR assessment. J Comput Assist Tomogr. 11(6):955-62, 1987

(Left) *Sagittal T1WI C+ FS MR shows granulation tissue enhancement in the dorsal margin of the L4-5 disc ⇗ at the site of a partial discectomy. This is a typical finding following discectomy.* **(Right)** *Axial T1WI C+ FS MR shows a small amount of enhancing peridural fibrosis at the site of a partial discectomy ⇗. The enhancement differentiates fibrosis from a recurrent disc herniation.*

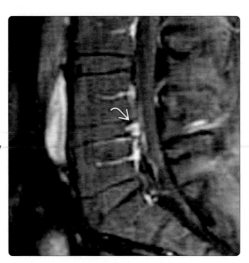
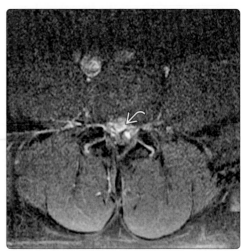

(Left) *Axial T1WI MR through a level of prior laminectomy ⇗ shows soft tissue flattening the ventral margin of the thecal sac, particularly prominent in the right anterolateral position ⇗, where the appearance is concerning for representing recurrent disc herniation.* **(Right)** *Axial T1WI C+ MR in the same patient shows enhancing peridural fibrosis and annulus ⇗. There is extensive enhancement of the disc margin ⇗ reflecting diffuse disc degeneration and annular fissures.*

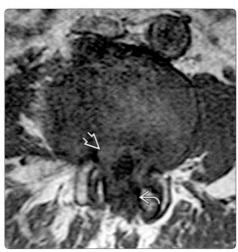
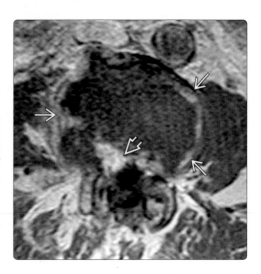

(Left) *Preoperative sagittal T1WI MR shows type I marrow changes ⇗ adjacent to degenerative spondylolisthesis of the L4-L5. The L4-5 and L5-1 discs are collapsed.* **(Right)** *Sagittal T1WI MR in the same patient demonstrates conversion of type I to type II marrow ⇗ adjacent to the L4-L5 disc space. The patient has undergone posterior instrumentation and fusion of L4-S1. Note the metallic artifact from a pedicle screw placement ⇗. The L5-S1 disc shows fatty marrow conversion ⇗.*

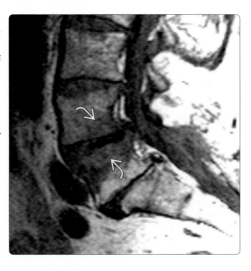
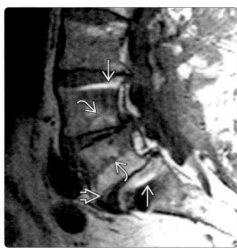

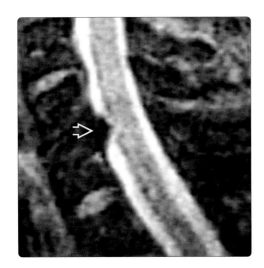

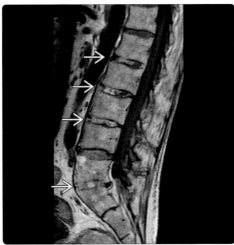

(Left) *Sagittal T2* GRE MR shows changes of a C4-C5 discectomy. Ventral extradural defect ➡ actually represents metallic susceptibility artifact and was not present on T1WI.* (Right) *Sagittal T1 MR shows diffuse hyperintensity within every lumbar intervertebral disc ➡, consistent with calcification &/or fatty marrow replacement. There is typical squaring of the lumbar vertebral bodies of ankylosing spondylitis.*

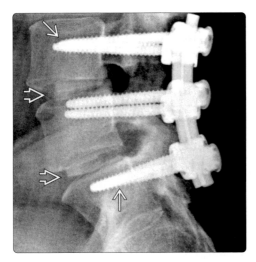

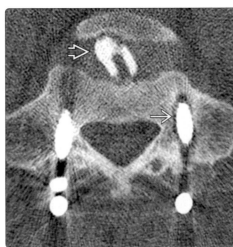

(Left) *Lateral radiograph shows a 2-level posterior ➡ PLIF with 3 levels of pedicle screws. Posterior rods show lucency around 1 of the L4 and 1 of the sacral screws ➡.* (Right) *Axial NECT in the same patient shows the interbody fusion graft ➡ and the lucency around the left sacral screw ➡ and normal appearance of the intervertebral graft. The degree of the lucency decreased on 1-year follow-up films.*

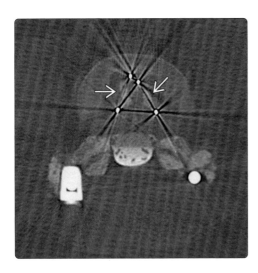

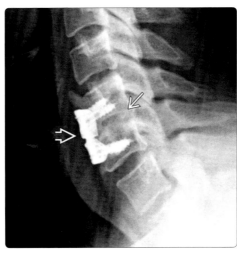

(Left) *Axial CT following myelography shows PLIF with 2 intervertebral grafts within the disc with radiopaque markers on each end ➡.* (Right) *Lateral radiograph of the cervical spine shows C5-C6 discectomy and solid anterior fusion ➡ (ADCF) with metallic plate and screw placement ➡. Hardware is intact and appears satisfactorily positioned without evidence of loosening, fracture, or subsidence.*

KEY FACTS

TERMINOLOGY

- Peridural fibrosis
  - Some degree of peridural fibrosis along margin of thecal sac is typical finding following discectomy
  - Edema and tissue disruption at discectomy site particularly conspicuous in first 6 weeks postoperatively
  - Can simulate disc residual/recurrent disc herniation
  - Scarring has been implicated with nerve root irritation in failed back surgery syndrome
- Postoperative fluid collection
  - Fluid collection in operative bed is not uncommon in immediate postoperative setting
  - May have complex signal
  - May have fluid-fluid levels
  - May demonstrate peripheral enhancement

IMAGING

- Utility of MR in postoperative epidural space related to timing since surgery

- If imaging within 4-6 weeks of surgery, normal postoperative changes may mimic epidural mass, residual disc herniation
- Acute imaging of postoperative spine best when limited to definition of epidural hemorrhage or CSF leak (pseudomeningocele)
- Definition of degree of thecal sac compression limited by poor correlation to patient's symptomatology
- Metal artifact due to disc space implant, posterior fusion hardware
  - Usually worth attempt at imaging with MR even in face of significant metal artifact
- MR: Best for epidural space evaluation
  - Hemorrhage
  - Pseudomeningocele
  - Scar vs. disc material

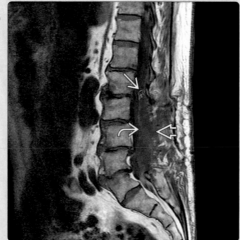
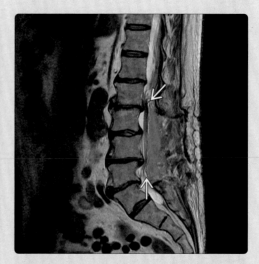

(Left) Sagittal T1WI C+ MR shows L2-L5 laminectomy with a postoperative fluid collection within the surgical bed ➡, effacing the dorsal thecal sac ➡. A small amount of enhancement is seen superiorly ➡. There was no clinical suspicion of infection, and the patient did well without further intervention. (Right) Sagittal T2WI MR in the same patient immediately following surgery shows effacement of the thecal sac ➡ and ventral displacement of the cauda equina from the laminectomy site fluid collection.

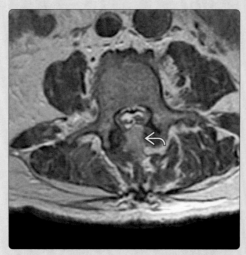
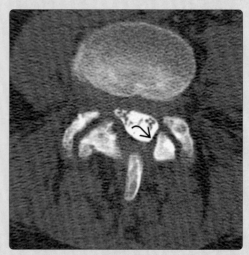

(Left) Axial T2WI MR shows an asymptomatic fluid collection in the laminectomy bed ➡, effacing the dorsal thecal sac. (Right) Axial image from a CT myelogram shows changes of a left hemilaminotomy. The actual bony defect is difficult to appreciate on this image. What is apparent is the absence of the left ligamentum flavum ➡ and mild distortion of the thecal sac.

TERMINOLOGY

Definitions

- Laminectomy
  - Removal of lamina to decompress spinal canal
    - Unilateral (hemilaminectomy) or bilateral
    - Partial removal of lamina and ligamentum flavum technically **laminotomy**, although terminology sometimes used interchangeably
- Posterior instrumentation
  - Including pedicle screws, paraspinous rods, transverse rods, laminar hooks
    - Translaminar or facet screws; can be inserted with minimally invasive techniques
- Posterolateral fusion
  - With severe loss of disc height, in lieu of interbody fusion
  - Lateral bone graft placement, fusion of transverse processes
  - Usually supplemented by posterior instrumentation
- Peridural fibrosis
  - Some degree of peridural fibrosis along margin of thecal sac is typical finding following discectomy
    - Edema and tissue disruption at discectomy site particularly conspicuous in first 6 weeks postoperatively
      - Can simulate disc residual/recurrent disc herniation
  - Scarring has been implicated with nerve root irritation in failed back surgery syndrome
- Postoperative fluid collection
  - Fluid collection in operative bed is not uncommon in immediate postoperative setting
    - May have complex signal
    - May have fluid-fluid levels
    - May demonstrate peripheral enhancement
  - Can be difficult to differentiate from postoperative hematoma, pseudomeningocele, infected collection
- Malpositioned pedicle screw
  - Pedicle screw should traverse pedicle and be securely positioned within vertebral body
  - Malpositioning includes
    - Perforation of anterior cortex of vertebral body
    - Perforation of cortex of pedicle
      - ± compromise of intervertebral neural foramen or spinal canal
- Lucency around pedicle screw
  - Clear zones (≥ 1 mm) around pedicle screws may be encountered on postoperative radiographs
    - Traditionally, concerning for loosening or infection
  - 1 longitudinal series describes majority (2/3) of clear zones as resolving over several years
    - Persistence 2 years postoperatively predictive of pseudoarthrosis

IMAGING

Imaging Recommendations

- Best imaging tool
  - CT: Best for definition of hardware, posterior element integrity
    - Little use in evaluation of epidural space, unless in conjunction with intrathecal contrast for definition of thecal sac compression
  - MR: Best for epidural space evaluation
    - Hemorrhage
    - Pseudomeningocele
    - Scar vs. disc material
  - Utility of MR in postoperative epidural space related to timing since surgery
    - If imaging within 4-6 weeks of surgery, normal postoperative changes may mimic epidural mass, residual disc herniation
    - Acute imaging of postoperative spine best when limited to definition of epidural hemorrhage or CSF leak (pseudomeningocele)
    - Definition of degree of thecal sac compression limited by poor correlation to patient's symptomatology
    - Metal artifact due to disc space implant, posterior fusion hardware
      - Usually worth attempt at imaging with MR even in face of significant metal artifact

SELECTED REFERENCES

1. Ghobrial GM et al: Iatrogenic neurologic deficit after lumbar spine surgery: a review. Clin Neurol Neurosurg. 139:76-80, 2015
2. Walsh KM et al: Spinal cord stimulation: a review of the safety literature and proposal for perioperative evaluation and management. Spine J. 15(8):1864-9, 2015
3. Yang H et al: MRI manifestations and differentiated diagnosis of postoperative spinal complications. J Huazhong Univ Sci Technolog Med Sci. 29(4):522-6, 2009
4. Tokuhashi Y et al: Clinical course and significance of the clear zone around the pedicle screws in the lumbar degenerative disease. Spine (Phila Pa 1976). 33(8):903-8, 2008
5. Rutherford EE et al: Lumbar spine fusion and stabilization: hardware, techniques, and imaging appearances. Radiographics. 27(6):1737-49, 2007
6. Williams AL et al: CT evaluation of lumbar interbody fusion: current concepts. AJNR Am J Neuroradiol. 26(8):2057-66, 2005
7. Carmouche JJ et al: Epidural abscess and discitis complicating instrumented posterior lumbar interbody fusion: a case report. Spine (Phila Pa 1976). 29(23):E542-6, 2004
8. Ross JS: Magnetic resonance imaging of the postoperative spine. Semin Musculoskelet Radiol. 4(3):281-91, 2000
9. Lonstein JE et al: Complications associated with pedicle screws. J Bone Joint Surg Am. 81(11):1519-28, 1999
10. Fritsch EW et al: The failed back surgery syndrome: reasons, intraoperative findings, and long-term results: a report of 182 operative treatments. Spine (Phila Pa 1976). 21(5):626-33, 1996
11. Larsen JM et al: Assessment of pseudarthrosis in pedicle screw fusion: a prospective study comparing plain radiographs, flexion/extension radiographs, CT scanning, and bone scintigraphy with operative findings. J Spinal Disord. 9(2):117-20, 1996
12. Ross JS: Magnetic resonance assessment of the postoperative spine. Degenerative disc disease. Radiol Clin North Am. 29(4):793-808, 1991
13. Ross JS et al: Lumbar spine: postoperative assessment with surface-coil MR imaging. Radiology. 164(3):851-60, 1987
14. Ross JS et al: Postoperative cervical spine: MR assessment. J Comput Assist Tomogr. 11(6):955-62, 1987

(Left) *Normal epidural space after laminectomy is shown. Sagittal T1WI MR shows the laminectomy site as intermediate signal at L4 and L5 levels ➡. There is mild mass effect on the dorsal thecal sac ➡. **(Right)** Sagittal T2WI FS MR in the same patient shows fluid within the L4-L5 laminectomy bed ➡ effacing the dorsal thecal sac. A small amount of extraarachnoid fluid tracks cephalad ➡ up to the L1 level.*

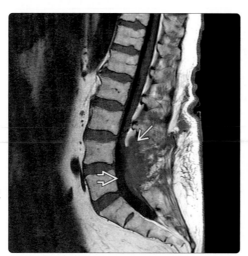 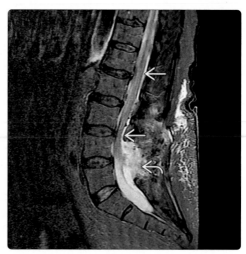

(Left) *Axial T2WI FS MR following lumbar laminectomy shows complex fluid collection in laminectomy bed ➡ as well as a small amount of subdural fluid ➡. The patient did well postoperatively. **(Right)** Axial T2WI MR shows a large posterior fluid collection ➡ following multilevel fixation and pedicle subtraction osteotomy. Note that the posterior rods by metal artifact ➡ and bone graft present posteriorly at the level of rods ➡. This degree of fluid is not uncommon in the immediate postoperative period.*

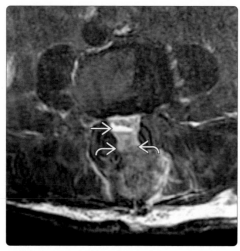 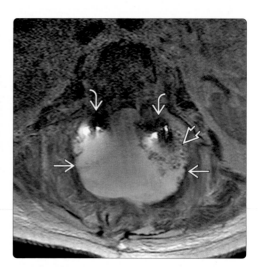

(Left) *Axial T1WI C+ FS MR shows pedicle screws ➡ and a laminectomy defect ➡. Diffusely increased signal probably reflects the effect of field inhomogeneity generated by the pedicle screws and resulting in poor fat saturation that obscures any potential enhancement due to underlying peridural fibrosis. **(Right)** Axial T1WI MR shows a defect in the right lamina and ligamentum flavum ➡ at the site of a left L5 hemilaminectomy.*

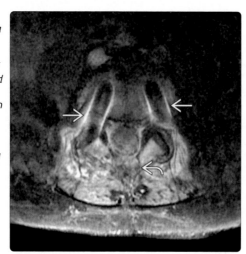 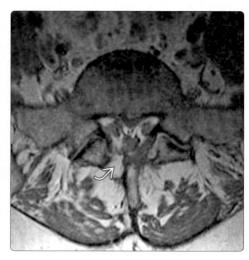

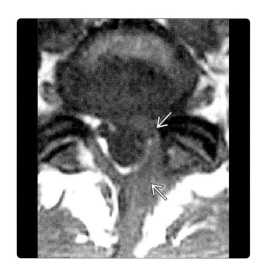

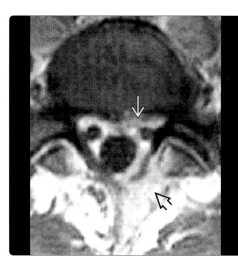

(Left) *Axial nonenhanced T1WI at L4-L5 demonstrates appearance of peridural fibrosis ➡ surrounding the left lateral aspect of thecal sac and exiting root.* (Right) *Axial T1WI C+ at L4-L5 demonstrates enhancing epidural fibrotic tissue ventral to the thecal sac ➡ and the traversing left L5 nerve root. Enhancing scar tissue is also present posteriorly at the laminectomy site ➡. The enhancing scar shows no mass effect upon the thecal sac and smoothly encompasses the exiting root.*

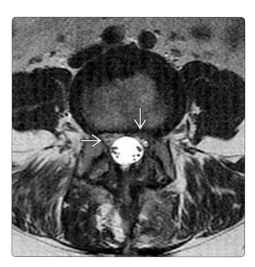

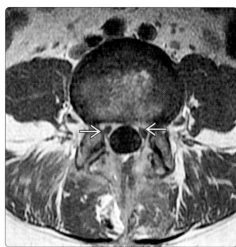

(Left) *In this postlaminectomy patient, peridural fibrosis is seen as intermediate signal on a T2-weighted image surrounding the thecal sac and exiting roots ➡.* (Right) *Postcontrast image in the same patient shows diffuse homogeneous enhancement of the peridural fibrosis. Rounded areas of no enhancement are exiting roots and root sleeves ➡, not to be confused with nonenhancing disc herniations.*

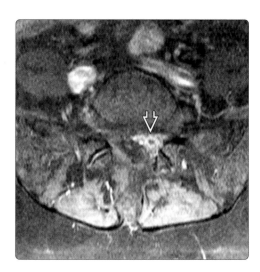

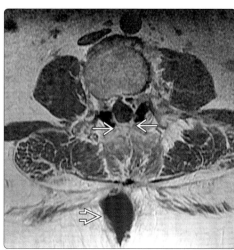

(Left) *Typical large extrusion and free fragment with peripheral enhancement are shown. T1WI C+ FS shows peripheral enhancement of the residual herniation ➡ within the left side of the epidural space.* (Right) *Axial T1WI C+ MR shows a modest-sized posterior fluid collection along the operative tract ➡, which is commonly present in the immediate postoperative period. Epidural fibrosis shows homogeneous enhancement ➡.*

TERMINOLOGY

- CT: Beam-hardening artifact and blooming artifact
- MR: Magnetic susceptibility artifact
- Image degradation related to metal prostheses/implants

IMAGING

- CT: Artifact from metal hardware related to image reconstruction algorithm, tube current, x-ray kilovolt peak, pitch, hardware composition, shape, & location
  - Beam-hardening artifact is dark banding between dense objects, such as bone
  - Bloom artifacts result of partial volume effects or areas of photon starvation propagated by high-density structures, such as metal, within scanned object
  - Materials with lower x-ray attenuation coefficients produce less artifactual distortions
    - Plastic (best) < titanium < < tantalum < stainless steel < cobalt chrome (worst)

- Metal composition, mass, orientation + position of implant are important factors that determine magnitude of image artifact
- MR susceptibility artifact due to geometric distortion + signal loss secondary to dephasing
- MR methods to minimize metal artifact
  - Fast spin-echo > conventional spin-echo > gradient-echo
  - Larger field of view
  - Smaller voxel size
  - Increase transmit and receive bandwidth
  - Frequency encoding direction along long axis of hardware
  - Lower magnet field strength
  - STIR sequences are alternative method of fat suppression and less dependent on homogeneity of main magnetic field

(Left) *Plain film shows right lateral fusion ➡ extending from the L2-L5 with vertebral body screws and longitudinal rods, interbody graft material, and lower lumbar posterior pedicle screw fixation from L4-S1 ➡. **(Right)** MR study in the same patient shows very little obscuration of the central canal by artifact, despite the amount of metal present. Metal artifact is present from lateral fusion ➡ and posterior fixation ➡. Solid fusion with incorporated graft is noted ➡ by fatty disc space signal.*

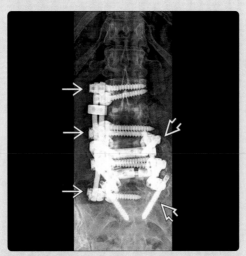

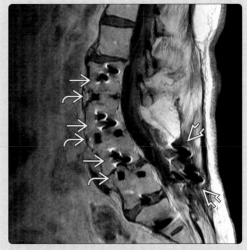

(Left) *Coronal CT reconstruction illustrates bloom hardening artifact ➡. Beam artifacts are a result of partial volume effects or underranging caused by areas of photon starvation propagated by high-density structures, such as metal, within the scanned object. When subtle, these artifacts appear as shading and, when severe, as high-intensity streaks and areas of photon starvation. **(Right)** Axial NECT shows star artifact along the margins of the right corporal screw, which has migrated out ➡.*

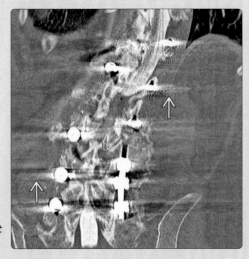

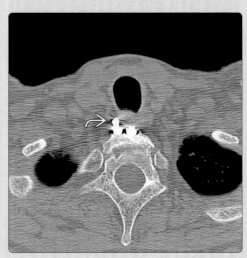

TERMINOLOGY

Definitions

- Magnetic susceptibility
  - Partial magnetization of material in presence of applied external magnetic field
  - Nonferromagnetic metals may produce local electrical currents induced by changing scanner magnetic field
  - Tissues with greatly different magnetic susceptibilities in uniform magnetic field lead to difference of susceptibilities, causing distortion in magnetic field → distortion on MR
  - Magnetic susceptibility artifact consists of 2 additive components

IMAGING

General Features

- Trade-off must occur in choice of metal
  - Titanium wires exhibit least artifact on CT when compared to cobalt chrome or stainless steel but are more susceptible to failure
  - Titanium screws + cages produce fewer artifacts than tantalum but may not have desirable biologic properties
- Use of high peak voltage (kilovolts peak), high tube charge (milliampere-seconds), narrow collimation, and thin sections helps reduce metal-related artifacts
  - Caution should always be exercised, particularly in children, young adults, and patients undergoing multiple examinations
  - Cone beam artifacts caused by geometry of multichannel CT scanners ↓ by using narrower x-ray beam collimation and low-pitch setting
- Reduce metal-related artifacts
  - Thick sections, lower kernel values (similar to standard reconstruction algorithm), and extended CT scale
- MR: Potential safety and biologic considerations
  - Stainless steel is safe but produces severe artifacts (especially with low nickel content)
  - Titanium = tantalum implant artifact; much less, relative to stainless steel
- Location
  - Intervertebral disc level related to fusion cages, anterior plates + screws, iatrogenic metal
  - Pedicles related to pedicle screws
  - Dorsal elements related to dorsal stabilization rods, interspinous process wiring
- Size
  - Variable
- Morphology
  - Central low signal, with indistinct margins, spatial mismapping of signal giving peripheral curvilinear high signal

Radiographic Findings

- Radiography
  - Visualize hardware malposition and alignment

CT Findings

- NECT
  - Missing data from metal attenuation cause classic "starburst" or streak artifacts

MR Findings

- T1WI
  - Focal central signal loss with peripheral "halo" of ↑ signal related to spatial mismapping
- T2WI
  - Focal central signal loss with peripheral "halo" of ↑ signal related to spatial mismapping
  - Artifact minimized with FSE technique
- T2* GRE
  - Blooming of susceptibility artifact with gradient-echo techniques, worse with increasing echo time

Nonvascular Interventions

- Myelography
  - May be necessary if extensive hardware precludes adequate MR examination
  - Fluoroscopic positioning will obtain most favorable projection with overlapping hardware

Imaging Recommendations

- Best imaging tool
  - MR best sequence choice: Fast spin-echo > conventional spin-echo > gradient-echo
- Protocol advice
  - CT: Thin-section spiral imaging has improved quality compared to conventional discrete slices
  - MR: Optimum sequence should not contain gradient-echoes
    - Preferably FSE technique
    - FSE: Maintain short echo spacing (short echo train less critical)
    - Single shot FSE sequences with half-Fourier (HASTE) useful
    - Hybrid imaging sequences that use both gradient-echo and spin-echo components should not be used
    - Frequency-selective fat saturation yields poor image quality with metal implants
    - Orienting frequency encoding direction along long axial of pedicle screws minimizes artifact (except in area just beyond tip of implant)

PATHOLOGY

General Features

- Etiology
  - In anterior cervical discectomies, sufficient metals to produce artifacts are deposited by contact of metal drill bits + suction tips

CLINICAL ISSUES

Presentation

- Most common signs/symptoms
  - Typically asymptomatic, ancillary finding of surgical procedure

DIAGNOSTIC CHECKLIST

Image Interpretation Pearls

- Minimize pedicle screw artifact by orienting frequency encoding gradient parallel to screw long axis, using FSE technique; slice thickness 3-4 mm is adequate; thinner sections yield little artifact reduction

SECTION 2
Devices and Instrumentation

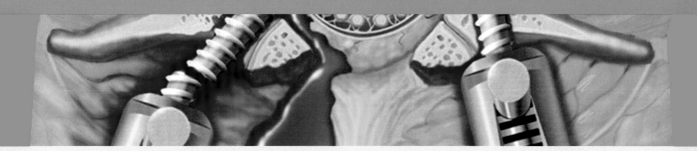

Regulation

Once a device becomes FDA approved and available, the physician can use the device in any manner (off-label) that he/she desires if it is in the best interest of the patient and supported by objective and appropriate peer-reviewed scientific and clinical information. This is termed the "practice of medicine." No investigational device exemption or institutional review board review is needed in these types of cases. A 2nd very different type of off-label use involves experimental or investigational devices. In these cases, clinical use requires an investigational device exemption and the implant can only be used in accordance with the device's approved investigation plan. The patient must provide a formal informed consent for that device. Finally, the device cannot be shared with other physicians outside the formal study plan.

Biomechanics and Function

Spinal implants are employed in a wide variety of indications and pathology, which includes (but is not limited to) trauma, tumor, infection, deformity correction, and degenerative disease. The goals of placing an implant are manifold, but implants typically reduce deformity, provide stabilization, share loading with adjacent tissues until healing occurs, and, most importantly, support and augment the fusion process. The average spine cycles around 3 million times per year. Without bone healing, all spinal implants will ultimately fail. Failure can occur at the anchor points within bone or within the device itself.

Spinal implants function in 1 or more of the following modes: Tension banding, buttressing, neutralization, lag screw, or deformity correction. The primary mode of function is determined by the location of the implant/device on the flexion or extension side of the spine and the type of loading that occurs. For example, cervical posterior lateral mass screws/rods are often used with a neutralization function to decrease strain across healing surfaces by shielding the tissues from axial and flexion forces. Buttressing is generally applied to prevent axial deformity.

Cages

Mesh cages have developed a wide variety of applications since their introduction for reconstructing large corpectomy defects. A wide variety of materials may be utilized, such as titanium, polyetheretherketone, carbon fiber, and trabecular metal. Cages offer the advantage of immediate structural support. Cages should be developed to resist subsidence and have a small footprint so as not to stress shield the graft material. By nature, these manufactured cages decrease or alleviate the morbidity of autograft harvest. Cages may have either a vertical or horizontal geometry. Vertical cage implants fill corpectomy defects. Horizontally oriented implants are generally used to reconstruct discectomy sites, by providing distraction-compression with restoration of annular tension.

Selected References

1. Mason A et al: The accuracy of pedicle screw placement using intraoperative image guidance systems. J Neurosurg Spine. 20(2):196-203, 2014
2. Tuschel A et al: Implant survival analysis and failure modes of the X STOP interspinous distraction device. Spine (Phila Pa 1976). 38(21):1826-31, 2013
3. Strube P et al: Stand-alone anterior versus anteroposterior lumbar interbody single-level fusion after a mean follow-up of 41 months. J Spinal Disord Tech. 25(7):362-9, 2012
4. Anderson DG et al: Anterior interbody arthrodesis with percutaneous posterior pedicle fixation for degenerative conditions of the lumbar spine. Eur Spine J. 20(8):1323-30, 2011
5. Denaro V et al: The best surgical treatment for type II fractures of the dens is still controversial. Clin Orthop Relat Res. 469(3):742-50, 2011
6. Fabrizi AP et al: Interspinous spacers in the treatment of degenerative lumbar spinal disease: our experience with DIAM and Aperius devices. Eur Spine J. 20 Suppl 1:S20-6, 2011
7. Kim DH et al: Occult spinous process fractures associated with interspinous process spacers. Spine (Phila Pa 1976). 36(16):E1080-5, 2011
8. Lindley EM et al: Complications of axial lumbar interbody fusion. J Neurosurg Spine. 15(3):273-9, 2011
9. Pimenta L et al: Lumbar total disc replacement from an extreme lateral approach: clinical experience with a minimum of 2 years' follow-up. J Neurosurg Spine. 14(1):38-45, 2011
10. Rodgers WB et al: Intraoperative and early postoperative complications in extreme lateral interbody fusion: an analysis of 600 cases. Spine (Phila Pa 1976). 36(1):26-32, 2011
11. Tamburrelli FC et al: Critical analysis of lumbar interspinous devices failures: a retrospective study. Eur Spine J. 20 Suppl 1:S27-35, 2011
12. Harrop JS et al: Optimal treatment for odontoid fractures in the elderly. Spine (Phila Pa 1976). 35(21 Suppl):S219-27, 2010
13. Isaacs RE et al: A prospective, nonrandomized, multicenter evaluation of extreme lateral interbody fusion for the treatment of adult degenerative scoliosis: perioperative outcomes and complications. Spine (Phila Pa 1976). 35(26 Suppl):S322-30, 2010
14. Kabir SM et al: Lumbar interspinous spacers: a systematic review of clinical and biomechanical evidence. Spine (Phila Pa 1976). 35(25):E1499-506, 2010
15. Lall R et al: A review of complications associated with craniocervical fusion surgery. Neurosurgery. 67(5):1396-402; discussion 1402-3, 2010
16. Nandakumar A et al: The increase in dural sac area is maintained at 2 years after X-stop implantation for the treatment of spinal stenosis with no significant alteration in lumbar spine range of movement. Spine J. 10(9):762-8, 2010
17. Rodgers WB et al: Early complications of extreme lateral interbody fusion in the obese. J Spinal Disord Tech. 23(6):393-7, 2010
18. Smoljanovic T et al: Six-year outcomes of anterior lumbar interbody arthrodesis with use of interbody fusion cages and recombinant human bone morphogenetic protein-2. J Bone Joint Surg Am. 92(15):2614-5; author reply 2615-6, 2010
19. Youssef JA et al: Minimally invasive surgery: lateral approach interbody fusion: results and review. Spine (Phila Pa 1976). 35(26 Suppl):S302-11, 2010
20. Shears E et al: Surgical versus conservative management for odontoid fractures. Cochrane Database Syst Rev. (4):CD005078, 2008
21. Vender JR et al: The evolution of posterior cervical and occipitocervical fusion and instrumentation. Neurosurg Focus. 16(1):E9, 2004
22. Haid RW et al: The Cervical Spine Study Group anterior cervical plate nomenclature. Neurosurg Focus. 12(1):E15, 2002

Instrumentation/Implants: Potential Early and Late Complications

Instrumentation/Implants	Early Complication (Days to Weeks)	Late Complication (Weeks to Years)
Thoracic or lumbar pedicle screws	Transverse placement: Medial or lateral cortical breach (> 1.2 mm)	Loosening
	AP placement: Tip breaches ventral cortex of vertebral body	Screw fracture
	Hematoma: Epidural or paravertebral	Pedicle stress fracture
		Screw separated from longitudinal rod
Dorsal occipitocervical constructs	Occipital screw placement: Inner table penetration with intradural extension	Occipitocervical rod fracture
	C1 lateral mass screw: Ventral C1 breach with carotid injury	Screw loosening
	C1 lateral mass screw: Transverse foramen penetration	
	C2 pars/pedicle screw: Vertebral artery injury	
Odontoid screw(s)	Placement: Screw tip penetrates distal aspect of odontoid (> 1 mm)	Screw fracture
	Inferior portion of screw not flush with C2 body but extends into C2-C3 interspace	Loosening: Windshield wiper motion of inferior aspect of screw
	Fracture angulation or distraction	
Lateral mass screw(s)	Placement: Penetration of transverse foramen	Screw fracture
	Penetration into neural foramen	Disconnection from longitudinal hardware
	Penetration into canal (rare)	Loosening
Transarticular screw(s)	C1-C2 with distal penetration of transverse foramen	Screw fracture
	C1-C2 medial penetration of canal	Disconnection from longitudinal hardware
	Subaxial cervical: Penetration into neural foramen	Loosening
Longitudinal rods	Detachment from ventral fixation device	Hardware fracture
Posterior sublaminar wires	Wire fracture/displacement	Wire fracture/displacement
	Mass effect on thecal sac from epidural component	
Posterior sublaminar hooks	Mass effect on thecal sac from epidural component	Hook displacement from lamina
		Disconnection from longitudinal hardware
Anterior vertebral body plate/screw	Placement: Penetration of transverse foramen or neural foramen	Screw fracture
	Penetration into adjacent disc space	Screw backout (rare with modern hardware)
		Loosening
Lateral vertebral body plate/screw	Distal penetration of cortex with extension into paravertebral soft tissues	Loosening
Laminotomy plate/screw	Plate or screw placement within canal	Loosening
Interbody cage	Position: Lateral or ventral displacement	Nonunion of graft material
	Dorsal displacement with thecal sac/root compression	Subsidence
		Rotation/migration of cage
Interbody graft	Position: Lateral or ventral displacement	Collapse/fragmentation
	Dorsal displacement with thecal sac/root compression	Nonunion
Total disc replacement	Placement: Specific for each device	Hardware failure/fracture
		Vertebral body fracture/subluxation
		Subsidence
		Ectopic bone formation
Axial interbody fusion screw	Placement off midline	Hardware fracture
		Nonunion
		Sacral fracture
Interspinous spacing devices	Position not on spinous process	Displacement
		Spinous process fracture

TERMINOLOGY

- Instrumentation in fusion surgery designed to stabilize, not replace, spinal bony elements

IMAGING

- Postoperative imaging: Assess progress of osseous fusion, confirm correct positioning & integrity of instrumentation, detect suspected complications (e.g., infection or hematoma), & detect new disease or disease progression
- Radiographs
  - Noninvasive, most common for assessment of fusion
  - Instrumentation break or periimplant lucency
- CT
  - Modality of choice for imaging bony detail to enable accurate assessment of degree of osseous fusion
- MR
  - Useful for detecting and monitoring infection or postoperative collections

CLINICAL ISSUES

- Complications
  - Pseudoarthrosis, instrumentation fractures
  - Surgical approach risks: Nerve or vascular injury, dural tear
  - Infection
  - Instrumentation malposition

DIAGNOSTIC CHECKLIST

- Compare current radiographs with multiple previous studies
  - Identify subtle progressive changes in spinal alignment & in position of instrumentation devices that may signify imminent failure of device or other complications

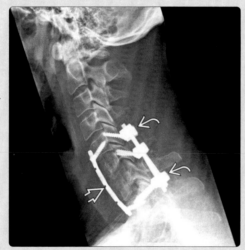

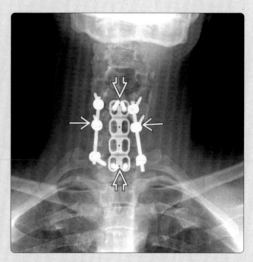

(Left) *Lateral radiograph shows multilevel anterior cervical discectomy and fusion spanning C5-T1 ➡. Lateral mass fixation is the gold standard in the presence of postlaminectomy instability and incompetency of posterior elements ➡. (Right) Dynamic plates ➡ allow some motion at screw-plate interface. By allowing the graft to subside, a higher fusion rate is obtained. Lateral mass plating ➡ resists rotational and extension forces more effectively than posterior cervical wiring techniques.*

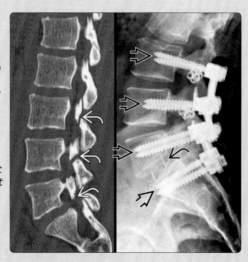

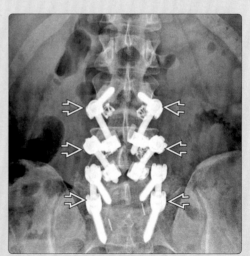

(Left) *Pars interarticularis defects ➡ are seen at L3-L4, L4-L5, and L5-S1. Repetitive hyperextension contributes to spondylolysis; ↑ incidence is in certain sports. Note repair of multiple-level spondylolysis by pedicle screws ➡. An interbody disc spacer is seen ➡. (Right) Patients with spondylolysis show higher incidence of spondylolisthesis or degenerative disc disease at the level of pars defects and at the upper adjacent level. AP plain film in the same patient shows pedicle screw-rod-hook constructs ➡.*

TERMINOLOGY

Synonyms

- Spine instrumentation, spine fusion surgery

Definitions

- Instrumentation in fusion surgery designed to stabilize, not replace, spinal bony elements
  - Intact osseous fusion is crucial

IMAGING

General Features

- Location
  - Cervical
    - Anterior cervical discectomy and fusion (ACDF) is standard treatment for degenerative disease
    - Posterior lateral mass plating
      - □ Laminoplasty
  - Thoracic
    - Pedicle screws connected by single or dual rods
  - Lumbar
    - Pedicle screws connected by plates or rods spanning single or multiple vertebral segments ± crossbars for additional strength

Radiographic Findings

- Noninvasive, most common for assessment of fusion
  - Instrumentation break or periimplant lucency
  - Interspinous distance ≥ 2 mm on dynamic radiographs is more reliable indicator of pseudarthrosis than angular motion of 2° based on Cobb angle measurements

CT Findings

- CT is reportedly more accurate than radiographs
  - Modality of choice for imaging bony detail to enable accurate assessment of degree of osseous fusion

MR Findings

- Best demonstrates intraspinal contents
- Useful for detecting and monitoring infection or postoperative collections
- Susceptibility artifact problematic, particularly with stainless steel devices
  - Implants made of titanium alloys less ferromagnetic → less severe susceptibility artifacts

PATHOLOGY

Staging, Grading, & Classification

- Cervical
  - ACDF
    - Inherent stability of bone graft in interspace
    - Instability of multiple level corpectomy (trauma or other pathology)
  - Posterior
    - Prevention or presence of postop instability
    - Laminoplasty developed to decompress spinal canal in patients with multilevel anterior compression caused by ossification of posterior longitudinal ligament or cervical spondylosis
- Lumbar

- For multilevel fusion, rods preferred over plates → rods can be individually cut & molded to facilitate maintenance of sagittal alignment
  - Tips of pedicle screws should be embedded in vertebral bone, should not breach anterior cortex
  - Sacral screws may be anchored in anterior cortex for additional stability
  - Translaminar facet screws: Alternative form of posterior instrumentation when posterior spinal elements are left intact
  - Posterior lumbar interbody fusion: Bilateral partial laminectomies, discectomy, interbody spacer(s), packing disc space with graft material
    - Posterior instrumentation provides rigid support until bone fusion occurs
  - Anterior lumbar interbody fusion: Remove degenerate disc material, replace disc height with large cages supplemented by screws & rods or plates placed either anteriorly or posteriorly, depending on access
    - At L5-S1 vertebrae, anterior fusion supplemented by instrumentation with posterior approach because iliac crests limit lateral access

CLINICAL ISSUES

Presentation

- Complications
  - Pseudoarthrosis
    - Recurrent pain in 5-50% of cervical fusion cases & up to 60% of lumbar fusion cases
  - Metal ion release secondary to corrosion occurs in implants, even those with successful fusion
  - Cervical anterior surgical approach risks
    - Graft migration, injury to superior or recurrent laryngeal nerves, esophageal perforation, persistent dysphagia, dysphonia, odynophagia, dural tear
  - Infection
  - Instrumentation misplacement
  - Perihardware fractures
    - Pedicle, facet breach

Natural History & Prognosis

- Surgical exploration remains reference standard for evaluating fusion
- Rate of fusion after anterior cervical intervertebral disc removal and fusions reported to be 97%
  - Average follow-up was 5.0 ± 3.3 years
  - Complete pain relief in 78%, partial in 18%, and little or no pain relief in 4%
- Long-term radiographic follow-up in patients with cervical anterior cervical discectomy → hypermobility & degenerative changes in nonfused segments: Disc space narrowing, endplate sclerosis, & osteophyte formation
- Cervical laminoplasty
  - Neurological outcome laminoplasty = laminectomy

SELECTED REFERENCES

1. Petscavage-Thomas JM et al: Imaging current spine hardware: part 1, cervical spine and fracture fixation. AJR Am J Roentgenol. 203(2):394-405, 2014
2. Murtagh RD et al: New techniques in lumbar spinal instrumentation: what the radiologist needs to know. Radiology. 260(2):317-30, 2011

(Left) *Lateral radiograph shows instrumentation for a plate and rod occiput-C4 fusion consisting of an occipital plate with bicortical screws ➡ and bilateral rods extending inferiorly, anchored by 3 levels of lateral mass screws ➡. **(Right)** Anteroposterior radiograph shows the instrumentation for the occiput to C4 fusion with occipital plate and bicortical screws ➡, left C2 pars screw ➡, and inferior C3 ➡ and C4 lateral ➡ mass screws.*

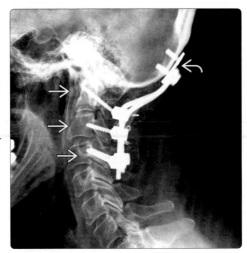
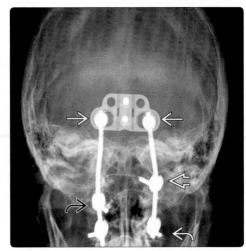

(Left) *C1 lateral mass screw malposition during C1-C2 fixation for an odontoid fracture is shown. The right C1 lateral mass screw is medial to the cortex of C1 and lies in between C1 and the odontoid process ➡. This required reoperation to correct. **(Right)** Anterior cervical plate subsides 1.0-1.5 mm per segment after procedure and may overlap disc space ➡. Rigid pedicle screw instrumentation with fixation plates ➡ ↑ probability of solid fusion but may be associated with ↑ postop morbidity.*

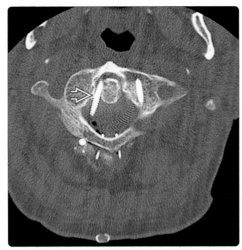
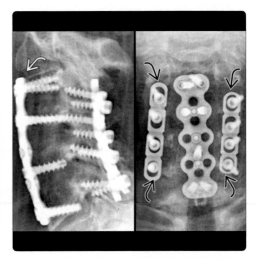

(Left) *Cervical laminoplasty ➡ decompresses the canal in patients with multilevel anterior compression due to posterior longitudinal ligament ossification or spondylosis. Laminoplasty can worsen alignment in ~ 35% with development of kyphosis in ~ 10% of patients at long-term follow-up. Cervical ROM is decreased substantially after laminoplasty. **(Right)** Laminoplasty with intralaminar grafts ➡ may be an alternative procedure for cervical myelopathy due to disc herniation.*

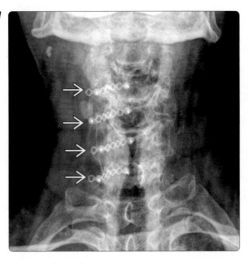
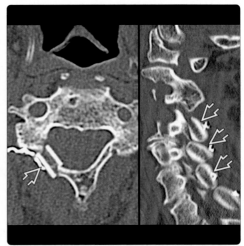

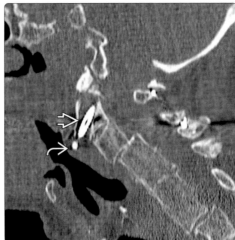

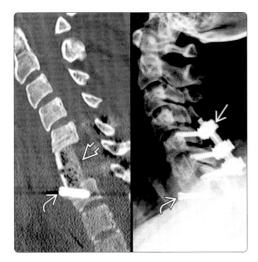

(Left) Sagittal CT shows C6 corpectomy with intervening allograft ⊠ secured in place by an interference screw ➔. The lateral radiograph demonstrates posterior lateral mass fusion ➔. (Right) Failure of single screw odontoid fixation with screw loosening is shown. CT study shows extensive loosening defined by the periscrew lucency within the C2 body ⊠. The screw has backed out with the screw head beyond the cortical margin, which distorts the mucosal surface of the oropharynx ➔.

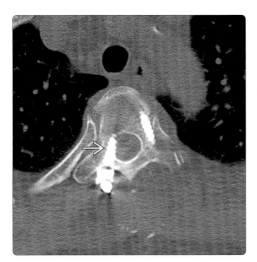

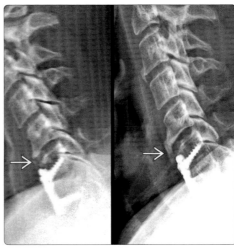

(Left) Axial NECT postoperatively shows the medial position of a right T4 pedicle screw ➔ through the right pedicle cortex. MR study (not shown) showed epidural hematoma at that level. (Right) Lateral radiographs in 2007 (L) and 2009 (R) demonstrate increase in heterotopic bone formation ⊠ due to suboptimal placement of an anterior fusion plate close to the disc space. Plates should be placed at least 1/2 a vertebral body height from adjacent disc space to prevent adjacent level ossification.

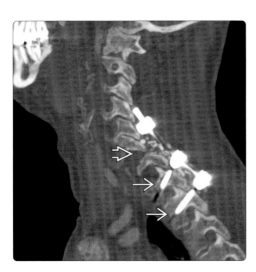

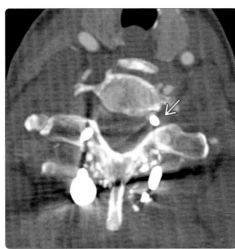

(Left) Sagittal CT reconstruction shows rod and screw fixation for a C6-C7 fracture dislocation ⊠. The correct position of pedicle screws is seen at T1 and T2 levels on the right ➔. (Right) Axial NECT in the same patient shows a left pedicle screw, which is malpositioned into the left neural foramen ➔.

KEY FACTS

TERMINOLOGY

- Cages used to reconstruct anterior spinal column after corpectomy
  - In vivo expansion of cage permits optimal fit and correction of deformity

IMAGING

- Cylindrical metallic prosthesis along craniocaudal span of vertebral body
- Radiography & CT
  - Difficult to assess fusion
  - Assess stability of expandable cages (EC)
  - Determine EC-related complications
- MR
  - Can be somewhat obscured by magnetic susceptibility artifact
  - Best to evaluate thecal sac and neural elements

CLINICAL ISSUES

- Indications for corpectomy or vertebrectomy: Tumors, trauma, degenerative disease, infection, deformity
  - Cage provides immediate segmental stability, correction of sagittal plane deformity, & restoration of anterior vertebral support
- Not designed as stand-alone device
  - Anterior instrumentation ± posterior instrumentation
- Complications
  - Migration, subsidence, structural failure of cage
  - Extensive distraction for cage placement may end up causing radicular pain due to stretching of nociceptive fibers in joint capsule

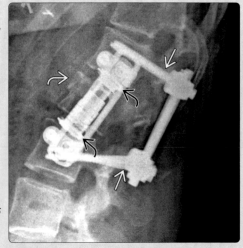

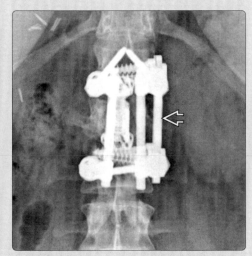

(Left) Lateral radiograph displays an L2 burst fracture ➡. Synex expandable cage ➡ extends from L1-L3 with bilateral L1 and L3 pedicle screws ➡. The goals of surgery include decompressing neural elements, restoring vertebral body height, correcting angular deformity, and stabilizing columns of spine. (Right) AP radiograph shows an expandable cage and lateral construct ➡, which provides intervertebral distraction, ↑ anterior column height, and ↓ additional stress across pedicle screw constructs.

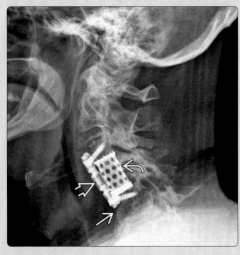

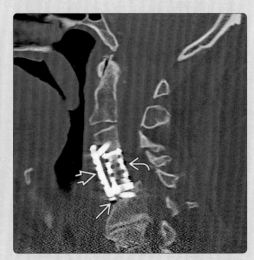

(Left) Lateral radiograph shows a nonexpandable cage across the C4 and C5 levels ➡. ACDF is noted from C3-C5 ➡. Titanium mesh cages have to be adjusted to the endplates and to the height of the defect. There is collapse of C5 vertebral body with subsidence of the anterior fusion plate and cage ➡. (Right) Sagittal CT shows cage spanning the C4-C5 levels ➡. ACDF is noted from C3-C5 ➡. There is collapse of the C5 endplate with subsidence of anterior plate/screw construct and cage ➡. Kyphosis is present at C6-C7.

TERMINOLOGY

Synonyms

- Expandable cage (EC), vertebral body (VB) replacement cage, VB prosthesis, distractible VB replacement

Definitions

- Cages used to reconstruct anterior spinal column after corpectomy

IMAGING

General Features

- Best diagnostic clue
  o Cylindrical metallic prosthesis along craniocaudal span of VB
- Location
  o Cervical, thoracic, lumbar
- Size
  o Variable depending on spinal segment

Radiographic Findings

- Difficult to assess fusion
- Assess stability of EC & related complications
- Important to determine degree of correction of kyphotic angle between pre- & postoperative phase
- Polyetheretherketone (PEEK) & carbon fiber cages are radiolucent
  o Upper & lower titanium pins identify cage position

CT Findings

- Due to beam-hardening artifact, difficult to assess fusion
- Assess stability of EC & related complications

MR Findings

- Best to evaluate thecal sac & neural elements
  o Can be somewhat obscured by magnetic susceptibility artifact
  o Little to no implant susceptibility artifact with PEEK cages
- Helpful to evaluate for postoperative collections

DIFFERENTIAL DIAGNOSIS

Interbody Fusion Devices

- Fusion across disc space to increase stability of operated segment(s)
- Substrate for fusion includes autograft, allograft, bone graft substitutes, & osteogenic factors

Plates & Screws

- Postop imaging to assess progress of osseous fusion, confirm correct positioning & integrity of instrumentation, & detect suspected complications

PATHOLOGY

General Features

- Following neural decompression, interbody replacement & bone fusion are main goals of spine surgery
  o Increase height & cross-sectional area of foramina

Staging, Grading, & Classification

- Most interbody fusion cages are made of titanium

- PEEK: Hard radiolucent plastic ± carbon fiber reinforcement
  o Provides strength & stiffness in disc space
  o Induces cell attachment & fibroblast proliferation & increases protein content of osteoblasts

CLINICAL ISSUES

Presentation

- Most common signs/symptoms
  o Indications for corpectomy or vertebrectomy: Tumors, trauma, degenerative disease, infection, deformity

Natural History & Prognosis

- Immediate segmental stability, correction of sagittal plane deformity, & restoration of anterior vertebral support
- Complications
  o Migration, structural failure of cage
  o Subsidence of cage into VB, leading to instrumentation failure
    – Particularly with mesh cages
    – Less with ECs because of their broader surface & duller edges
  o Extensive distraction for cage placement may end up causing radicular pain due to stretching of nociceptive fibers in joint capsule
  o Anterior approach: Vessel injury (5.8% reported) & internal organ injury
  o Retroperitoneal approach: Injury to ureter, lumbosacral plexus, or sympathetic chain
  o Adjacent-level VB fractures can occur in coronal plane

Treatment

- Reconstruction of VB with allograft, carbon fiber, mesh cages, tricortical autograft, ECs
  o Autograft: Gold standard but morbidity
  o Allograft: Long fusion times, possible immunological rejection
  o Carbon fiber: Radiolucent, inflammatory reaction, brittleness → breakage
  o Mesh cages: Must be cut to perfect size
    – Sharp edges anchor into adjacent VB → torsional stability
  o ECs: Expand to appropriate size after placement, reduce kyphotic deformity, & restore height loss
- ECs
  o Classically require anterior approach
    – Can be placed via extracavitary approach
  o Graft material can be used to fill EC
  o Not designed as stand-alone device → anterior plate or posterior rod construct

SELECTED REFERENCES

1. Epstein NE: Iliac crest autograft versus alternative constructs for anterior cervical spine surgery: pros, cons, and costs. Surg Neurol Int. 3(Suppl 3):S143-56, 2012
2. Sasani M et al: Single-stage posterior corpectomy and expandable cage placement for treatment of thoracic or lumbar burst fractures. Spine (Phila Pa 1976). 34(1):E33-40, 2009
3. Chou D et al: Adjacent-level vertebral body fractures after expandable cage reconstruction. J Neurosurg Spine. 8(6):584-8, 2008

(Left) *Subsidence of the superior aspect of interbody cage graft with instability demonstrates that the initial sagittal CT shows an expandable cage position at the L3 corpectomy site with the inferior margin engaged with the posterior-superior L4 body and the superior margin engaged with the anterior-inferior L2 body* ➡️. **(Right)** *Four-month follow-up study shows rotation of the cage and subsidence of the superior margin of the cage into the L2 body* ➡️. *The inferior aspect of the cage has rotated into the canal* ➡️.

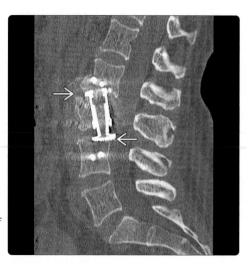
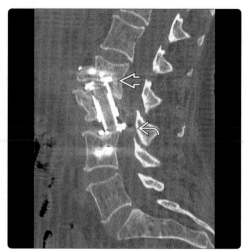

(Left) *Subsidence of the superior aspect of interbody cage graft with instability demonstrates that initial T1WI MR shows the extensive signal loss related to the cage but suggests abnormal position of the cage due to a metal artifact extending into the spinal canal* ➡️. **(Right)** *Sagittal T2WI MR shows the less extensive signal loss related to the cage, increasing confidence that the posterior position of the cage is abnormal due to the metal artifact extending into the spinal canal at the inferior L3 level* ➡️.

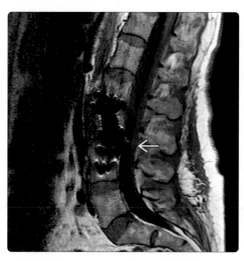
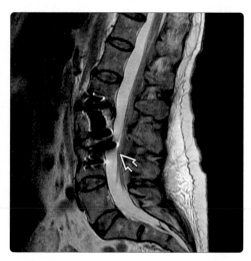

(Left) *In this sagittal CT after C5 and C6 corpectomies and partial C4 and C7 corpectomies for traumatic burst fractures, note the titanium mesh cage* ➡️ *with bone graft material* ➡️, *ACDF from C4-C7* ➡️, *and hardware failure with anterior displacement* ➡️. **(Right)** *AP radiograph displays different interbody fusion devices: Allografts with radiodense markers* ➡️ *and interbody lumbar cage* ➡️. *The latter is composed of porous titanium cylinders placed in the disc space, allowing bone graft to fuse adjacent vertebral bodies.*

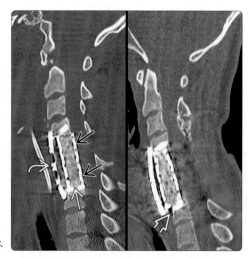
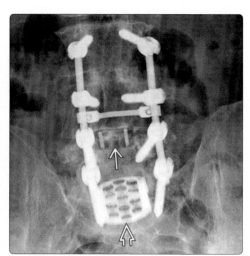

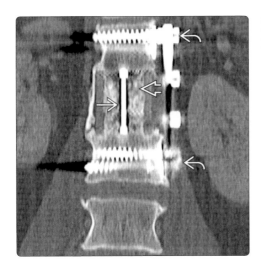

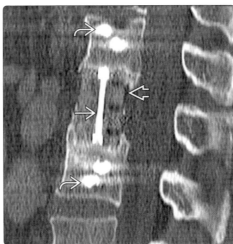

(Left) *Coronal CT reconstruction demonstrates a lumbar vertebral replacement prosthesis with a central metallic rod* ➡ *and outer PEEK radiolucent core* ⮕. *Lateral fusion construct* ⮑ *provides additional stability after total vertebrectomy.* (Right) *Sagittal CT reconstruction in the same patient shows a lumbar prosthesis with a central rod* ➡ *and outer PEEK core* ⮕. *Note the graft position within the anterior 2/3 of disc space. The corporal screw of a lateral fusion construct* ⮑ *provides additional stability.*

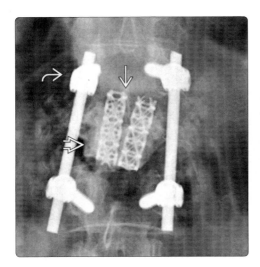

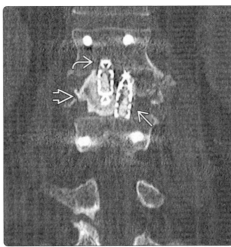

(Left) *AP plain film shows paired Pyramesh cages spanning the L2 level for vertebral collapse* ➡ *with bilateral pedicle screw fixation* ⮑. *Methylmethacrylate is noted surrounding the cages* ⮕. (Right) *Coronal CT demonstrates paired Pyramesh cages* ➡ *spanning the L2 level for vertebral collapse. The superior aspect of the cage had subsided into the endplate* ⮑. *Methylmethacrylate is noted surrounding the cages* ⮕.

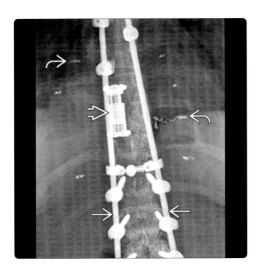

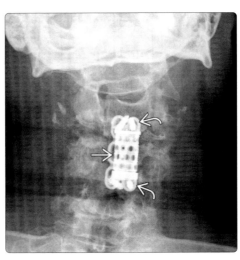

(Left) *Anteroposterior radiograph illustrates an expandable cage* ⮕ *and posterior instrumentation* ➡. *This patient underwent preoperative embolization of vertebral lesions at the T9 and T10 levels and of bilateral T8-T12 intercostal arteries* ⮑. *An expandable cage allows restoration and preservation of vertebral body height and alignment after anterior tumor resection.* (Right) *Anteroposterior radiograph exhibits a titanium mesh cervical cage* ➡. *ACDF from C3-C5 is also noted* ⮑.

Devices and Instrumentation

TERMINOLOGY

- Methods to stabilize subaxial cervical spine with posterior element constructs

PROCEDURE

- Interspinous wiring (Rogers 1942)
  - Simple and low risk
- Sublaminar wiring
  - Attach to onlay graft material or rods
- Facet wiring (Callahan 1977)
  - Facet capsules opened and holes drilled at each level
- Clamps (Tucker 1975)
  - Narrows spinal canal similar to sublaminar wires
- Lateral mass screws and plates (Roy-Camille)
  - Immediate stability with no need for external halo fixation
  - Usually oriented in superior and lateral direction to avoid VA and exiting nerve roots
- Transarticular screws
  - Used in C1-C2 interspace but also described for subaxial spine
- Lateral mass screws and rods
  - Very useful for multilevel disease
- Cervical pedicle screws (Abumi 1994)
  - Excellent stability and fixation
  - Resistant to pullout
  - Technically challenging since verterbal artery injury can occur

OUTCOMES

- Lateral mass screw: Incidence of facet joint violation as high as 20%
- Pedicle screw: 1.7% neurovascular complications
  - 7% cortical perforation rate for cervical pedicle screws
  - Pedicles should be at least 4.5 mm in diameter for safe screw placement
- Dural tear: Related to sublaminar wire placement

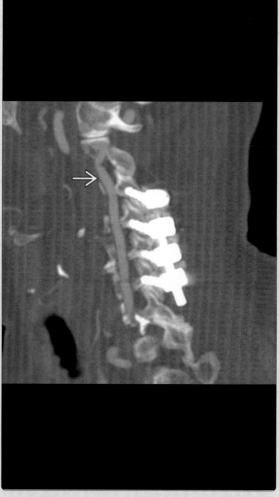

Lateral Mass Screws

Screw Position Relative to Vertebral Artery

Axial NECT shows laminectomy with bilateral-lateral mass fixation with polyaxial screws.

Sagittal CT angiogram shows the position of the 4-level lateral mass screws angled cephalad and the relationship to the ventral dominant vertebral artery ➡.

TERMINOLOGY

Abbreviations

- Vertebral artery (VA)

Synonyms

- Posterior cervical fusion
- Posterior cervical stabilization

Definitions

- Methods to stabilize subaxial cervical spine with posterior element constructs

PROCEDURE

Procedure Steps

- **Interspinous wiring** (Rogers 1942)
  - Simple and low risk
  - Holes drilled into spinous processes with wires passing through
  - Single point of fixation
  - Bohlman triple-wire variation used to stabilize 1 or more levels
- **Sublaminar wiring**
  - Can be used in subaxial spine
  - Difficulty related to narrowing of spinal canal with wires at spinal levels with normally small bony canal and maximum cervical cord size
  - Attach to onlay graft material or rods
- **Facet wiring** (Callahan 1977)
  - Facet capsules opened and holes drilled at each level
  - Wires passed through drilled holes in superior to inferior direction
  - Exiting joint space
  - Wires then wrapped around graft material secured to decorticated articular masses
- **Clamps** (Tucker 1975)
  - Introduced for C1-C2 arthrodesis
  - Claw-type construct
    - Allowing immediate fixation without risk of direct neural injury of sublaminar wire
  - Bone graft placed into interlaminar spaces bilaterally
  - Utilized for subaxial spine at any single level
  - Requires intact lamina
- **Lateral mass screws and plates** (Roy-Camille technique)
  - Immediate stability with no need for external halo fixation
  - Various modifications with slightly different entrance points and screw direction
  - Usually oriented in superior and lateral direction to avoid VA and exiting nerve roots
    - **Magerl** method
      - Axial plane: 25° lateral
      - Sagittal plane: Parallel to facet joint
      - Incidence of nerve root injury higher than with Roy-Camille technique
    - **Anderson** method
      - Axial plane: 10° lateral
      - Sagittal plane: 30-40° rostral
    - **An** method
      - Axial plane: 30° lateral
      - Sagittal: 15° rostral
      - Decreased neurovascular injury with this technique
  - **Transarticular screws**
    - Used in C1-C2 interspace but also described for subaxial spine
    - VA location simplifies screw placement relative to complexity at C1-C2
    - Screw direction is anterior and caudal
  - **Lateral mass screws and rods**
    - Various manufacturers including
      - Cervifix™ system (Synthes; Solothurn, Switzerland)
      - Summit™ and Mountaineer™ systems (DePuy; Raynham, MA)
      - Vertex® system (Medtronic; Fridley, MN)
      - S4® cervical system (Aesculap; Center Valley, PA)
      - Minit™ posterior cervical & upper thoracic fixation system (Zimmer; Warsaw, IN)
    - Allow for precise placement of screws with realignment
    - Very useful for multilevel disease
  - **Cervical pedicle screws** (Abumi 1994)
    - Excellent stability and fixation
    - Resistant to pullout
    - Technically challenging since VA injury can occur
    - Pedicle diameter smaller than thoracolumbar pedicle
    - Pedicle axis more inclined in transverse plane
      - Fluoroscopic-assisted pedicle axis view technique allows high success rate

OUTCOMES

Complications

- Lateral mass screws
  - With long 20-mm bicortical screws
    - Higher potential for injury has been documented with **Magerl** method than **An** method
  - Incidence of facet joint violation as high as 20%
- Pedicle screws have been recommended due to problems with mechanical loosening and avulsions at upper and lower construct margins
  - 7% perforation rate for cervical pedicle screws
  - 1.7% neurovascular complications
  - Screw perforation highest at C4 and C7
  - Pedicles should be at least 4.5 mm in diameter for safe screw placement
- Patients with severe cervical spondylotic myelopathy at risk of postoperative weakness and cord contusion from posterior decompression
  - Even without intraoperative difficulties and with stable somatosensory-evoked potentials monitoring
- Dural tear
  - Related to sublaminar wire placement

SELECTED REFERENCES

1. Liu G et al: Anatomical considerations for the placement of cervical transarticular screws. J Neurosurg Spine. 14(1):114-21, 2011
2. Memtsoudis SG et al: Increased in-hospital complications after primary posterior versus primary anterior cervical fusion. Clin Orthop Relat Res. 2011 Mar;469(3):649-57. Erratum in: Clin Orthop Relat Res. 469(5):1502-4, 2011
3. Zhao L et al: Comparison of two techniques for transarticular screw implantation in the subaxial cervical spine. J Spinal Disord Tech. 24(2):126-31, 2011

TERMINOLOGY

- Pedicle screw: Most common implant in spine surgery
  - High rigidity and resistance to pullout
  - Engages all 3 columns of spine
  - Resists motion in all 3 directions
- Used in wide variety of procedures
  - Maintain spine alignment while fusion occurs
  - Maintain reduction after fracture
  - Maintain correction of deformity

PROCEDURE

- 3 common techniques
  - Free hand
  - Fluoroscopy based
  - Computer assisted (navigation) either 2D or 3D
    - Safe and reproducible
    - Incidence of exposed screws outside of pedicle decreased with 3D navigation from 12% to 7%

OUTCOMES

- CT is gold standard for assessment of pedicle screw position
- Screw malposition rates vary widely (0.5-13%)
- **Medial wall penetration**
  - Pedicle wall penetration (10-20% overall incidence)
  - Neural injury to root or cord (< 1%)
  - CSF leak if dural laceration
- **Anterior or lateral penetration**
  - Visceral injury, esophageal perforation
  - Pneumothorax
  - Aortic or segmental vessel penetration
  - Some canal intrusion is asymptomatic (< 2 mm)
- **Pedicle fracture**
- **Pedicle plow**
  - Occurs during vertebral rotation in scoliosis surgery
  - May cause aortic abutment of screw

Complication Graphic

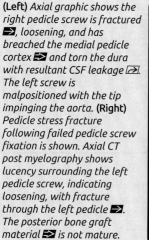

Stress Fracture

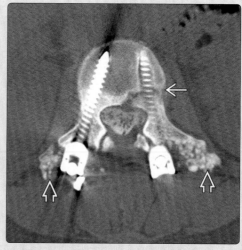

(Left) *Axial graphic shows the right pedicle screw is fractured ➡, loosening, and has breached the medial pedicle cortex ➡ and torn the dura with resultant CSF leakage ➡. The left screw is malpositioned with the tip impinging the aorta.* (Right) *Pedicle stress fracture following failed pedicle screw fixation is shown. Axial CT post myelography shows lucency surrounding the left pedicle screw, indicating loosening, with fracture through the left pedicle ➡. The posterior bone graft material ➡ is not mature.*

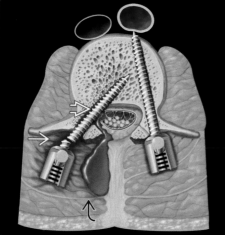

Screw Malposition and Loosening

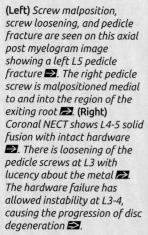

Screw Loosening

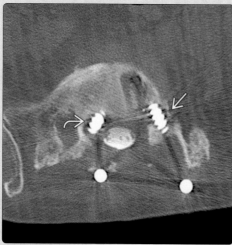

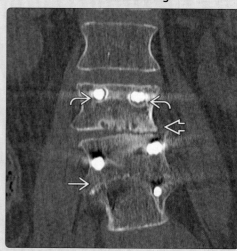

(Left) *Screw malposition, screw loosening, and pedicle fracture are seen on this axial post myelogram image showing a left L5 pedicle fracture ➡. The right pedicle screw is malpositioned medial to and into the region of the exiting root ➡.* (Right) *Coronal NECT shows L4-5 solid fusion with intact hardware ➡. There is loosening of the pedicle screws at L3 with lucency about the metal ➡. The hardware failure has allowed instability at L3-4, causing the progression of disc degeneration ➡.*

TERMINOLOGY

Synonyms

- Pedicle screw
- Pedicle fixation

Pedicle Screw

- Most common implant in spine surgery
  o High rigidity and resistance to pullout
  o Engages all 3 columns of spine
  o Resists motion in all 3 directions

PROCEDURE

Techniques

- 3 common techniques
  o Free hand
  o Fluoroscopy based
  o Computer assisted (navigation)
- Fluoroscopy
  o Not 100% accurate (80-90%)
  o Risk of radiation exposure
- Navigation system theoretically most accurate
  o Safe and reproducible
  o Incidence of exposed screws outside of pedicle decreased with 3D navigation from 12% to 7%

OUTCOMES

Problems

- Screw malposition rates vary widely (0.5-20%)
- Malpositioned instrumentation may have acute and chronic morbidity
  o Can cause delayed instability
  o Accelerate degenerative change in adjacent segment
- **Perioperative**
  o Pedicle wall penetration (10-20% overall incidence)
  o Medial wall penetration
    – Neural injury to root or cord (< 1%)
    – CSF leak if dural laceration
  o Anterior or lateral penetration
    – Visceral injury
    – Pneumothorax
    – Esophageal perforation
    – Aortic or segmental vessel penetration
    – Injury can occur due to screw itself; may also be related to taps and guidewire manipulation intraoperatively
      □ If screw or taps inserted at different angle than wire, wire can kink and be driven further into body
    – Some canal intrusion is asymptomatic
    – Medial violation must be > 3 mm to approach same volumetric intrusion as largest pedicle hook footplate
  o Pedicle fracture
  o Pedicle plow
    – Occurs at time of direct vertebral rotation in scoliosis surgery
    – Axial plane plow is medial &/or lateral translation of pedicle screw through cortical boundaries of pedicle &/or vertebral body
    – May cause aortic abutment of screw

- **Delayed postoperative**
  o Wound infection
  o Loosening of screw
  o Disconnection of screw from rod

Complications

- Most feared complication(s)
  o Medial cortical penetration by screw with cord injury
- Radiograph evaluation
  o Guidelines for detecting medial or lateral wall violation on plain films (Kim et al, 2005)
    – Violation of harmonious segmental change of tips of inserted screws with reference to vertebral rotation using posterior upper spinolaminar junction in PA radiograph (medial or lateral out)
    – No crossing of medial pedicle wall by tip of pedicle screw inserted with reference to vertebral rotation using posterior upper spinolaminar junction in PA radiograph (lateral out)
    – Violation of imaginary midline of vertebral body using posterior upper spinolaminar junction in PA radiograph by position of tip of inserted pedicle screw (medial out)
- CT is gold standard for assessment of pedicle screw position
  o Intraoperative CT can reduce revision rate
  o ↑ radiation dose
  o CT shows 10x more screws violating pedicle cortex than plain radiographs
- MR evaluation limited due to metal artifact
  o Adjusting direction of frequency encode can minimize screw artifact
  o Frequency encode in AP direction minimizes right-to-left artifact for pedicle screws
- EMG
  o Screw malposition can be detected by intraoperative triggered EMG after screw insertion in lumbar spine

SELECTED REFERENCES

1. Ponnusamy KE et al: Instrumentation of the osteoporotic spine: biomechanical and clinical considerations. Spine J. 11(1):54-63, 2011
2. Cho W et al: The biomechanics of pedicle screw-based instrumentation. J Bone Joint Surg Br. 92(8):1061-5, 2010
3. Hicks JM et al: Complications of pedicle screw fixation in scoliosis surgery: a systematic review. Spine (Phila Pa 1976). 35(11):E465-70, 2010
4. Samdani AF et al: Accuracy of free-hand placement of thoracic pedicle screws in adolescent idiopathic scoliosis: how much of a difference does surgeon experience make? Eur Spine J. 19(1):91-5, 2010
5. Samdani AF et al: Learning curve for placement of thoracic pedicle screws in the deformed spine. Neurosurgery. 66(2):290-4; discussion 294-5, 2010
6. Heary RF et al: Decision making in adult deformity. Neurosurgery. 63(3 Suppl):69-77, 2008
7. Kakkos SK et al: Delayed presentation of aortic injury by pedicle screws: report of two cases and review of the literature. J Vasc Surg. 47(5):1074-82, 2008
8. Lehman RA Jr et al: Computed tomography evaluation of pedicle screws placed in the pediatric deformed spine over an 8-year period. Spine (Phila Pa 1976). 32(24):2679-84, 2007
9. Shah SA: Derotation of the spine. Neurosurg Clin N Am. 18(2):339-45, 2007
10. Macagno AE et al: Thoracic and thoracolumbar kyphosis in adults. Spine (Phila Pa 1976). 31(19 Suppl):S161-70, 2006
11. Foster MR: A functional classification of spinal instrumentation. Spine J. 5(6):682-94, 2005
12. Kim YJ et al: Evaluation of pedicle screw placement in the deformed spine using intraoperative plain radiographs: a comparison with computerized tomography. Spine (Phila Pa 1976). 30(18):2084-8, 2005

Devices and Instrumentation

TERMINOLOGY

- Artificial disc replacement, total cervical disc replacement, artificial intervertebral disc arthroplasty
- Insertion of prosthetic total disc replacement after anterior decompression with aim of preserving normal range and type of intervertebral motion
- Preventing complications associated with rigid arthrodesis & subsequent segmental loss of motion

IMAGING

- Radiographs with flexion and extension views
- CT to assess for adjacent level disease and heterotopic ossification
- Postoperative MR may be helpful in cases of persistent pain to assess for inadequate decompression or myelopathy

CLINICAL ISSUES

- Ideal patient has soft disc herniation causing neuro signs/symptoms, motion at involved segment, no evidence of osteoporosis or infection
- Worldwide indication is 1-2-level radiculopathy or myelopathy; however, FDA indication is limited to single-level disease in levels C3 to C7
- Candidates: Those who failed conservative therapy + evidence of symptomatic nerve root ± spinal cord compression
- Complications
  - Device wear, subsidence or displacement, segmental hypermobility, and excessive disc space distraction to accommodate prosthesis, consequent facet joint separation, and screw breakage
  - Facet arthrosis, adjacent level degeneration
  - Paravertebral heterotopic ossification may be prevented with NSAIDs

(Left) *Lateral radiograph illustrates a ProDisc-C cervical disc ➡. It has cobalt-chromium endplates with a central keel for anchorage to the vertebral body and a locking core of ultra high molecular weight polyethylene that provides a ball-and-socket articulation.* (Right) *Lateral radiograph shows a Prestige LP total cervical disc replacement (TCDR) ➡. This titanium ceramic device is composed of articulating ball and trough components. Screws attach it to the cervical vertebrae.*

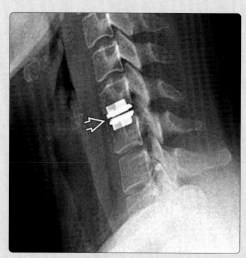
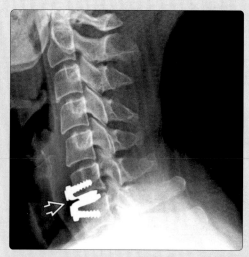

(Left) *Radiograph shows a grade 2 heterotopic ossification ➡, a complication of TCDR. Ossification along the lateral aspect of the device may result in fusion, causing reduced movement, whereas anterior ossification allows continued mobility.* (Right) *Lateral radiograph shows a Bryan cervical disc ➡, which is composed of porous, coated, clamshell-shaped, titanium endplates and a polycarbonate, polyurethane core. This prosthesis provides elasticity and compressibility.*

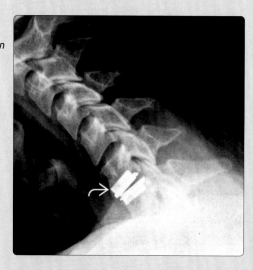
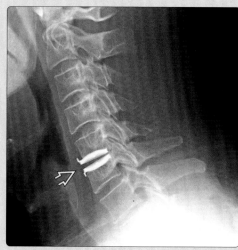

Lumbar Artificial Disc

TERMINOLOGY

- Total lumbar disc replacement, arthroplasty
- Treatment of degenerative disc disease restoring normal mobility of diseased segments & improving clinical outcomes by decreasing risk of adjacent-level disease

IMAGING

- Endplate keel, fixation spikes, and inlay may help identify individual devices
- Radiography helpful to identify midline placement, AP positioning, and degree of vertebral body penetration or subsidence
- CT best for evaluating extent of vertebral body penetration
- CT and MR helpful to evaluate adjacent vertebral bodies, particularly in detecting fractures and degenerative changes at adjacent disc space and facet levels

CLINICAL ISSUES

- Lumbar disc arthroplasty indicated for 1- or 2-level discogenic mechanical back pain primarily in absence of radiculopathy
- Complications
  - Heterotopic ossification incidence in 1.4-15.0%
  - Adjacent level degenerative disease, facet arthrosis
  - Device migration, extrusion of inlay
  - Subsidence: 3-10% incidence
  - Segmental lordosis alterations
  - Vertebral fractures
- Indications
  - Skeletal maturity
  - Degenerative disc disease at 1 level from L4 through S1
  - No relief of pain after 6 months or more of nonsurgical treatment

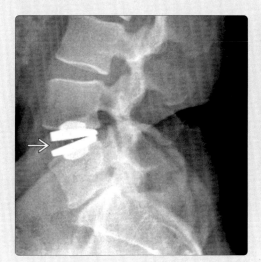

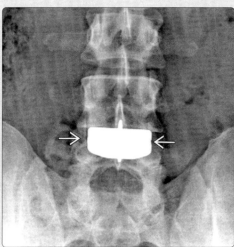

(Left) *Lateral radiograph shows Activ-L lumbar artificial disc* ➡. *Although arthrodesis is the gold standard for surgical treatment of lumbar degenerative disc disease, solid fusion can cause increased motion in adjacent segments. This may initiate &/or accelerate the adjacent segment disease process.* (Right) *Activ-L* ➡ *allows for maintenance/restoration of physiologic movement at affected segments. Restoring and maintaining normal motion of the segment reduces stresses and loads on adjacent levels.*

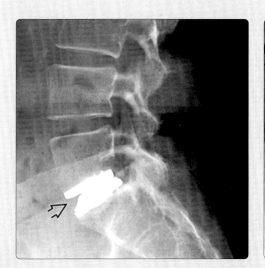

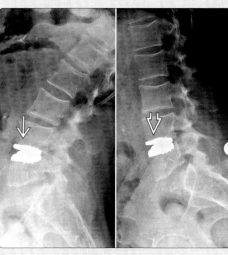

(Left) *Lateral radiograph shows the FlexiCore TLDR* ➡. *Current indications for lumbar disc arthroplasty are young, nonosteoporotic patients with 1- or 2-level symptomatic disc degeneration without severe facet arthropathy, segmental instability, or neural element compression requiring a posterior decompression.* (Right) *Extension* ➡ *and flexion* ➡ *views show relatively preserved range of motion. The normal spinal mobility and biomechanics are thought to reduce adjacent spinal deterioration.*

TERMINOLOGY

- Synonyms: Interspinous posterior decompression, interspinous distraction device, interspinous spacer device (ISD), interspinous implant
- Dynamic stabilization alters movement & load transmission of spinal motion segment without fusion of segment
- Interspinous spacing device places stenotic segment in slight flexion while preventing extension

IMAGING

- Radiographs & CT helpful to evaluate interspinous location
  - Assess for fractures

PATHOLOGY

- Lumbar neurogenic claudication symptoms are exacerbated during extension, relieved during flexion
  - Dimensions of canal & foramen ↑ in flexion, ↓ in extension
  - Facet loading ↑ during extension, ↓ during flexion

CLINICAL ISSUES

- ISD helpful for treatment of spinal stenosis with neurogenic claudication
  - Causes focal flexion at applied level, resulting in increased canal & foramen dimensions
- Complications
  - ISD malposition, migration, dislocation, spinous process fracture
- Indications
  - Lumbar stenosis ± facet joint hypertrophy & subarticular recess stenosis, foraminal stenosis
  - 1- to 2-level lumbar stenosis from L1-L5 in patients with at least moderate impairment in function
- Patients anatomy may influence outcomes
  - Decreased accessible distance between laminospinous plane and tip of spinous process
- Osteoporosis is contraindication

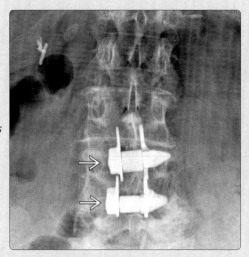
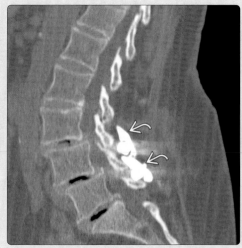

(Left) *X-Stop implants ⇒ at L4-L5 & L5-S1 are titanium alloy devices placed between spinous processes to reduce canal & foraminal narrowing that occurs in extension, thus reducing the symptoms of neurogenic intermittent claudication.* (Right) *Sagittal bone CT shows an interspinous spacing device (ISD) ⇒, which may increase the foraminal area & height as well as spinal canal diameter in extension. ISDs may improve recurrent facet joint pain in clinical short- and midterm settings but do not exceed outcome of denervated patients.*

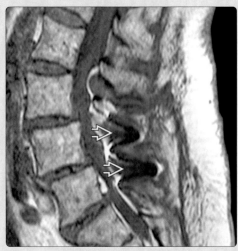
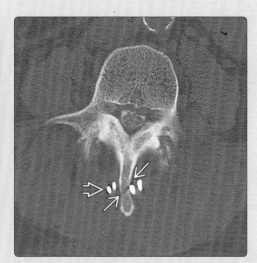

(Left) *Sagittal T1WI MR shows the susceptibility artifact from the ISDs ⇒. X-Stop is the most commonly used ISD in patients with neurogenic intermittent claudication due to lumbar stenosis.* (Right) *Axial CT myelographic image of spinous process fractures at 2 levels following placement of X-Stop devices for canal stenosis shows fractures through the L4 spinous processes ⇒. Note the overlap of the wings of the adjacent level devices ⇒.*

IMAGING

General Features

- Location
  - Interspinous soft tissues of lumbar spine
    - Extradural

Radiographic Findings

- Free-floating prosthesis in interspinous region

CT Findings

- Implant is not rigidly attached to bony anatomy
  - Restricted from migrating posteriorly by supraspinous ligament, anteriorly by laminae, cranially & caudally by spinous process (SP), & laterally by 2 wings or stops on implant

MR Findings

- Susceptibility artifact may obscure detailed delineation of hardware & its appropriate orientation in interspinous soft tissues

Imaging Recommendations

- Best imaging tool
  - Radiograph helpful for interspinous location (flexion & extension views useful to detect abnormal motion of hardware)
  - CT: Assess vertebral bodies & posterior elements for fractures

PATHOLOGY

Staging, Grading, & Classification

- Static (noncompressible)
  - X-Stop (Medtronic Sofamor Danek; Minneapolis, MN): Titanium oval spacer with 2 lateral wings to prevent lateral migration
  - Wallis implant (Abbott Spine; Austin, TX): Polyetheretherketone (PEEK) spacer placed between SPs & secured with 2 Dacron ligaments wrapped around SPs
    - Good 13-year clinical outcome in 1 study, obviated arthrodesis in 80% of patients
    - Current indications
      - Following discectomy for large herniated disc in which there is significant loss of disc material
      - Redo discectomy for recurrent herniation
      - Discectomy for herniation of transitional disc with sacralization of L5
      - Degenerative disc adjacent to fused segment
      - Isolated Modic 1 lesion attributable to chronic low back pain
  - Aperius PercLID system (Medtronic Sofamor Danek): Percutaneous device insertion
  - ExtenSure (NuVasive; San Diego, CA): Cylinder-shaped allograft device
- Dynamic (compressible)
  - Coflex Interspinous U (Paradigm Spine; New York, NY)
  - Diam (Medtronic Sofamor Danek): Silicone interspinous spacer covered by polyethylene coat, secured in place with 2 ligatures around superior & inferior SPs

CLINICAL ISSUES

Presentation

- Most common signs/symptoms
  - Standard surgical treatment of spinal stenosis or lateral recess stenosis: Laminectomy or bilateral hemilaminotomies & foraminotomies
    - Extensive soft tissue dissection for laminectomy, longer surgical time, & more blood loss
      - Procedures less attractive for frail elderly patients
  - Osteoporotic fractures may result only in loss of height or stooped posture
    - With spinal stenosis & narrowed lateral recess & foramina, extension of back from brace & axial loading from weight of standing causes nerve root compression
    - Extension of lumbar spine shown to decrease cross-sectional area of neural foramen by ~ 15%
- Complications
  - Postoperative complication rate 10.1% & reoperation rate 6-7.2%
  - Interspinous distraction device (ISD) malposition
  - Migration: Device remains between SP, function is preserved, & patient is asymptomatic
  - Dislocation: Device moved outside interspinous area but contained by detached supraspinous ligament or associated with ruptured supraspinous ligament
    - Nonfunctional with recurring symptoms requiring revision surgery
  - SP fissures & fractures
  - Rare stress fracture of facet joints

Treatment

- Indications
  - Lumbar stenosis ± facet joint hypertrophy & subarticular recess stenosis, foraminal stenosis, ± stable grade I spondylolisthesis or equivalent retrolisthesis
  - Limited to use in 1-2 level lumbar stenosis from L1-L5 in patients with at least moderate impairment
  - Dynamic stabilization attractive option (compared to fusion) for younger patients who would bear greater burden on adjacent segments during their prolonged follow-up
- Exclusion criteria in some studies
  - Unable to sit for prolonged periods without pain; unremitting spinal pain in any position; cauda equina syndrome; pathologic fractures of vertebrae; active infection; Paget disease at involved segments or spinal metastases; spinal anatomy, such as ankylosing spondylitis or fusion, at affected level
- ISD shown to have extremely high failure rate (defined as surgical reintervention) after short-term follow-up in patients with spinal stenosis caused by degenerative spondylolisthesis
- Implants are not favorable or currently recommended for use at L5-S1
- ISD does not restrict or eliminate any potential future therapeutic options that are currently being developed, such as arthroplasty

Devices and Instrumentation

TERMINOLOGY

- Spinal fusion surgery recommended when curve magnitude > 40-45° for adolescent idiopathic scoliosis
- Adult scoliosis presents with lumbar back ± leg pain, L3-L4 rotatory subluxation, L4-L5 tilt, and L5-S1 disc degeneration on radiographs

IMAGING

- Radiographs
  - Main thoracic, thoracolumbar, and lumbar curves should be assessed for structural characteristics
  - 36" standing anteroposterior & lateral radiographs & supine side-bending radiographs
  - In adult scoliosis, assess for degenerated changes and rotatory ± lateral listhesis
- CT
  - Assess integrity of hardware
  - Look for osseous bridging at levels of interbody fusion and lucency along screw tracks

- MR
  - Preoperative planning to evaluate for central &/or foraminal stenosis and disc degeneration

CLINICAL ISSUES

- Adult bones tend to be weaker or osteoporotic, making instrumentation and fusion more difficult
- Degenerative disc changes, spinal stenosis, and facet arthropathy can be exacerbated and in turn exacerbate scoliosis, leading to more rigid spines
- Goals: Prevent progression, restore acceptability of clinical deformity, reduce curvature, prevent neurologic deficit
  - Resolve pain ± make it more controllable with medications
  - Fuse spine in as normal anatomical position as possible

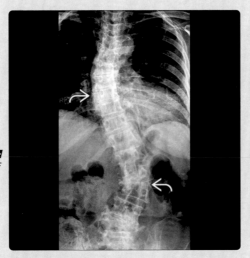

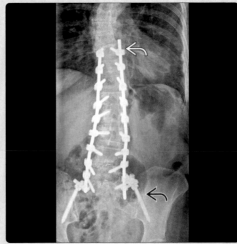

(Left) Anteroposterior radiograph shows sigmoid scoliosis of the thoracic and lumbar spines ➔. Fusion is extended to L5 if there is fixed tilt or subluxation at L4-L5, or to the sacrum if L5-S1 central or foraminal decompression is needed. (Right) Anteroposterior radiograph depicts posterior fusion from the thoracolumbar junction ➔ to the sacrum ➔. Extension of the fusion to the sacrum increases the incidence of pseudarthrosis and reoperation.

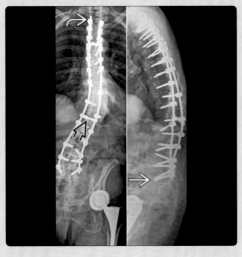

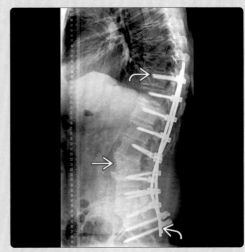

(Left) AP and lateral radiographs show fusion from the thoracic spine ➔ to the L5 level ➔. Fusion is not terminated next to a severely degenerated segment. Proximal extension of the fusion should not stop distal to a proximal thoracic curve. Cross-links ➔ improve torsional stiffness. (Right) Lateral radiograph shows posterior fusion ➔ and L3 pedicle subtraction osteotomy ➔ to restore lumbar lordosis. Lumbar scoliosis results in loss of lumbar lordosis with positive sagittal balance.

TERMINOLOGY

Abbreviations

- Scoliosis instrumentation (SI)

Synonyms

- Scoliosis surgery, long spinal fusion surgery (> 4 vertebral segments)

Definitions

- Spinal fusion surgery recommended when curve magnitude > 40-45° for adolescent idiopathic scoliosis (AIS)
- Adult scoliosis patient presents with lumbar back ± leg pain, L3-L4 rotatory subluxation, L4-L5 tilt, and L5-S1 disc degeneration on radiographs
  - Goals: Prevent progression, restore acceptability of clinical deformity, reduce curvature, correct positive sagittal malalignment, prevent neurologic deficit and pain reduction

IMAGING

Radiographic Findings

- Main thoracic, thoracolumbar, and lumbar curves should be assessed for structural characteristics
  - 36" standing AP & lateral radiographs and supine side-bending radiographs
  - ± 36" supine lateral or hyperextension lateral radiograph over bolster
    - Supine evaluation is helpful to determine curve flexibility
  - From Lenke classification system for AIS, structural curve is defined by Cobb angle 25° on side-bending radiographs
  - Overall flexibility is important to note → indicates expected curve correction
  - Coronal & sagittal balance, including center sacral vertical line and C7 plumbline
  - Shoulder height, apical vertebral translation of thoracic and lumbar curves, and relative curve magnitudes
  - In adult scoliosis, assess for degenerated changes and rotatory &/or lateral listhesis

CT Findings

- Look for osseous bridging at levels of interbody fusion and lucency along screw tracks
- Assess integrity of instrumentation
- May be helpful in delineating congenital osseous abnormalities (such as hemivertebrae or fused vertebrae)
- 3D reformations may be helpful for preoperative planning and postoperative evaluation

MR Findings

- Preoperative planning to evaluate for central &/or foraminal stenosis and disc degeneration

DIFFERENTIAL DIAGNOSIS

Plates and Screws

- Instrumentation in fusion surgery used to stabilize bony elements

Flat Back Syndrome

- Loss of lumbar lordosis after lumbar or scoliosis distraction instrumentation, vertebral fracture, ankylosing spondylitis, degenerative disease

CLINICAL ISSUES

Natural History & Prognosis

- **Complications**
  - Surgical: Severe blood loss, UTI, pancreatitis, obstructive bowel dysfunction due to bowel immobilization, neurological damage
    - Retroperitoneal approach: Abdominal visceral, great vessel, and superior hypogastric nerve plexus injury
    - Transthoracic approach: Injury to great vessels, pulmonary complications, chylothorax, and post-thoracotomy pain syndrome
  - Migration of graft, implant breakage
  - Penetration of implants into canal or dorsally into cutaneous tissues
  - Compression of nerve roots by implant components
- Pseudoarthrosis
  - Can occur years after surgery
  - Most likely to occur at thoracolumbar junction
  - Reported in 15-27% of cases
- Irreversible loss of normal active range of movement of spinal column, including nonfused segments
- Strain on unfused skeletal framework
  - Postsurgical degenerative changes within 2 years
  - Higher degree of correction results in higher rate of degenerative osteoarthritis
- Curvature progression: Crank shaft phenomenon described in children: Spinal growth causes rotation around fusion
- Pain at iliac graft site, rib resection site
- Infections reported in 5-10% of patients at 11-45 months after surgery
- Venous thromboembolism (pulmonary embolism and deep vein thrombosis)

Treatment

- Goal of surgery in adult scoliosis
  - Resolve pain ± make it more controllable with medications
  - Fuse spine in as normal anatomical position as possible
  - Biggest operative decision is to determine proximal and distal extent of instrumentation and fusion
    - Operative levels include fusion of Cobb angle, typically L3 or L4, and extending to L5 when there is lateral or rotatory listhesis present
    - Restoration of sagittal balance reported to be primary parameter associated with outcome
- SI recommended when magnitude of curvature exceeds 40-45° in AIS
  - Approaches: Posterior instrumentation & fusion alone, anterior instrumentation & fusion alone, & anterior release (to restore spinal flexibility) combined with posterior fusion, posterior only
  - Fusion often extended to sacrum if
    - L5-S1 spondylolisthesis, or prior laminectomy
    - L5-S1 stenosis
    - Severe L5-S1 disc degeneration

Devices and Instrumentation

TERMINOLOGY

- Intrathecal baclofen (ITB)
- Intraspinal drug delivery (IDD)
- Malfunction or malposition of pump or catheter delivery system

PATHOLOGY

- ITB used for treatment of spasticity
  - Typically used in children with severe quadriplegic pattern cerebral palsy
- IDD system therapy widely utilized in patients with intractable, nonmalignant, and malignant pain
  - Epidural analgesia trial may be conducted to document efficacy prior to implantation of permanent intrathecal drug delivery pump

CLINICAL ISSUES

- **ITB** rate of complications varies widely, range: 8-30%

- o **Baclofen** complications relate to withdrawal and overdose
- o **Infection** rates: 8-10%
- o **Hardware**-related complications from 5-20%
- o Majority of complications requiring reoperation involve the catheter
- **IDD** systems
  - o Granuloma formation at catheter tip relatively common
  - o Effects include loss of analgesia or new/progressive neurologic symptoms

DIAGNOSTIC CHECKLIST

- Malfunction must be evaluated from pump level to distal aspect of catheter
  - o CT abdomen following baclofen side port contrast injection extending cephalad beyond intradural catheter tip

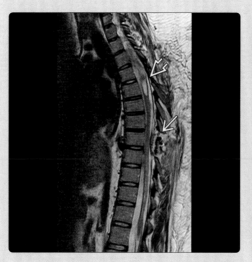
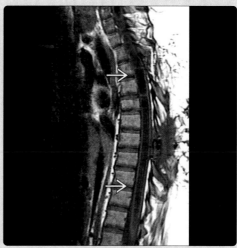

(Left) *This is a syringopleural shunt failure due to formation of a pseudocyst at the catheter site in the chest. Initial T2W MR study after placement of the shunt shows postoperative change* ➡ *with a small epidural fluid collection in the midthoracic spine and syrinx in the upper thoracic cord* ➡. (Right) *Sagittal T1WI MR in the same patient 1 year later now shows marked expansion of the syrinx throughout the thoracic cord* ➡.

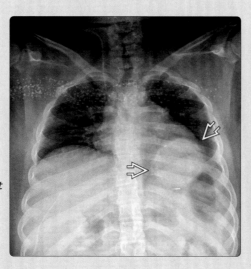
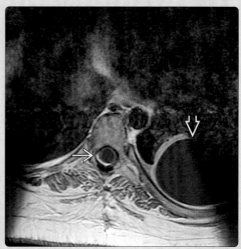

(Left) *AP chest film in the same patient shows a loculated pleural collection at the site of the coiled shunt catheter* ➡. (Right) *This is a syringopleural shunt failure with expansion of the extensive cord syrinx due to formation of a pseudocyst at the catheter site in the chest. Axial T1 MR in the same patient shows the large thoracic cord syrinx* ➡ *and a large fluid collection in the left chest at the site of catheter placement* ➡.

TERMINOLOGY

Abbreviations

- Intrathecal baclofen (ITB)
- Intraspinal drug delivery (IDD)

Definitions

- Malfunction or malposition of pump or catheter delivery system

IMAGING

General Features

- Best diagnostic clue
  - Abnormal contrast accumulation after pump side port injection
- Location
  - Anywhere along course of pump and catheter

DIFFERENTIAL DIAGNOSIS

Intrathecal or Epidural Catheter Granuloma

- May mimic epidural neoplasm or abscess

PATHOLOGY

General Features

- Etiology
  - ITB used for treatment of spasticity
    - Decrease level of spasticity to improve range of motion, facilitate movement, reduce contractures, and improve quality of life
    - Typically used in children with severe quadriplegic pattern cerebral palsy
  - IDD system therapy widely utilized in patients with intractable, nonmalignant, and malignant pain
    - Epidural or intrathecal
    - Epidural analgesia trial may be conducted to document efficacy prior to implantation of permanent intrathecal drug delivery pump

CLINICAL ISSUES

Presentation

- Most common signs/symptoms
  - **ITB** rate of complications varies widely, range: 8-30%
  - **Related to (a) baclofen, (b) infection, (c) hardware**
  - **Baclofen** complications relate to withdrawal and overdose
  - **Infection** rates: 8-10%
    - Common reason for infection is skin breakdown or dehiscence over pump
    - Subfascial implantation provides greater soft tissue coverage over pump
  - **Hardware**-related complications from 5-20%
    - Majority of complications requiring reoperation involve catheter
    - CSF leak from site of catheter penetration of dura
    - Catheter fracture or disconnection
    - Low rate of pump failure
  - **IDD** systems
    - Granuloma formation at catheter tip relatively common

- Multiple agents, including morphine, may cause formation
  - □ Dose escalation and increased dosage increase risk of formation
- Effects include loss of analgesia or new/progressive neurologic symptoms
- Other signs/symptoms
  - Pump malfunction may present with spinal/abdominal fluid collection/effusion

DIAGNOSTIC CHECKLIST

Consider

- Malfunction must be evaluated from pump level to distal aspect of catheter
  - CT abdomen following baclofen side port contrast injection extending cephalad beyond intradural catheter tip

SELECTED REFERENCES

1. Haranhalli N et al: Intrathecal baclofen therapy: complication avoidance and management. Childs Nerv Syst. 27(3):421-7, 2011
2. Lawson EF et al: Current developments in intraspinal agents for cancer and noncancer pain. Curr Pain Headache Rep. 14(1):8-16, 2010
3. Maugans TA: Intracranial migration of a fractured intrathecal catheter from a baclofen pump system: case report and analysis of possible causes. Neurosurgery. 66(2):319-22, 2010
4. Myers J et al: Intraspinal techniques for pain management in cancer patients: a systematic review. Support Care Cancer. 18(2):137-49, 2010
5. Stetkarova I et al: Procedure- and device-related complications of intrathecal baclofen administration for management of adult muscle hypertonia: a review. Neurorehabil Neural Repair. 24(7):609-19, 2010
6. Fukuhara T et al: Tangled catheter as a rare cause of baclofen pump malfunction. Surg Neurol. 72(1):80-2; discussion 82, 2009
7. van Rijn MA et al: Intrathecal baclofen for dystonia of complex regional pain syndrome. Pain. 143(1-2):41-7, 2009
8. Borowski A et al: Baclofen pump implantation and spinal fusion in children: techniques and complications. Spine (Phila Pa 1976). 33(18):1995-2000, 2008
9. Caird MS et al: Outcomes of posterior spinal fusion and instrumentation in patients with continuous intrathecal baclofen infusion pumps. Spine (Phila Pa 1976). 33(4):E94-9, 2008
10. Ruan X et al: Edema caused by continuous epidural hydromorphone infusion: a case report and review of the literature. J Opioid Manag. 4(4):255-9, 2008
11. Kallweit U et al: Successful treatment of methicillin-resistant Staphylococcus aureus meningitis using linezolid without removal of intrathecal infusion pump. Case report. J Neurosurg. 107(3):651-3, 2007
12. Markman JD et al: Interventional approaches to pain management. Med Clin North Am. 91(2):271-86, 2007
13. Motta F et al: The use of intrathecal baclofen pump implants in children and adolescents: safety and complications in 200 consecutive cases. J Neurosurg. 107(1 Suppl):32-5, 2007
14. Narouze SN et al: Erosion of the inferior epigastric artery: a rare complication of intrathecal drug delivery systems. Pain Med. 8(5):468-70, 2007
15. Vender JR et al: Identification and management of intrathecal baclofen pump complications: a comparison of pediatric and adult patients. J Neurosurg. 104(1 Suppl):9-15, 2006
16. Amar AP et al: Percutaneous spinal interventions. Neurosurg Clin N Am. 16(3):561-8, vii, 2005
17. Hassenbusch SJ et al: Polyanalgesic Consensus Conference 2003: an update on the management of pain by intraspinal drug delivery– report of an expert panel. J Pain Symptom Manage. 27(6):540-63, 2004
18. Gooch JL et al: Complications of intrathecal baclofen pumps in children. Pediatr Neurosurg. 39(1):1-6, 2003
19. McMillan MR et al: Catheter-associated masses in patients receiving intrathecal analgesic therapy. Anesth Analg. 96(1):186-90, table of contents, 2003

SECTION 3
Congenital and Genetic Disorders

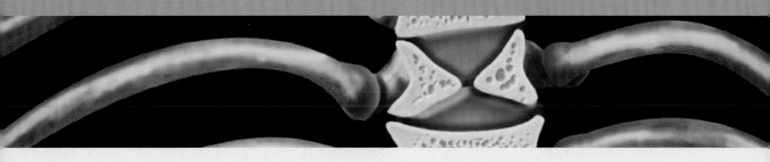

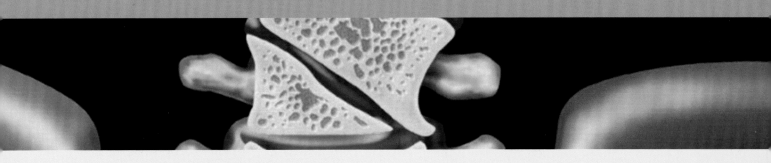

Genetic

KEY FACTS

TERMINOLOGY

- Congenital C2-C3 vertebral segmentation failure

IMAGING

- Rudimentary C2-C3 intervertebral disc space with narrow "waist"
  - C2-C3 disc space smaller than normal disc spaces in remainder of cervical spine
  - ± facet fusion
- Chiari 1 malformation may be present
- Spinal cord compression, syringomyelia unusual

TOP DIFFERENTIAL DIAGNOSES

- Juvenile inflammatory arthritis
- Surgical fusion
- Chronic sequelae of discitis

PATHOLOGY

- Congenital cervical fusion
  - Secondary to failure of normal cervical somite segmentation (3rd → 8th weeks)
- C2-C3 fusion (type II Klippel-Feil spectrum) → autosomal dominant with variable penetrance

CLINICAL ISSUES

- Usually asymptomatic
  - Identified incidentally during spinal imaging for other reasons
- Predisposition for accelerated degenerative changes below fused level

DIAGNOSTIC CHECKLIST

- C2-C3 segmentation failure is usually incidental finding discovered while imaging for other reasons
- Less often it is associated with multiple vertebral segmentation anomalies (Klippel-Feil spectrum)

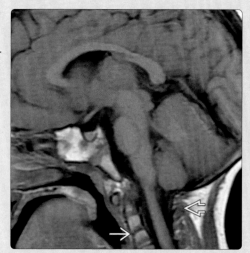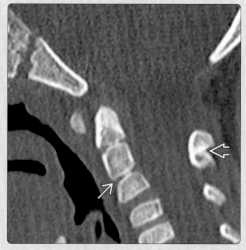

(Left) Sagittal T1WI MR of the craniovertebral junction demonstrates the characteristic rudimentary C2-C3 disc space ➡ with normal vertebral body marrow and intervertebral disc signal. The fused C2 and C3 spinous processes ➡ are relatively inapparent on MR. (Right) Sagittal bone CT of the craniovertebral junction depicts incomplete vertebral segmentation at C2-C3 ➡, with characteristic rudimentary intervertebral disc space (narrow "waist") and fusion of the spinous processes ➡.

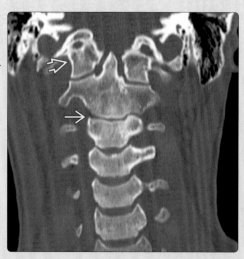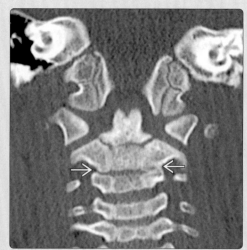

(Left) Coronal bone CT shows congenital fusion of C2-C3 with a small and rudimentary disc margin ➡. Note the normal-sized discs at the lower levels. There is also assimilation of C1 into the occiput ➡. (Right) Coronal bone CT of the craniovertebral junction in a child shows asymmetric, incomplete C2-C3 segmentation ➡ that results in mild upper cervical curvature convex to the right. The atlantooccipital and atlantoaxial articulations are normal.

C1 Assimilation

KEY FACTS

TERMINOLOGY

- Synonyms: Atlantooccipital assimilation, atlantal assimilation, "occipitalization"
- Nonresegmentation of proatlas sclerotome → failure of C1 to correctly segment from occipital bone

IMAGING

- Partial or complete atlas assimilation into occipital bone
  - ± C1 ring hypoplasia → canal stenosis
  - ± posterior C2 arch hypertrophy → canal stenosis
- ± posterior fossa, spinal cord anomalies

TOP DIFFERENTIAL DIAGNOSES

- Juvenile idiopathic arthritis
- Craniovertebral junction surgical fusion

PATHOLOGY

- Inappropriate *PAX1* repression (humans) probably contributory, not sole mechanism

- Associated anomalies include
  - Atlantoaxial instability (up to 60%)
  - C2/3 segmentation failure
  - Klippel-Feil syndrome
  - Basilar invagination
  - Chiari 1 malformation

CLINICAL ISSUES

- May remain asymptomatic throughout life
- Symptomatic patients report neck pain, stiffness, myelopathy
  - Neurological deficits usually begin in 3rd-4th decade, worsen with age

DIAGNOSTIC CHECKLIST

- Clinical symptoms related to presence of atlantoaxial instability, cervical stenosis, and severity of associated anomalies

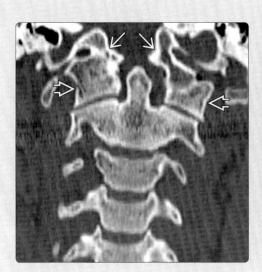

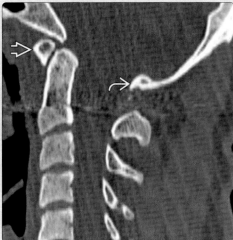

(Left) Coronal bone CT confirms segmentation failure of the occipital condyles ➡ and C1 lateral masses ➡ (zone 2 assimilation). Formation of the proatlas is asymmetric, producing a mild head tilt to the right. (Right) Sagittal bone CT obtained in the midline shows normal alignment of clivus and odontoid tip. The anterior C1 ring ➡ is in normal position, but the posterior C1 ring ➡ is fused to the foramen magnum opisthion (zone 3 assimilation).

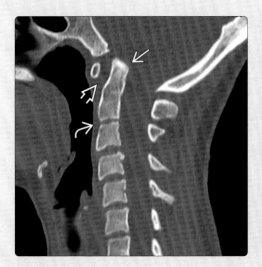

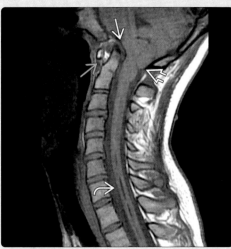

(Left) Sagittal midline bone CT shows no posterior C1 arch due to C1 assimilation to occiput. The odontoid is upwardly placed (basilar invagination) ➡, and the atlantodental interval is widened ➡. There is a rudimentary disc at C2-C3 ➡. (Right) Sagittal T1WI MR shows basilar invagination with mass effect on the cervicomedullary junction ➡. There is a Chiari 1 malformation ➡ and cervical cord syrinx ➡ as well as widening of the atlantodental interval ➡.

KEY FACTS

TERMINOLOGY

- Latin: "Little posterior bridge"
- Synonyms: Arcuate foramen, sagittale foramen, canalis vertebralis, retroarticular canal, retroarticular/retrocondylar vertebral artery ring, upper retroarticular foramen, and atlantal posterior foramen

IMAGING

- Osseous roof along superior C1 arch covers C1 vertebral artery foramen
  - Vertebral artery passes through osseous tunnel
- May be partial or complete
- Unilateral or bilateral

TOP DIFFERENTIAL DIAGNOSES

- Broad C1 posterior arch
  - Mistaking ponticulus posticus for broad posterior C1 arch → vertebral artery injury during C1 lateral mass screw placement

PATHOLOGY

- Postulated to arise from ossification of lateral segment of posterior atlantooccipital ligament or joint capsule
- Morphologically normal bone

CLINICAL ISSUES

- Most common: Asymptomatic
- Other symptoms
  - Vertebrobasilar ischemia or infarction
  - Vertigo
  - Headache
  - Neck pain

DIAGNOSTIC CHECKLIST

- Vertebral arteries predisposed to surgical injury during lateral mass screw placement
- Multiplanar bone CT with 3D reformats best demonstrate ponticulus posticus

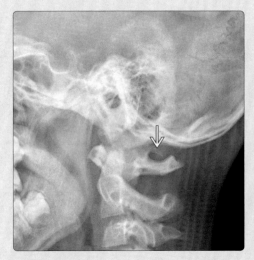
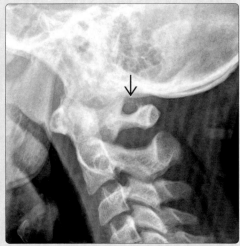

(Left) *Lateral radiograph of the upper cervical spine demonstrates a partial osseous roof* ➡ *over the C1 vertebral artery foramen, characteristic of ponticulus posticus (incomplete variant).* (Right) *Lateral radiograph of the upper cervical spine reveals a complete osseous roof* ➡ *over the C1 vertebral artery foramen, typical of classic ponticulus posticus (complete variant).*

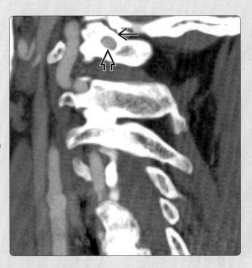
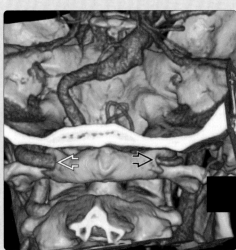

(Left) *Sagittal CTA depicts a complete C1 arch with a robust osseous covering (complete ponticulus posticus)* ➡ *over the vertebral artery* ➡ *along the superior aspect of the C1 arch.* (Right) *Anteroposterior view of a CTA 3D reformat shows a dominant left vertebral artery* ➡ *and smaller (nondominant) right vertebral artery* ➡. *Both are covered by a complete osseous bridge along the superior aspect of the C1 arch.*

Ossiculum Terminale

KEY FACTS

TERMINOLOGY

- Synonym: Ossiculum terminale persistens
- Persistence of unfused odontoid tip ossification center into adulthood

IMAGING

- Separate ossicle with intact cortical margin positioned above normal-sized odontoid process in adolescent or adult
  - May be dystopic or orthotopic
- Soft tissue pannus suggests atlantoaxial instability
- Myelomalacia, brainstem compression in rare cases

TOP DIFFERENTIAL DIAGNOSES

- Os odontoideum
- Type I or II odontoid fracture
- Normal unfused odontoid tip synchondrosis
- Degenerative remodeling of odontoid process

PATHOLOGY

- Terminal ossicle normally appears by age 3, fuses with odontoid body by age 12
- Terminal ossicle located above transverse ligament
  - Atlantoaxial instability less common than with os odontoideum
  - Unstable ossiculum terminale usually dystopic

CLINICAL ISSUES

- Usually asymptomatic
- Uncommonly, neck pain or myelopathy related to CVJ instability

DIAGNOSTIC CHECKLIST

- Consider ossiculum terminale in patients > 12 years with persistent terminal ossicle at odontoid tip
- Evaluate for atlantoaxial instability if dystopic ossicle, excessive soft tissue pannus, or trisomy 21 patient

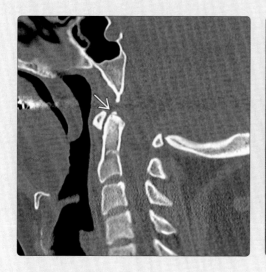
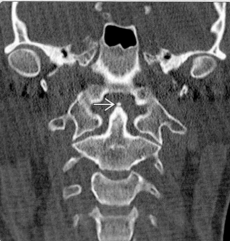

(Left) Sagittal bone CT demonstrates a small ossiculum terminale ➡ located adjacent to the odontoid tip. The ossicle is in orthotopic position, and CVJ alignment is normal. (Right) Coronal bone CT confirms orthotopic placement of a small orthotopic ossiculum terminale ➡. Note that there is minimal flattening of the odontoid tip adjacent to the ossicle, supporting classification as a persistent terminal odontoid ossicle.

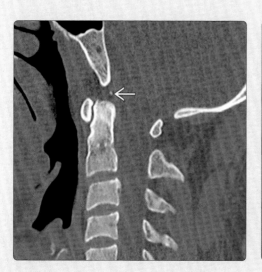
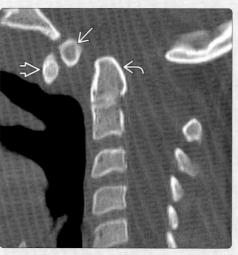

(Left) Sagittal bone CT reveals a small dystopic ossiculum terminale ➡ positioned between the odontoid tip and clivus. The odontoid tip has remodeled. (Right) Sagittal bone CT shows subluxation of the anterior C1 ring ➡ relative to the nearly normal-sized odontoid process ➡. There is a large dystopic ossiculum terminale ➡. Although debatable, the nearly normal size of the odontoid process favors classification as an ossiculum terminale rather than os odontoideum.

KEY FACTS

TERMINOLOGY

- Paramastoid process, paroccipital process, jugular process, parajugular process
- Enlarged bony process of cranial base projecting caudally to transverse process of atlas (C1)
- Uncommon variant (~ 0.5%)

IMAGING

- Many variants, ranging from small hump of bone (paracondylar tuberculum) to free-ended process or jointed with transverse process of C1
  - If not attached to occipital bone, process is isolated rod-like bony element called massa paracondylica
  - Portions may be pneumatized from mastoid air cells

TOP DIFFERENTIAL DIAGNOSES

- Assimilation of C1 into occiput
  - Bony fusion across occipital condyles and lateral masses of C1

- Klippel-Feil syndrome
  - Variable fusions of multiple cervical vertebral bodies and posterior elements
- Proatlas segmentation abnormality
  - Shelf-like bony projection arising from ventral foramen magnum or occipital condyle

CLINICAL ISSUES

- Typically asymptomatic
- May cause limitation of neck movement and restricted range of motion
- Rare cases of chronic headache pain relieved by surgical resection of paracondylar process
- Rare reports of associated vertebral stenosis
- May be associated with other abnormalities
  - Assimilation of anterior arch of C1 with anterior foramen magnum
  - C2-C3 fusion

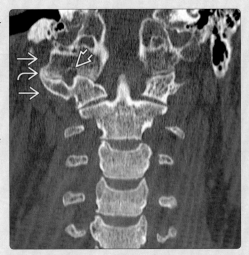
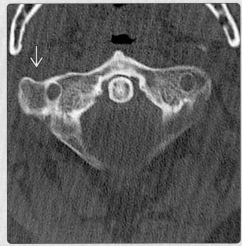

(Left) Coronal NECT shows a large bony mass projecting off the right occipital condyle ➡️ and merging with an enlarged right transverse process of C1 with a neoarticulation ➡️. The vertebral artery has a well-defined canal through the bony mass ➡️. (Right) Axial NECT shows the junction of the right paracondylar process with the markedly enlarged right transverse process of C1 ➡️. The paracondylar process shows considerable variation, ranging from a small tubercle to a large bony process.

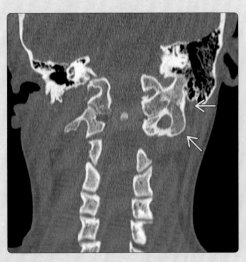
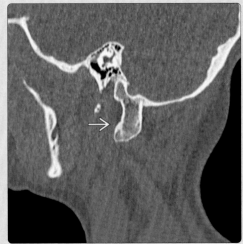

(Left) Coronal NECT shows a large, well-defined, and corticated bony fusion that has occurred on a congenital basis connecting the mastoid region to the transverse process of C1 ➡️. This is usually asymptomatic, although there are rare reports of associated vertebral artery stenosis. (Right) Sagittal NECT shows the paracondylar process as a large, cone-shaped, corticated bony mass extending inferiorly from the occipital condylar region ➡️.

Condylus Tertius

TERMINOLOGY

- **Condylus tertius**
  - Bony process in median line at front rim of foramen magnum, articulated with tip of dens or anterior C1 arch
  - Uncommon variation = 0.5-5.0% incidence
  - Medial residue of hypochordal arch of proatlas (4th occipital sclerotome)
  - Forms joint or pseudojoint with clivus, odontoid process, or anterior arch of C1
- **Basilar process** (processus basilaris)
  - Bony variant in similar region as condylus tertius but with slightly different imaging features and different embryology
  - Also known as mammillary or papillary processes
  - Uncommon = 4% incidence
  - Unilateral or bilateral, paramedian, sphere-shaped bony projections off of anterior inferior margin of foramen magnum
  - Lateral residue of hypochordal arch of proatlas

TOP DIFFERENTIAL DIAGNOSES

- Proatlas segmentation abnormality
  - Larger horizontal bony excrescence with significant cord or cervicomedullary junction compression
- Os odontoideum
  - Rounded, corticated, separate bony density with no normal odontoid process
- Os avis
  - Failure of fusion of odontoid tip to remainder of C2
- Degenerative osteoarthritis of C1-C2
- Condylar fracture with displacement

CLINICAL ISSUES

- Typically incidental finding
- Rarely may be cause of limitation of range of motion of craniovertebral junction due to joint or pseudojoint with C1 arch

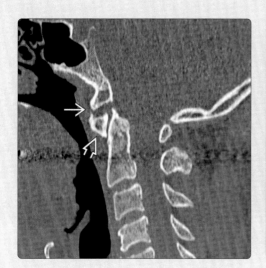
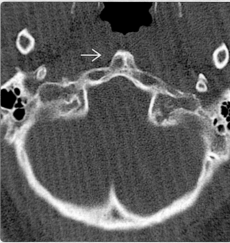

(Left) Sagittal NECT shows a condylus tertius as a well-corticated bony projection arising off of the inferior midline aspect of the clivus ➡, which articulates with the superior aspect of the odontoid process and the superior aspect of the anterior arch of C1 ➡. (Right) Axial NECT shows a midline, well-corticated bony projection from an anterior aspect of the clivus ➡. The midline position differentiates this condylus tertius from the basilar process, which has a position that is off of the midline.

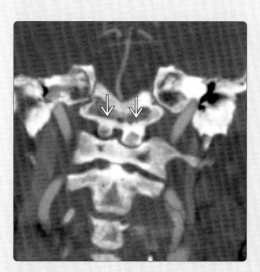
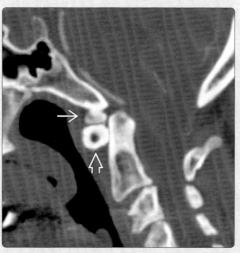

(Left) Coronal CTA demonstrates the typical appearance of basilar processes ➡, which are seen as paired spherical bony projections to either side of the midline of the clivus that extend inferior to articulate with the superior aspect of the C1 arch. (Right) Sagittal CTA shows the orientation of the basilar process ➡, just off of midline, with its articulation with the superior aspect of the C1 arch ➡.

TERMINOLOGY

- Synonym: Incomplete C1 posterior ring
- Definition: Posterior C1 arch is incompletely formed with midline or paramidline osseous defect(s)

IMAGING

- Partial or complete absence of posterior C1 arch
  - Osseous defect may be midline or paramidline
  - Partial agenesis may be unilateral or bilateral

TOP DIFFERENTIAL DIAGNOSES

- Normal immature ossification of cartilaginous posterior C1 arch

PATHOLOGY

- Commonly isolated anomaly; seen infrequently in conjunction with anterior C1 ring, other CVJ anomalies
  - Posterior C1 arch deficiency 10x more common than anterior arch defect
- Currarino classification

- Type A: Median clefts of posterior C1 arch
- Type B: Unilateral posterior arch defect
- Type C: Bilateral posterior arch defects
- Type D: Absent posterior arch + present posterior tubercle
- Type E: Total agenesis of posterior arch including tubercle

CLINICAL ISSUES

- Most commonly asymptomatic, incidental finding
  - Observational management
- Expectant treatment directed toward symptomatic associated anomalies

DIAGNOSTIC CHECKLIST

- Posterior C1 ring rachischisis usually incidental finding
- Generally stable if isolated, requires no specific treatment

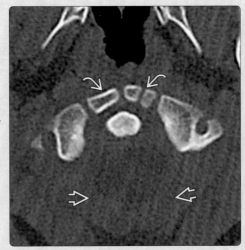

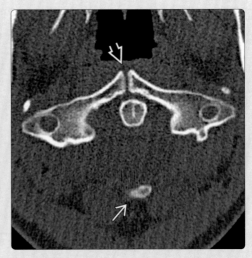

(Left) Axial bone CT demonstrates complete absence of the posterior C1 ring ➡. There is abnormal formation of the anterior C1 ring with 3 dysplastic anterior ring ossification centers ➡ instead of the usual 1 ossification center. (Right) Axial bone CT shows failure of fusion of the right and left C1 hemirings, resulting in a split atlas ➡. There is near complete lack of formation of the posterior ring with only a small ossicle near the posterior midline ➡.

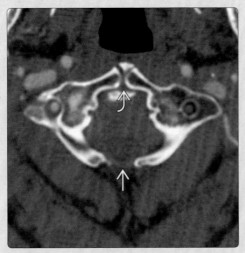

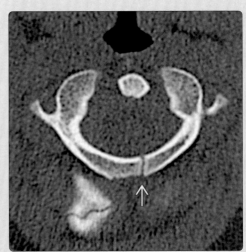

(Left) Axial CECT shows failure of fusion of the right and left C1 hemirings, resulting in a split atlas. The midline posterior C1 arch ➡ gap is larger than the anterior arch cleft ➡. (Right) Axial bone CT depicts an asymmetric cleft ➡ through the posterior C1 ring. The corticated margins confirm that this represents asymmetric development of the posterior C1 ring, resulting in asymmetric location of the posterior synchondrosis, rather than acute fracture.

Split Atlas

KEY FACTS

TERMINOLOGY

- Synonym: Split C1

IMAGING

- Anterior, posterior C1 arch defects → 2 C1 hemirings
  - Defects usually midline but may be paramedian
  - Wider gaps suggest independent lateral migration of C1 hemirings, instability
- ± hypoplastic ring → spinal canal stenosis, cord compression, myelomalacia, syrinx

TOP DIFFERENTIAL DIAGNOSES

- Jefferson C1 fracture
- Isolated anterior C1 arch defect
- Isolated posterior C1 arch defect

PATHOLOGY

- Simultaneous hypoplasia of C1 hypochordal bow, lateral C1 sclerotomes → combined anterior, posterior C1 arch defects

- Ring defects usually contain fibrous connective tissue, not cartilage
- Connective tissue more fragile than cartilage → hemirings may split

CLINICAL ISSUES

- May be asymptomatic in adult
  - Simple bifid atlas (minimal gaps) usually asymptomatic, discovered incidentally
- Prognosis largely depends on severity of ring defects, CVJ stability, C1 ring hypoplasia
- Split atlas with larger arch defects more likely to be unstable → neck pain, torticollis, myelopathy

DIAGNOSTIC CHECKLIST

- Split atlas is rare congenital anomaly
  - Stability depends on anomaly severity, transverse atlantal ligament integrity
- Search for associated skull base, CVJ anomalies

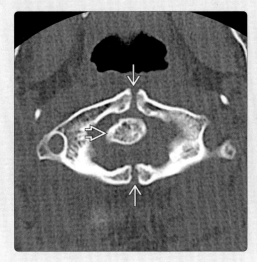

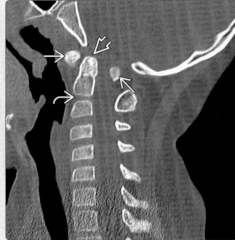

(Left) Axial bone CT demonstrates short AP dimension of the hypoplastic C1 ring as well as a split ring configuration characterized by midline defects ➡ in both anterior and posterior rings. The dens ➡ is thickened and dysplastic. (Right) Sagittal bone CT in patient with a split C1 ring shows mildly dysplastic dens ➡ formation and abnormal hypoplastic C1 ring ➡, resulting in severe spinal canal stenosis. Note associated C2/3 segmentation failure ➡.

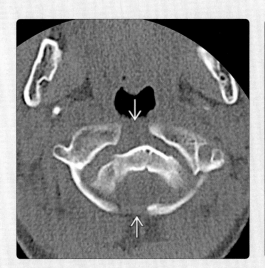

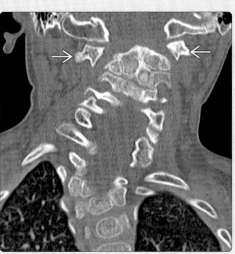

(Left) Axial bone CT reveals large midline osseous defects ➡ in both the anterior and posterior C1 rings. The wide gaps suggest instability. (Right) Coronal bone CT shows congenital scoliosis and extensive cervicothoracic vertebral segmentation failure. The C1 lateral masses ➡ are independently displaced laterally in opposite directions, permitted by the split atlas configuration. This is a very unstable configuration necessitating surgical fusion.

TERMINOLOGY

- Congenital small or absent odontoid process

IMAGING

- Reduced size of odontoid process
  - Odontoid process is small, blunted
  - Hypoplasia > > aplasia
- ± enlargement of anterior C1 ring
- ± spinal cord myelomalacia, syringomyelia

TOP DIFFERENTIAL DIAGNOSES

- Os odontoideum
- Odontoid C2 fracture
- Surgical odontoid resection

PATHOLOGY

- Developmental abnormality
  - More common in patients with skeletal dysplasias, trisomy 21

- Generally nonfamilial, although some reports of autosomal dominant inheritance
- Associated anomalies: Segmentation failure, CVJ dynamic instability
- Status of transverse atlantal ligament (TAL), other stabilizing ligaments variable

CLINICAL ISSUES

- Most commonly asymptomatic
- Symptomatic patients report neck pain, myelopathy
  - Variable depending on severity, presence of dynamic instability, other associated anomalies
- Asymptomatic patients may be amenable to expectant observation

DIAGNOSTIC CHECKLIST

- More common in skeletal dysplasias, trisomy 21
- Severity, status of TAL, & associated anomalies determine CVJ stability

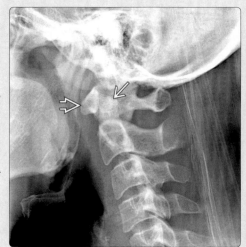

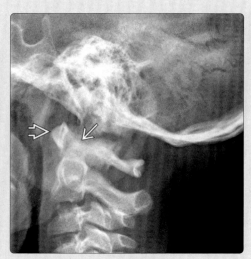

(Left) Lateral cervical radiograph demonstrates a congenital hypoplastic odontoid process ➡ with normal C1/2 alignment. The anterior C1 ring ⇒ is mildly enlarged, likely compensatory hypertrophy. No other cervical spine abnormalities were present. (Right) Lateral cervical radiograph reveals mild congenital hypoplasia of the dens process ➡. There is compensatory enlargement of the anterior C1 ring ⇒. Craniovertebral junction alignment is normal, and no additional anomalies are present.

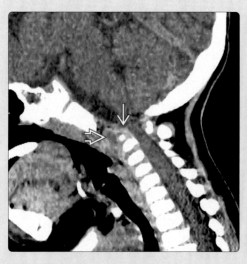

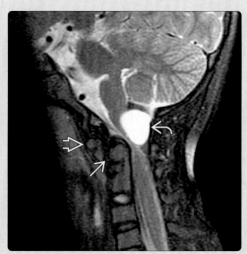

(Left) Sagittal CECT (spondylometaphyseal dysplasia) confirms odontoid process hypoplasia ➡ and hypoplastic C1 ring, resulting in cervical canal stenosis. The anterior atlas arch ⇒ is cartilaginous, representing abnormal delayed ossification. (Right) Sagittal T2WI MR (neurenteric cyst, ➡) demonstrates congenital CVJ osseous anomalies, including a short, dysplastic odontoid process ➡. The anterior C1 ring ⇒ is anteriorly displaced, reflecting atlantoaxial instability.

C1 Dysmorphism/Hypoplastic Arch

KEY FACTS

TERMINOLOGY

- Synonyms: Hypoplastic C1, hypoplastic atlas

IMAGING

- Hypoplastic posterior C1 ring with decreased AP dimension of central canal
  - Posterior C1 ring anteriorly positioned on midline lateral, sagittal imaging
- May be associated with spinal cord compression, myelomalacia, syringomyelia, other CVJ osseous anomalies

TOP DIFFERENTIAL DIAGNOSES

- Posterior arch rachischisis
- Split atlas
- Atlantoaxial instability
- Achondroplasia

PATHOLOGY

- Hypoplasia of complete posterior arch secondary to premature fusion of cartilaginous neurocentral synchondrosis, which leads to spinal canal stenosis at C1 level
  - Less common than atlas arch clefts and defects
- Associated with skull-base osseous anomalies, Klippel-Feil spectrum, skeletal dysplasias

CLINICAL ISSUES

- May be asymptomatic
- Symptomatic patients present with transient quadriparesis, myelopathy, syrinx

DIAGNOSTIC CHECKLIST

- C1 ring hypoplasia relatively uncommon
  - Less common than C1 arch clefts, defects
- Associated with Klippel-Feil spectrum, skeletal dysplasias

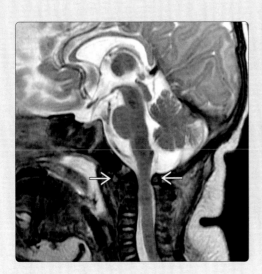
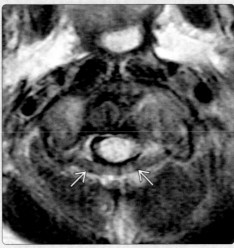

(Left) Sagittal T2WI MR (VACTERL) demonstrates moderately severe central spinal canal stenosis at the C1 level secondary to C1 ring ➡ hypoplasia. There is subtle spinal cord T2 hyperintense signal and volume loss at that level, indicating myelomalacia. (Right) Axial T1WI MR (VACTERL) confirms moderately severe central canal stenosis related to C1 ring hypoplasia ➡. The stenosis is usually most pronounced in the anteroposterior dimension, as demonstrated in this patient.

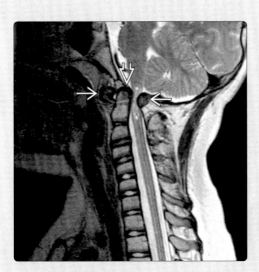
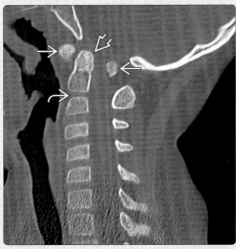

(Left) Sagittal T2WI MR (Klippel-Feil syndrome) shows dysplastic formation of the dens ➡ as well as an abnormal hypoplastic C1 ring ➡, resulting in severe canal narrowing, spinal cord compression, and focal syringomyelia at the C1/2 level. (Right) Sagittal bone CT confirms thickened dysplastic appearance of the dens ➡ and C1 ring ➡, with the hypoplastic posterior C1 ring severely narrowing the central spinal canal. There is also segmentation failure at C2/3 ➡.

Chiari 1

TERMINOLOGY

- Synonyms: Chiari 1 malformation (CM1), Arnold-Chiari 1 malformation

IMAGING

- Pointed cerebellar tonsils extend ≥ 5 mm below foramen magnum ± syringohydromyelia, scoliosis, hydrocephalus

TOP DIFFERENTIAL DIAGNOSES

- Normal low-lying tonsils below foramen magnum
- Acquired tonsillar herniation (acquired Chiari 1)

PATHOLOGY

- Etiology not fully understood
  - Postulated mechanisms include hydrodynamic theory and posterior fossa underdevelopment theory
- May present as isolated finding or in conjunction with syndromic (4th occipital sclerotome) or nonsyndromic skull base and CVJ anomalies

CLINICAL ISSUES

- Up to 50% of CM1 asymptomatic
  - Surgical treatment for asymptomatic patients controversial
- Symptomatic patients
  - Surgical goal is restoration of normal CSF flow at foramen magnum
  - Posterior fossa decompression and resection of posterior C1 arch ± duraplasty, cerebellar tonsil resection
- Clinical CM1 syndrome: Headache, pseudotumor-like episodes, Ménière disease-like syndrome, lower cranial nerve and spinal cord signs

DIAGNOSTIC CHECKLIST

- Tonsillar herniation > 12 mm usually symptomatic
- Probably not clinically significant CM1 unless tonsils > 5 mm &/or pointed

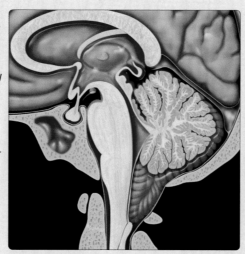

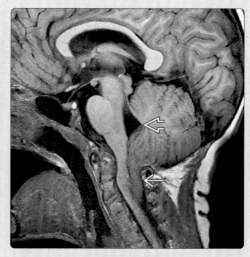

(Left) Sagittal graphic demonstrates pointed peg-like tonsils extending below the foramen magnum, elongating the normally positioned 4th ventricle. (Right) Sagittal T1WI MR shows the normal position and appearance of the 4th ventricle. The fastigium ⇒ is in normal position, helping to distinguish from Chiari 2 malformation. There is inferior displacement of the ectopic cerebellar tonsils ⇒ through the foramen magnum with ventral spinal cord displacement.

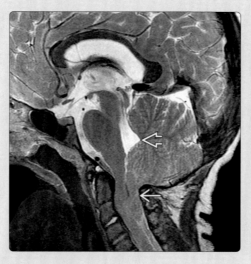

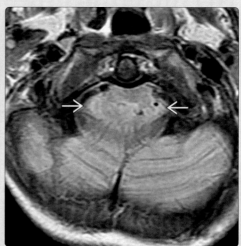

(Left) Sagittal T2WI MR shows the normal position and appearance of the 4th ventricle. The fastigium ⇒ is in normal position, helping to distinguish from the Chiari 2 malformation. Note inferior displacement of the ectopic elongated cerebellar tonsils ⇒ through the foramen magnum that produces mass effect on the upper cervical spinal cord. (Right) Axial T2WI MR shows inferior displacement of the ectopic cerebellar tonsils ⇒ through the foramen magnum with crowding of the foramen magnum.

Complex Chiari

KEY FACTS

TERMINOLOGY

- Complex Chiari malformation (CCM), Chiari 1.5

IMAGING

- Cerebellar tonsillar herniation with low obex, dorsal medullary "bump"
  - "Bump" thought to represent aberrant clava, used as marker for cervicomedullary junction
  - Abnormal tonsillar "pistoning" motion, reduced CSF flow around foramen magnum and cerebellar tonsils
- ± syringohydromyelia, ventral cervicomedullary compression
- ± odontoid retroflexion, small posterior fossa, clival anomalies, platybasia

TOP DIFFERENTIAL DIAGNOSES

- Chiari 1 malformation
- Chiari 2 malformation

PATHOLOGY

- Medullary pyramid decussation anatomic border between spinal cord, medulla oblongata
  - Normal obex level is 10-12 mm above foramen magnum
  - Obex displaced to or below foramen magnum level in CCM patients

CLINICAL ISSUES

- Headaches, myelopathy, bulbar symptoms, lethargy, failure to thrive

DIAGNOSTIC CHECKLIST

- Consider CCM in context of cerebellar tonsillar herniation + low obex, dorsal medullary "bump"
- CCM considered subgroup of Chiari 1 malformation with more severe clinical phenotype

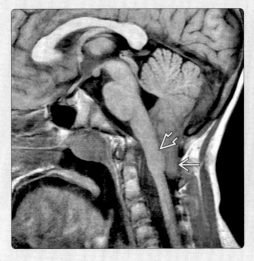

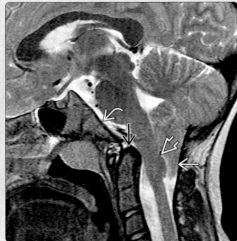

(Left) *Sagittal T1WI MR shows classic features of a complex Chiari malformation, including marked cerebellar tonsil ectopia ➡ and inferior displacement of the obex ➡. The 4th ventricle is in normal position.* (Right) *Sagittal T2WI MR reveals characteristic tonsillar ectopia ➡ and inferior displacement of the cervicomedullary junction, marked by position of the obex ➡ below the foramen magnum. There is also mild retroflexion of the odontoid process ➡ and mild clivus ➡ foreshortening.*

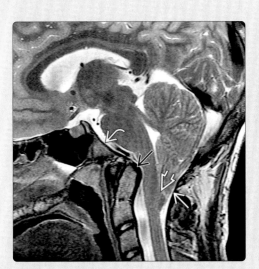

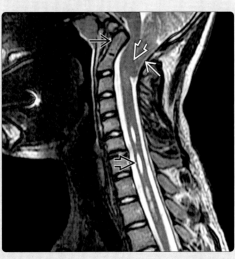

(Left) *Sagittal T2WI MR (different patient) shows a prominent obex ➡ and pointed, ectopic cerebellar tonsils ➡. The odontoid process ➡ is retroflexed, and the clivus ➡ is foreshortened, with a reduced craniocervical angle with platybasia.* (Right) *Sagittal T2WI MR (different patient) reveals striking odontoid ➡ retroflexion. Note also severe cerebellar tonsillar ectopia ➡ extending inferiorly to the C3 level and cervical syringohydromyelia ➡. The prominent, inferiorly displaced obex ➡ confirms a complex Chiari malformation.*

TERMINOLOGY

- Synonyms: Chiari 2 malformation 2, Chiari II
- Complex hindbrain malformation
- Virtually 100% associated with neural tube closure defect, usually lumbar myelomeningocele

IMAGING

- Cerebellum "wraps" around medulla and "towers" through incisura, with "beaked" tectum and heart-shaped midbrain
- Virtually 100% have neural tube closure defect

TOP DIFFERENTIAL DIAGNOSES

- Chiari 1 malformation
- Chiari 3 malformation
- Intracranial CSF hypotension
- Severe, chronic shunted hydrocephalus (congenital)

PATHOLOGY

- Secondary to sequelae of CSF leakage through open spinal dysraphism during gestation (4th fetal week)
- Methylenetetrahydrofolate reductase (*MTHFR*) mutations → abnormal folate metabolism
- Spine- and brain/skull-associated anomalies common

CLINICAL ISSUES

- Chiari 2 malformation most common cause of death in myelomeningocele patients
  - Brainstem compression/hydrocephalus, intrinsic brainstem "wiring" defects

DIAGNOSTIC CHECKLIST

- Towering cerebellum, downward vermian displacement, ± brainstem compression diagnostic for Chiari 2

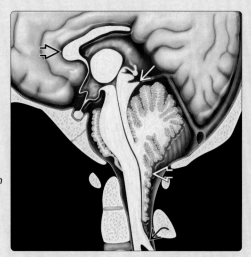

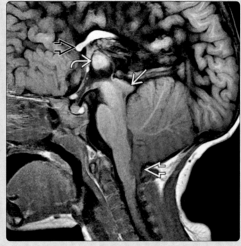

(Left) Sagittal graphic of the posterior fossa and upper cervical spine demonstrates characteristic findings of Chiari 2 malformation, including callosal dysgenesis ⟹, tectal beaking ➡, small posterior fossa, vermian ectopia ⟹, and medullary kinking ⟹. (Right) Sagittal T1WI MR reveals characteristic Chiari 2 malformation findings. Note tectal beaking ➡ and vermian displacement ⟹ through the foramen magnum, large massa intermedia ➡, and dysplastic corpus callosum ⟹.

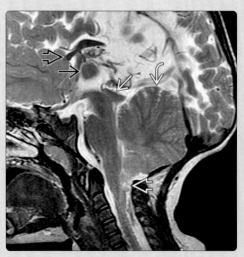

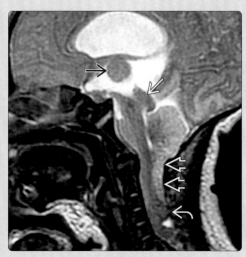

(Left) Sagittal T2WI MR confirms characteristic findings of Chiari 2 malformation including tectal beaking ➡, vermian displacement through the foramen magnum ⟹, "towering cerebellum" ⟹, large massa intermedia ➡, and dysplastic corpus callosum ⟹. (Right) Sagittal T2WI MR depicts marked vermian ectopia ⟹ and a prominent medullary kink ➡ positioned lower than typically seen at the C4 level. Note also the dysplastic "beaked" tectum ➡ and prominent massa intermedia ➡.

KEY FACTS

TERMINOLOGY

- Chiari 3 malformation
- Synonyms: Chiari III, rhombencephalocele

IMAGING

- Low occipital or high cervical meningoencephalocele containing cerebellum ± brainstem, meninges, vessels, CSF
- Midline bone defect within supraoccipital bone, opisthion

TOP DIFFERENTIAL DIAGNOSES

- Isolated occipital encephalocele
- Other occipital encephaloceles
  - Iniencephaly
  - Syndromic occipital encephalocele

PATHOLOGY

- Severity classified by sac contents
- Cephalocele contents: Meninges, cerebellum, brainstem ± cervical cord, occipital poles, vasculature

- Disorganized (neuronal migration anomalies, cortical dysplasias) and gliotic brain tissue
- Lining of sac may show gray matter heterotopias
- Associated abnormalities: Corpus callosum anomalies, gray matter heterotopia, syringohydromyelia, tethered cord

CLINICAL ISSUES

- Microcephaly, severe developmental delay, spasticity, hypotonia, seizures
- Mechanical brainstem traction, respiratory deterioration, lower cranial nerve dysfunction

DIAGNOSTIC CHECKLIST

- Occipitocervical cephalocele containing cerebellum ± brainstem in conjunction with C1-C2 spina bifida = Chiari 3 malformation
- Distinct malformation; not just Chiari 2 malformation with encephalocele

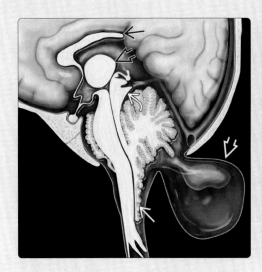

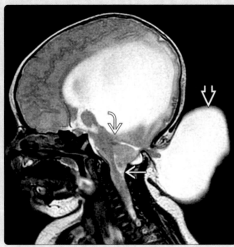

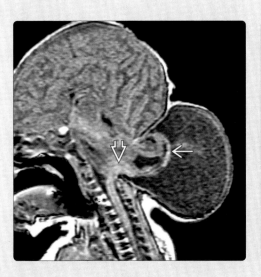

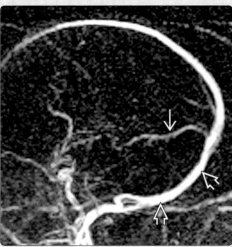

(Left) Sagittal graphic shows typical Chiari 3 features of Chiari 2 plus meningocele. Note callosal hypoplasia ➡, prominent massa intermedia ➡, beaked tectum ➡, and inferiorly displaced cerebellar tissue ➡. There is a supraoccipital bone defect with protruding skin-covered cephalocele ➡ containing gliotic tissue and meninges. (Right) Sagittal T2WI MR shows a large cephalocele ➡ containing gliotic cerebellum and meninges. Tectal beaking ➡ and tonsillar descent ➡ confirmed Chiari 3 malformation.

(Left) Sagittal T1WI MR shows a large meningoencephalocele composed of meninges, CSF, cerebellum ➡, brainstem ➡, and upper cervical spinal cord herniated through a bone defect in the lower occiput and upper cervical spine. (Right) Sagittal MRV demonstrates typical venous abnormalities of Chiari 3. The straight sinus ➡ and vein of Galen are severely hypoplastic. Large occipital sinuses ➡, rather than transverse sinuses, are present.

TERMINOLOGY

- Posterior spinal defect lacking skin covering → neural tissue, CSF, and meninges exposed to air
- Synonyms: Meningomyelocele, open spinal dysraphism, spina bifida aperta, spina bifida cystica

IMAGING

- Lumbosacral (44%) > thoracolumbar (32%) > lumbar (22%) > thoracic (2%)
- Preoperative: Posterior spinal defect lacking skin covering → neural tissue, CSF, and meninges exposed to air
- Postoperative: Dysraphism, low-lying cord/roots, postoperative skin closure changes

TOP DIFFERENTIAL DIAGNOSES

- Dorsal meningocele
- Closed (occult) spinal dysraphism
- Postoperative pseudomeningocele

PATHOLOGY

- Failure of neural tube closure
  - Placode may be segmental or terminal
- Association with maternal folate deficiency or abnormal folate metabolism
- Usually accompanied by multiple neurological and orthopedic complications

CLINICAL ISSUES

- Stable neurological deficits expected following closure
- Subsequent neurological deterioration prompts imaging evaluation for tethered cord, dural ring constriction, cord ischemia, or syringohydromyelia

DIAGNOSTIC CHECKLIST

- Cord retethering is most common spinal cause of delayed deterioration
- Low-lying cord on MR does not always equate to clinical tethering

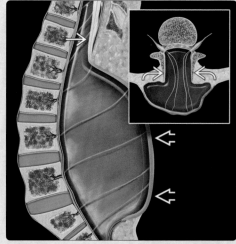

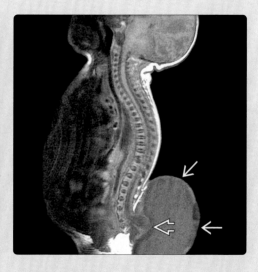

(Left) Sagittal graphic shows ballooning of the meninges through a dysraphic spinal defect with a low-lying cord ⇥ terminating in the red neural placode ⇥. Axial insert shows the origin of spinal roots from ventral placode and protrusion of the meninges and placode through the dysraphic posterior elements ⇥. (Right) Sagittal T1WI MR shows a large unrepaired lumbosacral myelomeningocele sac ⇥ protruding through a posterior dysraphic defect. Neural elements are seen protruding into the sac ⇥.

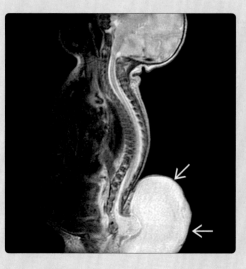

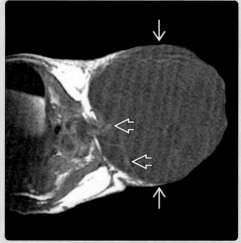

(Left) Sagittal T2WI MR shows typical posterior fossa Chiari 2 malformation changes. The large myelomeningocele lumbosacral sac ⇥ has not been surgically repaired, and it protrudes dorsally through a large posterior dysraphic defect. (Right) Axial T1WI MR of an unrepaired lumbosacral myelomeningocele confirms an exophytic meningeal sac ⇥ and extension of dysplastic neural elements ⇥ through the osseous spinal dysraphic defect into the myelomeningocele.

Lipomyelomeningocele

KEY FACTS

TERMINOLOGY

- Lipomyelomeningocele, lipomyelocele, spinal lipomatous malformation

IMAGING

- Subcutaneous fatty mass contiguous with neural placode/lipoma through posterior dysraphism
  - Size varies from nearly imperceptible to large
- Posterior spinal dysraphism, enlarged canal at placode level
- Tethered, low-lying spinal cord ± meningocele inserts into lipoma through dysraphic defect

TOP DIFFERENTIAL DIAGNOSES

- Terminal lipoma
- Intradural (juxtamedullary) lipoma
- Dorsal meningocele
- Myelocele/myelomeningocele

PATHOLOGY

- Premature disjunction of neural ectoderm from cutaneous ectoderm → induction of mesenchyme to form fat (lipoma)
- Spinal cord always tethered
- Association with vertebral segmentation anomalies, sacral dysgenesis, anorectal and genitourinary abnormalities

CLINICAL ISSUES

- Soft midline or paramedian skin-covered mass above buttocks
- Back/leg pain, scoliosis, lower extremity paraparesis, bladder/bowel dysfunction
- Incidence not impacted by folate supplementation to pregnant women (unlike myelomeningocele)
- Closed dysraphism, so no Chiari II malformation

DIAGNOSTIC CHECKLIST

- Diagnosis of postoperative retethering primarily clinical; use imaging to search for complications

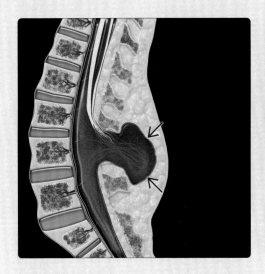

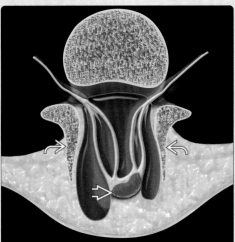

(Left) Sagittal graphic of the lumbosacral spine demonstrates classic lipomyelomeningocele anatomy. The low-lying spinal cord and cauda equina nerve roots protrude through the dysraphic posterior elements into a dorsal meningocele sac ➡ covered by skin and subcutaneous fat. (Right) Axial graphic of the lower lumbar spine shows protrusion of the nerve roots and neural placode ➡ through the dysraphic posterior elements ➡ into a skin-covered sac.

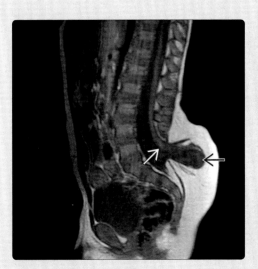

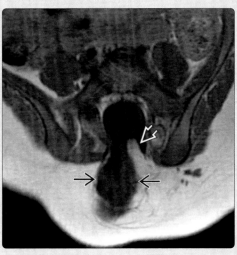

(Left) Sagittal T1WI MR shows the low-lying tethered spinal cord ➡ extending through a dorsal dysraphic defect into the subcutaneous fat to terminate in a skin-covered cyst ➡. (Right) Axial T1WI MR demonstrates protrusion of the lipomyelomeningocele sac ➡ with eccentric lipoma ➡ through the parallel-oriented dysraphic posterior elements into the subcutaneous fat (clinically evident as a skin-covered fatty mass).

Lipoma

TERMINOLOGY

- Intradural (juxtamedullary, subpial) or terminal lipoma

IMAGING

- Lipoma intimately associated with spinal cord (intradural) or distal cord/filum insertion (terminal)
- Lipoma follows fat signal intensity, density, and echogenicity

TOP DIFFERENTIAL DIAGNOSES

- Lipomyelocele/lipomyelomeningocele
- Filum fibrolipoma
- Dermoid cyst

PATHOLOGY

- Follows premature separation (premature disjunction) of cutaneous ectoderm from neuroectoderm during neurulation

- ○ Surrounding mesenchyme enters ependyma-lined central spinal canal, impedes neural tube closure open placode
- Skin closed over malformation (closed neural tube defect)
- Proposed (2009) classification scheme proposes dividing lipomas into 2 groups of lipomatous malformations based on presence or absence of dural defect
  - ○ Lipomas without dural defect
    - Filum lipoma, caudal lipoma without dural defect, intramedullary lipoma
  - ○ Lipomas with dural defect
    - Dorsal lipoma, caudal lipoma with dural defect, transitional lipoma, lipomyelocele, lipomyelomeningocele

CLINICAL ISSUES

- Symptoms referable to lipoma level, presence of spinal cord compression
- Small lipomas may grow dramatically during infancy

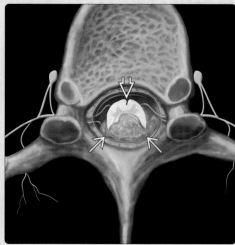

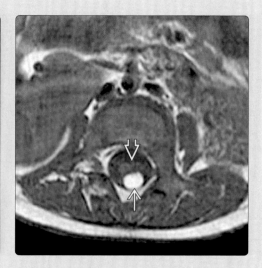

(Left) Axial graphic of the thoracic spine demonstrates incomplete closure of the dorsal spinal cord ➡ around a dorsal juxtamedullary conus lipoma ➡, encompassing the dorsal spinal nerve roots. (Right) Axial T1WI MR reveals the typical hyperintense appearance of a conus juxtamedullary (subpial) lipoma ➡. Note the intradural location and close relationship with the dorsal conus ➡ surface.

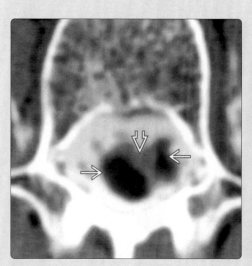

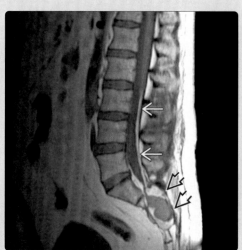

(Left) Axial NECT following intrathecal myelography reveals a typical markedly hypodense dorsal juxtamedullary (subpial) lipoma ➡. The lipoma encircles and distorts the spinal cord conus tip ➡. Note mild scalloping of the posterior vertebral body. (Right) Sagittal T1WI MR demonstrates a low-lying spinal cord with long hyperintense filum lipoma ➡ that inserts into a heterogeneous intraspinal sacral dermoid tumor ➡.

Dorsal Dermal Sinus

TERMINOLOGY

- Synonyms: Dermal sinus tract (DST)
- Midline/paramedian stratified squamous epithelial-lined sinus tract
- Extends inward from skin surface for variable distance

IMAGING

- Sinus tract easily identified superimposed on background of cutaneous fat
- Terminus usually conus medullaris (lumbosacral) or central spinal canal (cervical, thoracic)

TOP DIFFERENTIAL DIAGNOSES

- Low coccygeal midline dimple
- Pilonidal sinus
- (Epi)dermoid tumor without dermal sinus

PATHOLOGY

- Focal incorporation of cutaneous ectoderm into neural ectoderm during disjunction at circumscribed point only → focal segmental adhesion
- Spinal cord ascends relative to spinal canal, stretches adhesion into long, tubular tract

CLINICAL ISSUES

- Infancy → 3rd decade
- Presentation either asymptomatic (incidentally noted skin dimple) or infection, neurological deficits 2° to cord tethering or compression

DIAGNOSTIC CHECKLIST

- Must differentiate DST from simple sacral dimple or pilonidal sinus
- Identify sinus course, termination for surgical planning

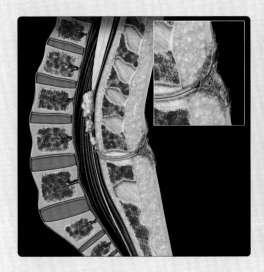

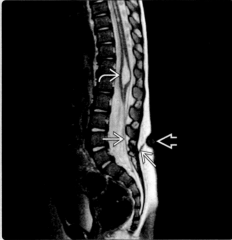

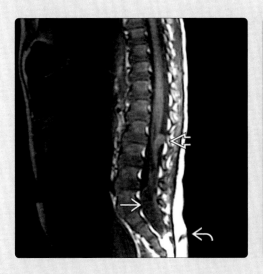

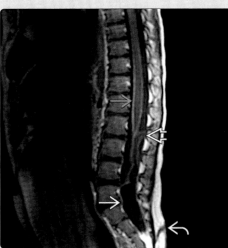

(Left) Sagittal graphic shows a dermal sinus extending from the skin surface into the spinal canal to terminate at conus with epidermoid cysts. A skin dimple with capillary angioma and hairy tuft (cutaneous marker) indicates sinus opening. (Right) Sagittal T2WI MR shows hypointense dermal sinus ➡ extending through L5 posterior elements and coursing intradural to tether the low-lying hydromyelic conus ➡ at L2-L3. A vitamin E capsule has been placed to mark the skin opening of the sinus ➡.

(Left) Sagittal T1WI MR shows low to isointense signal intradural masses (epidermoid cysts) at L2-L3 ➡ and L5-sacrum ➡. There is a dermal sinus tract extending dorsally from the low sacral region ➡. (Right) Sagittal T1WI C+ MR in a patient with a dorsal dermal sinus tract ➡ and clinical meningitis demonstrates diffuse abnormal pial and cauda equina enhancement ➡ Note minimal rim enhancement of the sacral ➡ and lumbar ➡ epidermoid cysts.

Congenital and Genetic Disorders

TERMINOLOGY

- Synonym: Sacral dimple

IMAGING

- Low sacral dimple connecting to coccyx by fibrous tract
  o Usually resides within intergluteal cleft
  o No intradural extension by definition
- Variable size; deeper dimples usually evoke more physician and parental concern

TOP DIFFERENTIAL DIAGNOSES

- Dorsal dermal sinus
- Pilonidal sinus

PATHOLOGY

- Congenital
- Tract usually atretic; may occasionally be patent with fluid in lumen

CLINICAL ISSUES

- Often asymptomatic discovery by parents during diaper change or bathing
  o Dimple becomes less conspicuous as patient grows
  o No specific treatment indicated; reassure parents
- Occasionally present with acute inflammation or purulent discharge

DIAGNOSTIC CHECKLIST

- Important to distinguish from dorsal dermal sinus, which requires surgical excision
  o Low dimple opening within intergluteal cleft usually but not always coccygeal dimple
  o High dimple position, leaking of fluid more likely dorsal dermal sinus
- Look for hypointense tract surrounded by bright fat on MR
- Always mark skin dimple ostium with MR visible marker

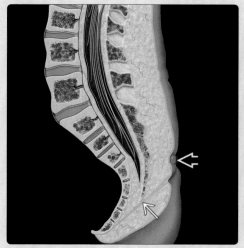
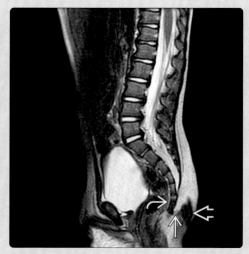

(Left) Sagittal graphic of the lumbosacral spine demonstrates a low sacral dimple (marked by a vitamin E capsule ➦), which is connected to the coccyx tip by a fibrous tract ➡. There is no intradural extension, and the conus/intradural structures are normal. (Right) Sagittal T2WI MR demonstrates a deep low sacral dimple with a vitamin E marker capsule ➥ placed. The conus terminates at normal L1 level. The dimple and tract ➡ connect directly to the coccyx ➦ with no intradural extension.

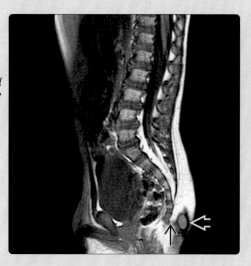
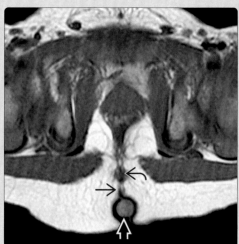

(Left) Sagittal T1WI MR reveals a deep sacral dimple marked for imaging with a vitamin E capsule ➥. The conus terminates at normal L1 level. The dimple shows typical "spot-welded" proximity to the coccyx via a short fibrous tract ➡. (Right) Axial T1WI MR confirms that the sacral dimple, marked with a vitamin E capsule ➥, and tract ➡ connect directly to the coccyx ➦ without intradural extension.

Dermoid Cysts

KEY FACTS

TERMINOLOGY

- Synonyms: Dermoid tumor, "dermoid"
- Benign spinal mass composed of cells embryologically comprising skin and its appendages

IMAGING

- Lumbosacral or cauda equina CSF isointense/isodense mass ± interspersed fat signal intensity/density
  - Lumbosacral (60%), cauda equina (20%)
- Focal osseous erosion, spinal canal widening, flattening of pedicles and laminae at spinal level of mass
- Less likely to show diffusion restriction than epidermoid cyst

TOP DIFFERENTIAL DIAGNOSES

- Arachnoid/meningeal cyst
- Neurenteric cyst
  - Intradural cyst; usually ventral to cord

PATHOLOGY

- Congenital or acquired origin
  - Congenital cysts arise from dermal rests or focal expansion of dermal sinus
- Cyst filled with thick cheesy, buttery, yellowish material (desquamated keratin, lipids)
- Associated anomalies include dermal sinus, vertebral segmentation anomalies, closed dysraphism

CLINICAL ISSUES

- Most commonly asymptomatic or presentation with slowly progressive compressive radiculopathy/myelopathy
- Infectious meningitis in association with dermal sinus
- Acute chemical meningitis 2° to rupture, discharge of inflammatory cholesterol crystals into CSF

DIAGNOSTIC CHECKLIST

- Often difficult to diagnose on CT and MR; presence of fat helpful to suggest diagnosis

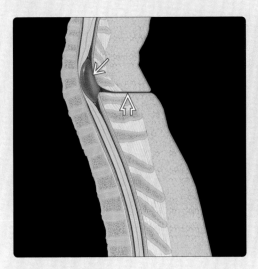

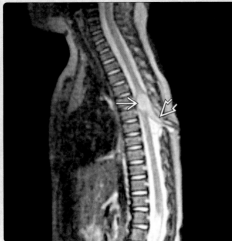

(Left) Sagittal graphic of the cervicothoracic spine demonstrates a large dorsal dermoid cyst ➡ in association with a dermal sinus tract ➡. There is marked spinal cord compression. (Right) Sagittal T2WI MR (myelopathy) demonstrates a hyperintense dermoid tumor with an intramedullary component ➡ contiguous with an extramedullary component following a dermal sinus tract ➡ to the skin surface.

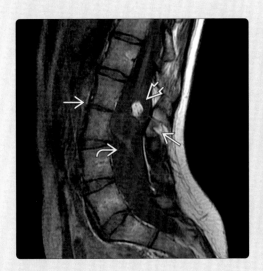

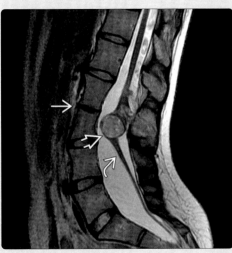

(Left) Sagittal T1WI shows a variant case of intradural teratoma ➡, with mixed fat and soft tissue mass at the level of multiple vertebral body segmentation abnormalities ➡. The conus is also low lying ➡. (Right) Sagittal T2WI shows an unusual case of mature intradural teratoma ➡ seen as a lobulated mass involving the distal thoracic cord. The teratoma occurs at the site of vertebral body segmentation abnormalities ➡. The tethered cord is apparent ➡.

Congenital and Genetic Disorders

TERMINOLOGY

- Benign nonneoplastic spinal mass embryologically derived from epidermal (skin) elements

IMAGING

- Lumbosacral or cauda equina CSF isointense/isodense mass
  - 40% intramedullary, 60% extramedullary
  - Acquired epidermoid cysts nearly always occur at cauda equina

TOP DIFFERENTIAL DIAGNOSES

- Arachnoid cyst
- Neurenteric cyst

PATHOLOGY

- Congenital (60%)
  - Arise from epidermal rests or dermal sinus
- Acquired (40%)

- Iatrogenic, follows implantation of viable epidermal elements after lumbar puncture or surgery (myelomeningocele closure)
- Striking white, pearly sheen capsule containing creamy, waxy, pearly material

CLINICAL ISSUES

- Asymptomatic or slowly progressive compressive radiculopathy/myelopathy
- Symptoms slowly progress if untreated
- Complete surgical resection offers best opportunity for good neurologic outcome

DIAGNOSTIC CHECKLIST

- Epidermoid cysts may be congenital or acquired
- Acquired epidermoid cysts nearly always occur in cauda equina

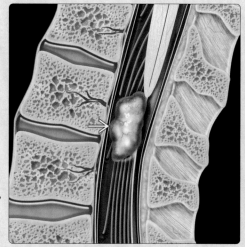
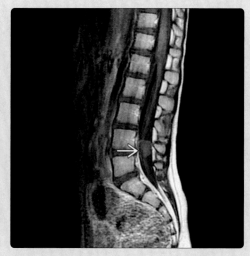

(Left) Sagittal graphic of the thoracolumbar spine shows a pearly white epidermoid cyst ➡ located within the cauda equina at the conus, a typical location for post lumbar puncture acquired epidermoid cyst. (Right) Sagittal T1WI MR demonstrates a hypointense intradural extramedullary mass ➡ within the cauda equina in a patient who previously had a lumbar puncture as an infant. Signal intensity is slightly hyperintense to CSF, and there is no hyperintense lipid content to indicate that dermoid cyst is conspicuous.

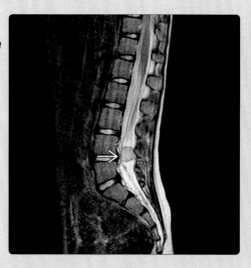
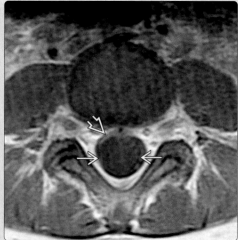

(Left) Sagittal T2WI MR in a patient who had a lumbar puncture as an infant reveals a well-circumscribed intradural extramedullary mass ➡ within the cauda equina. The cauda equina is distorted and anteriorly displaced by the cyst. Signal intensity is slightly hypointense to CSF. (Right) Axial T1WI MR demonstrates that the epidermoid cyst ➡ nearly fills the spinal canal and displaces the cauda equina ➡ anteriorly. This location is typical of a post lumbar puncture acquired epidermoid cyst.

Tethered Spinal Cord

KEY FACTS

TERMINOLOGY

- Synonyms: Tethered cord syndrome, tight filum terminale syndrome

IMAGING

- Stretched, thinned cord with low-lying conus, thickened filum
- ± fibrolipoma/terminal lipoma, dysraphism, vertebral segmentation anomalies
- ↓ spinal cord motion

TOP DIFFERENTIAL DIAGNOSES

- Normal variant low-lying conus
- Open or closed spinal dysraphism
- Postsurgical low-lying conus

PATHOLOGY

- Tethering stretches nerve fibers, arterioles, and venules → impairs oxidative metabolism of conus and nerve roots → syringohydromyelia, myelomalacia

- Tethered filum histologically abnormal, even if conus terminates at normal level

CLINICAL ISSUES

- Low back and leg pain, gait and sensory abnormalities, urinary bladder dysfunction
- Symptomatic presentation most common during rapid somatic growth (adolescent growth spurt, school age 4-8 years), or 2° to kyphosis (elderly)
- Gait spasticity, weakness, muscular atrophy

DIAGNOSTIC CHECKLIST

- Tethered cord syndrome is clinical diagnosis
  - Imaging role is detection of low-lying conus/thick filum, associated anatomic abnormalities for surgical decision making
  - Clinical tethering may be present despite normal conus level

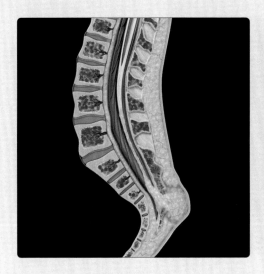

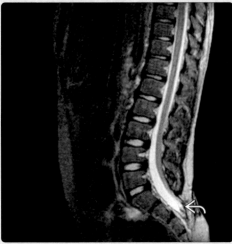

(Left) Sagittal graphic of the lumbosacral spine depicts composite tethered cord syndrome (TCS) findings of low-lying, hydromyelic tethered cord with thickened filum and fibrolipoma inserting into a terminal lipoma that is contiguous with subcutaneous fat through dorsal dysraphism. (Right) Sagittal T2WI MR (clinical TCS) demonstrates an elongated low-lying spinal cord extending to the S2 level, where it ends in a small terminal lipoma ⮞. Focal sacral posterior dysraphism is also present.

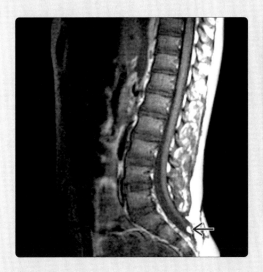

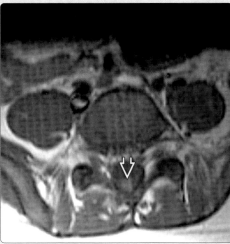

(Left) Sagittal T1WI MR (clinical TCS symptoms) confirms an elongated low-lying spinal cord extending to the S2 level and ending in a small terminal lipoma ⮞. Focal sacral posterior dysraphism is also conspicuous. In general, lipomas are considerably more conspicuous on T1WI than T2WI. (Right) Axial T1WI MR at the lumbosacral transition reveals that the abnormal elongated, low-lying spinal cord ⮞ continues to the sacral level.

KEY FACTS

TERMINOLOGY

- Segmental spinal dysgenesis (SSD), caudal regression syndrome (CRS)

IMAGING

- Localized segmental lumbar or thoracolumbar vertebral, spinal cord dysgenesis or agenesis
- Congenital acute angle kyphosis or kyphoscoliosis
- Distal spinal osseous architecture usually normal (unless concurrent CRS)

TOP DIFFERENTIAL DIAGNOSES

- Multiple vertebral segmentation disorders
- Congenital vertebral displacement
- Medial spinal aplasia
- Caudal regression syndrome

PATHOLOGY

- Characteristic segmental vertebral, cord anomalies

- ○ Normal upper spinal cord
- ○ Hypoplastic or absent spinal cord, vertebral dysgenesis at gibbus apex
- ○ Bulky, thickened, low-lying cord segment within spinal canal below dysgenesis

CLINICAL ISSUES

- Thoracic or lumbar kyphosis
- Palpable bone spur at gibbus apex
- Spastic paraparesis or paraplegia
- Rarely present with normal or mildly impaired lower extremity function → subsequent deterioration

DIAGNOSTIC CHECKLIST

- SSD and CRS probably represent 2 different phenotypes along single malformation spectrum
- Morphologic severity correlates with residual spinal cord function, severity of clinical deficit

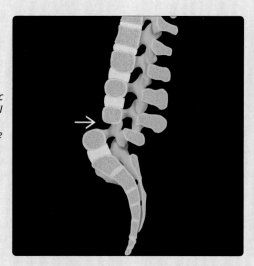

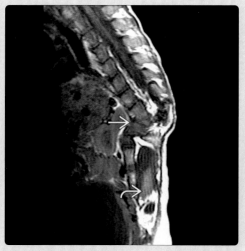

(Left) Sagittal graphic demonstrates lower lumbar segmental spinal dysgenesis (SSD) with posterior subluxation of the upper lumbar spine relative to the segment below the dysgenetic level ➡. (Right) Sagittal T1WI MR (lumbosacral SSD) depicts complete disconnection of the spinal canal at the dysgenetic level ➡. Note that the distal spinal cord ➡ is separate from, not connected to, the proximal thoracic spinal cord.

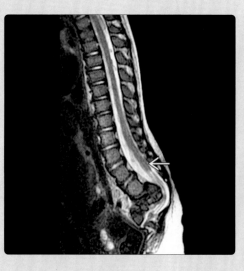

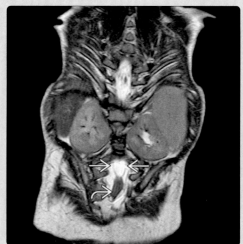

(Left) Sagittal T2WI MR (mixed SSD, caudal regression) shows relatively low dysgenetic level. The dysmorphic vertebral bodies produce acute angle focal kyphosis. Note the truncated, squared-off conus ➡. (Right) Coronal T2WI MR (severe lumbosacral SSD) shows separation of the distal spinal cord component ➡ from the thoracic spinal cord (not shown) above the dysgenetic level. The cephalad-directed nerve roots ➡ are commonly observed in lumbosacral SSD.

KEY FACTS

TERMINOLOGY

- Caudal regression syndrome, sacral agenesis, lumbosacral hypogenesis

IMAGING

- Constellation of caudal developmental growth abnormalities and associated soft tissue anomalies
- Spectrum ranges in severity from absent coccyx to lumbosacral agenesis
- 2 main types
  - Group 1: Distal spinal cord hypoplasia, severe sacral osseous anomalies
  - Group 2: Tapered, low-lying, distal cord elongation with tethering, less severe sacral anomalies

TOP DIFFERENTIAL DIAGNOSES

- Tethered spinal cord
- Closed spinal dysraphism
- Occult intrasacral meningocele

PATHOLOGY

- Group 1: More severe caudal dysgenesis with high-lying, club-shaped cord terminus (decreased number of anterior horn cells)
- Group 2: Less severe dysgenesis with low-lying, tapered, distal cord tethered by tight filum, lipoma, lipomyelomeningocele, or terminal myelocystocele

CLINICAL ISSUES

- Clinical spectrum ranges from neurologically normal → severely impaired
- Symptomatic patient presentation spans mild foot disorders → complete lower extremity paralysis and distal leg atrophy

DIAGNOSTIC CHECKLIST

- Look for caudal spine anomalies in patients with genitourinary or anorectal anomalies

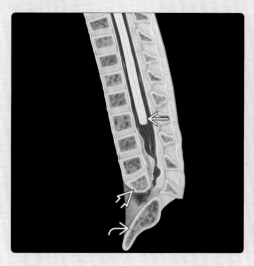

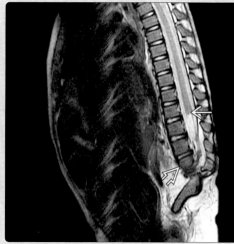

(Left) Sagittal graphic of the lumbosacral spine in severe group 1 caudal regression syndrome (CRS) shows high truncation of the sacrum ⇒ and medial position of the iliac wing ⇗. The conus ➡ terminates abnormally high in a blunt wedge shape. (Right) Sagittal T2WI MR (group 1 CRS) reveals severe truncation of the sacrum ⇒ and abnormally high termination of the spinal cord at the T12-L1 vertebral body level with a typical blunted, wedge-shaped conus ➡.

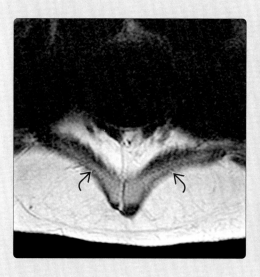

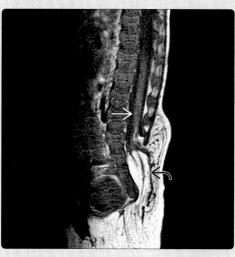

(Left) Axial T2WI MR of the pelvis (severe group 1 CRS) demonstrates bilateral abnormal hypoplastic iliac wings ⇗ closely approximated in the midline secondary to complete absence of a normal sacrum at this level. (Right) Sagittal T1WI MR (group 2 CRS) depicts mild sacral dysgenesis and posterior spinal dysraphism, with the abnormal low-lying tapered spinal cord terminating ➡ into a large terminal lipoma ⇗.

Congenital and Genetic Disorders

TERMINOLOGY

- Synonym: Terminal syringocele

IMAGING

- Complex spinal malformation → closed spinal dysraphism, large skin-covered back mass
- Hydromyelic, low-lying tethered spinal cord traverses dorsal meningocele and terminates in dilated terminal cyst (myelocystocele)
- Multiplanar MR best demonstrates constellation of abnormalities

TOP DIFFERENTIAL DIAGNOSES

- Anterior sacral meningocele
- Simple dorsal meningocele
- Sacrococcygeal teratoma
- Myelomeningocele

PATHOLOGY

- Results from deranged secondary neurulation of caudal cell mass
- Associated malformations: Cloacal exstrophy, imperforate anus, omphalocele, pelvic deformities, equinovarus, ambiguous hypoplastic genitalia, and renal abnormalities

CLINICAL ISSUES

- Presents at birth with large skin-covered back mass
- Usually neurologically intact at birth; may later develop lower extremity sensorimotor deficits

DIAGNOSTIC CHECKLIST

- Early diagnosis and surgery → best chance for normal neurological outcome
- Nonneurological prognosis largely linked to severity of associated anomalies

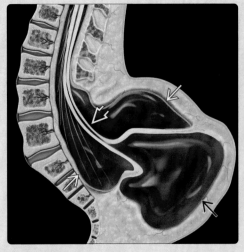

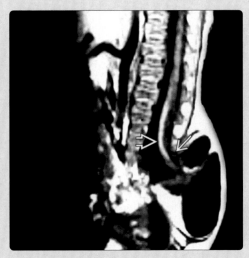

(Left) Sagittal graphic displays a low-lying, hydromyelic spinal cord ➡ piercing an expanded subarachnoid space (meningocele ➡), terminating in a myelocystocele ➡. (Right) Sagittal T1WI MR depicts a low-lying hydromyelic spinal cord ➡ traversing a meningocele and expanding into a large terminal cyst. Note the dorsal fibrous band ➡. Note that the back mass is caused by both the meningocele and myelocystocele in this case.

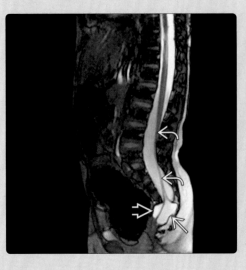

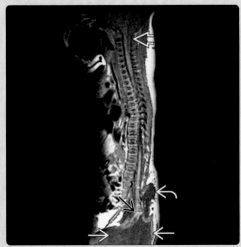

(Left) The spinal cord is low lying with caudal extension of the attenuated cord ➡ through a sacral cyst ➡ (meningocele). The terminal spinal cord flares into a 2nd terminal cyst ➡ within the meningocele, completing the terminal myelocystocele malformation. (Right) Sagittal T1WI MR shows a central canal of low-lying cord traversing the meningocele ➡ before expanding into a large terminal cyst ➡. Note "trumpet" splaying ➡ of the terminal spinal cord. There is an associated Chiari 1 malformation ➡.

Anterior Sacral Meningocele

KEY FACTS

TERMINOLOGY

- Anterior sacral meningocele (ASM)
- Sacral meninges herniate anteriorly into pelvis through focal erosion or hypogenesis of sacral ± coccygeal vertebral segments

IMAGING

- Presacral cyst, contiguous with thecal sac through anterior osseous defect
- Deficient sacrum ± curved (scimitar) shape

TOP DIFFERENTIAL DIAGNOSES

- Sacrococcygeal teratoma
- Sacral chordoma
- Neurenteric cyst
- Cystic neuroblastoma
- Ovarian cyst

PATHOLOGY

- Currarino triad: Anorectal anomalies, caudal regression syndrome, epidermoid/dermoid tumor or other tethering lesion
- Associated with conditions where dural ectasia is prominent (neurofibromatosis type 1, Marfan syndrome, homocystinuria)

CLINICAL ISSUES

- Constipation, urinary frequency, incontinence, dysmenorrhea, dyspareunia, low back/pelvic pain

DIAGNOSTIC CHECKLIST

- Continuity of cyst with thecal sac necessary to ensure ASM diagnosis
- Soft tissue mass or calcification implies tumor
- Imaging recommendations
  - Ultrasound for NICU infant screening; MR to confirm presacral cyst location and characterize contents

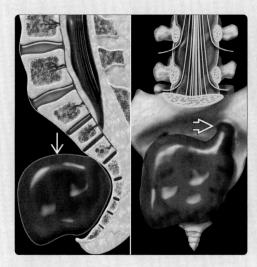
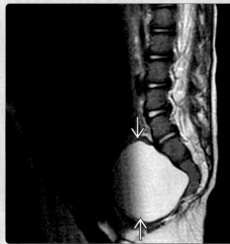

(Left) Sagittal graphic (L) depicts the characteristic anterior sacrum "scimitar" remodeling by a large anterior meningocele cyst ➡. Coronal graphic (R) shows an anterior sacral meningocele cyst origin through an enlarged neural foramen ➡. (Right) Midline sagittal T2WI MR demonstrates the classic relationship of characteristic "scimitar sacrum" configuration with the adjacent anterior sacral meningocele ➡.

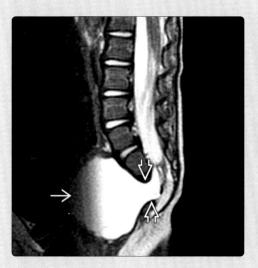
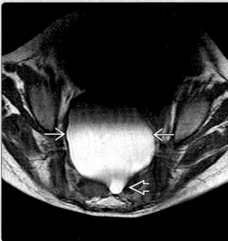

(Left) Sagittal T2WI MR obtained off-midline parasagittal shows a large anterior presacral cyst ➡ contiguous with the meninges, extending from the thecal sac into the pelvis through an enlarged neural foramen ➡. (Right) Axial T2WI MR confirms unilateral left sacral neural foraminal enlargement ➡ permitting ventral herniation of the meninges into the pelvis to form a classic anterior sacral meningocele ➡.

TERMINOLOGY

- Spinal extradural arachnoid cyst (AC) located within sacrum, caudal to thecal sac termination
  - Sacral meningeal cyst, type IB meningeal cyst
- Synonym: Occult intrasacral meningocele

IMAGING

- Smooth enlargement of sacral spinal canal
  - Expands but does not transgress sacrum margins
  - No expansion or remodeling of neural foramina
- Posterior sacral vertebral scalloping characteristic
- No cyst wall enhancement

TOP DIFFERENTIAL DIAGNOSES

- Tarlov cyst
- Dorsal spinal meningocele
- Dural dysplasia

PATHOLOGY

- Diverticulum of sacral subarachnoid space expands into sacral cyst with secondary remodeling of sacral canal
- Extradural arachnoid cyst; no meningeal herniation (not true meningocele)
- Cyst is connected to thecal sac by thin pedicle
- No neuronal elements within cyst

CLINICAL ISSUES

- Usually asymptomatic; incidental discovery on MR
  - Asymptomatic patients need no specific treatment
  - Indications for operation include ↑ cyst size on serial exams, onset of symptoms referable to cyst

DIAGNOSTIC CHECKLIST

- AC centered in midline; cyst center over neural foramen implies Tarlov cyst

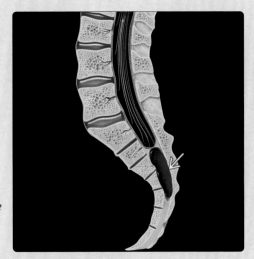
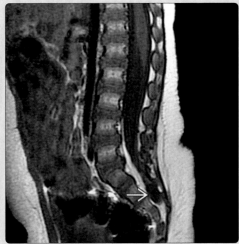

(Left) Sagittal graphic of the lumbosacral spine demonstrates an extradural cyst ➔ within the sacral spinal canal below the thecal sac termination at S2. Note osseous remodeling of the sacral spinal canal margins. (Right) Sagittal T1WI MR demonstrates a small fluid signal extradural cyst in the sacral spinal canal ➔. The location is typical for occult sacral meningocele, now designated an extradural arachnoid cyst. No solid tissue or fat is detected within the cyst.

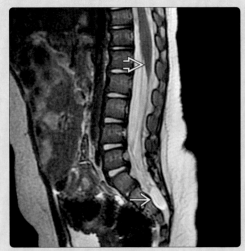
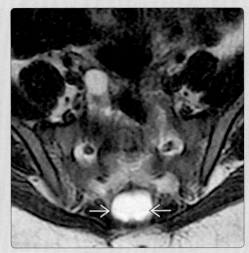

(Left) Sagittal T2WI MR demonstrates a small extradural sacral arachnoid cyst ➔ at the caudal end of the spinal canal. The conus termination ➔ is normal. Note that the cyst signal intensity is slightly brighter than CSF within the dural sac, reflecting increased proteinaceous content. (Right) Axial T2WI MR through the sacrum at the level of the arachnoid cyst ➔ confirms mild expansile remodeling of the caudal osseous spinal canal by the cyst at the sacral level.

Sacrococcygeal Teratoma

KEY FACTS

TERMINOLOGY
- Congenital sacral tumor containing elements of all 3 germ layers

IMAGING
- Large, heterogeneous sacral mass in infant
  - Variably contains calcifications, mixed solid and cystic components, fat-debris levels, bone, hair, teeth, or cartilage
- Usually large at diagnosis

TOP DIFFERENTIAL DIAGNOSES
- Anterior sacral meningocele
- Chordoma
- Dermoid tumor
- Exophytic rhabdomyosarcoma

PATHOLOGY
- Tumor originates from totipotential cell rests at caudal spine/notochord (Hensen node)

- Altman/AAP classification: 4 surgical subtypes
  - Type I: Primarily external (47%) → best prognosis
  - Type II: Dumbbell shape, equal external/internal portions (34%)
  - Type III: Primarily internal within abdomen/pelvis (9%)
  - Type IV: Entirely internal (10%) → worst prognosis

CLINICAL ISSUES
- Back/pelvic mass in newborn
  - Exophytic masses (AAP types I, II) easily diagnosed, but internal (types III, IV) occult → delayed diagnosis
- In utero presentation
  - Polyhydramnios, high-output cardiac failure with hydrops, hepatomegaly, placentomegaly

DIAGNOSTIC CHECKLIST
- Heterogeneous sacral tumor ± calcification, cysts, hemorrhage in infant strongly suggest diagnosis
- AAP type influences prognosis and treatment approach

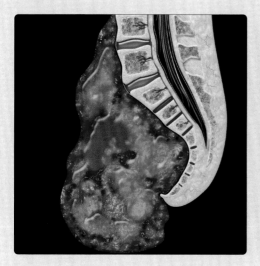

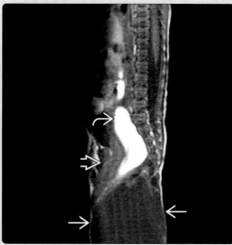

(Left) Sagittal graphic (AAP II) depicts a typical large, heterogeneous, partially cystic sacrococcygeal teratoma located anterior to the sacrum with both internal and external components. (Right) Sagittal T1WI MR (AAP type I) demonstrates a predominately cystic sacrococcygeal teratoma ➡ contiguous with the coccyx tip. The tumor is nearly entirely external. The urinary bladder ➡ is not displaced. Hyperintense rectal contents ➡ probably reflect meconium.

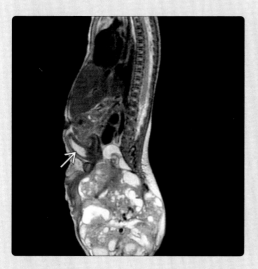

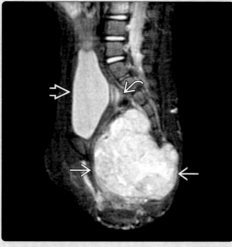

(Left) Sagittal T2WI MR (AAP type II) reveals a large, heterogeneous exophytic sacral mass with relatively equal internal and external distribution. The mass displaces the urinary bladder ➡ anteriorly and superiorly. (Right) Sagittal STIR MR (AAP type III, older female infant) reveals a heterogeneous, predominantly internal pelvic mass ➡. The tumor anteriorly and upwardly displaces the rectum ➡ and urinary bladder ➡. No sacral osseous destruction is apparent.

TERMINOLOGY

- Synonyms: Klippel-Feil syndrome (KFS)
- Congenital spinal malformation characterized by segmentation failure of ≥ 2 cervical vertebrae ± thoracic, lumbar segmentation failure

IMAGING

- Single- or multiple-level congenital cervical segmentation and fusion anomalies
- C2-3 (50%) > C5-6 (33%) > CVJ, upper thoracic spine
- Vertebral bodies usually smaller than normal
- Vertebral body narrowing ("wasp waist") at fused rudimentary disc space ± fusion of posterior elements

TOP DIFFERENTIAL DIAGNOSES

- Juvenile idiopathic arthritis
- Surgical fusion
- Chronic sequelae of discitis
- Ankylosing spondylitis

PATHOLOGY

- Sporadic; familial genetic component with variable expression identified in many patients
- Type 1 (9%): Massive fusion of cervical, upper thoracic spine → severe neurological impairment, other abnormalities
- Type 2 (84%): Fusion of ≥ 1 cervical vertebral interspace
- Type 3 (7%): Fusions involve cervical and lower thoracic/lumbar vertebra

CLINICAL ISSUES

- Classic triad (33-50%): Short neck, low posterior hairline, and limited cervical motion
- Wide variation in clinical and anatomical expression

DIAGNOSTIC CHECKLIST

- Much KFS morbidity and nearly all mortality related to visceral system dysfunction
- Look for instability, progressive degenerative changes, cord/brainstem compression

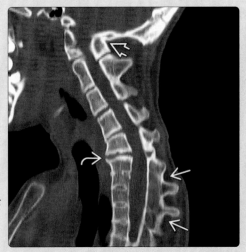 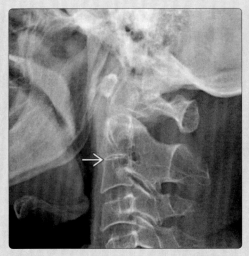

(Left) *Sagittal CT of the cervicothoracic spine shows lack of segmentation of the cervical and thoracic spinal column. Note C1 spinous process fused to the occiput* ⇒ *and fusion of bodies and posterior elements* ➡ *of C6-T4. Note accelerated disc degeneration at C5-C6* ⇗. (Right) *Lateral radiograph [Klippel-Feil spectrum type 2 (KFS 2)] demonstrates typical C2/3 congenital segmentation failure ("fusion") with characteristic rudimentary disc space* ➡ *and fusion of the facets and spinous processes.*

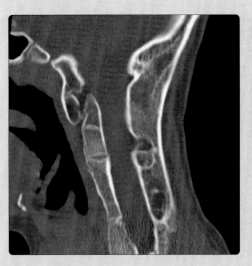 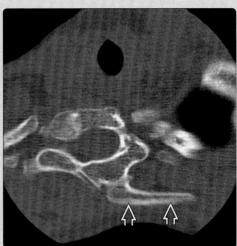

(Left) *Sagittal bone CT (KFS 1) reveals extensive fusion of all cervical vertebrae and posterior elements, with the characteristic hypoplastic appearance of the vertebrae and intervertebral disc spaces. In this patient, there is additionally incorporation of C1 into the skull base ("occipitalization of the atlas"). (Right) Axial bone CT (KFS 1, severe segmentation anomalies) demonstrates the vertebral articulation of a unilateral left omovertebral bone* ➡.

KEY FACTS

TERMINOLOGY

- Vertebral dysplasia, segmentation and fusion anomaly, "disorganized spine"
- Partial or complete failure of vertebral formation

IMAGING

- Sharply angulated, single curve, or focal (kypho)scoliosis
- Hemivertebra, butterfly vertebra generally smaller than normal vertebra

TOP DIFFERENTIAL DIAGNOSES

- Vertebral fracture, history critical
- Inherited spinal dysplasias

PATHOLOGY

- Deranged *PAX1* gene expression in developing vertebral column
- Many syndromes manifest vertebral dysplasia

- Associated anomalies include dysraphism, split notochord syndromes, visceral anomalies (61% of congenital scoliosis patients)

CLINICAL ISSUES

- Many asymptomatic or detected during scoliosis evaluation
- Syndromal patients usually detected in infancy
  - Abnormal spine curvature ± neural deficits, limb or visceral abnormalities
  - Respiratory failure (impeded chest movement 2° to fused ribs, kyphoscoliosis)

DIAGNOSTIC CHECKLIST

- Important to look for and characterize associated visceral anomalies
- Type of deformity determines propensity for scoliosis progression

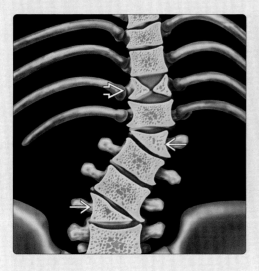

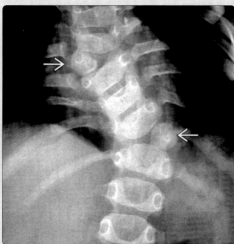

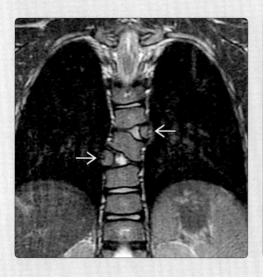

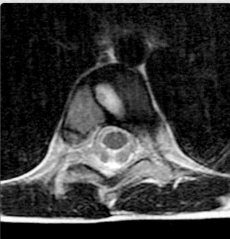

(Left) Coronal graphic of the thoracolumbar spine demonstrates several different types of vertebral formation failure, with segmented "balanced" L1 and L4 hemivertebrae ➡ and a T11 butterfly vertebra ⮑. (Right) Anteroposterior radiograph shows segmented right T7 and left T11 hemivertebrae ➡ producing focal scoliotic curves. Because they mostly cancel each other's curve, this configuration is considered "balanced" for the purposes of prognostic and treatment planning.

(Left) Coronal T2WI MR demonstrates left T6 and right T8 hemivertebrae ➡. There is only minimal resultant leftward curvature because the 2 hemivertebrae "balance" each other, and this curvature would not be expected to be rapidly progressive. (Right) Axial T2WI MR depicts the abnormal intervertebral disc space appearance in the presence of a hemivertebra. Diagnosing hemivertebra is most straightforward in the coronal plane and often difficult in the sagittal and axial planes.

TERMINOLOGY

- Synonyms: Segmentation anomaly, segmentation and fusion anomaly, "block vertebra"

IMAGING

- Sharply angulated focal scoliotic curvature with abnormal "fused" vertebra
  o Ranges single level → extensive multilevel involvement
  o Lumbar > cervical > thoracic
- May have scoliosis, kyphosis, cord compression
- Search for related fused pedicles, ribs, posterior elements

TOP DIFFERENTIAL DIAGNOSES

- Juvenile chronic arthritis
- Surgical vertebral fusion
- Chronic sequelae of discitis
- Ankylosing spondylitis

PATHOLOGY

- Deranged *PAX1* gene expression → abnormal notochord signaling in developing vertebral column
- Many syndromes associated with segmentation fusion anomalies
- Associations include other neuraxis anomalies, renal, gastrointestinal, congenital cardiac defects

CLINICAL ISSUES

- Usually asymptomatic or present with kyphoscoliosis
- Less commonly neural deficit, limb or visceral anomalies, respiratory failure
- Scoliosis frequently progressive

DIAGNOSTIC CHECKLIST

- Clinical manifestations variable, determined by type of segmentation anomaly and syndromal association
- Block vertebra usually larger than single normal vertebral body

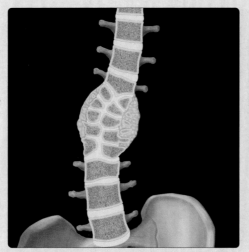
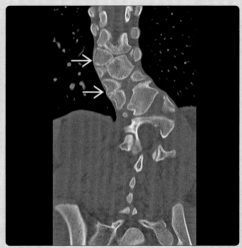

(Left) Coronal graphic of the thoracolumbar spine demonstrates multilevel failure of vertebral segmentation producing congenital scoliosis. Space between the dysplastic vertebra is filled with cartilage and aberrant disc material. *(Right) Coronal bone CT (congenital scoliosis) shows multiple examples of vertebral segmentation failure with several right-sided hemivertebra ➡ that have failed to successfully segment, producing a jumble of malformed vertebra and multiple curve scoliosis.*

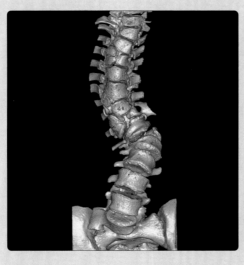
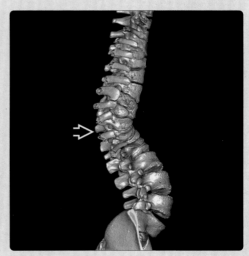

(Left) Coronal 3D bone CT reformat shows multiple curve scoliosis with convex right thoracic and convex left thoracolumbar kyphoscoliosis resulting from multiple levels of vertebral segmentation failure. 3D CT is best for fully characterizing contribution of the various anomalous vertebra to scoliosis and kyphosis for treatment planning. (Right) Sagittal 3D CT reformat demonstrates focal kyphosis at the thoracolumbar junction ➡ related to multilevel vertebral segmentation failure.

Diastematomyelia

KEY FACTS

TERMINOLOGY

- Synonyms: Split cord malformation (SCM), "diastem"

IMAGING

- Sagittal division of spinal cord into 2 hemicords, each with 1 central canal, dorsal horn, and ventral horn
  - Hemicords usually reunite above and below cleft
  - ± fibrous or osseous spur
- Frequently associated vertebral segmentation anomalies
- Imaging evaluation
  - Consider ultrasound to screen infants with skin dimple or cutaneous marker
  - MR most definitive for characterization
  - Supplement with bone CT ± myelography to optimally define spur anatomy for surgical planning

TOP DIFFERENTIAL DIAGNOSES

- Duplicated spinal cord (diplomyelia)

PATHOLOGY

- "Split notochord syndrome" is spectrum of diastematomyelia, dorsal enteric fistula/sinus, and dorsal enteric cysts/diverticula
- Spinal cord split into symmetric or asymmetric hemicords
- Either 1 (type II) or 2 (type I) dural tubes

CLINICAL ISSUES

- May be clinically indistinguishable from other causes of tethered spinal cord in absence of cutaneous stigmata
  - Cutaneous stigmata indicate diastematomyelia level (> 50%); "fawn's tail" hair patch most common

DIAGNOSTIC CHECKLIST

- Search for diastematomyelia in patients with cutaneous stigmata, intersegmental fusion of posterior elements, clinical tethered cord
- Presence of spur = type I SCM; more severe symptoms and anomalies, worse prognosis

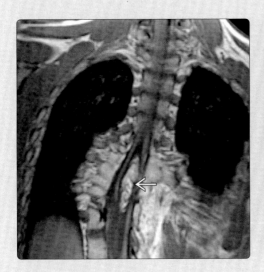

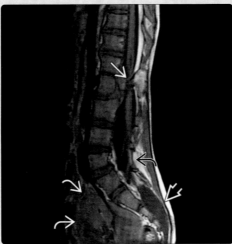

(Left) Coronal T1WI MR [type I split cord malformation (SCM)] shows multiple vertebral segmentation anomalies, with large midline osseous spur ➡ that splits the thoracic spinal cord into 2 hemicords. Note associated multiple posterior element and rib fusions. (Right) Sagittal T1WI MR (type I SCM) shows a large osseous spur ➡ extending from the L2 vertebral body to the dysplastic posterior elements. The spinal cord is low lying and tethered by a lipoma ➡ and extradural arachnoid cyst ➡. Note solitary pelvic kidney ➡ anterior to the sacrum.

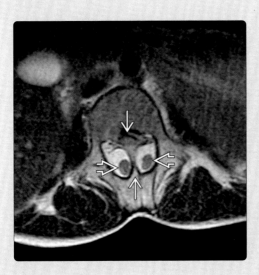

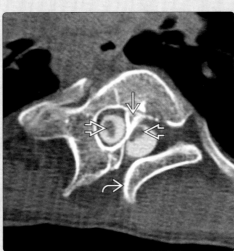

(Left) Axial T2WI MR confirms characteristic "splitting" of the abnormal spinal cord into 2 symmetric hemicords ➡. The prominent osseous spur ➡ classifies this patient as a type I SCM. (Right) Axial bone CT following myelography (type I SCM) shows dural tube division by an osseous septum ➡. Two hemicords ➡ are produced. The left spinal lamina ➡ is dysraphic.

Congenital and Genetic Disorders

TERMINOLOGY

- Synonyms: Spinal enterogenous cyst, spinal enteric cyst, spinal dorsal enteric cyst

IMAGING

- Intraspinal cyst ± vertebral abnormalities (persistent canal of Kovalevsky, vertebral anomalies)
- Thoracic (42%) > cervical (32%) > > lumbar spine, intracranial/basilar cisterns (rare)

TOP DIFFERENTIAL DIAGNOSES

- Arachnoid cyst
- (Epi)dermoid cyst
- Anterior thoracic meningocele

PATHOLOGY

- Subgroup of split notochord syndrome spectrum
  - Sporadic or syndromic (Klippel-Feil, VACTERL, OEIS syndromes)

- Association with vertebral anomalies, diastematomyelia, lipoma, dermal sinus tract, and tethered spinal cord

CLINICAL ISSUES

- Most common symptoms: Back/radicular pain, paraparesis/paresthesias, gait disturbance, meningitis
  - Children usually present with cutaneous stigmata, spinal dysraphism symptoms
  - Adults present primarily with pain, myelopathy
- Some asymptomatic, but most show progressive neurological deterioration
- Primary treatment goal is complete surgical excision
  - Drainage, partial resection if complete excision not possible

DIAGNOSTIC CHECKLIST

- Imaging appearance reflects cyst composition
- Look for associated mediastinal or abdominal cysts, connecting fistulae, or vertebral anomalies

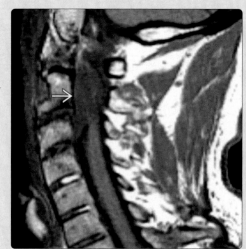
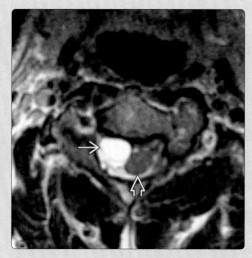

(Left) Sagittal T1WI MR demonstrates a large ventral extradural cystic mass ➡ (neurenteric cyst) producing spinal cord compression. CVJ segmentation anomalies are better demonstrated on other slices (not shown). (Courtesy M. Brandt-Zawadzki, MD.) (Right) Axial T2WI MR confirms a ventral, extradural neurenteric cyst ➡ that displaces the spinal cord and dura to the left, resulting in mild spinal cord compression ⇧. (Courtesy M. Brandt-Zawadzki, MD.)

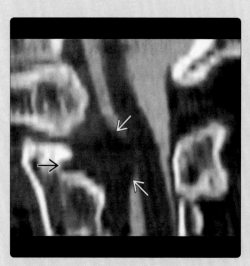
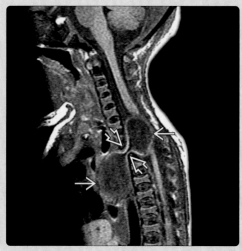

(Left) Sagittal bone CT (Klippel-Feil syndrome) after myelography shows a sagittal vertebral cleft ➡ in conjunction with a ventral extradural neurenteric cyst ➡. The cyst produces mild spinal cord displacement. (Right) Sagittal T1WI MR demonstrates a large, dumbbell-shaped neurenteric cyst ➡ extending from the mediastinum into the central canal through a patent canal of Kovalevsky ➡, producing marked spinal cord compression. (Courtesy S. Blaser, MD.)

Os Odontoideum

TERMINOLOGY

- Corticated oval or round ossicle (os) at odontoid process tip

IMAGING

- Well-defined round or oval ossicle at dens tip with smooth, uniform cortex
- ± hypertrophy of anterior C1 (atlas) arch
- ± spinal cord contusion, myelomalacia (if craniocervical instability)

TOP DIFFERENTIAL DIAGNOSES

- Ossiculum terminale
- Odontoid C2 fracture (type II)

PATHOLOGY

- 2 types based on os position
  - Orthotopic: Os in anatomic position
  - Dystopic: Os in any position other than orthotopic (considered less stable)

- Incompetence of transverse atlantal ligament → C1/2 instability

CLINICAL ISSUES

- Commonly asymptomatic
  - Os incidentally detected on imaging obtained for other reasons (e.g., trauma)
  - Nonoperative management recommended for most patients incidentally diagnosed with os odontoideum
- Symptomatic patients
  - Local mechanical neck pain, torticollis, headache, or other neurological symptoms
  - Surgical stabilization for spinal instability, neurologic decline, or intractable pain
- Prognosis variable; depends in large part on CVJ ligamentous stability

DIAGNOSTIC CHECKLIST

- Evaluate dynamic CVJ stability when os odontoideum is identified

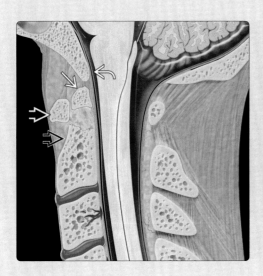

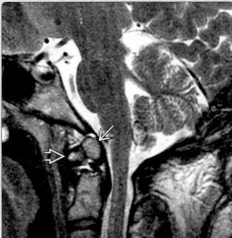

(Left) Sagittal graphic of the cervical spine demonstrates an orthotopic os odontoideum ➡. There is mild separation of the os away from the odontoid process ➡ toward the clivus ➡. Note the maintenance of normal os distance to the mildly enlarged anterior C1 ring ➡. (Right) Sagittal T2WI MR of the craniovertebral junction depicts an orthotopic os odontoideum ➡ with close os approximation to the anterior C1 arch ➡. The cervical spinal cord is normal.

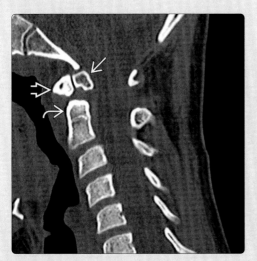

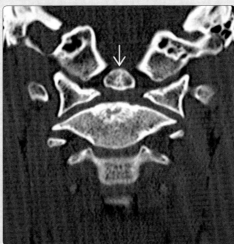

(Left) Sagittal bone CT reveals enlargement of the C1 anterior ring ➡ in conjunction with mildly dystopic os odontoideum ➡ that is discontiguous with the dysplastic, rounded odontoid process ➡. Note maintenance of os alignment with C1 and the clivus. (Right) Coronal bone CT confirms discontinuity of the rounded os odontoideum ➡ with the C2 vertebral body. The os is mildly displaced to the left. Alignment of the occipital condyles and C1 lateral masses is normal.

KEY FACTS

TERMINOLOGY

- Lateral thoracic meningocele, lateral lumbar meningocele

IMAGING

- CSF-filled dural/arachnoidal sac protrudes laterally through neural foramen
- Pedicular erosion, foraminal enlargement, dural dysplasia
- Bilateral meningoceles: Consider neurofibromatosis type 1 (NF1), Marfan syndrome

TOP DIFFERENTIAL DIAGNOSES

- Nerve sheath tumor
- Radicular (meningeal) cyst
- Foregut duplication cyst

PATHOLOGY

- Etiology secondary to primary meningeal dysplasia
  o Strong association with NF1 (85%)
  o Less common with Ehlers-Danlos, Marfan syndromes

- o Occasionally isolated finding
- Scalloping of pedicles, laminae, and vertebral bodies adjacent to meningocele
- Enlarged central spinal canal, neural foramina

CLINICAL ISSUES

- Asymptomatic (most common) or nonspecific motor or sensory symptoms referable to cord/nerve root compression
- Most remain asymptomatic unless very large or scoliosis causes symptoms
  o Most static in size; occasionally grow slowly
  o Very large meningoceles may → respiratory embarrassment (meningocele fills hemithorax)

DIAGNOSTIC CHECKLIST

- Lateral meningocele prompts search for history/stigmata of NF1 or connective tissue disorder

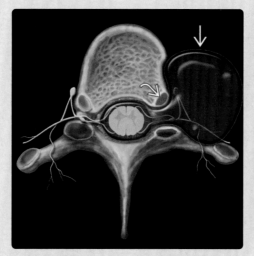

(Left) Axial graphic depicts a large left lateral thoracic meningocele ➡ producing pedicular erosion ⮥, transverse process remodeling, and widening of the neural foramen.

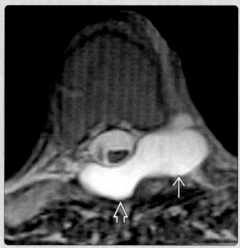

(Right) Axial T2WI MR (Marfan syndrome) demonstrates a large left lateral thoracic meningocele ➡ extending through an enlarged, remodeled neural foramen. The contiguous intraspinal extradural component of the meningocele ➡ displaces the thecal sac anteriorly.

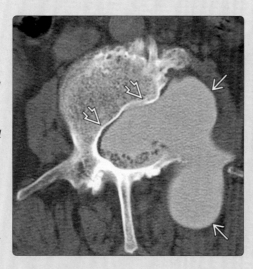

(Left) Axial NECT following myelography (neurofibromatosis type 1) reveals a large left lateral lumbar meningocele ➡ and extensive vertebral scalloping from dural dysplasia ➡, resulting in marked left pedicular erosion and enlargement of the ipsilateral neural foramen.

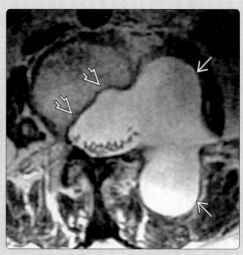

(Right) Axial T2WI MR (neurofibromatosis type 1) shows a large left lateral lumbar meningocele ➡ in conjunction with extensive dural dysplasia, vertebral remodeling ➡, and marked left pedicular erosion.

TERMINOLOGY

Synonyms

- Lateral thoracic meningocele, lateral lumbar meningocele

IMAGING

General Features

- Location
  - Thoracic > lumbar spine
  - R > L; 10% bilateral
    - Bilateral meningoceles usually associated with neurofibromatosis type 1 (NF1) but may be seen in Marfan syndrome
- Size
  - Typical size 2-3 cm; range from tiny to huge
- Morphology
  - CSF signal/density "cyst" adjacent to spine
    - Contiguous with neural foramen
    - ± sharply angled scoliosis at meningocele level

CT Findings

- CECT
  - CSF density mass extends through enlarged neural foramen
  - No enhancement; useful to distinguish from nerve sheath tumor, nerve inflammation (CIDP)
- CTA
  - ± aortic aneurysm, dissection in context of systemic connective tissue disorder
- Bone CT
  - Wide neural foramen; ± pedicular thinning, posterior vertebral scalloping (usually)
  - Reformatted images may show focal scoliosis (coronal plane) and dural ectasia (sagittal plane)

MR Findings

- T1WI
  - CSF signal intensity (hypointense) mass in contiguity with thecal sac; pedicular thinning, neural foraminal widening ± posterior vertebral scalloping
- T2WI
  - CSF signal intensity (hyperintense) mass in contiguity with thecal sac; rarely see neural elements within meningocele
- T1WI C+
  - No enhancement; distinguishes from nerve sheath tumor or inflammation (CIDP)

Ultrasonographic Findings

- Grayscale ultrasound
  - Posterior mediastinal or lumbar hypoechoic paraspinal cystic mass contiguous with expanded spinal canal
    - Displaces and compresses adjacent spinal cord
  - Ultrasound is primary diagnostic tool in utero, screening newborn infants
- Pulsed Doppler
  - No vascular flow pattern
- Color Doppler
  - Avascular hypoechoic mass

Imaging Recommendations

- Best imaging tool
  - MR
- Protocol advice
  - Consider sonography for newborn screening; follow-up with MR to clarify positive ultrasound study; MR for diagnosis, preoperative planning; bone CT to evaluate pedicles, vertebral bodies (particularly if surgery is contemplated)

DIFFERENTIAL DIAGNOSIS

Nerve Sheath Tumor

- Less hyperintense than CSF on T2WI, higher signal intensity than CSF on T1WI

Radicular (Meningeal) Cyst

- CSF signal intensity/density cyst within neural foramen
  - Cyst separate from dural sac, unlike meningocele

Foregut Duplication Cyst

- Bronchogenic most common; may contain gastrointestinal mucosa
- Proximity to spinal canal ± vertebral anomalies = neurenteric cyst

PATHOLOGY

General Features

- Etiology
  - Meningocele 2° to primary meningeal dysplasia
    - Meningeal weakness permits dural sac to focally stretch in response to repetitive CSF pulsation → enlarged neural foramina
    - Secondary osseous remodeling permits further herniation
  - Posterior vertebral scalloping with dural dysplasia → same etiology
- Associated abnormalities
  - Occasionally isolated finding
  - ± coexistent lumbar and thoracic lateral meningoceles
  - ± findings specific to hereditary disorder
    - NF1: Dural ectasia, nerve sheath tumors, CNS neoplasms, pheochromocytomas, interstitial pulmonary fibrosis, skin, and subcutaneous neurofibromas
    - Marfan syndrome: Dural ectasia, vascular dissection/aneurysm, lens dislocation, joint laxity
- Dural sac diverticulum, pedicular erosion, neural foraminal widening, and posterior vertebral scalloping

Gross Pathologic & Surgical Features

- Scalloping of pedicles, laminae, and vertebral bodies adjacent to meningocele
- Enlarged central spinal canal, neural foramina
- Cord position variable; usually displaced away from meningocele
- Scoliosis convex toward meningocele

Congenital and Genetic Disorders

TERMINOLOGY

- Synonyms: von Recklinghausen disease, peripheral neurofibromatosis
- Mesodermal dysplasia with neurofibromas (NFs), spinal deformity, neoplastic and nonneoplastic brain lesions, and cutaneous stigmata

IMAGING

- Kyphoscoliosis ± multiple nerve root tumors, plexiform NF, dural ectasia/lateral meningocele
- Tumors range from tiny to very large

TOP DIFFERENTIAL DIAGNOSES

- Neurofibromatosis type 2 (NF2, central neurofibromatosis)
- Chronic inflammatory demyelinating polyneuropathy
- Congenital hypertrophic polyradiculoneuropathies

PATHOLOGY

- Autosomal dominant

- Characteristic lesion is plexiform NF, although 3 types of spinal NF seen in NF1
  - Localized NF (90% of all NF)
  - Diffuse NF
  - Plexiform NF (pathognomonic for NF1)

CLINICAL ISSUES

- Pigmentation anomalies (café au lait, axillary freckling, Lisch nodules)
- Focal or acute angle kyphoscoliosis ± myelopathy
- Palpable spinal or cutaneous masses

DIAGNOSTIC CHECKLIST

- Multiple nerve sheath tumors, ≥ 1 NF, bizarre kyphoscoliosis with deformed vertebra → consider NF1
- Absence of visible stigmata does not exclude NF1
- Characteristic plexiform NF imaging appearance best displayed using fat-saturated T2WI or STIR MR

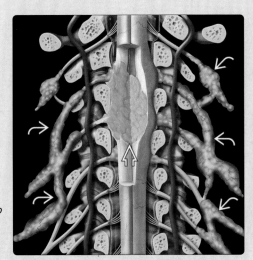
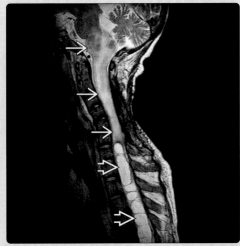

(Left) Coronal graphic of the cervical spine demonstrates multiple manifestations of neurofibromatosis type 1 (NF1), including a large intramedullary spinal cord tumor ⇒ and bilateral brachial plexus plexiform neurofibromas ⇉. (Right) Sagittal T2WI MR demonstrates a large expansile intramedullary primary spinal cord neoplasm ⇒ expanding into the brainstem. A large neoplastic syrinx ⇒ is present. Note also cervical lordosis reversal, probably secondary to laminectomy for cord biopsy.

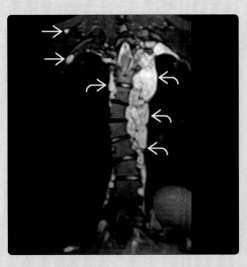
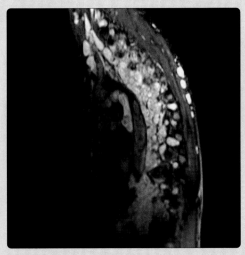

(Left) Coronal STIR MR reveals extensive plexiform neurofibromas ⇒ involving the bilateral paraspinal sympathetic chains, as well as involvement of multiple intercostal nerves ⇉. (Right) Sagittal STIR MR obtained off-midline demonstrates innumerable T2 hyperintense plexiform neurofibromas involving the spinal nerves, sympathetic chains, bilateral brachial plexus, as well as multiple cutaneous nerves.

TERMINOLOGY

Abbreviations

- Neurofibromatosis type 1 (NF1), nerve root neurofibroma (NF), plexiform neurofibroma (PNF), malignant peripheral nerve sheath tumor (MPNST)

Synonyms

- von Recklinghausen disease, peripheral neurofibromatosis

Definitions

- Autosomal dominant mesodermal dysplasia characterized by PNFs and nerve root NFs, spinal deformity, neoplastic and nonneoplastic brain lesions, and cutaneous stigmata

IMAGING

General Features

- Best diagnostic clue
  - Kyphoscoliosis ± multiple nerve root tumors, PNF, dural ectasia/lateral meningocele
- Location
  - Entire craniospinal axis
- Size
  - Tumors range from tiny to very large
- Morphology
  - Kyphosis/kyphoscoliosis often severe and bizarre
  - Neurogenic tumors localized to nerve roots as well as within plexiform nerve masses, cutaneous lesions

Radiographic Findings

- Radiography
  - Kyphosis/scoliosis, scalloped vertebra, hypoplastic pedicles and posterior elements, "ribbon" ribs

CT Findings

- NECT
  - Hypodense fusiform or focal nerve root enlargement ± heterogeneous spinal cord expansion (glial tumor)
  - Dural ectasia ± CSF density lateral meningocele(s)
- CECT
  - Variable mild/moderate tumor enhancement
- Bone CT
  - Vertebral findings similar to radiography; canal, foraminal widening 2° to dural ectasia ± spinal cord tumor

MR Findings

- T1WI
  - Nerve root NF: Intramedullary glial cord tumors hypo- to isointense to normal spinal cord, nerve roots, muscle
- T2WI
  - Nerve root NF: Cord tumors hyperintense to normal spinal cord, nerve roots
    - Target sign (hyperintense rim, low/intermediate signal intensity center) suggests neurogenic tumor; PNF > NF > MPNST
- STIR
  - Nerve root NF: Cord tumors hyperintense to normal nerve root, cord, muscle
- T1WI C+
  - Variable mild to moderate NF, cord tumor enhancement

Nuclear Medicine Findings

- PET
  - FDG standard uptake value MPNST > benign tumors

Imaging Recommendations

- Best imaging tool
  - MR
- Protocol advice
  - Radiography to quantitate and follow kyphosis, scoliosis
  - Multiplanar enhanced MR (especially STIR, fat-saturated T2WI, and T1 C+ MR) to evaluate cord, nerve pathology
  - Bone CT to optimally define osseous anatomy for surgical planning

DIFFERENTIAL DIAGNOSIS

Neurofibromatosis Type 2 (Central Neurofibromatosis)

- Multiple intracranial schwannomas and meningiomas, spinal schwannomas and meningiomas
- Spinal deformity uncommon
- Clinical, laboratory, and genetic testing findings distinguish from NF1

Chronic Inflammatory Demyelinating Polyneuropathy

- Repeated episodes of demyelination, remyelination → "onion skin" spinal, peripheral nerve enlargement
- Mimics PNF on imaging studies
- No cutaneous stigmata of NF1

Congenital Hypertrophic Polyradiculoneuropathies

- Charcot-Marie-Tooth, Dejerine-Sottas disease
- Nerve root enlargement mimics PNF on imaging studies
- No cutaneous stigmata of NF1

PATHOLOGY

General Features

- Etiology
  - Postulated that NF1 tumor suppression gene "switched off" → tissue proliferation, tumor development
- Genetics
  - Autosomal dominant; chromosome 17q12, penetrance → 100%
    - NF gene product (neurofibromin) is tumor suppressor
  - ~ 50% new mutations (paternal germ line; paternal age 35 years → 2x ↑ in new mutations)
- Associated abnormalities
  - Brain abnormalities: Macrocephaly, focal areas of signal abnormality, sphenoid wing dysplasia, glial tumors, intellectual handicap, epilepsy, hydrocephalus, aqueductal stenosis
  - ↑ risk of other neuroendocrine tumors (pheochromocytoma, carcinoid tumor), chronic myelogenous leukemia
  - Congenital bowing, pseudoarthrosis of tibia and forearm, massive extremity overgrowth
  - ↑ fibromuscular dysplasia, intracranial aneurysms, multiple sclerosis
- PNF is hallmark of NF1

- Kyphoscoliosis is most common NF1 osseous abnormality; variable severity mild, nonprogressive → severe curvature
  - Dystrophic scoliosis: Short segment, sharply angulated, < 6 spinal segments, tendency → severe deformity
  - Nondystrophic scoliosis: Similar to adolescent idiopathic curvature, usually 8-10 spinal segments, right convex
  - Severe cervical kyphosis highly suggestive of NF1
- Dural ectasia: 1° bone dysplasia, some cases 2° pressure erosion from intraspinal tumors
- "Ribbon" ribs 2° to bone dysplasia ± intercostal NF

Staging, Grading, & Classification
- Consensus Development Conference on Neurofibromatosis (NIH, 1987)
  - 2 or more of the following criteria
    - > 6 café au lait spots measuring ≥ 15 mm in adults or 5 mm in children
    - ≥ 2 NFs of any type or ≥ 1 PNF
    - Axillary or inguinal freckling
    - Optic glioma
    - 2 or more Lisch nodules (iris hamartomas)
    - Distinctive osseous lesion (sphenoid wing dysplasia, thinning of long bone ± pseudoarthrosis)
    - 1st-degree relative with NF1

Gross Pathologic & Surgical Features
- 3 types of spinal NF recognized in NF1
  - Localized NF (90% of all NF)
    - Most common NF in both NF1, non-NF1 patients
    - Cutaneous and deep nerves, spinal nerve roots
    - NF1: Larger, multiple, more frequently involve large deep nerves (sciatic nerve, brachial plexus)
    - Malignant transformation rare
  - Diffuse NF
    - Infiltrating subcutaneous tumor; rarely affects spinal nerves, majority (90%) unassociated with NF1
  - PNF (pathognomonic for NF1)
    - Diffuse enlargement of major nerve trunks/branches → bulky rope-like ("bag of worms") nerve expansion with adjacent tissue distortion
    - Commonly large, bilateral, multilevel with predilection for sciatic nerve, brachial plexus
    - ~ 5% risk malignant degeneration → sarcoma

Microscopic Features
- Neoplastic Schwann cells + perineural fibroblasts grow along nerve fascicles
  - Collagen fibers, mucoid/myxoid matrix, tumor, nerve fascicles intermixed
  - S100-positive, mitotic figures rare unless malignant degeneration

CLINICAL ISSUES

Presentation
- Most common signs/symptoms
  - Skeletal deformity common (25-40%)
    - Focal or acute angle kyphoscoliosis ± myelopathy
    - Extremity bowing or overgrowth
  - Palpable spinal or cutaneous mass
  - Pigmentation anomalies (café au lait, axillary freckling, Lisch nodules) ≥ 90% NF1 patients

- Clinical profile
  - Severity of clinical appearance highly variable
  - Classic NF1 triad: Cutaneous lesions, skeletal deformity, and mental deficiency

Demographics
- Age
  - Childhood diagnosis; minimally affected patients may be diagnosed as adults
- Gender
  - M = F
- Ethnicity
  - ↑ frequency in Arab-Israeli populations
- Epidemiology
  - Common (1:4,000)

Natural History & Prognosis
- Kyphosis, scoliosis frequently progressive
- NF growth usually slow; rapid growth associated with pregnancy, puberty, or malignant transformation

Treatment
- Conservative observation; intervention dictated by clinical symptomatology, appearance of neoplasm
- Surgical resection of symptomatic localized NF, spinal cord tumors
- PNF invasive, rarely resectable; observation ± biological or chemotherapeutic (thalidomide, antihistamines, maturation agents, antiangiogenic drugs) intervention
- Spinal fusion reserved for symptomatic or severe kyphoscoliosis

DIAGNOSTIC CHECKLIST

Consider
- Multiple nerve sheath tumors, ≥ 1 NF, bizarre kyphoscoliosis with deformed vertebra → consider NF1
- Absence of visible stigmata does not exclude NF1

Image Interpretation Pearls
- Characteristic PNF imaging appearance best displayed using fat-saturated T2WI or STIR MR

SELECTED REFERENCES

1. Nguyen R et al: Characterization of spinal findings in children and adults with neurofibromatosis type 1 enrolled in a natural history study using magnetic resonance imaging. J Neurooncol. 121(1):209-15, 2015
2. Pourtsidis A et al: Malignant peripheral nerve sheath tumors in children with neurofibromatosis type 1. Case Rep Oncol Med. 2014:843749, 2014
3. Jett K et al: Clinical and genetic aspects of neurofibromatosis 1. Genet Med. 12(1):1-11, 2010
4. Wasa J et al: MRI features in the differentiation of malignant peripheral nerve sheath tumors and neurofibromas. AJR Am J Roentgenol. 194(6):1568-74, 2010
5. Scalzone M et al: Neurofibromatosis type 1 clinical features and management. Pediatr Med Chir. 31(6):246-51, 2009
6. Van Meerbeeck SF et al: Whole body MR imaging in neurofibromatosis type 1. Eur J Radiol. 69(2):236-42, 2009

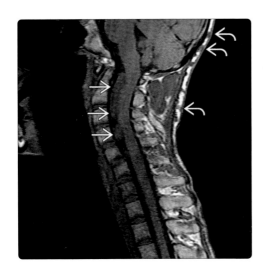 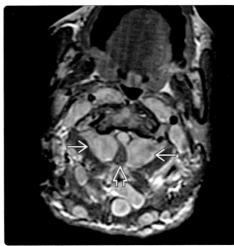

(Left) *Sagittal T1WI MR shows extensive intradural extramedullary neurofibromas* ➡ *located ventral to the spinal cord, displacing the cord posteriorly. Numerous subcutaneous soft tissue neurofibromas are also present posteriorly (several indicated with* ➡*).* (Right) *Axial T1 C+ MR of the upper cervical spine demonstrates marked extent of involvement by innumerable soft tissue and spinal neurofibromas. Note severe spinal cord* ➡ *compression produced by bilateral C2 neurofibromas* ➡*.*

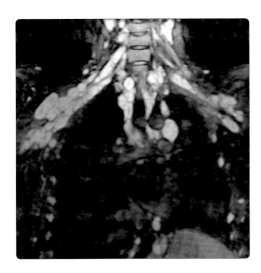 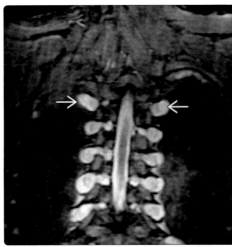

(Left) *Coronal STIR MR reveals innumerable plexiform neurofibromas involving the bilateral spinal nerves, sympathetic chains, and bilateral brachial plexus, as well as extensive involvement of multiple intercostal nerves.* (Right) *Coronal STIR MR depicts bilateral thoracic nerve root neurofibromas* ➡*, extending through the neural foramina into the paraspinal tissues. Neurofibromas are moderately hyperintense on STIR MR.*

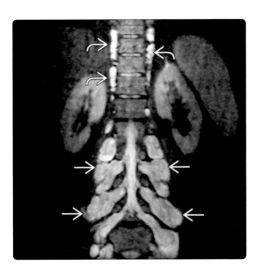 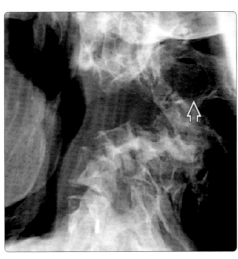

(Left) *Coronal STIR MR demonstrates multiple bilateral lumbar nerve root neurofibromas* ➡ *extending through the neural foramina into the adjacent paraspinal soft tissues. Small plexiform neurofibromas* ➡ *of the sympathetic chain are also detected.* (Right) *Lateral radiograph of the cervical spine depicts bizarre acute angle cervical kyphosis with marked dural ectasia and neural foraminal enlargement* ➡*, highly characteristic of NF1.*

KEY FACTS

TERMINOLOGY

- Rare autosomal dominant disease from chromosomal 22 defect in which all patients develop CNS tumors
- Mnemonic for NF2 tumors: **M**ultiple **i**nherited **s**chwannomas, **m**eningiomas, and **e**pendymomas (MISME)

TOP DIFFERENTIAL DIAGNOSES

- Metastases
- Hemangioblastomas
- Nonsyndromic schwannoma
- Nonsyndromic meningioma
- Nonsyndromic ependymoma
- Lymphoma

PATHOLOGY

- 22q12 deletion correlates with loss of *NF2* gene product "merlin" (a.k.a. schwannomin)
- Definite diagnosis of NF2
    - Bilateral CNVIII (vestibular) schwannomas

- 1st-degree relative with NF2 and either unilateral early-onset vestibular schwannoma (age < 30 years) or any 2: Meningioma, glioma, schwannoma, juvenile posterior subcapsular lenticular opacity
- Presumptive diagnosis of NF2
    - Early-onset unilateral CNVIII schwannomas (age < 30 years) and 1 of the following
    - Meningioma, glioma, schwannoma, juvenile posterior subcapsular lenticular opacity
    - Multiple meningiomas (> 2) and unilateral vestibular schwannoma
    - Or 1 of these: Glioma, schwannoma, juvenile posterior subcapsular lenticular opacity

DIAGNOSTIC CHECKLIST

- Screen using MR C+ of brain and entire spine
- Imaging follow-up of patients with spinal tumors should be based on knowledge of tumor location, number, and suspected histologic type

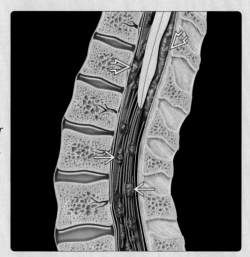
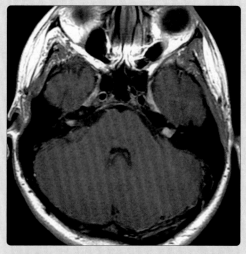

(Left) *Sagittal graphic illustrates multiple rounded schwannomas (brown)* ➡ *along the cauda equina, as well as flat dural-based meningiomas (red)* ➡ *impinging the conus.* (Right) *Axial T1WI C+ MR shows bilateral cerebellopontine angle masses due to vestibular schwannomas in this patient with neurofibromatosis type 2 (NF2).*

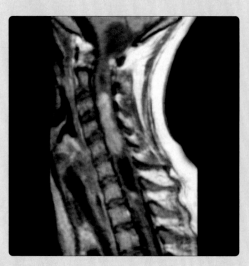
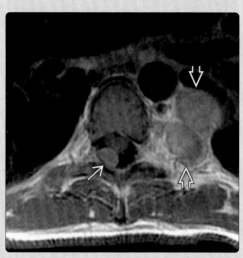

(Left) *Sagittal T1WI C+ MR demonstrates multiple intramedullary enhancing ependymomas. The largest is at the C3-C5 level, with associated inferior cyst, with a smaller 2nd tumor at C7-T1 level.* (Right) *Axial T1 C+ MR shows heterogeneous enhancement of paraspinal schwannomas* ➡*, as well as an intradural extramedullary tumor with a broad dural base consistent with meningioma* ➡*.*

TERMINOLOGY

Abbreviations

- Neurofibromatosis type 2 (NF2), nonsyndromic (NS)

Synonyms

- Bilateral acoustic neurofibromatosis, central neurofibromatosis (both obsolete)

Definitions

- Autosomal dominant disease from chromosomal 22 defect in which all patients develop CNS tumors
- Mnemonic for NF2 tumors: **M**ultiple **i**nherited **s**chwannomas, **m**eningiomas, and **e**pendymomas (MISME)

IMAGING

General Features

- Best diagnostic clue
  - Multiple spinal tumors of various histologic types

MR Findings

- T1WI C+
  - Schwannomas: Enhance intensely; homogeneously when small, heterogeneously when large and cystic
  - Meningiomas: Enhance intensely (often to lesser degree than schwannomas) and homogeneously
  - Ependymomas: Enhancing, centrally located mass

DIFFERENTIAL DIAGNOSIS

Metastases

- Cord lesions tend to have extensive edema
- Eccentrically placed, rarely within center of cord

Hemangioblastomas

- Often associated with von Hippel-Lindau
- Originate from leptomeninges, associated cyst

Nonsyndromic Schwannoma

- Focal, usually solitary lesion

Nonsyndromic Meningioma

- Isolated dura-based mass

Nonsyndromic Ependymoma

- Usually solitary, with imaging identical to syndromic tumors

Lymphoma

- May coat spinal cord surface

PATHOLOGY

General Features

- Etiology
  - Chromosomal 22 deletion with eventual inactivation of merlin functionality
- Genetics
  - Inherited autosomal dominant syndrome
  - 22q12 deletion correlates with loss of *NF2* gene product "merlin" (a.k.a. schwannomin)

Staging, Grading, & Classification

- Definite diagnosis of NF2
  - Bilateral CNVIII (vestibular) schwannomas

- 1st-degree relative with NF2 and either unilateral early onset vestibular schwannoma (age < 30 years) or any 2 of the following
  - Meningioma, glioma, schwannoma, juvenile posterior subcapsular lenticular opacity
- Presumptive diagnosis of NF2
  - Early-onset unilateral CNVIII schwannomas (age < 30 years) and 1 of the following
    - Meningioma, glioma, schwannoma, juvenile posterior subcapsular lenticular opacity
  - Multiple meningiomas (> 2) and unilateral vestibular schwannoma or 1 of the following
    - Glioma, schwannoma, juvenile posterior subcapsular lenticular opacity
- 3 features of intramedullary ependymomas
  - Central location within cord parenchyma
  - Intense enhancement
  - Multiplicity, often too many to count

CLINICAL ISSUES

Presentation

- Most common signs/symptoms
  - Nearly half initially present with hearing loss
  - Up to 45% with extramedullary tumors exhibit signs/symptoms of cord compression
    - Varies depending on location
    - Weakness and sensory loss at or below level
    - Spasticity, pain, loss of bowel/bladder control

Demographics

- Age
  - Genetic disease present at conception
  - Become symptomatic 2nd-3rd decades
- Epidemiology
  - 1 in 50,000 live births worldwide
  - Intradural spinal tumors are present in up to 65% of patients at initial presentation for imaging
    - 84% have intramedullary tumors
    - 87% have intradural extramedullary tumors

Natural History & Prognosis

- Many have relatively normal lifespans
- Few patients require therapeutic intervention for intramedullary tumors, which often remain quiescent
- Intradural extramedullary tumors frequently lead to surgical intervention
  - Percentage of patients with extramedullary tumors who undergo surgery is about 5x higher than percentage of patients with intramedullary tumors
  - Higher surgical rate is result of high number of tumors and frequent occurrence of cord compression
  - Schwannomas are present more often and in higher numbers than meningiomas and have more surgical procedures overall
  - Meningiomas account for disproportionate number of symptomatic lesions

Treatment

- Tumor resection is mainstay of NF2 treatment

(Left) *Axial T1WI C+ MR of the brain reveals bilateral vestibular schwannomas ➡ and a left trigeminal schwannoma ➡, confirming the diagnosis of NF2.* **(Right)** *Parasagittal T1WI C+ MR of the cervical spine shows enhancing foraminal schwannomas ➡.*

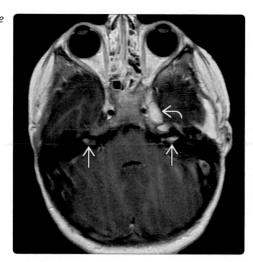

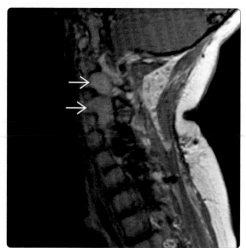

(Left) *Sagittal T1 C+ MR of the lumbar spine in a typical case of spinal NF2 demonstrates numerous nodules arising within the cauda equina with avid tumor enhancement, characteristic of schwannoma.* **(Right)** *Sagittal T1WI C+ MR of the lumbar spine shows enhancement of multiple intradural masses scattered along the cauda equina, characteristic of schwannoma.*

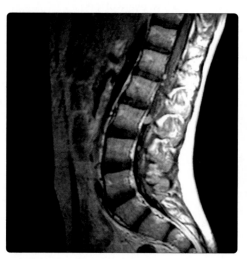

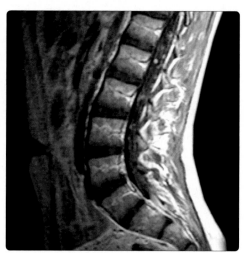

(Left) *Axial T1WI C+ MR of the cervical spine shows both intramedullary ependymoma enhancement ➡ and an intradural extramedullary lesion ➡, which is a schwannoma.* **(Right)** *Axial T1WI C+ MR of the lumbar spine demonstrates the origin of the schwannomas to be from the cauda equina nerve roots.*

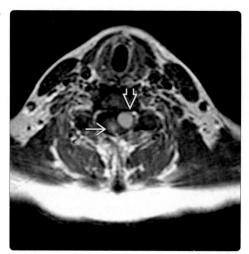

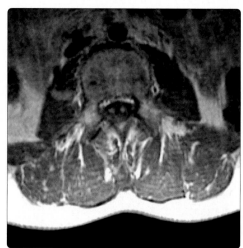

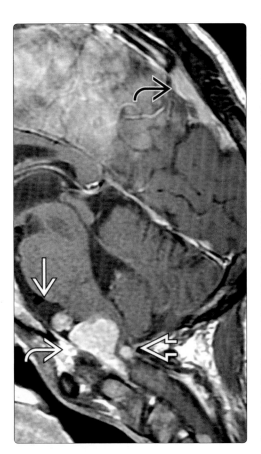

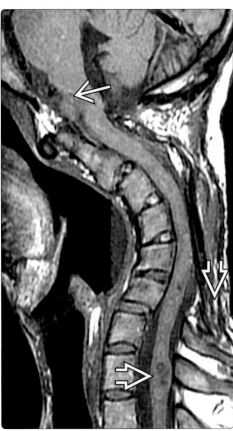

(Left) *Sagittal T1WI C+ MR shows multiple intradural extramedullary masses at the cervicomedullary junction, reflecting a mixture of meningioma ⇗ and schwannomas ➡. There is also an enhancing intramedullary ependymoma ➡. Recurrent meningioma is seen at the parietooccipital junction ⇗.* (Right) *Sagittal T1WI MR shows a "swan neck" deformity from prior multilevel laminectomy. Multiple intramedullary lesions within the spinal cord are biopsy-proven ependymomas ➡, vaguely seen as slightly diminished signal. Meningioma is also present at skull base ➡.*

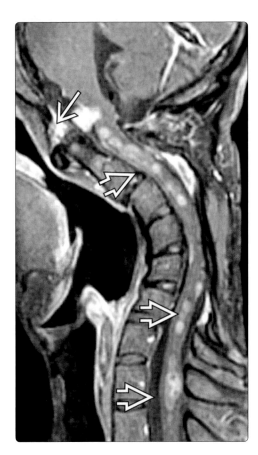

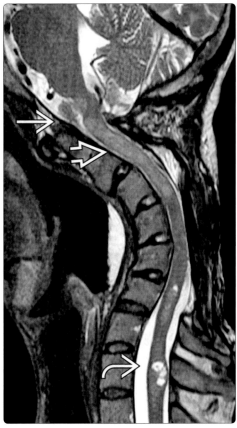

(Left) *Sagittal T1WI C+ MR shows multiple enhancing intramedullary masses throughout the cervical and thoracic cord due to ependymomas ➡ in this patient with NF2. Note the enhancing meningioma at the foramen magnum ➡. Patient shows severe "swan neck" deformity as complication of prior multilevel laminectomies for tumor resection.* (Right) *Sagittal T2WI MR shows variable signal intensity from the multiple intramedullary tumors throughout the cervical and thoracic cord in this patient with NF2. These vary from near isointense ➡ to hyperintense ➡ signal. Meningioma is also present at the foramen magnum, seen as a near-cord isointense signal ➡. "Swan neck" deformity is present from prior multilevel laminectomy with significant narrowing of subarachnoid space at the laminectomy site.*

Down Syndrome

TERMINOLOGY

- Synonym: Trisomy 21

IMAGING

- Ranges normal CVJ to CVJ bone anomalies ± atlantooccipital instability (AOI), atlantoaxial instability (AAI)
- ± myelomalacia, syringomyelia, cervicomedullary compression
- Imaging recommendations
  - Static radiographs to identify CVJ anomalies
  - Dynamic radiographs for CVJ stability assessment
  - Bone CT to evaluate CVJ osseous structures
  - Multiplanar MR for cord compression, syringomyelia

TOP DIFFERENTIAL DIAGNOSES

- Achondroplasia
- Mucopolysaccharidoses

PATHOLOGY

- Most common cervical anomalies in Down syndrome patients
  - Occipital condyle hypoplasia
  - AOI (8–63% of Down syndrome patients)
  - C1 ring hypoplasia (6.7% in small series)
  - Odontoid hypoplasia
  - Os odontoideum
  - AAI (10–30% of Down syndrome patients)
  - Cervical spondylosis

CLINICAL ISSUES

- Hypotonia (infants)
- Asymptomatic (older Down syndrome children)
- Myelopathy, torticollis

DIAGNOSTIC CHECKLIST

- Evaluate for dynamic CVJ instability

(Left) Lateral radiograph of the cervical spine obtained in extension shows notable posterior displacement of the occipital condyle ⇒ relative to the C1 lateral mass superior articular surface ⇒, reflecting atlantooccipital instability. (Right) Lateral radiograph of the cervical spine obtained in flexion shows anterior translation of the C1 anterior ring ⇒ relative to the odontoid process ⇒. The odontoid process is also mildly hypoplastic. Note flattened occipital condyles ⇒.

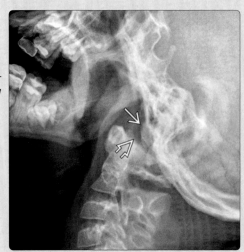 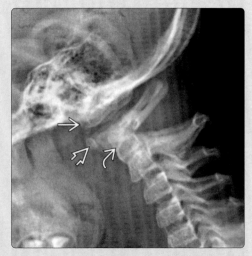

(Left) Sagittal T1WI MR reveals mild C1 ⇒ posterior ring hypoplasia and anterior translation of the C1 anterior ring. The odontoid process ⇒ is mildly dysplastic. Note also abnormal craniofacial proportions reflecting microcephaly. (Right) Sagittal T2WI MR of the cervical spine demonstrates a mildly dysplastic odontoid process ⇒ as well as accelerated degenerative changes (cervical spondylosis) at C2/3 ⇒.

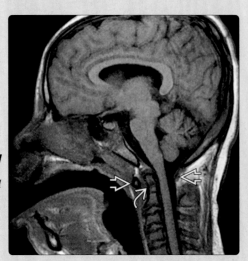 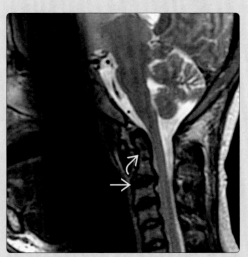

Mucopolysaccharidoses

KEY FACTS

TERMINOLOGY

- Mucopolysaccharidoses (MPS) are inherited lysosomal storage disorders
- MPS I: Hurler; MPS II: Hunter; MPS III: Sanfillipo; MPS IV: Morquio

IMAGING

- Craniocervical spine
  - CVJ stenosis, dens hypoplasia, ligamentous laxity, atlantoaxial instability, thickened dural ring at foramen magnum
- Thoracolumbar spine
  - Kyphoscoliosis, platyspondyly, anterior vertebral beaking, ± thoracolumbar gibbus deformity

TOP DIFFERENTIAL DIAGNOSES

- GM1 gangliosidosis
- Mucolipidosis III (pseudo-Hurler polydystrophy)
- Achondroplasia

- Trisomy 21 (Down syndrome)
- Spondyloepiphyseal dysplasia

PATHOLOGY

- Inherited lysosomal enzyme deficiency → storage disorder
  - Autosomal recessive (except MPS II, Hunter; X-linked recessive)
- Glycosaminoglycan (GAG) accumulates in organs and ligaments

CLINICAL ISSUES

- Gradual progressive myelopathy
- Clinical neurologic symptoms attributable to brain GAG deposition, myelination abnormalities, spinal deformities, peripheral nerve entrapment

DIAGNOSTIC CHECKLIST

- Successful diagnosis requires combination of clinical, imaging, and genetic/biochemical information

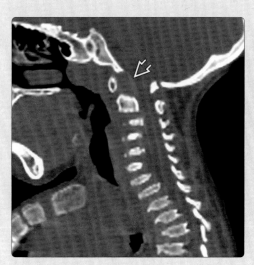
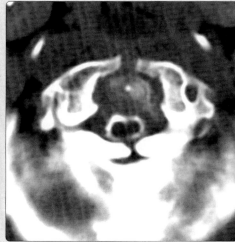

(Left) Sagittal bone CT (MPS IV) shows flattening and anterior beaking of all vertebra, consistent with Morquio syndrome. The central beak placement is said to be more characteristic of Morquio syndrome than Hurler syndrome. The odontoid process ➡ is hypoplastic and nonossified. (Right) Axial bone CT (MPS IV) following myelography confirms moderate central canal narrowing at the craniovertebral junction secondary to osseous abnormalities as well as ligamentous thickening.

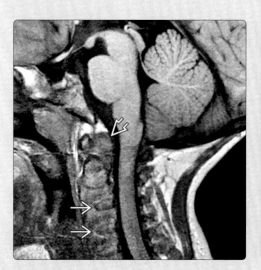
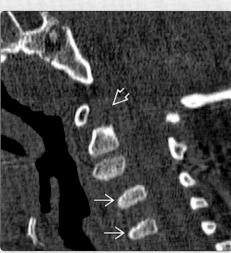

(Left) Sagittal T1WI MR (MPS IV: Morquio) demonstrates an unossified odontoid process ➡. There is no platybasia or basilar invagination. Characteristic hypoplasia of the subaxial vertebral bodies ➡ is also demonstrated. (Right) Sagittal bone CT (MPS IV: Morquio) confirms nonossification of the odontoid process ➡ as well as mild hypoplasia of the C3 and C4 vertebral bodies ➡.

KEY FACTS

IMAGING

- Shortened vertebral pedicles
  - Decreasing interpediculate distance toward lower levels of lumbar spine
- Mildly flattened &/or anteriorly wedged vertebral bodies
- Thoracolumbar kyphosis
- Lumbar hyperlordosis
- Small foramen magnum
- T2W: Compression of cervicomedullary junction, spinal cord, nerve roots → myelopathic hyperintensity in cord
- Other
  - Growth disturbance more obvious in proximal limbs (rhizomelic dwarfism)
  - "Champagne glass" pelvis: Pelvic inlet is flat and broad
  - Squared iliac wings
  - Short ribs

TOP DIFFERENTIAL DIAGNOSES

- Pseudoachondroplasia
- Hypochondroplasia
- Diastrophic dysplasia
- Spondyloepiphyseal dysplasia
- Osteogenesis imperfecta

PATHOLOGY

- Usually spontaneous mutation (80%)
  - Results in defective enchondral bone formation
- Autosomal dominant transmission
- Defect in *FGFR3*, responsible gene mapped to 4p16.3

CLINICAL ISSUES

- Most common nonlethal skeletal dysplasia
- High morbidity from spinal stenosis
  - Surgical correction of progressive/unresolving kyphosis
  - Surgical decompression of foramen magnum in severe cases; usually symptoms resolve
  - Surgical decompression of stenosis

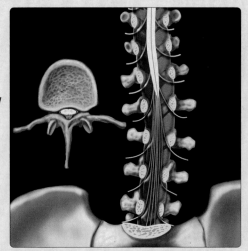

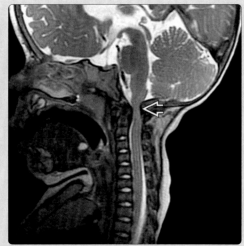

(Left) *Graphic shows progressive narrowing of the interpediculate distance in a caudad direction. Axial insert image shows spinal stenosis related to short pedicles and decreased interpediculate distance.* (Right) *Sagittal T2WI MR shows a constricted skull base relative to the visualized cranial vault. Stenosis of the foramen magnum ⇒ compresses the cervicomedullary junction, with mildly increased signal in the upper cervical cord due to myelopathic changes.*

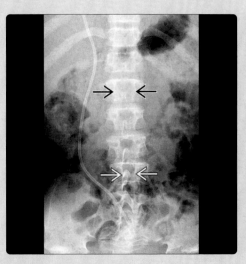

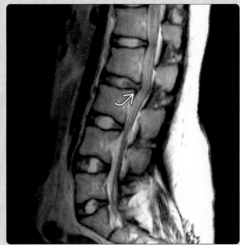

(Left) *AP radiograph of the lumbar spine shows narrowing of the interpediculate distance and progressive interpedicular narrowing between L1 ⇨ and L4 ⇨, causing narrowing of the lumbar canal in the transverse dimension.* (Right) *Sagittal T2WI MR shows a diffusely narrowed AP dimension of the lumbar spinal canal, reflecting shortened vertebral pedicles. Congenital canal stenosis is further narrowed by a small disc protrusion ⇨ at L2-L3.*

Osteogenesis Imperfecta

KEY FACTS

TERMINOLOGY

- Genetic disorder of type I collagen resulting in bone fragility
- Classified into 4 types based on clinical, genetic, and radiographic criteria

IMAGING

- Severe osteopenia
- Vertebral fractures, kyphoscoliosis
- Multiple long bone, rib fractures
- Enlarged epiphyses, "popcorn" metaphyseal calcifications
- Medullary cavity nearly entirely filled with fat
  - Primary trabeculae sparse but normally oriented
  - Secondary trabeculae nearly absent

TOP DIFFERENTIAL DIAGNOSES

- Nonaccidental trauma
- Congenital dwarfism
- Osteoporosis

PATHOLOGY

- Numerous type I collagen mutations → brittle bone
  - Most autosomal dominant
  - Inherited or spontaneous mutation
- Associated anomalies include blue sclerae, early hearing loss, brittle teeth, thin fragile skin, joint laxity

CLINICAL ISSUES

- Short stature secondary to multiple spinal and extremity fractures, kyphoscoliosis, growth plate abnormalities
- Diagnosis suggested by radiographs, confirmed with ancillary testing

DIAGNOSTIC CHECKLIST

- Important to differentiate from nonaccidental trauma
- Basilar impression and other spinal complications may be difficult to detect on radiographs
  - Consider MR or CT

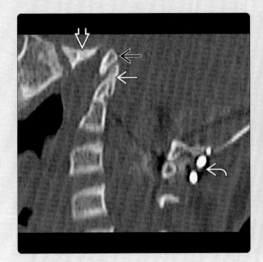

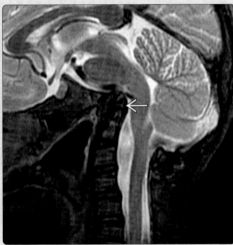

(Left) Sagittal bone CT demonstrates platybasia and severe basilar impression with upward displacement of the remodeled odontoid process and anterior C1 ring through the foramen magnum. Metallic posterior spinal hardware has been placed to arrest basilar impression. (Right) Sagittal T2WI MR reveals severe cranial settling and platybasia with basilar impression of the odontoid process into the foramen magnum, producing ventral cervicomedullary compression.

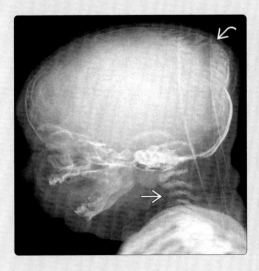

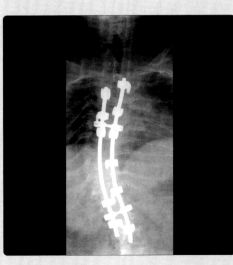

(Left) Lateral skull radiograph in a newborn shows an abnormal head shape with numerous wormian bones in the lambdoid suture. Also detected was an abnormal swan neck deformity of the cervical spine. (Right) Anteroposterior radiograph of the thoracic spine shows convex right neuromuscular scoliosis with spinal rods. There are also osteopenia and ribbon-like ribs, characteristic findings of osteogenesis imperfecta.

Spondyloepiphyseal Dysplasia

TERMINOLOGY

- Spondyloepiphyseal dysplasia (SED)
- Group of generalized skeletal dysplasias primarily involving vertebrae, proximal epiphyseal centers
- Affected patients demonstrate short trunk, neck, and limbs with normal hand and foot size

IMAGING

- Platyspondyly, vertebral hypoplasia & underossification, abnormal epiphyses
- ± pannus at C1/C2, os odontoideum
- Delayed ossification of capital femoral epiphysis → femoral head flattening, premature osteoarthritis

TOP DIFFERENTIAL DIAGNOSES

- Spondylometaphyseal dysplasia
- Spondyloepimetaphyseal dysplasia
- Multiple epiphyseal dysplasia

PATHOLOGY

- SED congenita
  - Abnormal type II collagen synthesis
- SED tarda
  - *SEDL* gene mutation (vesicular transport protein)

CLINICAL ISSUES

- SED congenita: Diagnosed at birth, short proximal limbs with normal hand, foot size
- SED tarda: Normal appearance at birth, subsequent identification of disproportionately short stature in adolescence or adulthood

DIAGNOSTIC CHECKLIST

- Consider SED congenita for platyspondyly, dysplastic epiphyses
- Consider SED tarda in adults with short trunk, early symmetric large joint osteoarthritis

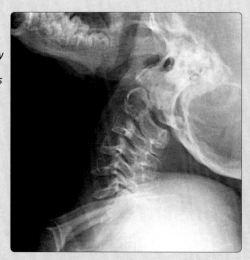
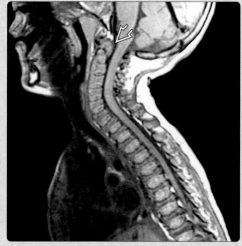

(Left) Lateral cervical radiograph (kyphosis, myelopathy) obtained in extension shows platyspondyly and delayed ossification status. The odontoid process is hypoplastic or underossified, rendering evaluation for atlantoaxial subluxation difficult. (Right) Sagittal T1WI MR (kyphosis, myelopathy) of the cervical spine reveals characteristic abnormal vertebral shape as well as a large odontoid process ➡ with delayed tip ossification. No spinal cord compression is demonstrated.

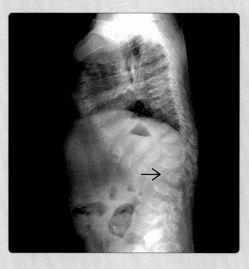
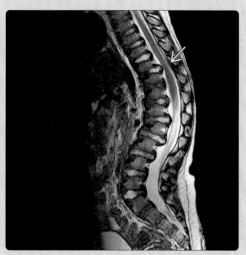

(Left) Lateral radiograph of the thoracolumbar spine (kyphosis, myelopathy) demonstrates characteristic platyspondyly in addition to focal kyphosis at the thoracolumbar junction secondary to a hypoplastic L2 vertebra ➡. (Right) Sagittal T2WI MR (kyphosis, myelopathy) of the thoracolumbar spine confirms significant stenosis of the lower thoracic spinal canal producing focal spinal cord compression and abnormal spinal cord T2 hyperintensity ➡.

IMAGING

General Features

- Location
  - Spine, large joints
- Morphology
  - Extent of osseous abnormalities diffusely distributed throughout skeleton
    - Severity of osseous abnormalities is variable

Imaging Recommendations

- Best imaging tool
  - Plain radiographs for screening
  - Multiplanar CT or MR for further evaluation, preoperative planning

Radiographic Findings

- Platyspondyly, vertebral hypoplasia, and underossification
- ± os odontoideum

CT Findings

- CECT
  - ± pannus at C1 to odontoid articulation
- Bone CT
  - Platyspondyly, vertebral hypoplasia, and underossification
  - ± os odontoideum

MR Findings

- T1WI
  - Same as bone CT
  - Improved detection of spinal cord and soft tissue (pannus) abnormalities
- T2WI
  - Same as T1WI
  - Better detection of spinal cord myelomalacia or syringohydromyelia

DIFFERENTIAL DIAGNOSIS

Spondylometaphyseal Dysplasia

- Generalized skeletal dysplasia featuring significant vertebral involvement; affects metaphyseal rather than epiphyseal portions of long bones

Spondyloepimetaphyseal Dysplasia

- Generalized skeletal dysplasia featuring significant vertebral involvement; affects both metaphyseal and epiphyseal regions of long bones

Multiple Epiphyseal Dysplasia

- Primarily affects (multiple) epiphyses
- Relatively mild clinical signs and symptoms

PATHOLOGY

General Features

- Etiology
  - Spondyloepiphyseal dysplasia (SED) congenita
    - Abnormal synthesis of type 2 collagen (α-1 chain)
      - Type 2 collagen is primary matrix protein of physeal and epiphyseal cartilage, major component of nucleus pulposus, vitreous (eye)
      - Other skeletal dysplasias affected by collagen 2 include achondrogenesis type 2, hypochondrogenesis, Kniest dysplasia, Stickler dysplasia, autosomal forms of SED tarda, and spondylometaepiphyseal (Strudwick) dysplasia
  - SED tarda
    - SEDL gene mutation encoding vesicular transport protein
- Genetics
  - SED congenita
    - COL2A1 gene mutation, mapped to long arm of chromosome 12 (12q14.3)
      - Most cases result from random new mutation
    - Autosomal dominant (M = F)
    - Rare autosomal recessive cases reported
  - SED tarda
    - Genetically distinct from SED congenita
    - Most commonly X-linked recessive (M > > F)
    - Rare autosomal forms described
    - Caused by mutation in SEDL (SED late) gene (Xp22)
      - Encodes vesicular transport protein
- Associated abnormalities
  - Cervical instability, spinal curvature (scoliosis, kyphosis, lordosis), vision (myopia, retinal detachment), hearing loss, extremity (coxa vara, genu valgum, equinovarus foot, 2° large joint degenerative disease), nephrotic syndrome

Staging, Grading, & Classification

- International Nomenclature and Classification of Osteochondrodysplasias
  - SED congenita, tarda most common
  - Other rare SED variants
    - SED Maroteaux type: Musculoskeletal system only
    - SED tarda Toledo type: Musculoskeletal + corneal opacification
    - SED tarda (Wynne-Davies): Progressive arthropathy (similar to juvenile inflammatory arthritis)
    - SED with brachydactyly
    - SED tarda Namaqualand type
    - Pseudo-Morquio disease
    - Pseudoachondroplasia SED

CLINICAL ISSUES

Natural History & Prognosis

- No increased mortality
- Osteoarthritis nearly inevitable 2° complication of skeletal dysplasia

Treatment

- Address musculoskeletal deformities, secondary complications

DIAGNOSTIC CHECKLIST

Consider

- SED congenita in context of platyspondyly, dysplastic epiphyses
- SED tarda in adults with short trunk and barrel chest in conjunction with early symmetric large joint osteoarthritis

SECTION 4
Disorders of Alignment

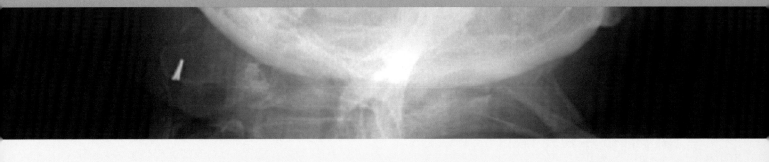

Terminology

Scoliosis is considered to be present when there is a coronal plane curvature of the spine measuring at least 10°. However, treatment is not generally instituted unless the curvature is > 20-25°. The curvature may be balanced (returning to midline) or unbalanced. The vertebrae at the ends of the curve are designated the terminal (or end) vertebrae, whereas the apical vertebra is at the curve apex.

Curvatures are described by the side to which they deviate. A dextroscoliosis is convex to the right, with its apex to the right of midline. A levoscoliosis is convex to the left, with its apex to the left of midline.

Curvatures can be categorized as flexible (normalizing with lateral bending toward the side of the curve) or structural (failing to correct).

Most scoliotic curvatures are associated with abnormal curvature in the sagittal plane. These are described as kyphosis (apex dorsal) or lordosis (apex ventral).

Morphology of the Curvature

Scoliosis due to fracture, congenital anomaly, or infection typically has an angular configuration. Other causes of scoliosis tend to have a smooth curvature. Scoliosis most commonly involves the thoracic spine, followed by the thoracolumbar spine. In the past, curves were categorized as primary and secondary (compensatory), but it is often difficult to make the distinction. Therefore, these designations are no longer commonly used.

Measurement of Scoliosis

The Cobb method is most commonly used to measure scoliosis. The vertebrae at each end of the curve (the terminal vertebrae) are chosen. These are the endplates with the greatest deviation from the horizontal. The curvature is the angle between a line drawn along the superior endplate of superior terminal vertebra and a line along the inferior endplate of the inferior terminal vertebra. In severe curvatures, the endplates are often difficult to see. In that case, the inferior cortex of the pedicle can be used as the landmark for making the measurement. If measurements are made on hard copy radiographs, it is usually necessary to draw lines perpendicular to the endplates and measure the angle between the perpendicular lines. On most PACS, the measurements can be made directly from the endplates.

The Ferguson method is another way to measure scoliosis. In this method, lines are drawn from the center of the apical vertebra to the center of each terminal vertebrae. The angle of the scoliosis is the angle between these 2 lines.

Scoliosis is almost always associated with abnormal curvature in the sagittal plane. The most common finding is loss of normal thoracic kyphosis. The Cobb method can be used to determine sagittal plane deformity. Rotational deformity is often present but can only be grossly assessed on radiographs. It can be measured on CT scan by superimposing the apical and terminal vertebra.

Normally, the T1 vertebra is centered over the L5 vertebra in both the coronal and sagittal planes. Coronal or sagittal plane imbalance can be measured as the horizontal distance between the center of the L5 vertebral body and a plumb line drawn through the center of the T1 vertebral body.

Rotational deformity is present in most types of scoliosis. This is difficult to measure. Measurement is most easily made by superimposing axial images of the terminal and apical vertebrae or by using 3D CT.

Risser Index

Because idiopathic scoliosis tends not to progress after skeletal maturity, it is useful to assess how close the young patient is to skeletal maturity. This is commonly assessed by the Risser method, based on the appearance of the apophysis of iliac wing. However, this has been shown to be less accurate than skeletal age assessed on hand radiographs.

- Apophysis not present = stage 0
- Apophysis covers lateral 25% of iliac wing = stage 1: Bone age 13 yr, 8 mo (F); 14 yr, 7 mo (M)
- Apophysis covers lateral 50% of iliac wing = stage 2: Bone age 14 yr, 6 mo (F); 15 yr, 7 mo (M)
- Apophysis covers 75% of iliac wing = stage 3: Bone age 15 yr, 2 mo (F); 16 yr, 2 mo (M)
- Apophysis covers entire iliac wing = stage 4: Bone age 16 yr, 2 mo (F); 17 yr, 0 mo (M)
- Apophysis fused = stage 5: Bone age 18 yr, 1 mo (F); 18 yr, 6 mo (M)

Radiology Reporting of Scoliosis

The radiology report should include measurements of all coronal and sagittal plane curvatures, using the Cobb method. If bending or supine films are obtained, the radiologist should report the change in the curvature from the upright film. Spondylolysis is a frequent finding below the scoliosis, and a routine search pattern should include evaluation for spondylolysis.

The radiographs should be evaluated for atypical findings: Are there any vertebral anomalies? Is the patient osteopenic, and are fractures visible? Is the thoracic curve to the right (typical) or to the left (atypical)? Are the curves balanced in the coronal and sagittal planes, i.e., is the spine centered over L5? Are the ribs, cardiac silhouette, and paraspinous soft tissues normal?

Role of Advanced Imaging

MR or CT are performed when there is concern for an underlying abnormality, such as syrinx, tethered spinal cord, congenital bony abnormality, or tumor.

Suspicion of syrinx is raised when the thoracic curve is convex to the left or when the thoracic curve does not exhibit lordosis at its apex. Tethered cord usually presents in childhood but can be seen in early adulthood, in which it presents with lower extremity symptoms or bowel and bladder dysfunction.

Treatment of Scoliosis

The goal of scoliosis treatment involves obtaining anchor points to allow for spine stabilization with potential correction. This can be accomplished with hooks, wires, pedicle screws, or cables. Infantile scoliosis (0-3 years) treatment is performed by casting (Mehta-Cotwel) for growth modulation (elongation, derotation, and flexion). Juvenile scoliosis (3-10 years) tends not to progress after skeletal maturity unless it is severe (> 50-60°). Therefore, minimal scoliosis is often treated with observation, especially if the patient is near skeletal maturity. Mild degrees of scoliosis (< 40°) are treated with bracing if continued growth remains. Bracing has a high rate of success in compliant patients who wear a brace > 16 hours per day. More severe curvatures are usually treated with fusion, either growing rod constructs for early onset scoliosis or fusion for those who have completed growth. Currently, most surgeons use paired posterior rods and transpedicular screws. Historically, an anterior transthoracic approach with fusion of the vertebral bodies and a lateral fusion rod was also common. Harrington rods, which have hooks at the ends but no pedicle screws, are rarely used today.

Postoperative Imaging

Imaging is performed after scoliosis surgery to evaluate the success of the operation. In general, it is irrelevant for the radiologist to name the brand of instrumentation used and a simple description is preferable. Postoperative radiographs must be evaluated first for correction of deformity in the coronal and sagittal planes. Then the instrumentation is assessed. On digital radiography, a thin lucent rim is typically seen surrounding screw threads and is not a sign of loosening. However, lucencies of > 1 mm suggest screw loosing. Screws may also back out from the vertebral body (in which case the screw heads are described as "proud"). Laminar hooks may become dislodged from the bone or detached from the fixation rod.

Instrumentation placed for correction of scoliosis provides rigid fixation as the bone fusion matures. If there is failure of bony fusion, the instrumentation will fail. CT scans with reformatted coronal and sagittal images are the most reliable method for assessing bony union. A CT scan will show gradual coalescence of bone graft over a several-month period postoperatively. By the end of 6 months, the graft should have developed a confluent mass with a well-defined cortex surrounding the trabecular bone. Facet joint fusion is seen as a loss of joint space and bridging trabeculae. Intervertebral body fusion will also show confluent bone.

If there is failure of bony fusion and consequent instrumentation failure, there may be loss of surgical correction of the scoliotic curvature. Crankshaft phenomenon results when the ends of the curvature are fixed but the intermediate portions are not, so the curve apex may continue to migrate. This can be seen in early-onset scoliosis (growth potential).

When reviewing postoperative imaging, a useful pattern is to evaluate the instrumentation and bone at the fused levels and then look for abnormalities above and below the fused levels. In addition to instrumentation failure, common problems include adjacent segment degeneration, infection, and insufficiency fractures.

Imaging Protocols

Radiographs are performed to include the entire thoracic and lumbar spine. If the patient has unequal limb lengths, a lift is used under the shorter limb. Frontal radiographs are usually obtained PA instead of AP in order to minimize radiation dose to the breasts.

A CT scan should always be performed with reformatted images. Angled reformatted images and 3D reformations are often useful in assessment of severe curvatures.

Some physicians find it useful to obtain both SPECT and CT images of degenerative scoliosis. An area of arthritis on a CT scan, which shows increased uptake on SPECT, is probably a pain generator.

MR can be difficult to interpret when scoliosis is severe. Angled axial images should be obtained based on both sagittal and coronal scout images and angled along the plane of the vertebral endplate on both scouts. Sagittal images should be angled along each segment of the curvature. The coronal plane is often the most useful for evaluating bony anomalies, spondylolysis, or degeneration of the discs and facet joints.

Differential Diagnosis

Idiopathic scoliosis is the most common type and may present in infancy, childhood, or adolescence. It may have a single curve or a balanced, S-shaped curve. The thoracic curvature is usually to the right. The vertebral bodies near the apex of the curve are often slightly wedged due to asymmetric stress during growth, but no anomalies are present.

Congenital scoliosis is scoliosis due to an abnormality of vertebral segmentation. It is associated with hemivertebrae, block (unsegmented) vertebrae, &/or fusions of the posterior elements. It often occurs as part of the VACTERL association: **V**ertebral anomalies, **a**nal atresia, **c**ardiac anomalies, **t**racheo-**e**sophageal fistula, **r**enal and other genitourinary anomalies, and **l**imb anomalies.

Congenital syndromes may cause scoliosis without vertebral anomalies. Collagen vascular disorders, neurofibromatosis, and osteogenesis imperfecta are the most common syndromes causing scoliosis. The curvatures are variable in appearance.

Neuromuscular scoliosis is seen in a variety of disorders, including muscular dystrophy and cerebral palsy. The curvature is most often a long, thoracolumbar C-shaped curve. It has a tendency to progress and can be very difficult to treat.

Osteoid osteoma and osteoblastoma may cause scoliosis. These tumors are very closely related, distinguished primarily by size and host response. Osteoid osteoma is < 1 cm in size and surrounded by dense reactive bone. Both tumors secrete prostaglandins, which stimulate a short-curve scoliosis, with the tumor on the concave side of the curvature. Prostaglandin release also often causes bone marrow edema involving bones not involved with tumor, pleural effusion, or soft tissue edema. Importantly, scoliosis due to osteoid osteoma/osteoblastoma is painful, whereas idiopathic scoliosis is not.

Adult scoliosis is divided into 3 types. The 1st is degenerative scoliosis, which usually involves the lumbar spine. Degenerative scoliosis often develops above a surgical fusion, especially if there is a mild preexisting curvature above the fused levels. The 2nd type is juvenile scoliosis, which continues to progress after skeletal maturity. The 3rd type is scoliosis due to an underlying abnormality, such as limb length inequality, asymmetric variants at the lumbosacral junction, or osteoporosis.

Trauma, infection, failure of surgical instrumentation, or neuropathic arthropathy may cause scoliosis. In each of these cases, the curvature is short, and the bony abnormality causing the scoliosis is visible on radiographs.

Chest wall anomalies or thoracic surgery in childhood are an uncommon cause of scoliosis. In the past, radiation therapy for Wilms tumor was an important cause of scoliosis, but changes in radiation therapy technique have rendered that a rare occurrence.

(Left) *PA radiograph shows idiopathic thoracic dextroscoliosis. The apical vertebra ➔ is the most displaced from the midline. Terminal vertebrae ➔ show the greatest deviation of the endplates from the horizontal.* **(Right)** *Lateral radiograph in the same patient shows reversal of usual thoracic kyphosis. Rotational component of the scoliosis can be grossly assessed by the degree of rotation of the ribs ➔.*

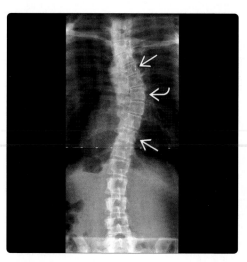
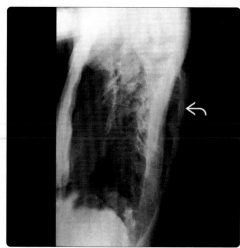

(Left) *Axial 3D reformation allows measurement of the rotational component of scoliosis. This is the angle between the terminal vertebra ➔ and the apical vertebra ➔.* **(Right)** *Coronal CT reconstruction shows measurement of severe neuromuscular scoliosis. The scoliotic curvature is the angle between the vertebrae with the greatest degree of inclination from the horizontal.*

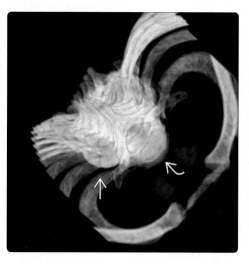
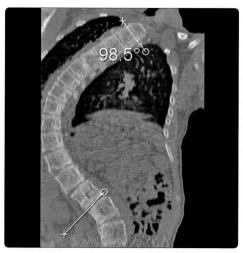

(Left) *PA radiograph shows a single, long sweeping curve thoracolumbar scoliosis typical of neuromuscular scoliosis. No vertebral anomalies are present.* **(Right)** *PA radiograph in the same patient shows only slight improvement in the curve when the patient bends to the right. Lateral bending films or supine films are used to assess the flexibility of a scoliotic curvature. Rigid curves are less amenable to reduction.*

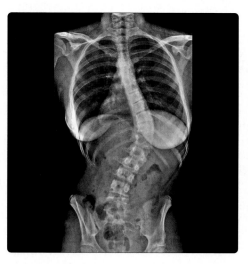
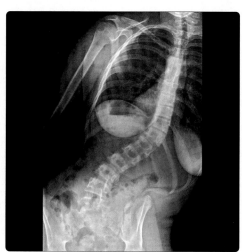

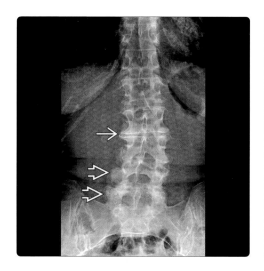

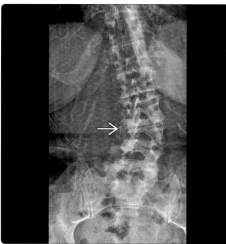

(Left) *Anteroposterior radiograph shows multilevel degenerative disc disease and only minimal leftward curvature in a 50-year-old woman. Disc disease is slightly asymmetric at the apex of the curve ➡, and facet osteoarthritis ➡ is more severe on the right (concave) side.* (Right) *Anteroposterior radiograph in the same patient 4 years later shows significant curve progression and progression of the asymmetric degenerative disc disease ➡ and facet osteoarthritis.*

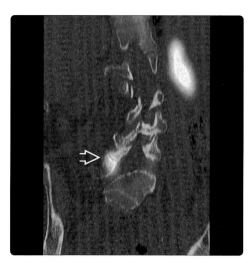

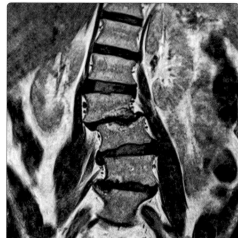

(Left) *Coronal CT reconstruction fused with SPECT bone scan shows abnormal uptake ➡ at facet joint at the concave aspect of degenerative scoliosis. Fusion of CT and SPECT is sometimes useful to pinpoint pain generators and guide joint injections.* (Right) *Coronal T2WI MR is useful in evaluating disc and facet abnormalities in degenerative scoliosis. In addition, it can be used as a scout to set angled images through the intervertebral discs.*

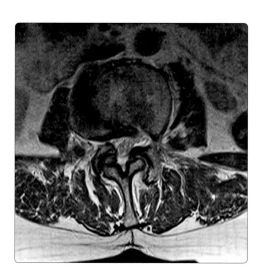

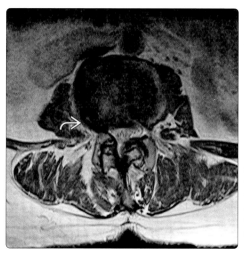

(Left) *Axial T2WI MR at the L2-L3 level was angled based on sagittal scout but not in reference to sagittal images. The disc is obliquely imaged, and, even though the scoliosis was mild, the image appears distorted.* (Right) *Axial T2WI MR at the same level, but angled with the disc orientation on the coronal image, shows an annular fissure ➡ on the right. Spinal stenosis appears more severe because the image is perpendicular to the canal rather than oblique as in the preceding image.*

Disorders of Alignment

TERMINOLOGY

- General term for any lateral curvature of spine (≥ 10°)

IMAGING

- Lateral curvature of spine
  - Returns to midline at ends of curve
  - Rotational component common
- Most commonly thoracic or thoracolumbar
- Imaging approach
  - Radiography for initial diagnosis
  - Multiplanar MR to screen for bone, cord abnormalities
  - CT for surgical planning, complications

TOP DIFFERENTIAL DIAGNOSES

- Idiopathic scoliosis
- Neuromuscular scoliosis
- Congenital scoliosis
- Scoliosis due to congenital syndromes without vertebral anomalies

- Degenerative scoliosis
- Scoliosis due to infection
- Scoliosis due to tumor
- Scoliosis due to trauma
- Curvature related to limb length inequality
- Positional scoliosis

CLINICAL ISSUES

- Usually presents in childhood or adolescence
- Idiopathic scoliosis usually asymptomatic
  - Painful scoliosis indicates underlying abnormality
- Surgical fusion for rapidly progressive curves, curves > 40°

DIAGNOSTIC CHECKLIST

- Short-curve or painful scoliosis usually has underlying abnormalities
- Curve may progress rapidly, especially during growth spurts

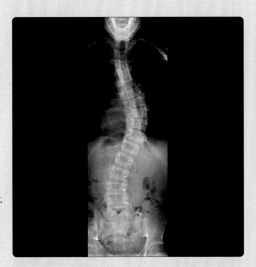

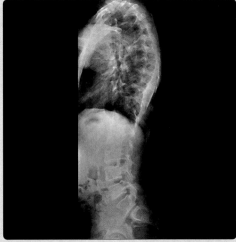

(Left) PA radiograph in an idiopathic scoliosis patient shows the typical curve of idiopathic scoliosis that is convex to the right in the thoracic spine and convex to the left in the lumbar spine. No vertebral anomalies are present, excluding congenital scoliosis. (Right) Lateral radiograph (idiopathic scoliosis) depicts the rotational component of scoliosis, leading to posterior position of the ribs on the left. Thoracic kyphosis is diminished, another characteristic finding.

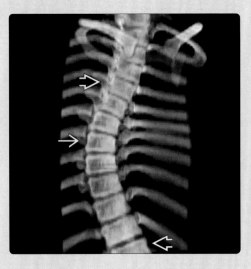

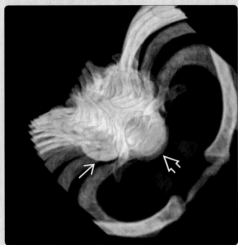

(Left) Anteroposterior 3D reformatted bone CT of idiopathic scoliosis shows rotation as well as scoliosis to be present on the apical vertebra ➡ and terminal vertebrae ⇥. (Right) Axial bone CT 3D reformation demonstrates the rotation of the apical vertebra ➡ compared to the terminal vertebrae ⇥. 3D CT is valuable in surgical planning to evaluate severity of rotation.

TERMINOLOGY

Definitions

- General term for any lateral spine curvature
- Dextroscoliosis: Curve convex to right
- Levoscoliosis: Curve convex to left
- Kyphoscoliosis: Scoliosis with component of kyphosis
- Rotoscoliosis (outdated term): Scoliosis that includes rotation of vertebrae
- S-curve scoliosis: 3 adjacent curves, 1 to right and 1 to left, 1 at lumbosacral junction
- C-curve scoliosis (outdated term): Long sweeping curvature
- Terminal vertebra: Most superior or inferior vertebra included in curve
- Transitional vertebra: Vertebra between 2 curves
- Apical vertebra: Vertebra with greatest lateral displacement from midline
- Primary curvature: Curvature with greatest angulation
- Secondary or compensatory curvature: Smaller curve that balances primary curvature

IMAGING

General Features

- Best diagnostic clue
  - Lateral curvature of spine that returns to midline at ends of curve
- Location
  - Most commonly thoracic or thoracolumbar
- Size
  - Curve > 10°
  - May be > 90°
- Morphology
  - S-curve scoliosis
    - Idiopathic
    - Congenital
    - Syndromic
  - C-curve scoliosis
    - Neuromuscular
    - Neurofibromatosis
    - Scheuermann disease
    - Congenital
    - Syndromic
  - Short-curve scoliosis
    - Tumor
    - Trauma
    - Infection
    - Radiation
    - Congenital
    - Neuropathic

Radiographic Findings

- Radiography
  - Standing PA radiograph of full thoracic and lumbar spine on single cassette (14" x 36")
    - PA projection gives lower radiation dose to breasts than AP
    - Lifts used to equalize limb lengths if needed
  - Method of Cobb is standard for measuring scoliosis
    - Draw lines parallel to endplates of terminal vertebrae
    - If endplates difficult to see, use pedicles as landmarks

- Cobb angle is between terminal endplates
  - Can also measure angle between 2 lines drawn perpendicular to endplates
  - 2nd method is easier with small curves
- Choosing correct vertebrae to measure scoliosis is critical to accuracy and monitoring
  - Terminal vertebra is one with greatest angle of endplate from horizontal
  - Rotoscoliosis: Terminal vertebra spinous process returns to midline
  - Interobserver variability 7-10°
- Coned-down radiographs for better definition of vertebral abnormalities and pedicles
- Lateral radiograph to show sagittal plane abnormalities
  - Usually alters normal thoracic kyphosis, lumbar lordosis
- Estimate rotational deformity by rib displacement on lateral radiograph

CT Findings

- Bone CT
  - Shows congenital bone anomalies, tumor, infection, postoperative complications
  - Not as useful for measuring curves compared with radiography

MR Findings

- Shows bone and spinal cord anomalies, syrinx, tumor, infection

Imaging Recommendations

- Best imaging tool
  - Radiography for initial diagnosis
- Protocol advice
  - Multiplanar MR to screen for bone, cord abnormalities
    - Coronal and sagittal T1WI and T2WI
    - Include craniocervical junction
    - Axial T2WI through areas of suspected abnormality
    - Axial T2WI through conus
  - CT for surgical planning
    - 1- to 3-mm multidetector CT with reformatted images
    - 3D helpful
  - CT for surgical complications
    - Thin, overlapping sections minimize artifact
    - Bone and soft tissue windows

DIFFERENTIAL DIAGNOSIS

Idiopathic Scoliosis

- Classic S-curve scoliosis

Neuromuscular Scoliosis

- Usually long sweeping curvature
- Neurologic disorders
- Muscular dystrophies

Congenital Scoliosis

- Morphology of curve highly variable
  - Focal short curves common
- Due to abnormal vertebral formation and segmentation

Scoliosis Due to Congenital Syndromes Without Vertebral Anomalies

- Often complex curvatures
- Neurofibromatosis
- Marfan
- Osteogenesis imperfecta
- Diastrophic dwarfism
- Ehlers-Danlos syndrome

Scoliosis Due to Infection

- Usually short curve
- Painful
- Systemic signs may be absent
- Pyogenic bacteria, tuberculosis, fungi

Scheuermann Disease

- 15% have scoliosis as well as kyphosis
- Scoliosis usually mild compared to kyphosis

Scoliosis Due to Tumor

- Short curve
- Painful
- Tumor may be occult on radiography
- Multiplanar MR most helpful for evaluation

Scoliosis Due to Trauma

- Usually see posttraumatic deformity
- Stress fracture may be occult cause

Scoliosis Due to Radiation

- Usually avoided today by radiation port placement
- Radiation to entire vertebra rather than portion preferred

Degenerative Scoliosis

- Develops in adults
- Degenerative disc disease, facet arthropathy seen
- Can also have secondary degenerative disease from idiopathic scoliosis

Neuropathic Spine

- Rapidly developing spine deformity
- Bony destruction seen on radiography

Compensatory Scoliosis

- Due to limb length inequality
- Can be diagnosed on frontal spine radiographs by position of iliac crests

Positional Scoliosis

- Poor positioning by radiology technologist
- Present on supine radiographs
- Resolves on upright radiographs

Iatrogenic Scoliosis

- Rib resection
- Level above lumbar fusion
- Hardware failure

PATHOLOGY

General Features

- Etiology
  - Variable, causes listed above

- Epidemiology
  - Common

Gross Pathologic & Surgical Features

- Deformity of trunk visible on physical examination

Staging, Grading, or Classification Criteria

- Etiology
- Direction of curve
- Severity of curve

CLINICAL ISSUES

Presentation

- Most common signs/symptoms
  - Visible truncal deformity
  - Idiopathic scoliosis asymptomatic
  - Painful scoliosis indicates underlying abnormality

Demographics

- Age
  - Usually presents in childhood or adolescence
- Gender
  - Idiopathic M:F = 1:7

Natural History & Prognosis

- Most scoliosis is mild
- May progress rapidly, especially during growth spurts
- Degenerative disc disease common
  - Greatest along concave aspect of scoliosis
- Severe scoliosis
  - Respiratory compromise
  - Neurologic symptoms
  - Instability

Treatment

- Options, risks, complications
  - Observation for minor curves
  - Bracing for curves > 25°
  - Fusion for rapidly progressive curves, curves > 40°

DIAGNOSTIC CHECKLIST

Consider

- Short-curve scoliosis usually has underlying abnormalities

SELECTED REFERENCES

1. Parnell SE et al: Vertical expandable prosthetic titanium rib (VEPTR): a review of indications, normal radiographic appearance and complications. Pediatr Radiol. 45(4):606-16, 2015
2. Ahmed R et al: Long-term incidence and risk factors for development of spinal deformity following resection of pediatric intramedullary spinal cord tumors. J Neurosurg Pediatr. 13(6):613-21, 2014
3. Harris JA et al: A comprehensive review of thoracic deformity parameters in scoliosis. Eur Spine J. 23(12):2594-602, 2014
4. Karami M et al: Evaluation of coronal shift as an indicator of neuroaxial abnormalities in adolescent idiopathic scoliosis: a prospective study. Scoliosis. 9:9, 2014
5. Presciutti SM et al: Management decisions for adolescent idiopathic scoliosis significantly affect patient radiation exposure. Spine J. 14(9):1984-90, 2014
6. Waldt S et al: Measurements and classifications in spine imaging. Semin Musculoskelet Radiol. 18(3):219-27, 2014
7. Arlet V et al: Congenital scoliosis. Eur Spine J. 12(5):456-63, 2003

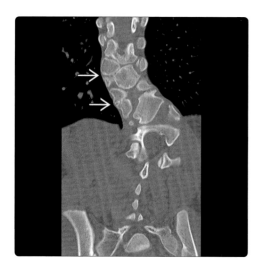

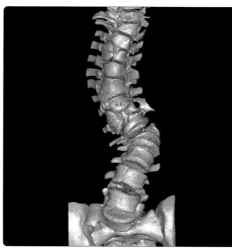

(Left) *Coronal bone CT reveals multiple examples of vertebral segmentation failure. Several right-sided hemivertebra* ➡ *have failed to successfully segment from the adjacent vertebra, producing a jumble of malformed vertebra and multiple-curve scoliosis.* (Right) *Frontal bone CT 3D surface rendering of congenital scoliosis, secondary to multiple vertebral anomalies (same patient), is helpful for fully characterizing contribution of the various anomalous vertebra to scoliosis and kyphosis to facilitate treatment planning.*

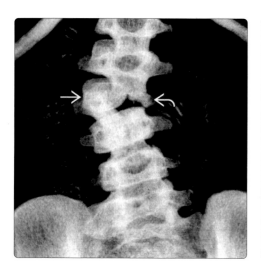

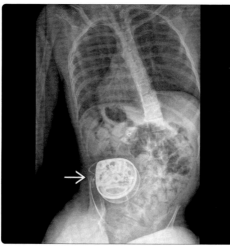

(Left) *Coronal 3D reformatted bone CT reveals a right L3 hemivertebra* ➡ *resulting in convex right congenital scoliosis. There are rudimentary left L3 pedicle and posterior elements* ➡. (Right) *PA radiograph of the thoracolumbar spine demonstrates a long sweeping curvature neuromuscular dextroscoliosis in a cerebral palsy patient. The intrathecal baclofen infusion pump* ➡ *and gastrostomy tube are clues to the diagnosis.*

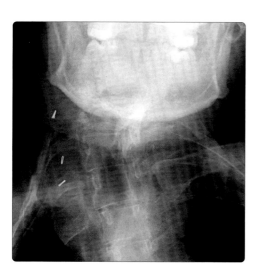

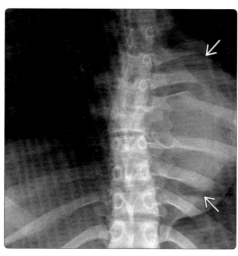

(Left) *Anteroposterior radiograph depicts focal high cervical short-curve scoliosis in a patient with neurofibromatosis type 1. Vascular clips in the right neck reflect the surgical site of prior neurofibroma resection.* (Right) *Anteroposterior radiograph demonstrates a large posterior paraspinal mass* ➡ *causing short-segment, tumor-related scoliosis. Note osseous remodeling of the ipsilateral ribs.*

TERMINOLOGY

- Accentuated thoracic ± reduced normal cervical, lumbar lordotic spinal curvature
- Normal 20-40°, hyperkyphotic if > 40°
- Curvature secondary to vertebral anomalies, degenerative spine disease, or idiopathic causes

IMAGING

- Accentuated dorsal thoracic curvature on lateral image
- Look for vertebral anomalies in patient with scoliosis or kyphosis
- Common in thoracic spine but can occur at any spinal level

TOP DIFFERENTIAL DIAGNOSES

- Scheuermann kyphosis
  - Wedging of 3 or more vertebral bodies, undulation of endplates
- Idiopathic kyphosis
  - Vertebral anomalies absent

- Kyphosis or scoliosis due to syndromes
  - Neurofibromatosis type 1
  - Marfan syndrome
  - Osteogenesis imperfecta
- Traumatic kyphosis
- Osteomyelitis, granulomatous

PATHOLOGY

- May be congenital or acquired
- Congenital abnormalities due either to failure of development &/or failure of segmentation

CLINICAL ISSUES

- May be isolated anomaly or associated with multisystem anomalies (VACTERL)

DIAGNOSTIC CHECKLIST

- Image entire spine (particularly in children) to exclude additional bone or cord abnormalities, Chiari 1 malformation

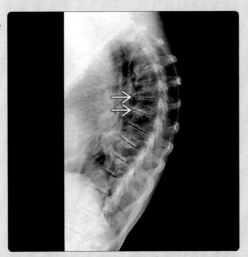
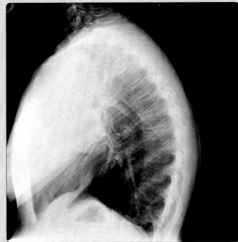

(Left) Lateral radiograph demonstrates smoothly curved thoracic kyphosis with premature upper thoracic degenerative disc disease ➡ in this patient with degenerative kyphosis. (Right) Lateral chest radiograph (idiopathic kyphosis) reveals diffuse upper thoracic kyphosis with a round-back deformity. There is no underlying cause of kyphosis (e.g., Scheuermann disease, prior trauma, congenital anomaly, or infection).

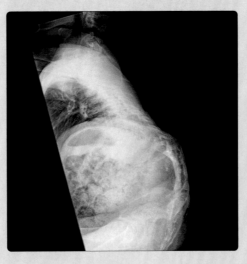
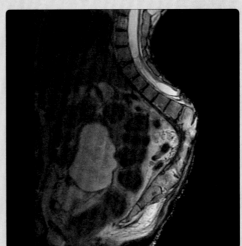

(Left) Lateral radiograph (repaired high myelomeningocele, congenital vertebral segmentation failure with kyphosis) depicts severe focal lumbosacral kyphotic curvature. There is also posterior spinal dysraphism and segmentation failure of the lumbar and sacral vertebra associated with kyphosis. (Right) Sagittal T2WI MR (same patient) reveals distal spinal cord attenuation at the thoracolumbar junction myelomeningocele repair site. Note extensive congenital vertebral anomalies.

TERMINOLOGY

Definitions

- Accentuated thoracic ± reduced normal cervical, lumbar lordotic spinal curvature
  - Spinal curvature secondary to vertebral anomalies, degenerative spine disease, or idiopathic causes

IMAGING

General Features

- Best diagnostic clue
  - Accentuated dorsal thoracic spine curvature on lateral image
  - Vertebral anomaly in patient with scoliosis or kyphosis
- Location
  - Most common in thoracic spine but can occur at any spinal level

Radiographic Findings

- Accentuated dorsal curvature of thoracic spine &/or reduced lordotic curvature of cervical, lumbar spine

CT Findings

- Improved visualization of anomalous vertebrae compared with radiographs
- Coronal and sagittal reformatted images essential
  - Helps confirm abnormal curvature and better demonstrates osseous abnormalities in osteopenic patients
  - 3D imaging helpful for surgical planning

MR Findings

- Similar to CT but better demonstrates spinal cord, soft tissues

Imaging Recommendations

- Best imaging tool
  - CT preferable for surgical planning in adults because of superior spatial resolution
  - Multiplanar MR best modality to evaluate full spine in children

DIFFERENTIAL DIAGNOSIS

Scheuermann Kyphosis

- Wedging of 3 or more vertebral bodies, undulation of endplates
- 15% have scoliosis as well as kyphosis

Idiopathic Kyphosis

- Vertebral anomalies absent

Kyphosis or Scoliosis Due to Syndromes

- Neurofibromatosis type 1
- Marfan syndrome
- Osteogenesis imperfecta
- Diastrophic dwarfism
- Ehlers-Danlos syndrome

Traumatic Kyphosis

- Short-curve kyphosis, vertebral body deformity

Osteomyelitis, Granulomatous

- Paraspinous cold abscess, endplate destruction
- Kyphosis may be severe (gibbus) deformity

PATHOLOGY

General Features

- Genetics
  - Sometimes associated with chromosomal abnormalities
- Associated abnormalities
  - Spinal cord abnormalities
    - Syringohydromyelia
    - Diastematomyelia
    - Tethered cord
  - Caudal regression
  - Component of VACTERL association

CLINICAL ISSUES

Presentation

- Most common signs/symptoms
  - Visible spinal axis deformity
- Clinical profile
  - May be isolated anomaly or associated with multisystem anomalies (VACTERL)

Demographics

- Age
  - Congenital kyphosis present at birth but may not be evident clinically until later in childhood or adolescence
  - Acquired kyphosis usually adolescence to adulthood
- Gender
  - M = F
- Epidemiology
  - Sporadic, relatively uncommon

Natural History & Prognosis

- Congenital kyphosis
  - Kyphosis tends to progress without treatment; fusion during childhood indicated
- Degenerative kyphosis frequently progressive
- Scheuermann kyphosis frequently progressive

Treatment

- Brace is of limited utility
- Fusion of congenital kyphosis to prevent paralysis

DIAGNOSTIC CHECKLIST

Image Interpretation Pearls

- Lateral radiography usually adequate to measure curvature
  - CT may be necessary in osteopenic patients
- Image entire spine to exclude additional bone or cord abnormalities, Chiari 1 malformation in children especially

SELECTED REFERENCES

1. Ansari SF et al: Dorsal midline hemivertebra at the lumbosacral junction: report of 2 cases. J Neurosurg Spine. 22(1):84-9, 2015
2. Cho W et al: The prevalence of abnormal preoperative neurological examination in Scheuermann kyphosis: correlation with X-ray, magnetic resonance imaging, and surgical outcome. Spine (Phila Pa 1976). 39(21):1771-6, 2014

Degenerative Scoliosis

TERMINOLOGY

- Lateral curvature in spine due to degenerative disc and facet disease in older patients
- Deformity in skeletally mature patient with Cobb angle of > 10° in coronal plane
- Predominance of lower lumbar curves

IMAGING

- Conventional standing full-length PA and lateral radiographs for monitoring curve progression
- Most common from L1 to L4
  - Lateral listhesis, vertebral rotation
  - Disc space loss, endplate sclerosis
  - Circumferential endplate spurring
  - Facet arthropathy
  - Spondylolisthesis, loss of lordosis

TOP DIFFERENTIAL DIAGNOSES

- Adult idiopathic scoliosis

- Neuromuscular
- Congenital scoliosis
- Posttraumatic, inflammatory, or neoplastic
- Dysplasias (neurofibromatosis type 1, Marfan)

PATHOLOGY

- Asymmetric degenerative change at multiple levels
  - Asymmetric loading of spinal segments gives 3-dimensional deformity
  - Spondylolisthesis &/or rotatory listhesis

CLINICAL ISSUES

- Low back pain, radiculopathy
  - Pain worse with prolonged spinal extension
  - Radiculopathy not reliably relieved by flexion
- Risk factors for curve progression
  - Cobb angle > 30°
  - Lateral listhesis > 6 mm
  - > 30° apical vertebral rotation

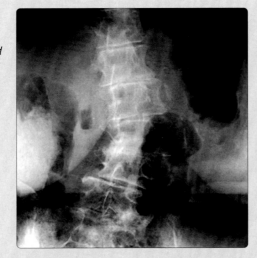
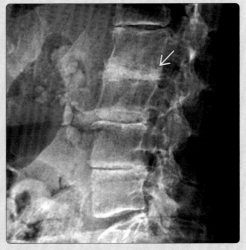

(Left) Anteroposterior radiography shows lumbar rotatory levoscoliosis with associated multilevel marked disc height loss and endplate sclerosis. There is left lateral listhesis of L4 on L5. (Right) Lateral radiography shows loss of lumbar lordosis with multilevel disc space height loss and degenerative endplate bony eburnation, worst at L2-L3 ➡.

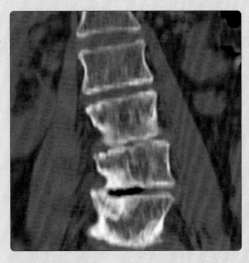
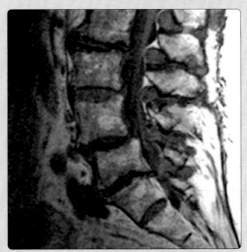

(Left) Coronal reformation of nonenhanced lumbar spine CT shows mild levoscoliosis at L4-L5 with vacuum disc phenomenon and right-sided endplate sclerosis. There is disc height loss at L3-L4 and L4-L5. (Right) Sagittal T1WI MR shows grade 1 anterolisthesis of L4 on L5 with severe disc degeneration and vacuum phenomenon. Degenerative disc and endplate disease is also present at L2-L3 and L5-S1. There is severe central stenosis at L4-L5 and L5-S1.

TERMINOLOGY

- Spinal fusion surgery recommended when curve magnitude > 40-45° for adolescent idiopathic scoliosis
- Adult scoliosis presents with lumbar back, ± leg pain, L3–L4 rotatory subluxation, L4–L5 tilt, and L5–S1 disc degeneration on radiographs

IMAGING

- Radiographs
  - Main thoracic, thoracolumbar, and lumbar curves should be assessed for structural characteristics
  - 36" standing AP and lateral radiographs and supine side-bending radiographs
  - In adult scoliosis, assess for degenerated changes and rotatory ± lateral listhesis
- CT
  - Assess integrity of instrumentation
  - Look for osseous bridging at levels of interbody fusion and lucency along screw tracks

- MR
  - Preoperative planning to evaluate for central &/or foraminal stenosis and disc degeneration

CLINICAL ISSUES

- Adult bones tend to be weaker or osteoporotic, making instrumentation and fusion more difficult
- Degenerative disc changes, spinal stenosis, and facet arthropathy can be exacerbated and in turn exacerbate scoliosis, leading to more rigid spines
- Goals: Prevent progression, restore acceptability of clinical deformity, reduce curvature
  - Resolve pain ± make it more controllable with medications
  - Fuse spine in as normal anatomical position as possible
  - Since degenerated lumbar curves present with loss of lordosis, surgical plan should specifically address this issue

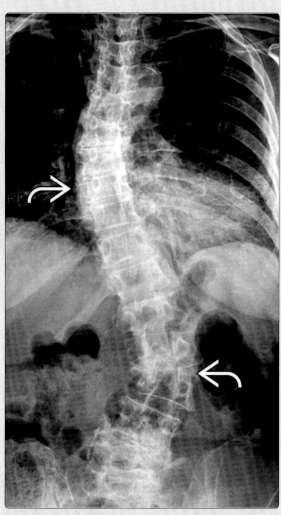

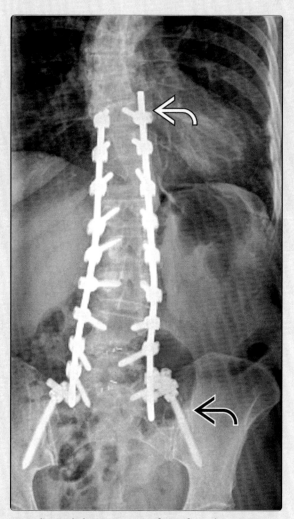

Anteroposterior radiograph shows sigmoid scoliosis of the thoracic and lumbar spines ➔. Fusion is extended to L5 if there is fixed tilt or subluxation at L4–L5, or to the sacrum if L5-S1 central or foraminal decompression is needed.

AP radiograph depicts posterior fusion from the thoracolumbar junction ➔ to sacrum. Extension of fusion to the sacrum increases the incidence of pseudarthrosis and reoperation. Instrumentation into iliac ➔ protects L5-S1 construct and decreases pseudoarthrosis.

Spondylolisthesis

TERMINOLOGY

- Anterolisthesis: Anterior displacement of vertebral body relative to one below
- Retrolisthesis: Posterior displacement of vertebral body relative to one below

IMAGING

- Lateral flexion and extension to evaluate for instability
  - Napoleon's hat sign on AP plain film
  - Instability uncommon in degenerative listhesis
    - 90% of normal volunteers show 1- to 3-mm translation on flexion-extension radiographs
- Spondylolysis may be difficult to identify on MR
  - T1-weighted sagittal images critical
  - CT for definitive diagnosis of subtle fracture

PATHOLOGY

- Degenerative (DS)
  - Degenerative retrolisthesis associated with disc degeneration
  - Sagittal oriented facets more likely to have DS
- Spondylolysis (isthmic)
  - Bilateral in 80%
- Postsurgical: Loss of posterior element stability
- Dysplastic: Small L5 body leading to pars lysis
- Trauma: Severe to produce vertebral body displacement
- Pathologic: Underlying tumor with instability

CLINICAL ISSUES

- **9.2% overall complication rate for treatment of spondylolisthesis**
  - Complications related to higher grade spondylolisthesis, DS > isthmic, older age (> 65)
- DS + stenosis treated surgically show greater improvement in pain and function over 4 years compared to nonsurgical treatment

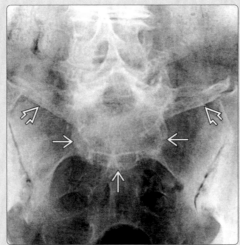

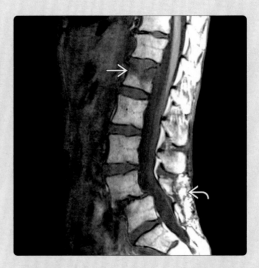

(Left) *Anteroposterior radiograph shows the Napoleon's hat sign. The hat is inverted with the crown* ➡ *representing the anterior cortex of the vertebral body and the brim* ➡ *being the transverse processes.* (Right) *Sagittal T1WI MR shows postoperative spondylolisthesis following lumbar laminectomy* ➡. *There is advanced degenerative changes of the L4-L5 intervertebral disc space with anterior subluxation of L4 on L5. Note the acute superior endplate compression fracture of L1* ➡.

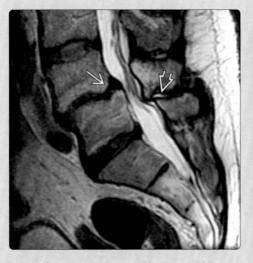

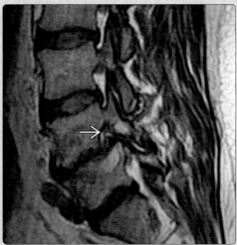

(Left) *Sagittal T2WI MR shows grade I spondylolisthesis of L4 on L5* ➡ *with intervertebral disc degeneration and associated fatty endplate change. There is also degeneration of the interspinous ligament* ➡. (Right) *Sagittal T2WI MR shows a grade I spondylolisthesis of L4 on L5 with resultant severe foraminal stenosis* ➡.

Instability

TERMINOLOGY

- Loss of spine motion segment stiffness, when applied force produces greater displacement than normal, with pain/deformity

IMAGING

- Deformity, which increases with motion and time
- Various parameters used for degenerative instability by plain films
  - Dynamic slip > 3 mm in flexion/extension
  - Static slip of ≥ 4.5 mm
  - Angulation > 10-15° suggests need for surgical intervention
- Flexion/extension plain films best for definition of motion

TOP DIFFERENTIAL DIAGNOSES

- Pseudoarthrosis
- Infection
  - Endplate destruction, disc T2 hyperintensity

- Tumor
  - Enhancing soft tissue mass
- Postoperative
  - Following multilevel laminectomy or facetectomy

PATHOLOGY

- Degenerative instabilities
  - Axial rotational
  - Translational; plain films show spondylolisthesis, traction spurs, vacuum phenomenon
  - Retrolisthesis; plain films show increased retrolisthesis with extension
  - Degenerative scoliosis
  - Post laminectomy; resection of 50% of bilateral facets alters segmental stiffness
  - Post fusion; altered biomechanics

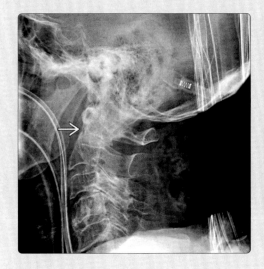

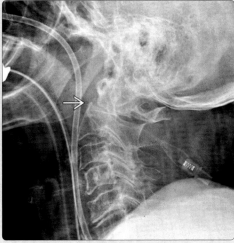

(Left) Lateral radiograph shows a fracture through the base of the odontoid ➡, which shows satisfactory alignment in the neutral position. (Right) Lateral radiograph shows a fracture through the base of the odontoid, which displaces posteriorly with slight extension ➡. This patient underwent occiput to C3 fusion.

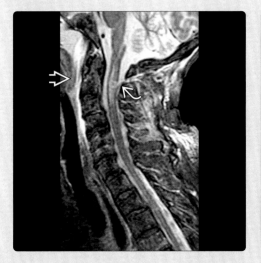

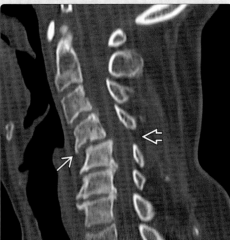

(Left) Sagittal STIR MR shows extensive prevertebral edema ➡ in this patient with a type II odontoid fracture. There is cord edema and focal cord hemorrhage seen as slight hypointensity ➡. (Right) CT study 3 months after trauma shows new instability and subluxation of C4 on C5 ➡ with a kyphotic deformity and widening of the posterior elements ➡. The initial study showed normal alignment.

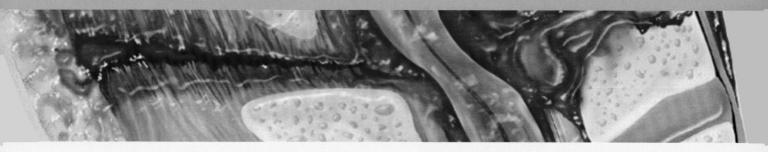

SECTION 5
Trauma

Vertebral Column, Discs

Cord, Dura, and Vessels

Craniocervical Junction

Occipital condyle fractures are classified into 3 types.
- Type I = comminuted fractures due to axial loading; stable if contralateral side is intact
- Type II = occipital condyle fracture with skull base fractures; most of these are stable
- Type III = avulsion fracture due to tensile force on alar ligaments; may show occipitocervical instability

Recent data (Maserati 2009) suggests that initial evaluation should be primarily concerned with identification of craniocervical malalignment. Fusion or halo used in patients with initial scans show fracture and malalignment with rigid cervical collar with delayed imaging follow-up for all others.

Atlantooccipital Disassociation (Dislocation)/C0-C1 Distraction Injury

Complete (disassociation) or partial (subluxation) ligamentous disruption between occiput and C1, which can occur in 1 of 3 directions: (1) Anterior superior displacement of cranium relative to spine most common; (2) pure distraction injury with superior displacement of cranium; or (3) posterior dislocation of cranium which is least common.

Numerous measurement techniques have been used to assess craniovertebral junction trauma, many of which were 1st defined in the plain film era. Many of these measurements have been superseded by the direct soft tissue visualization afforded by CT and MR. There is reasonable literature support for use of the following measurements.

Basion-dental interval (BDI) is abnormal if > 10 mm on sagittal CT.

Summed condylar displacement (sum of the bilateral distances between midpoint of occipital condyle and C1 condylar fossa) is abnormal if > 4.2 mm.

Single side condylar distance measurement of > 2 mm is also considered abnormal in adults. The 2-mm upper limit of C0-C1 spacing also applies to children up to 18 years of age.

Other measurements such as the Powers ratio and Lee lines do not have sufficient sensitivity and specificity to recommend their use. The Harris "rule of 12" for the BDI and basion-axial interval are for plain film use only and so are very limited given the use of CT for acute trauma evaluation.

C1 Fractures
- Anterior arch = vertical or transverse with avulsion from longus colli
- Anterior arch bilateral fractures with posterior atlantoaxial dislocation = plow fracture
- Lateral mass = stable if lateral ring intact; rare
- Posterior arch = common
- Jefferson = combined lateral mass displacement relative to C2 of 6.9 mm indicates disruption of transverse ligament and potential for instability

Atlantoaxial Instability
- Nonphysiologic motion between C1-C2
- Wide variety of causes
- → transverse ligament rupture (most common)
- → odontoid fracture
- → unstable Jefferson fracture
- → fracture of lateral mass of C1 or C2
- → unilateral alar ligament rupture
- → alar and tectorial membrane rupture

Classification of Atlantoaxial Rotatory Fixation (Fielding 1977)
- Type I = rotation about dens without anterior translation [no increase in atlantodental interval (ADI)]
- Type II = rotation about 1 lateral mass with anterior translation of 3-5 mm (ADI) (transverse ligament injury)
- Type III = rotation about lateral mass with anterior translation > 5 mm (transverse and alar ligament injury)
- Type IV = posterior dislocation of C1 behind dens (rare, usually fatal)

Odontoid
- Type I = avulsion at tip of odontoid
- Type II = transverse fracture of dens above C2 body
- Type III = fracture involving superior portion of C2 body

C2 Ring Fractures (Effendi 1981)
- Type I = bilateral pars fractures with < 3-mm anterior subluxation (stable)
- Type II = displacement of pars fracture + anterior translation of C2 with discoligamentous injury
- Type III = pars fractures with C2-C3 facet dislocations

C2 Body Fractures (Fujimura 1996)
- Type I = extension teardrop fracture of anterior inferior endplate of C2
- Type II = horizontal shear fracture through body (more caudal than type III odontoid fracture)
- Type III = C2 body burst fracture
- Type IV = unstable sagittal cleavage fractures

Cervical Fracture Classification

Hyperflexion
- Simple compression fracture
- Anterior subluxation = posterior ligament disruption
- Bilateral interfacetal dislocation = unstable
- Flexion teardrop fracture = unstable
- Clay shoveler's fracture: Avulsion of spinous process of C7-T1

Hyperflexion and Rotation
- Unilateral facet dislocation (locked facet)
- May have associated facet fracture
- Radiograph shows forward displacement of vertebra < 1/2 AP diameter of cervical vertebral body

Hyperextension and Rotation
- Pillar fracture

Vertical Compression
- Jefferson fracture = fractures of both anterior and posterior rings with 2, 3, or 4 parts with radial displacement
- Burst fracture = middle column involvement with bony retropulsion

Hyperextension
- Hyperextension dislocation
- C1 anterior arch avulsion fracture = longus colli insertion around anterior tubercle of C1
- Extension teardrop fracture of C2
- C1 posterior arch fracture = compressed between occiput and C2 spinous process
- Lamina fracture = between articular mass and spinous process
- Hangman's fracture = bilateral pars fractures of C2
- Hyperextension fracture: Dislocation = bilateral facet fracture ± dislocation

Lateral Flexion
- Uncinate process fracture

Subaxial Cervical Spine Injury Classification (Vaccaro 2007)
- 3 major components including morphology of spinal column disruption, integrity of discoligamentous complex, and neurologic status
- Within each component, subgroups are graded from least to most severe

Thoracolumbar Fracture Classification

Holdsworth 2 Column Model (1963)
- Superseded by Denis classification
- Anterior column = anterior longitudinal ligament (ALL), vertebral body, disc, posterior longitudinal ligament (PLL)
- Posterior column = skeletal and ligamentous structures posterior to PLL

Denis 3 Column Model (1983)
- Anterior = ALL, anulus, anterior vertebral body
- Middle = posterior wall of vertebral body, anulus, PLL
- Posterior = facets, posterior elements, posterior ligaments
- 3 column model also relevant to lower cervical injuries

Denis Subclassification of Burst Fracture (1984)
- **Denis type A**
- Axial load force; anterior and middle columns involved, unstable
- Upper and lower endplates involved
- **Denis types B and C**
- Flexion and axial load, anterior and middle columns, possibly unstable
- B upper endplate involved (most common)
- C lower endplate involved
- **Denis type D**
- Axial load and rotation, all columns, unstable
- Atlas modification of D injuries (1986)
- D1 burst lateral translation, D2 burst sagittal translation
- **Denis type E**
- Lateral compression, all columns, possibly unstable

Magerl AO Pathomorphologic System (1994)
- A, B, C types reflecting common injury patterns
- Each type has 3 groups, each with 3 subgroups (3-3-3 scheme)
- Type A vertebral compression fractures due to axial loading without soft tissue disruption in transverse plane (66%)
- Type B distraction of anterior and posterior elements with soft tissue disruption in axial plane (14.5%)
- Type C with axial torque forces giving anterior and posterior element disruption with rotation (19%)
- Severity progresses through types A to C as well as within types, groups, and subdivisions
- Stable type A1 most common (wedge fracture)
- A3 corresponds to burst fracture of Denis classification
- Unstable = A3.2, A3.3, B, C types

McCormack "Load-Sharing" Classification (1994)
- Specifically designed to evaluate need for anterior column reconstruction following pedicle screw stabilization
- Also useful as more generic guide to magnitude of comminution and biomechanical instability
- Comminution graded

- → amount of vertebral of body damage
- → fragment of spread at fracture site
- → degree of corrected kyphosis

Thoracolumbar Injury Classification and Severity Score (TLICS) (Vaccaro 2006)
- 3 components give final numeric score that directs treatment
- Injury mechanism, integrity of posterior ligamentous complex, and neurologic status

Unstable Fractures

Cervical
- Atlantoaxial dissociation
- Atlantooccipital dislocation
- Occipital condyle fracture with malalignment
- Jefferson fracture where combined offset of C1 lateral masses > 7 mm or > 7 mm separation of fracture fragments
- Hangman II, III
- Odontoid types I, II
- Subaxial anterior subluxation of > 3.5 mm
- Hyperflexion fracture dislocation
- Hyperflexion teardrop
- Hyperextension fracture dislocation
- Burst

Selected References

1. Pizones J et al: Prospective analysis of magnetic resonance imaging accuracy in diagnosing traumatic injuries of the posterior ligamentous complex of the thoracolumbar spine. Spine (Phila Pa 1976). 38(9):745-51, 2013
2. Walters BC et al: Guidelines for the management of acute cervical spine and spinal cord injuries: 2013 update. Neurosurgery. 60 Suppl 1:82-91, 2013
3. Vaccaro AR et al: The subaxial cervical spine injury classification system: a novel approach to recognize the importance of morphology, neurology, and integrity of the disco-ligamentous complex. Spine (Phila Pa 1976). 32(21):2365-74, 2007
4. Vaccaro AR et al: Reliability of a novel classification system for thoracolumbar injuries: the Thoracolumbar Injury Severity Score. Spine (Phila Pa 1976). 31(11 Suppl):S62-9; discussion S104, 2006
5. Vaccaro AR et al: A new classification of thoracolumbar injuries: the importance of injury morphology, the integrity of the posterior ligamentous complex, and neurologic status. Spine (Phila Pa 1976). 30(20):2325-33, 2005
6. Leone A et al: Occipital condylar fractures: a review. Radiology. 216(3):635-44, 2000
7. Oner FC et al: MRI findings of thoracolumbar spine fractures: a categorisation based on MRI examinations of 100 fractures. Skeletal Radiol. 28(8):433-43, 1999
8. Brandser EA et al: Thoracic and lumbar spine trauma. Radiol Clin North Am. 35(3):533-57, 1997
9. Vollmer DG et al: Classification and acute management of thoracolumbar fractures. Neurosurg Clin N Am. 8(4):499-507, 1997
10. Dickman CA et al: Injuries involving the transverse atlantal ligament: classification and treatment guidelines based upon experience with 39 injuries. Neurosurgery. 38(1):44-50, 1996
11. Fujimura Y et al: Classification and treatment of axis body fractures. J Orthop Trauma. 10(8):536-40, 1996
12. Noble ER et al: The forgotten condyle: the appearance, morphology, and classification of occipital condyle fractures. AJNR Am J Neuroradiol. 17(3):507-13, 1996
13. Benzel EC et al: Fractures of the C-2 vertebral body. J Neurosurg. 81(2):206-12, 1994
14. Magerl F et al: A comprehensive classification of thoracic and lumbar injuries. Eur Spine J. 3(4):184-201, 1994
15. McCormack T et al: The load sharing classification of spine fractures. Spine (Phila Pa 1976). 19(15):1741-4, 1994
16. Atlas SW et al: The radiographic characterization of burst fractures of the spine. AJR Am J Roentgenol. 147(3):575-82, 1986
17. Denis F: The three column spine and its significance in the classification of acute thoracolumbar spinal injuries. Spine (Phila Pa 1976). 8(8):817-31, 1983

Subaxial Cervical Spine Injury Classification

	Description	Points
Morphology		
	No abnormality	0
	Compression	1
	Burst	+ 1 = 2
	Distraction (perched facet, hyperextension)	3
	Rotation/translation (facet dislocation, unstable teardrop)	4
Discoligamentous Complex		
	Intact	0
	Indeterminate (MR signal abnormality only, isolated interspinous widening)	1
	Disrupted	2
Neuro Status		
	Intact	0
	Root injury	1
	Complete cord injury	2
	Incomplete cord injury (most urgent situation so higher value than complete injury	3
	Continuous cord compression in setting of neuro deficit (modifier)	+ 1

Surgical vs. nonsurgical is determined by the total score: 1-3 nonoperative treatment, ≥ 5 operative treatment recommended. (Vaccaro 2007.)

Thoracolumbar Injury Severity Score

	Description	Qualifier	Points
Injury Mechanism			
	Compression		
		Simple	1
		Lateral angulation >15°	1
		Burst	1
	Transitional/rotational		3
	Distraction		4
Posterior Ligamentous Complex			
	Intact		0
	Suspected/indeterminate for disruption		2
	Injured		3
Neuro Status			
	Nerve root involvement		2
	Cord, conus involvement (incomplete)		3
	Cauda equina involvement		3
	Cord, conus involvement (complete)		2

The score is a total of 3 components. A score ≤ 3 suggests nonoperative treatment, while a score of 4 is indeterminate. A score ≥ 5 suggests operative treatment. For injury mechanism, the worst level is used, and the injury is additive. An example is distraction injury with burst without angulation is 1 (simple compression) + 1 (burst) + 4 (distraction) = 6 points. (Vaccaro 2006.)

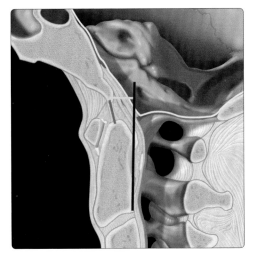

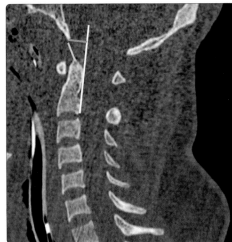

(Left) *Sagittal graphic shows a normal basion-dental interval (BDI) (red line) and basion-posterior axial line interval (BAI) (yellow line). BAI is the distance from the basion to posterior axial line (black line). BDI is abnormal if > 10 mm on sagittal CT. BAI is abnormal if > 12 mm on plain films.* (Right) *Sagittal NECT of a trauma patient with atlantooccipital dislocation shows abnormal distance between basion & dens (yellow) & abnormal separation of basion from posterior axial line (orange). Posterior axial reference line is white.*

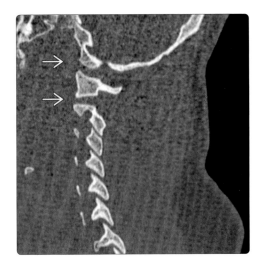

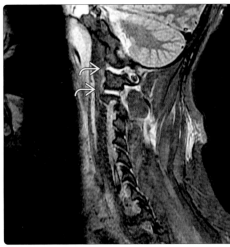

(Left) *Parasagittal NECT in a patient with atlantooccipital dislocation shows widening of both C0-C1 and C1-C2 articulations ➡. Summed condylar displacement (sum of the bilateral distances between midpoint of occipital condyle and C1 condylar fossa) is abnormal if > 4.2 mm.* (Right) *Sagittal STIR MR shows abnormally widened and hyperintense C0-C1 and C1-C2 articulations ➡. This patient underwent occiput to C3 posterior fusion for atlantooccipital and atlantoaxial dislocation.*

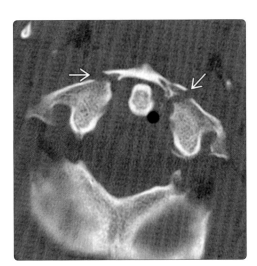

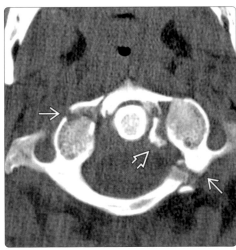

(Left) *Axial NECT shows multiple fracture sites involving the C1 ring ➡ without canal compromise.* (Right) *Axial NECT shows fractures involving both anterior and posterior rings of C1 ➡ and an additional avulsion fracture off of the mesial C1 ring at the level of attachment of transverse ligament ➡.*

(Left) *Coronal graphic of the C2 vertebra shows the schematic for the location of types I, II, and III odontoid fractures.* **(Right)** *Coronal NECT shows an oblique type III fracture extending across the base of odontoid and the upper body of C2* ➡ *with fragmentation of the left lateral mass of C2.*

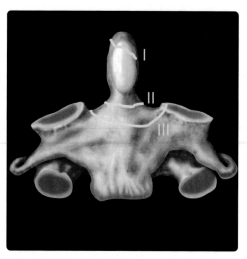
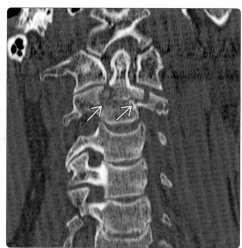

(Left) *Sagittal NECT shows a C2 pars fracture* ➡ *without significant offset, angulation, or distraction.* **(Right)** *Axial bone CT shows a typical case of traumatic C2 pars fractures in a classic hangman configuration. This patient demonstrates the mildest class of injury (type I) using the Levine and Edwards modification of the Effendi classification system and would be considered a stable fracture.*

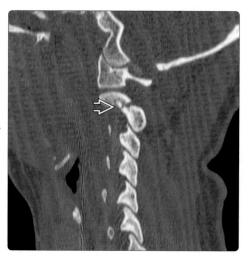
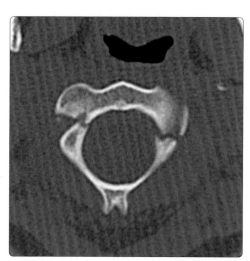

(Left) *Sagittal graphic shows an unstable cervical hyperflexion injury involving anterior* ➡ *and posterior longitudinal ligaments* ➡, *a disc, and interspinous ligaments* ➡ *with epidural hemorrhage and cord compression.* **(Right)** *Lateral radiograph shows C4-C5 flexion facet dislocation with bilateral "jumped" facets. There is disruption of all 3 columns by this injury.*

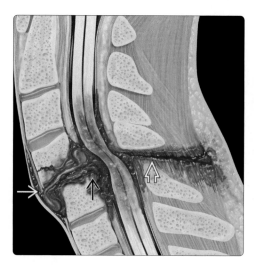
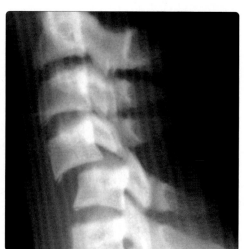

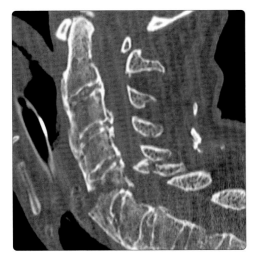

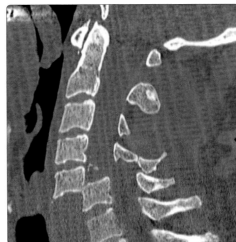

(Left) *Sagittal NECT of transverse extension fracture in a patient with ankylosing spondylitis (AS) shows a horizontal fracture line extending through the C5 body into the base of the spinous process with posterior displacement of the superior aspect of the fracture, indicating hyperextension mechanism. Note typical anterior ossification of AS.* (Right) *Sagittal NECT shows complete dislocation of the upper cervical spine at the C5-C6 level. There is over 100% listhesis of the C5 body relative to C6.*

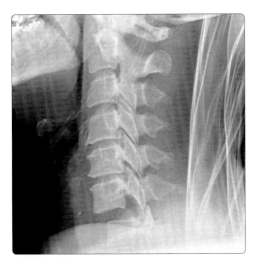

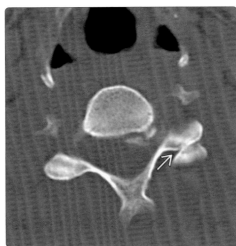

(Left) *Lateral radiograph shows a hyperflexion injury with bilateral locked facets, a widened disc space, anterior subluxation of C6 on C7 of 50%, and a widened spinous process distance.* (Right) *Axial bone CT shows unilateral left facet dislocation ➡. There is reversed relationship of the facets with the inferior articular facet of C6 lying anterior to the superior articular facet of C7 (back-to-back apposition).*

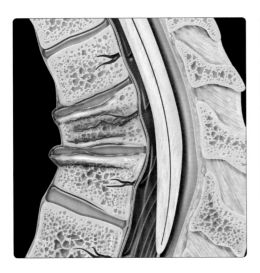

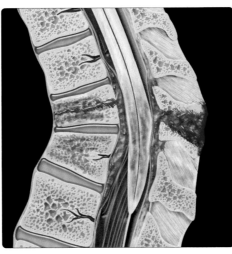

(Left) *Sagittal graphic of the thoracolumbar junction shows compression (wedge) fractures involving primarily the anterior column with normal middle and posterior columns.* (Right) *Sagittal graphic shows a Chance (seat belt) fracture of the thoracolumbar junction extending in the horizontal plane through the body and posterior elements (3-column involvement).*

TERMINOLOGY

- Disruption of stabilizing ligaments between occiput and C1

IMAGING

- Widened prevertebral soft tissues (nonspecific)
- Condylar sum > 4.2 mm has 100% sensitivity, 69% specificity, and 76% accuracy
- Increased basion-dens interval (BDI) distance > 8.5 mm (CT in adults)
- Widened unilateral atlantooccipital interval > 2 mm
  - Widened, fluid-filled facet joints between condyles and C1
- STIR/T2WI MR best show ligamentous injury

TOP DIFFERENTIAL DIAGNOSES

- Occipital condyle fracture
- C1 Jefferson fracture
- Odontoid fracture
- Rheumatoid arthritis, adult

PATHOLOGY

- High-speed motor vehicle accident
- Associated injuries
  - Brainstem and cranial nerve injury
  - Fractures of occipital condyles, C1 and C2

CLINICAL ISSUES

- < 1% of acute cervical spine injuries
- Often immediately fatal; however, may have good outcome with recognition and fixation

DIAGNOSTIC CHECKLIST

- No imaging sign 100% sensitive
- Condylar sum > 4.2 mm most sensitive CT sign of atlantooccipital dislocation
- Powers ratio not recommended (has low sensitivity and specificity)
- Detection of subarachnoid hemorrhage at craniocervical junction should direct search for atlantooccipital injuries

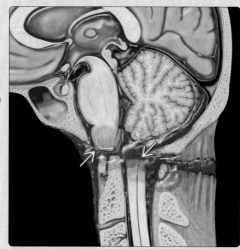
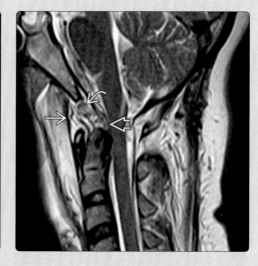

(Left) Sagittal graphic depicts fatal atlantooccipital dissociation with cord transection ➡ at the craniocervical junction. Stretch injury to the spinal cord may occur, resulting in neurologic dysfunction. (Right) Sagittal T2WI MR exhibits extensive abnormality with thinning and irregularity of the tectorial membrane ➡. The anterior atlantooccipital membrane is irregular and stretched anteriorly ➡. Abnormal soft tissue in the supraodontoid space ➡ suggests injury to the apical & alar ligaments.

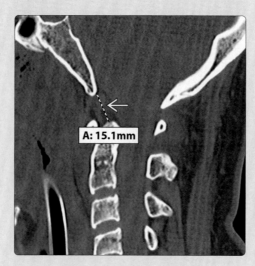
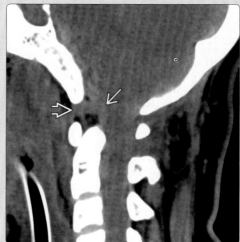

(Left) Sagittal CT reconstruction illustrates an increase in the basion-dens interval (BDI) ➡. The normal distance by CT is ≤ 8.5 mm in adults, or 12 mm on lateral radiographs. (Right) Sagittal CT in a soft tissue algorithm exhibits hyperdense blood products in the ventral epidural space ➡. Abnormal soft tissue is also observed in the supraodontoid space ➡, compatible with hemorrhage along the ligaments. Rupture of both the tectorial membrane and alar ligament are necessary for AOD to occur.

A: 15.1mm

TERMINOLOGY

Abbreviations

- Atlantooccipital dislocation (AOD)

Definitions

- Disruption of stabilizing ligaments between occiput and C1 ± between C1 and C2

IMAGING

General Features

- Best diagnostic clue
  - Widening between occipital condyles and C1
  - Increased distance between basion and dens
- Location
  - Axial distraction across craniocervical junction (CCJ) can produce either atlantooccipital or atlantoaxial dislocation

CT Findings

- Widened unilateral atlantooccipital interval > 2 mm
  - Normal range 0.5-1.8 mm in adults (wider in children)
    - 1.4 mm (max for 97.5% of population)
  - Condylar sum > 4.2 mm has 100% sensitivity, 69% specificity, and 76% accuracy
- Midline occiput to C1 spinolaminar line > 4.2 mm
  - May be artifactually shortened due to extension positioning in collar
- Basion-dens interval (BDI) range 1.4-9.1 mm
  - Normal < 8.5 mm (max for 97.5% of population) in adults
- Anterior or posterior position of C1 relative to basion
  - Incongruity of occiput-C1 facet joints well seen on sagittal images
- Avulsion fracture of occipital condyle or anterior arch of C1
- Subarachnoid hemorrhage at CCJ is associated with AOD, & its detection should direct search for atlantooccipital injuries

MR Findings

- STIR, T2WI best shows ligamentous injury
  - Tectorial membrane disruption seen in 71% of 1 series of 16 pediatric patients
  - Nonvisualization of apical, alar, and anterior atlantoaxial ligaments
- Widened, fluid-filled facet joints between condyle and C1 > 2 mm
  - May be unilateral
- Vertebral artery injury
- Prevertebral hematoma

Imaging Recommendations

- Best imaging tool
  - CT useful for rapid triage
  - MR better shows extent of ligament injury

DIFFERENTIAL DIAGNOSIS

Occipital Condyle Fracture

- Condyle avulsions may be associated with AOD

Jefferson Fracture of C1

- Often see lateral displacement of C1 lateral masses

Odontoid C2 Fracture

- Type 2 odontoid fracture often results in posterior displacement of dens

Atlantoaxial Rotatory Fixation

- Occiput-C1 facet joints and atlantodental interval are normal

Rheumatoid Arthritis, Adult

- Nontraumatic atlantooccipital instability
  - Pannus destabilizes joints and ligaments

PATHOLOGY

General Features

- Etiology
  - High-speed motor vehicle accident

Staging, Grading, & Classification

- Longitudinal AOD
  - Vertical displacement
- Anterior AOD
  - Skull positioned anterior to C1
- Posterior AOD
  - Skull positioned posterior to C1

CLINICAL ISSUES

Presentation

- Most common signs/symptoms
  - Respiratory failure, cranial nerve and motor deficits
  - 20% have no neurological deficit, need high index of suspicion

Demographics

- Age
  - More common in children
    - Due to relatively large head, horizontal orientation of condyles
- Epidemiology
  - < 1% of acute cervical spine injuries

Natural History & Prognosis

- Often immediately fatal
  - However, with recognition and fixation may have good outcome
- Poor outcomes if basion-dens distance ≥ 16 mm

Treatment

- Occiput to C2 fusion required

DIAGNOSTIC CHECKLIST

Consider

- No imaging sign 100% sensitive
- Condylar sum > 4.2 mm most sensitive CT sign of AOD
- All patients with upper cervical prevertebral soft tissue swelling should undergo CT scan

SELECTED REFERENCES

1. Theodore N et al: The diagnosis and management of traumatic atlanto-occipital dislocation injuries. Neurosurgery. 72 Suppl 2():114-26, 2013
2. Chaput CD et al: Defining and detecting missed ligamentous injuries of the occipitocervical complex. Spine (Phila Pa 1976). 36(9):709-14, 2011

IMAGING

- Conventional radiographs insensitive to ligamentous injury
- CT: Ligamentous disruption may be inferred with varying degrees of success by observing disruption of normal vertebral alignment
- Best imaging method is T2W FS or STIR MR
  - Abnormal T2 hyperintensity or gross discontinuity of spinal ligamentous structure
- Flexion-extension films: Segmental instability
  - > 3.5-mm subluxation
- STIR and T2WI FS to evaluate spinal ligamentous injury
  - Normal ligament should be thin, contiguous, and low in signal intensity on both T1 and T2WI
  - Increased signal within ligamentous structure indicative of edema, hemorrhage, or inflammation (stretch injury, strain, partial tear)
  - Complete discontinuity of ligamentous structure on T2WI indicative of disruption

PATHOLOGY

- Forced motion of vertebral segment beyond limits of tissue elasticity
- Associated abnormalities
  - Spinal instability
  - Traumatic disc herniation
  - Vertebral fractures

CLINICAL ISSUES

- Spinal instability predisposing to progressive deformity or to impingement on spinal cord, nerve roots
  - Instantaneous (instability immediately following injury)
  - Delayed (> 20 days after injury)

DIAGNOSTIC CHECKLIST

- Ventral ligamentous injury of cervical spine without fracture is rare (< 0.7%)

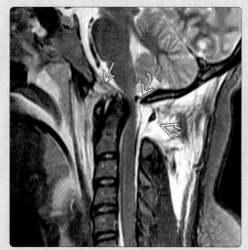
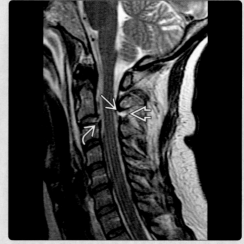

(Left) Sagittal STIR MR shows atlantooccipital dislocation with disruption of the tectoral membrane & alar ligaments ➡ & extensive disruption & edema of posterior interspinous ligaments ➡. Note cord compression due to cranial dislocation ➡. (Right) Sagittal T2 MR of cervical hyperflexion-distraction injury shows hyperintensity of the interspinous ligament ➡ & disruption of both the ligamentum flavum ➡ & posterior longitudinal ligament (PLL) ➡. Thickening & increased signal are seen in prevertebral soft tissues.

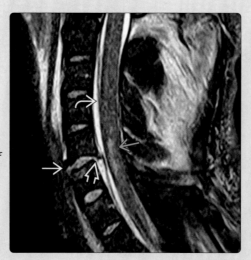
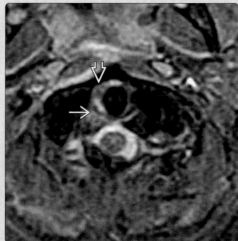

(Left) Sagittal STIR MR shows disruption of the anterior longitudinal ligament ➡ and PLL ➡ as well as posterior displacement of the ventral dural margin ➡ due to epidural hemorrhage. Cord contusion is also present as increased cord signal ➡. (Right) Axial T2* GRE MR at the C1 arch level shows increased signal to the right of the midline in the transverse ligament ➡ due to disruption with mild asymmetric widening of the right dens-lateral mass interval ➡.

Occipital Condyle Fracture

TERMINOLOGY

- Bony disruption of occipital condyle

IMAGING

- Linear, comminuted, or avulsion-type fracture
  - Radiography insensitive
  - CT: Lucency in occipital condyle ± displaced fragment
  - MR: Marrow edema on T1, STIR MR
    - Prevertebral or nuchal ligament edema

TOP DIFFERENTIAL DIAGNOSES

- Accessory ossification center(s)
- Osteomyelitis
- Primary or secondary skull base neoplasm
- Rheumatoid arthritis

PATHOLOGY

- High-energy blunt trauma, most often motor vehicle accident

- Anderson & Montesano classification (1988)
  - Type I: Comminuted condylar fracture without displacement (uncommon)
  - Type II: Extension of linear basilar skull fracture
  - Type III: Avulsion of inferomedial condyle (most common type 75%)

CLINICAL ISSUES

- Presenting symptoms usually related to severity of head injury
  - Most patients have mild/moderate ↓ GCS due to intracranial injury
  - Head injury is main determinant of outcomes
- CN deficit(s) (up to 30%)
- Spasmodic torticollis from concomitant atlantoaxial rotatory fixation

DIAGNOSTIC CHECKLIST

- Easy fracture to overlook in severely injured trauma patients

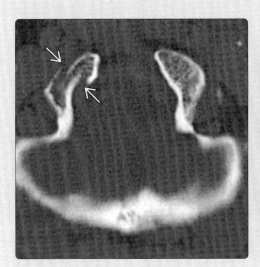
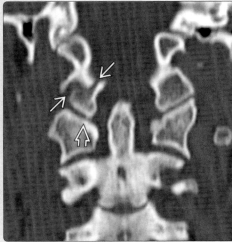

(Left) Axial bone CT shows a mildly displaced fracture of the right occipital condyle with cortical break ➡ and medial movement of the fracture fragment. (Right) Coronal reformatted bone CT in the same patient shows a lucent fracture line ➡ with minimal displacement. Articulation with C1 is preserved ➡.

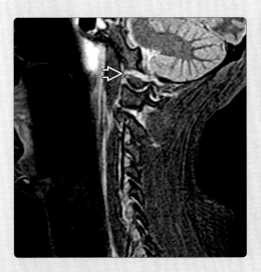
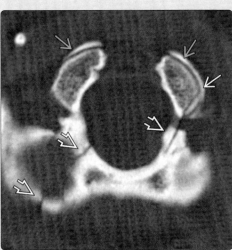

(Left) Sagittal STIR MR shows hyperintense signal through a horizontal fracture ➡ of the occipital condyle. Signal in the adjacent marrow spaces is normal. (Right) Axial bone CT shows a nondisplaced left occipital condyle fracture ➡ as involvement from a skull base fracture ➡. Note the normal C0-1 joint space appearance ➡.

Jefferson C1 Fracture

TERMINOLOGY

- Fracture(s) of C1 ring

IMAGING

- Multiple fractures of C1 arch (2-, 3-, and 4-part fractures)
- Combined offset of lateral masses of C1 relative to lateral margins of C2 ≥ 7 mm suggests interruption of transverse ligament
- Avulsion fragment off inner C1 pillar at insertion of transverse ligament indicates unstable fracture
- Widening of atlantoaxial interval
  - ≥ 4 mm concerning for interruption of transverse ligament
  - ≥ 7 mm presumed interruption of transverse ligament
- Associated C2 fracture (hangman's fracture, odontoid fracture)
  - Fractures at lower levels not uncommon
- May see T2 hyperintense edema if cord contusion present

TOP DIFFERENTIAL DIAGNOSES

- Congenital variants, clefts, malformations of atlas
- Rotational malalignment of atlas, axis pillars
- Pseudospread of atlas in children

PATHOLOGY

- Force transmitted down through occipital condyles onto sloped C1 pillars with head and neck rigidly erect
- Transverse ligament often intact
- If transverse ligament is interrupted, stability of fracture depends on integrity of alar ligaments

CLINICAL ISSUES

- Neurologic signs uncommon unless unstable fracture, injury at another level, or vascular injury

DIAGNOSTIC CHECKLIST

- Important to evaluate lower levels for additional fractures

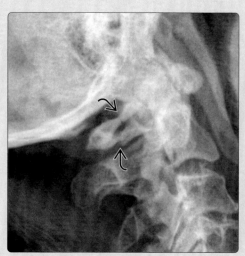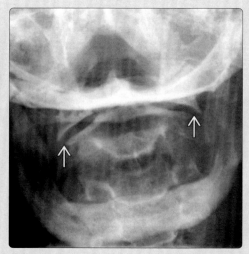

(Left) Lateral radiograph of the craniovertebral junction shows faint lucencies ⤳ in the posterior arch of C1. (Right) Coronal radiograph, in which the interval between the dens and the lateral masses of C1 is obscured by the occipital bone, shows lateral displacement of the outer margins ➡ relative to C2.

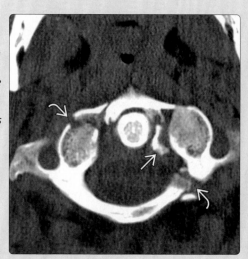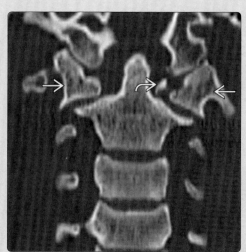

(Left) Axial NECT shows fractures ➡ extending through the anterior and posterior arches of C1. A small bony fragment demonstrates the site of an avulsion fracture ➡ at the attachment of the transverse ligament. (Right) Coronal reformatted CT shows lateral displacement of both C1 lateral masses ➡ relative to the occipital condyles and C2 lateral masses. Also seen is a bony fragment due to transverse ligament tubercle avulsion ➡.

IMAGING

General Features
- Best diagnostic clue
  - Lateral displacement of both articular masses of C1 relative to margins of C2 on open mouth radiograph

Radiographic Findings
- Radiography
  - Bony defects of C1
  - Widening of distance between odontoid and C1 lateral masses on open mouth view
    - Normal rotation may produce apparent offset of pilar, simulating fracture
    - Combined offset of lateral masses of C1 relative to lateral margins of C2 ≥ 7 mm suggests interruption of transverse ligament
      - Potentially unstable fracture

Fluoroscopic Findings
- Subluxation if unstable

CT Findings
- NECT
  - Axial CT defines components of fracture to best advantage
  - May demonstrate various patterns of arch disruption; may demonstrate hyperdensity in epidural space if bleeding occurs
- CTA
  - Loss of vertebral artery integrity if vertebrobasilar vascular syndrome present

MR Findings
- T1WI
  - Prevertebral soft tissue swelling anterior to C1; disruption of cortical margins of C1
- T2WI
  - Edema in prevertebral soft tissues
  - May see hyperintense cord edema if contusion is present
- MRA
  - Vertebral artery injury, if present, with dissection or occlusion

Angiographic Findings
- Useful if CTA/MRA equivocal or for persistent concern for vertebral artery injury; endovascular intervention

Imaging Recommendations
- Best imaging tool
  - Unenhanced multidetector CT scan
- Protocol advice
  - Any lateral spread of C1 pillars on open mouth x-ray view requires CT
  - Thin-slice (≤ 1 mm) axial CT in bone reconstruction algorithm
  - Evaluate entire cervical spine as well as upper thoracic spine
  - Axial and sagittal T1WI and T2WI, sagittal STIR to evaluate fracture morphology, displacement, ligamentous injury, soft tissue edema

DIFFERENTIAL DIAGNOSIS

Congenital Variants, Clefts, Malformations of Atlas
- May show 1-2 mm offset of C1 pillars from those of C2
- Various deficiencies of arch development can be seen
- Most are partial hemiaplasias of posterior arch
- Clefts, congenital defects show smooth or well-corticated edges

Rotational Malalignment of Atlas, Axis Pillars
- Generally seen unilaterally, with rotation and abduction of head

Pseudospread of Atlas in Children
- Common finding in children 3 months to 4 years of age evaluated for minor trauma
- Caused by disparity in growth rates of atlas and axis

PATHOLOGY

General Features
- Etiology
  - Axial compressive force applied to skull vertex

CLINICAL ISSUES

Presentation
- Most common signs/symptoms
  - Upper neck pain after compression trauma (e.g., diving); cervical muscle spasm; limited range of motion; head tilt
- Clinical profile
  - Trauma victim; upper neck pain

Natural History & Prognosis
- Stable fracture
  - Healing with conservative therapy in majority of cases

Treatment
- Nondisplaced isolated anterior or posterior atlas arch fractures and fractures of atlas lateral mass
  - External cervical immobilization; rigid collars, suboccipital mandibular immobilizer braces, and halo ring-vest orthoses; 8-12 weeks; 96% rate of healing
- Combined anterior and posterior arch fractures of atlas with intact transverse ligament
  - Rigid collar, suboccipital mandibular immobilizer brace, or halo orthosis; 10-12 weeks
- Combined anterior and posterior arch fractures of the atlas with transverse ligament disruption; halo orthosis for 12 weeks or surgical stabilization and fusion

DIAGNOSTIC CHECKLIST

Consider
- Routine CT of cervical spine in trauma victims with severe neck pain
- Evaluate for extension of fracture into foramina transversarium

Image Interpretation Pearls
- Well-corticated edges of midline C1 arch defects are likely congenital clefts
- 1-2 mm offset of C1 lateral masses vs. C2 on open mouth view in infants may be normal variant

Atlantoaxial Rotatory Fixation

IMAGING

- Abnormal rotatory motion of C1 with respect to C2 defined by 3-position CT scan

TOP DIFFERENTIAL DIAGNOSES

- **Etiologies of atlantoaxial rotatory fixation (AARF)**
  - ○ Trauma
  - ○ Nasopharyngeal infection (Grisel syndrome)
  - ○ Prior head and neck surgery

PATHOLOGY

- **Pang type I AARF**: Unaltered or locked C1-C2 coupled configuration regardless of corrective counter-rotation
- **Pang type II AARF**: Reduced C1-C2 separation angle with forced correction but C1 does not cross C2
- **Pang type III AARF**: Show C1-C2 crossover but only with head turned far to opposite side

CLINICAL ISSUES

- Persistently rotated head that is painful during attempts at correction (painful torticollis)
- Head typically laterally flexed on side opposite to pointing chin (cock-robin appearance)
- Treatment in acute phase gives best outcome (Pang type I-III)

DIAGNOSTIC CHECKLIST

- **Fielding-Hawkins** type III, IV involve traumatic rupture of transverse atlantal and other stabilizing ligaments
  - ○ Emergent and serious injuries require immediate surgical intervention to protect cord
  - ○ These more serious injuries are separate from pure rotatory fixations, which are never acutely unstable (as in Pang type I-III AARF)

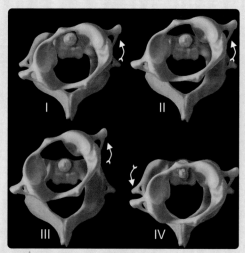

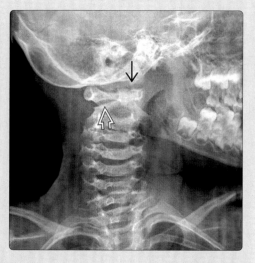

(Left) Fielding-Hawkins classification of atlantoaxial fixation shows type I rotatory displacement of C1 without ligamentous abnormality; type II 3- to 5-mm anterior displacement of C1; type III shows > 5-mm anterior displacement associated with deficiency of transverse ligament; type IV shows C1 displacement posteriorly. (Right) In Fielding-Hawkins type I fixation, radiograph shows rotation of head to the left. Note typical appearance of rotated C1 applied to left side of C1 ➡ with widening of right C1-C2 spacing ➡.

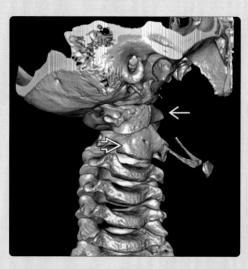

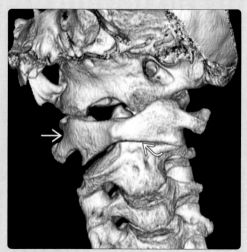

(Left) Fielding-Hawkins type I atlantoaxial rotatory fixation on this 3D CT reconstruction nicely visualizes the markedly left rotated C1 ➡ with respect to the mildly rotated C2 ➡. (Right) Fielding type I rotatory fixation is seen on this anterior view from a volume-rendered CT reconstruction showing the morphology of the rotated C1 ➡ and morphologically normal odontoid. The axis of rotation is about the anterior atlantodental joint ➡, which is consistent with intact ligamentous complex.

TERMINOLOGY

Abbreviations

- Atlantoaxial rotatory fixation (AARF)

Synonyms

- Atlantoaxial rotatory subluxation, rotary subluxation

Definitions

- Rotatory fixation or subluxation: Persistent rotational deformity of C1-C2 complex with resultant torticollis and head in cock-robin position; normal atlantodental interval (ADI)
- Rotatory dislocation: More severe injury with anterior displacement of lateral mass of C1 relative to C2 with widening of ADI

IMAGING

General Features

- Best diagnostic clue
  o Abnormal rotatory motion of C1 with respect to C2 defined by 3-position CT scan

Imaging Recommendations

- Protocol advice
  o 3 separate scans covering occiput to C2
    – Head in presenting position, undisturbed (designated as P position)
    – Head turned to zero position by examiner (designated as P0 position)
    – Head turned to side opposite to presenting position as far as tolerable (designated as P_)

DIFFERENTIAL DIAGNOSIS

Etiologies of Atlantoaxial Rotatory Fixation

- **Trauma**
  o More severe forms caused by violent trauma
  o Frequent coexistence of fractured clavicle on opposite side of chin
- **Nasopharyngeal infection (Grisel syndrome)**
  o Many purported mechanisms, including spread of infection to CV joints; synovial inflammation
- **Prior head and neck surgery**
  o Head rotated or hyperextended with otopharyngeal inflammation; general anesthesia and muscle relaxants
- **Mimics**
  o Muscular torticollis related to overactivity or contracture of sternomastoid muscle on side opposite to chin
  o CV junction segmentation anomalies with instability

PATHOLOGY

Staging, Grading, & Classification

- **Fielding-Hawkins (1977)**
  o **Type I**: Rotatory fixation without anterior displacement of atlas (displacement of < 3 mm)
    – Most common type
  o **Type II**: Rotatory fixation with anterior displacement of atlas from 3-5 mm
    – Associated with abnormality of transverse ligament
  o **Type III**: Rotatory fixation with displacement > 5 mm

    – Associated with deficiency of transverse and alar ligaments
  o **Type IV**: Rotatory fixation with posterior displacement
    – Rare
- **Pang (2005)**
  o **5 distinct groups** based on motion curves obtained from 3-position CT
    – Does not include cases of concomitant acute translational instabilities of C1 on C2 as in Fielding-Hawkins types III, IV
  o **Type I AARF**: Unaltered or locked C1-C2 coupled configuration regardless of corrective counter-rotation
    – Motion curve is horizontal in upper 2 quadrants of C1-C2 motion template
  o **Type II AARF**: Reduced C1-C2 separation angle with forced correction but C1 does not cross C2
    – Motion curve slopes downward from right to left in upper quadrants but does not traverse x-axis
  o **Type III AARF**: Shows C1-C2 crossover but only with head turned far to opposite side
    – Motion curve traverses x-axis left of C1 = -20°
  o **Group IV**: Normal dynamics in muscular torticollis without injury to C1-C2 joints
  o **Group V**: Diagnostic gray zone
    – Motion curve shows features between normal and type III AARF

CLINICAL ISSUES

Presentation

- Most common signs/symptoms
  o Persistently rotated head that is painful during attempts at correction (painful torticollis)
  o Head typically laterally flexed on side opposite to pointing chin (cock-robin appearance)

Demographics

- Age
  o Childhood (18 months to 18 years)

Natural History & Prognosis

- Treatment in acute phase gives best outcome (Pang type I-III)
- 1 study showed no acute patients required halo fixation or surgical fusion with short treatment duration of < 4 months
- Subacute patients have worse outcome with longer treatment course; many of these patients require halo fixation
- Chronic patients have worst prognosis with Pang type I, II AARF, with high percentage of persistent abnormal motion requiring fusion
- Best overall outcome with Pang acute type III AARF and worst outcome chronic type I AARF

DIAGNOSTIC CHECKLIST

Consider

- Fielding-Hawkins type III, IV involve traumatic rupture of transverse atlantal and other stabilizing ligaments
  o Emergent and serious injuries requiring immediate surgical intervention to protect cord
  o These more serious injuries are separate from pure rotatory fixations, which are never acutely unstable

Odontoid C2 Fracture

TERMINOLOGY

- Type I: Avulsion fracture from tip of odontoid at insertion of alar ligament
  - Usually stable injury
  - Usually seen in conjunction with more extensive craniocervical injury
- Type II: Transverse fracture through base of odontoid
  - Most likely to progress to nonunion without surgical fusion
- Type III: Oblique fracture extending from base of odontoid into body of C2

IMAGING

- Direct visualization of fracture line on radiography
  - Soft tissue swelling anterior to C2 in acute cases
  - Displacement of dens, C1 on lateral film
- CT protocol: Thin-slice (1 mm or less) multidetector CT, fast scan time to minimize motion
  - Sagittal and coronal reformatted images mandatory

- MR
  - Effacement of thecal sac on MR due to displaced fracture
  - Cord injury, if present, hyperintense on T2WI
  - Fractures without compression &/or fractures with distraction do not reliably generate marrow edema and can lead to false-negative MR imaging

TOP DIFFERENTIAL DIAGNOSES

- Os odontoideum
- Congenital variation: 3rd occipital condyle (condylus tertius)
- Rheumatoid arthritis: C1/C2 subluxation
- Pathologic C2 fracture
- Ossiculum terminale persistens

PATHOLOGY

- Osteoporosis in elderly predisposes to type II fracture and nonunion

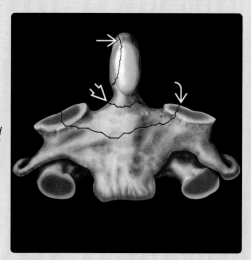

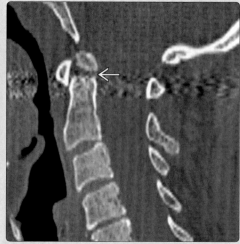

(Left) Anterior graphic shows an avulsion fracture through the tip of the odontoid ➡ (type I), transverse fracture at the base of the odontoid ➡ (type II), and an odontoid fracture extending through the body of C2 ➡ (type III). (Right) Sagittal reformatted bone CT shows a nondisplaced fracture ➡ through the tip of the odontoid (type I odontoid fracture).

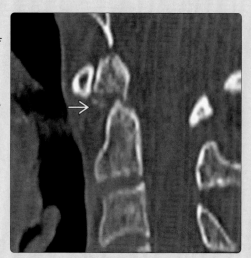

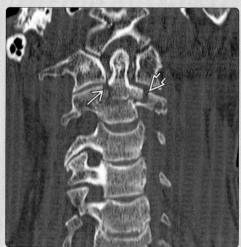

(Left) Sagittal reconstructed CT shows a fracture ➡ extending through the base of the dens (type II). The dens is moderately displaced anteriorly. (Right) Coronal reformatted CT shows a type III fracture extending from the right of the base of the odontoid ➡ through the C2 body and into the left lateral mass ➡.

TERMINOLOGY

Synonyms

- Dens fracture

Definitions

- Type I: Avulsion fracture from tip of odontoid at insertion of alar ligament
- Type II: Transverse fracture through base of odontoid
- Type III: Oblique fracture extending from base of odontoid into body of C2

IMAGING

General Features

- Best diagnostic clue
  - Lateral radiograph: Anterior or posterior displacement of C1 arch vs. C2 with prevertebral soft tissue swelling
  - Fracture visible on open mouth (dens) view

Radiographic Findings

- Radiography
  - Type I: Oblique fracture fragment at rostral aspect of odontoid on frontal view
  - Type II: Fracture line through base of odontoid
  - Type III
    - Fracture line through base of odontoid extending into C2 body
    - Fracture may extend into superior articular surfaces of C2
  - All: Swelling of prevertebral soft tissues

CT Findings

- NECT
  - Soft tissue swelling anterior to C2 in acute cases
  - Lucent fracture line through tip of odontoid (type I) or base of odontoid (type II) ± extent into C2 body (type III)

MR Findings

- T1WI
  - Abnormal low T1 marrow signal due to osseous edema
  - Cortical disruption
  - May directly appreciate cortical defect at fracture site
  - Thickened prevertebral soft tissues
- T2WI
  - Variable and inconsistent hyperintense signal in C2 marrow due to osseous edema
  - Hyperintense soft tissue edema
  - Effacement of thecal sac due to displaced fracture

DIFFERENTIAL DIAGNOSIS

Os Odontoideum

- Odontoid replaced by ossicle with no continuity to C2 body
- Corticated margins on radiography, CT
- No soft tissue swelling

Pathologic C2 Fracture

- Can produce pathologic odontoid fracture
- Metastases, infection, other inflammatory arthritidis

Rheumatoid Arthritis: C1/C2 Subluxation

- Laxity, subluxation

Ossiculum Terminale Persistens

- Nonfusion of ossiculum terminal (apical odontoid epiphysis) to body of dens beyond 12 years of age

Congenital Variation: 3rd Occipital Condyle (Condylus Tertius)

- Midline bony peg off anterior lip of foramen magnum may articulate to dens, simulate odontoid type I fracture

PATHOLOGY

Staging, Grading, & Classification

- Anderson and D'Alonzo (1974)
  - Type I fracture: Oblique fracture through upper portion of odontoid process
  - Type II fracture: Fracture across base of odontoid process near junction with axis body
  - Type III fracture: Fracture that includes odontoid and extends into axis body
- Hadley modification (1988)
  - Type IIA: Comminuted fracture of base of odontoid with associated free fracture fragments
    - Highly unstable
- Grauer modification (2005)
  - Type IIA: Minimally/nondisplaced fracture with no comminution; treated with external immobilization
  - Type IIB: Displaced odontoid fracture that extends from anterior-superior to posterior-inferior or transverse; treated with anterior screw fixation if reducible
  - Type IIC: Fracture extending from anterior-inferior to posterior-superior or with significant comminution; considered for posterior internal fixation and fusion

CLINICAL ISSUES

Natural History & Prognosis

- Fusion produces stability
- Nonunion common in elderly without primary fusion
  - May stabilize by fibrous union with prolonged immobilization

Treatment

- Fracture pattern dictates management
- Type I fracture
  - Usually stable injury
  - Treated with simple immobilization
- Type II fracture
  - Most likely to progress to nonunion
- Type III fracture
  - Nonunion uncommon after treatment with traction followed by bracing

DIAGNOSTIC CHECKLIST

Consider

- STIR to show soft tissue edema in prevertebral space (missing in chronic nonunion)
  - Marrow edema an unreliable sign for presence of fracture in distraction injuries
- Flexion/extension films or fluoroscopy for evaluating stability

TERMINOLOGY

- Comminuted fracture through C2 vertebral body
- Displacement of fragments in AP direction

IMAGING

- AP displacement of fracture fragments
- Fat C2 sign
- Often see associated hangman's fracture, unstable injury
- Displaced fracture fragments may encroach on spinal canal
- CTA or MRA for screening vertebral artery injury
  - Especially if fracture extends to foramen transversarium

TOP DIFFERENTIAL DIAGNOSES

- Flexion teardrop fracture of C2
- Other nonodontoid, non-hangman's C2 body fracture
- Pathologic fracture

PATHOLOGY

- High-energy mechanisms cause most C2 fractures

- Fujimara (1996) classification of C2 body fractures (non-hangman's, nonodontoid C2 fractures)
  - Avulsion fracture
  - Transverse fracture
  - Burst fracture
  - Sagittal fracture

CLINICAL ISSUES

- High-energy, high-velocity trauma
- May have concomitant head injury
- Often managed with conservative/nonoperative treatment
- Surgical management for inability to reduce fragments, associated hangman's fracture, malalignment of atlantoaxial articulation

DIAGNOSTIC CHECKLIST

- C2 burst fractures can involve body, pedicle, lateral mass, and transverse foramina

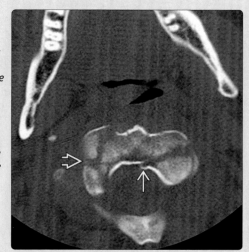
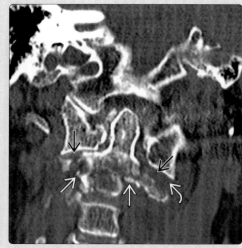

(Left) Axial NECT shows a comminuted C2 body fracture with fragmentation of the right lateral mass ⊟. There is slight posterior displacement of fragments ⊟ flattening the thecal sac. C2 burst injuries may occur as a result of isolated or combined hyperflexion or hyperextension forces. (Right) Coronal CT illustrates a highly comminuted C2 burst fracture ⊟. The fracture extends into the superior articular facets ⊟ with widening of the C1-2 facet joint on the left ⊟.

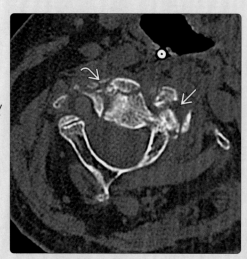
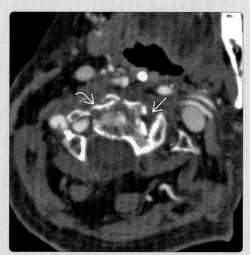

(Left) Axial bone CT demonstrates a comminuted burst fracture of C2 ⊟ involving the left transverse foramen ⊟. Primary hyperflexion mechanism predominantly disrupts the anterior margin, while primary hyperextension is suggested if the posterior margin is disrupted. Combined hyperextension-hyperflexion injuries may result in the interruption of both margins. (Right) Axial CTA exhibits occlusion of the left vertebral artery ⊟ due to C2 burst fracture ⊟ involving the left transverse foramen.

Hangman's C2 Fracture

TERMINOLOGY

- Traumatic spondylolisthesis of axis
- Bilateral C2 pars interarticularis fractures

IMAGING

- Fracture through pars interarticularis of C2
  - Fracture may extend into C2 vertebral body
  - Anterior displacement of C2 body relative to C3
  - C1 arch and skull ride forward with C2 vertebral body
  - Posterior elements and spinolaminar line of C2 and C3 remain aligned
  - Flexion exaggerates C2-C3 subluxation
  - Involvement of vertebral artery foramen would be concerning for vertebral artery injury
  - Additional fracture levels seen in 33% of cases, C1 most common
- Imaging: Thin-section (1-mm) helical CT with sagittal and coronal reformations

- Any anterior subluxation of C2 vs. C3 on lateral x-ray warrants CT

PATHOLOGY

- Hyperextension with axial loading or forced hyperflexion with axial loading
- Effendi classification
  - Type I: Hairline fracture, nondisplaced; no disruption of C2-C3 disc
  - Type II: Fracture with ≥ 3-mm anterior translation of C2 on C3, abnormal C2-C3 disc
  - Type IIA: Minimal C2-C3 displacement but severe angulation associated with flexion distraction
  - Type III (rare): Displaced anterior fracture fragment with dislocated or subluxed facet joints

CLINICAL ISSUES

- Type I: Stable lesion, no permanent deficits
- Types II, III: Higher rates of sequelae, disability

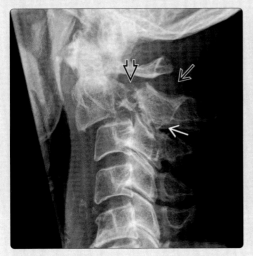
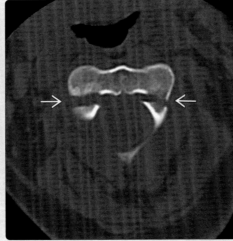

(Left) Lateral radiograph shows fractures of bilateral C2 pars interarticularis with distraction ➡ and anterolisthesis of C2 on C3. The C2-C3 spinolaminar line ➡ is preserved with interruption at C2 ➡. (Right) Axial NECT shows posteriorly displaced fractures of bilateral C2 pars interarticularis ➡ in this adolescent with hyperextension injury.

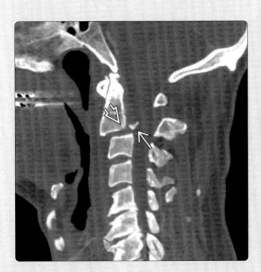
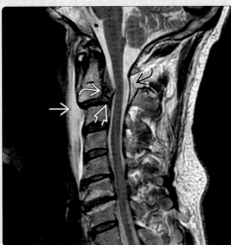

(Left) Sagittal bone CT shows anterolisthesis of C2 on C3 ➡ with a bone fragment from the inferior posterior C2 body extending into the canal and compressing the cord ➡. (Right) Sagittal T2W MR shows disruption of the posterior longitudinal ➡ and interspinous ligaments ➡ with C2-C3 anterolisthesis. Prevertebral soft tissue edema is noted ➡ and there is a ventral epidural hematoma ➡ and bone fragment causing canal stenosis and cord compression.

Apophyseal Ring Fracture

TERMINOLOGY

- Fracture or avulsion of vertebral ring apophysis following injury in immature skeleton

IMAGING

- Concentric bone fragment displaced from vertebral endplate margin in skeletally immature patient
- Inferior or superior endplate may be involved
  - Limbus vertebra usually superior
- Fractured apophyseal fragment usually midline

TOP DIFFERENTIAL DIAGNOSES

- Flexion teardrop fracture of anterior endplate corner
- Schmorl node
- Calcified disc fragment; posterior osteophyte
- Disc herniation

PATHOLOGY

- Limbus vertebra: Herniation of nucleus pulposus between ring apophysis and vertebral body
- Posterior apophyseal fracture: 2 mechanisms described
  - Same as limbus vertebra
  - Herniating nucleus spares Sharpey fibers, avulses ring apophysis

CLINICAL ISSUES

- Back pain in acute (adolescent) cases
- Adolescent athlete with acute low back pain
- Majority of patients report engagement in sporting activities

DIAGNOSTIC CHECKLIST

- MR more sensitive than radiographs or CT in young children since ring apophysis not ossified
- T2WI FS/STIR MR essential to assess for associated ligamentous injury

(Left) Sagittal graphic demonstrates an acute lumbar apophyseal ring fracture ⇒ involving the posterior inferior vertebral body corner ⇒ with displacement and associated hemorrhage. There is compression of the adjacent thecal sac. (Right) Sagittal nonenhanced T1W MR shows a focal area of fat signal within the posterior disc margin ⇒, which is the old ring apophyseal avulsion. Note the endplate irregularity involving L5 ⇒.

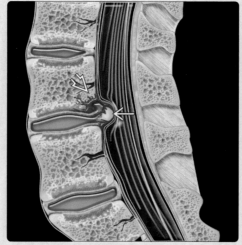
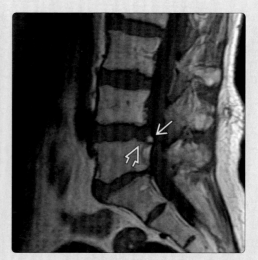

(Left) Sagittal T1WI MR in this case of posterior ring apophysis fracture demonstrates herniation of the L5-S1 disc ⇒ and fracture with displacement of the L5 ring apophysis ⇒. Note marrow edema and endplate irregularity. (Right) Axial T2WI MR shows posterior displacement of the fractured apophysis ⇒, narrowing the central spinal canal and both lateral recesses.

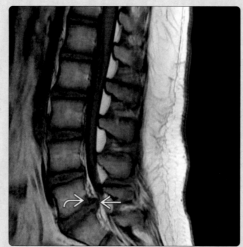
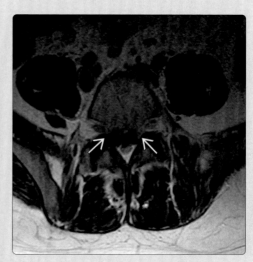

TERMINOLOGY

- Injury from cervical hyperflexion with compression or hyperflexion with distraction/shearing

IMAGING

- Hyperflexion with compression
  - Forced flexion of cervical spine with axial loading vector slightly anterior to vertebral column
  - Primary injury to anterior and (later) middle columns
- Hyperflexion with distraction
  - Forced flexion of cervical spine with rostrally oriented force vector nearly perpendicular to trunk
  - Primary failure of posterior and (later) middle columns
  - Focal kyphosis, ↑ space between spinous processes; distracted, perched, or jumped facets
- Mid or lower cervical spine more common
- Best imaging modality
  - Thin-slice (≤ 1-mm) helical CT with sagittal and coronal reformations
  - MR (especially STIR and GRE) to evaluate soft tissue structures, spinal cord

TOP DIFFERENTIAL DIAGNOSES

- Burst fracture
- Flexion-rotation injury
- Whiplash fracture

PATHOLOGY

- Spinal instability
- Spinal cord injury, radiculopathy
- Associated with closed head injury, polytrauma

CLINICAL ISSUES

- Immobilization, axial traction, surgical fusion
- Surgical decompression for spinal cord injury
- Methylprednisolone for treatment of acute spinal cord injury **not** recommended

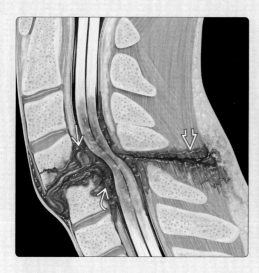
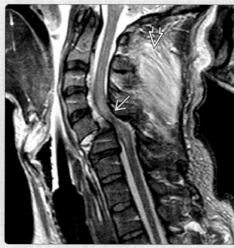

(Left) Sagittal graphic shows flexion injury at C4-C5 with subluxation, disc disruption, disc herniation ➡, ligamentous disruption ➡, cord compression, and epidural hemorrhage ➡. (Right) Sagittal T2WI MR shows severe flexion injury with subluxation of C5 on C6, flexion deformity and severe cord compression ➡, and cord edema. Note the posterior ligamentous injury ➡.

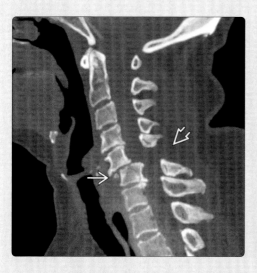
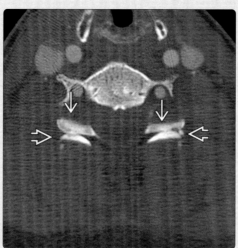

(Left) CT angiogram shows the typical CT and MR appearance of severe hyperflexion injury with vertebral C5-C6 subluxation with C6 corner fracture ➡ and severe widening of the spinous processes, reflecting interspinous ligament disruption ➡. (Right) Axial CECT in a flexion injury with jumped facets shows inferior facets of the C6 ➡ anterior to superior facets of C7 ➡ (known as naked facets sign or hamburger sign).

Cervical Hyperextension Injury

TERMINOLOGY

- Injury from cervical hyperextension with compression or hyperextension with distraction/shearing

IMAGING

- Hyperextension injury with axial compression
  - Unilateral or bilateral fracture of posterior elements
  - Traumatic anterolisthesis with more severe injury; ligamentous disruption ± superior endplate impaction fracture of subjacent vertebral body
- Hyperextension injury with distraction or shear
  - May have minimal radiographic findings even with significant injury
  - Anterior longitudinal ligament (ALL) rupture, widening of anterior disc space
  - Minimally displaced fracture of anterior margin of inferior vertebral body (extension teardrop) without retrolisthesis
- Best imaging modality
  - Thin-slice helical CT with sagittal and coronal reformations
  - MR (especially STIR) to evaluate ligaments, cord
    - STIR MR
      - Disruption of ALL, widened and ↑ signal in disc space anteriorly
      - Marrow edema if bone contusion, fracture
      - ↑ signal in cord, if cord injury present

TOP DIFFERENTIAL DIAGNOSES

- Flexion teardrop fracture
- Clay shoveler fracture
- Whiplash injury

PATHOLOGY

- Spinal cord injury
  - Especially central cord syndrome
  - Potential for injury increased with congenital spinal stenosis

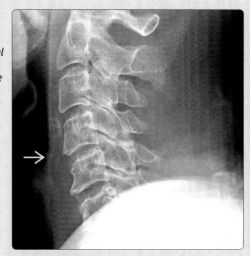

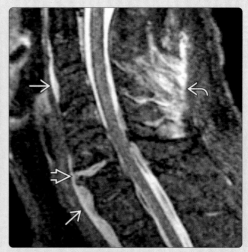

(Left) Lateral radiograph shows mild prevertebral soft tissue swelling ➡. Mild changes of preexisting cervical spondylosis are also noted. (Right) Sagittal STIR MR in the same patient shows prevertebral edema ➡ and disruption of the ALL ➡. A nonphysiologic hyperintense signal within the C6-C7 disc space reflects disruption of the discovertebral unit by hyperextension-distraction injury at this level. Posterior soft tissue edema is also present ➡.

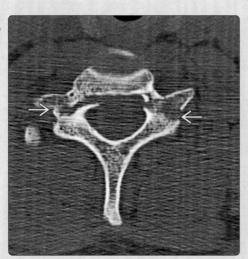

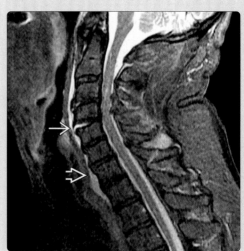

(Left) Axial NECT shows mildly displaced fractures of bilateral C7 articular pillars ➡ due to a hyperextension-compression type of injury. (Right) Sagittal STIR MR in this patient with a normal cervical spine CT shows an abnormal increased signal from the disrupted ALL ➡ at the C4-C5 level and disc. Note the prevertebral edema ➡.

Cervical Burst Fracture

TERMINOLOGY

- Comminuted fracture of cervical vertebral body due to axial loading
- Vertical compression fracture

IMAGING

- Loss of vertebral body height
- Vertically oriented fracture planes
  - Extending to endplates and posterior cortex
- Centrifugal displacement of fragments
  - Compromise of spinal canal
  - Cord injury on MR
- Typically mid or lower cervical spine
- Prevertebral soft tissue swelling

TOP DIFFERENTIAL DIAGNOSES

- Flexion teardrop fracture
- Hyperextension teardrop fracture
- Benign compression fracture
- Pathologic compression fracture

PATHOLOGY

- Axial loading with neck in neutral position
- Centrifugal displacement of comminuted fracture fragments
- Displacement into spinal canal → cord injury
  - Spinal cord injury common
- Spinal cord injury common with retropulsion

CLINICAL ISSUES

- Variable neurologic symptoms, from no deficit to tetraparesis
- Treatment
  - May be able to be managed conservatively
    - Traction, immobilization
  - Unstable injury may need surgical stabilization
    - ± surgical decompression of canal if cord injury present

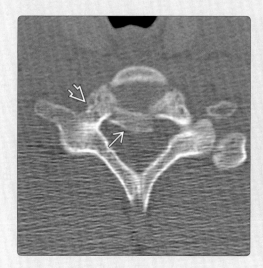

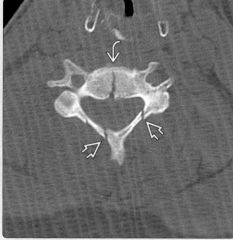

(Left) Axial bone CT shows a vertebral body fragment ⟹ displaced into the spinal canal. Fracture of the right pedicle ⟹ is also seen. This is the classic CT appearance of burst fracture, which causes loss of vertebral body height and posterior displacement of bone fragment into the spinal canal. (Right) Axial NECT shows a burst fracture in the sagittal fracture plane ⟹. There is widening of the interpedicular width and multiple fractures of the neural arch ⟹.

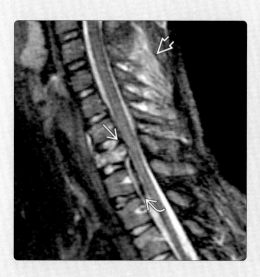

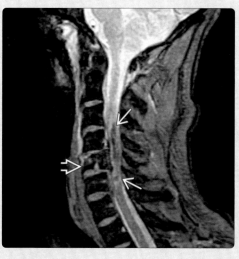

(Left) Sagittal STIR MR shows a C7 burst fracture with posterior displacement of a fracture fragment ⟹ into the spinal canal, contacting the spinal cord. There are no signal changes in the cord. A small amount of ventral epidural hemorrhage ⟹ is seen. Edema of the dorsal soft tissue is also present ⟹. (Right) Sagittal T2* GRE MR shows extensive edema and low-signal hemorrhage ⟹ within the cervical cord in this patient with a C5 burst fracture ⟹. There is moderate retropulsion of the posterior aspect of the C5 body.

TERMINOLOGY

- Traumatic disruption of annularis fibrosis with associated displacement of nucleus pulposus

IMAGING

- Location: Cervical > thoracic > > lumbar
- Radiographs insensitive for disc pathology
  - Cause of spinal cord injury without radiographic abnormality
- Associated with spinal fracture, facet subluxation
- MR is modality of choice to evaluate intervertebral discs, soft tissue contents of spinal canal
  - Disc material effacing anterior CSF ± cord or nerve root compression
  - ± cord edema if cord compressed

TOP DIFFERENTIAL DIAGNOSES

- Nontraumatic intervertebral disc herniation
- Epidural abscess, phlegmon

- Epidural tumor

CLINICAL ISSUES

- Anterior cord syndrome highly associated with traumatic disc herniation
- Cauda equina syndrome with lumbar herniation: Pain, incontinence 2° to compression of lumbosacral spinal nerve roots
- 5-54% incidence of herniation with cervical spine trauma
- Cord compression from herniation is reported complication of reduction of cervical facet dislocation without discectomy

DIAGNOSTIC CHECKLIST

- Consider MR prior to reduction of facet dislocation
- MR to exclude anterior cord compression from herniated disc or hematoma prior to aggressive attempts at closed reduction

(Left) Sagittal T2WI MR shows hyperflexion-compression injury with focal kyphosis of C6-C7, disruption of the posterior longitudinal ligament ➡, narrowing of the anterior disc space, and a posterior disc protrusion ➡ causing canal stenosis. There is splaying of the spinous processes and a small amount of dorsal epidural hematoma ➡. (Right) Sagittal T2WI MR shows a flexion teardrop fracture of C2 ➡, increased kyphosis at C2-C3, and a traumatic disc protrusion ➡ effacing the thecal sac at C2-C3.

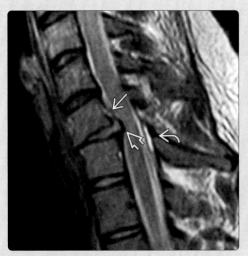
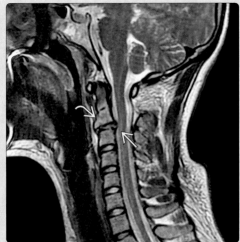

(Left) Sagittal T1WI MR shows C5-C6 flexion injury with subluxation, prevertebral hemorrhage ➡, and disc extrusion touching ventral cord ➡. (Right) Sagittal STIR MR in this trauma patient shows a large disc extrusion at C6-C7 ➡ that compresses the cord. There is disruption of the anterior longitudinal ligament ➡ and endplate marrow edema ➡ from axial loading. Note the extensive dorsal soft tissue edema ➡.

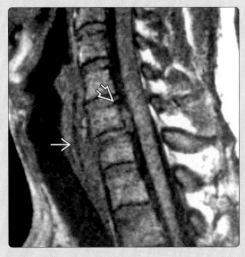
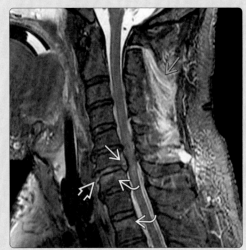

Thoracic and Lumbar Burst Fracture

TERMINOLOGY

- Vertebral body fracture due to axial load, involving anterior & middle, ± posterior columns
  - Anterior: Anterior longitudinal ligament, anterior 1/2 vertebral body, & anterior anulus fibrosis
  - Middle: Posterior longitudinal ligament, posterior 1/2 vertebral body, & posterior anulus fibrosis
  - Posterior: Neural arch, facet ligaments, ligamentum flavum, inter- & supraspinous ligaments

IMAGING

- Thoracolumbar junction with loss of vertebral height
- Fracture involves posterior vertebral body cortex
  - ± retropulsion of posterior cortex
  - ± vertically oriented posterior element fractures
- Cord contusion best seen on T2WI MR

TOP DIFFERENTIAL DIAGNOSES

- Compression fracture

- Chance fracture
- Pathologic fracture due to tumor
- Fracture-dislocation

PATHOLOGY

- Associated with other spine fractures, pelvic/lower extremity fractures

CLINICAL ISSUES

- Surgical indications include neural compression and kyphosis

DIAGNOSTIC CHECKLIST

- Orientation of posterior element fractures distinguish between Chance and burst fractures
  - Burst: Vertically oriented posterior element fractures reflect axial load force
  - Chance: Horizontally oriented posterior element fractures reflect distraction force

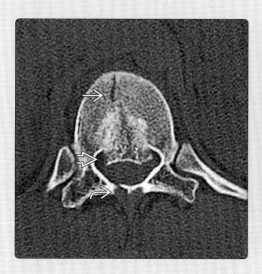

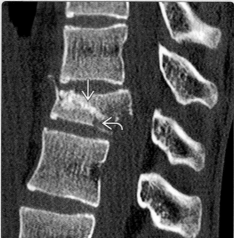

(Left) Axial bone CT shows a sagittal fracture line ➜ through the vertebral body. The axial load force has continued through the right lamina ➜. The posterior vertebral body cortex is displaced posteriorly ➜. (Right) Sagittal bone CT in the same patient shows a sclerotic line ➜ reflecting trabecular impaction. There is also a coronal fracture line ➜ extending to the inferior vertebral body cortex.

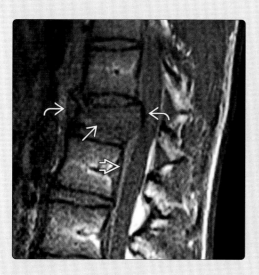

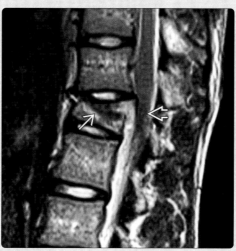

(Left) Sagittal T1WI MR in the same patient shows the body deformity ➜ and epidural hematoma ➜. However, the fracture line ➜ is difficult to see because of the surrounding red marrow. (Right) Sagittal T2WI MR in the same patient better shows the low signal intensity fracture line ➜ outlined by marrow hematoma. The tip of the conus ➜ is displaced posteriorly.

Trauma

TERMINOLOGY

- Transversely applied force vector, resulting in shearing injury ± flexion &/or rotation

IMAGING

- Traumatic spondylolisthesis with fracture(s) of posterior elements &/or vertebral body
  - Vertebral column discontinuity/listhesis at level of injury, involving 3 columns
  - Complete disruption of disc or horizontal fracture through vertebral body with displacement &/or rotation
  - Soft tissue edema associated with ligamentous disruption
- Spinal cord injury common

TOP DIFFERENTIAL DIAGNOSES

- Chance fracture
  - Distracted, horizontal fracture through pedicles, no listhesis

- Burst fracture
  - Comminuted fracture of vertebral body extending to posterior cortex

PATHOLOGY

- Force vector perpendicular to vertebral column, ± rotation &/or flexion
- Shear injury, failure of all 3 columns
- High-energy mechanisms

CLINICAL ISSUES

- Severely injured trauma patient
- Lower extremity paralysis, sensory deficit
- Spinal shock with hypotension

DIAGNOSTIC CHECKLIST

- Fracture-dislocation injuries have high rate of paraplegia, instability

(Left) Sagittal CT reconstruction shows a widened T10-T11 disc space ➡ with mild traumatic anterolisthesis. The inferior T10 facet is fractured ➡ and perched. There is a fragmented fracture of the anterior T11 vertebral body ➡. (Right) Sagittal T2WI MR in the same patient shows abnormal signal and widening of the T10-T11 disc space ➡ and fracture of the T10 spinous process and lamina ➡. Traumatic anterolisthesis causes spinal canal stenosis and spinal cord contusion ➡.

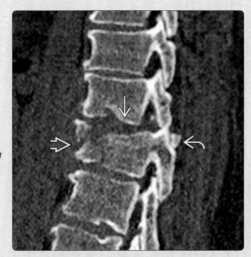
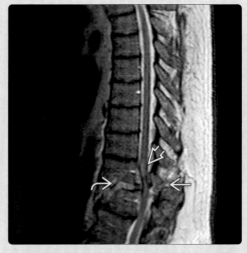

(Left) Sagittal reconstructed bone CT shows anterior fracture-dislocation of T10-T11 ➡ with comminuted fracture of the T11 vertebral body. There is severe canal stenosis due to 75% anterior translation and bone fragment ➡ displaced into the spinal canal. Mild compression fractures are noted at T5 and T7 ➡. (Right) Axial NECT (bone window) in the same patient shows the margin of T10 ➡ anteriorly displaced relative to T11 ➡. Thickening of the paravertebral soft tissues is due to hematoma.

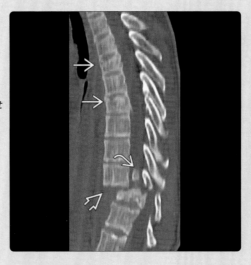
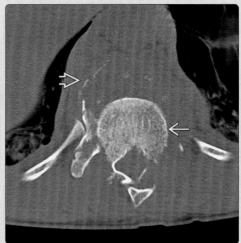

Chance Fracture

TERMINOLOGY

- Flexion-distraction injury, seat belt fracture
- Compression injury of anterior column with distraction of middle and posterior columns

IMAGING

- Usually occurs at T11-L3, occasionally midthoracic
- Wedging of anterior vertebral body
- Focal kyphosis ± fracture
- Bony or ligamentous injury to posterior column
  - Transversely oriented posterior element fracture &/or
    - Separation of facet joints
    - Increased interspinous distance
    - Ligament disruption on MR
- No subluxation of vertebral body

TOP DIFFERENTIAL DIAGNOSES

- Shear injury
- Distraction injury

- Burst fracture
- Traumatic compression fracture
- Pathologic vertebral fracture

PATHOLOGY

- Anterior compression, posterior distraction around fulcrum
- 15-80% have significant abdominal injuries (bowel and mesentery most common)

CLINICAL ISSUES

- Traumatic back pain ± neurologic injury

DIAGNOSTIC CHECKLIST

- MR evidence of hematoma between spinous processes is not sufficient to diagnose ligament disruption
  - Hematoma may occur due to compression force
  - Look for discontinuity of ligament on MR
- Chance fracture may have retropulsion of posterior vertebral body cortex mimicking burst fracture

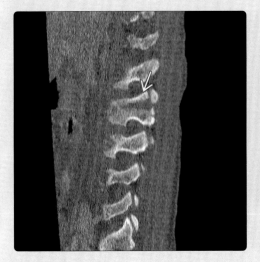
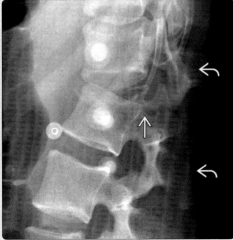

(Left) Sagittal NECT in a child shows the typical horizontal pedicle fracture of the Chance morphology ➡. There is distraction of the posterior elements with a compressive component anteriorly. (Right) Lateral radiograph shows a different variant in the osteoligamentous pattern. Wide separation of the spinous processes ➡ indicates rupture of supraspinous and interspinous ligaments. A fracture ➡ extends through the pedicle and superior articular facet into the vertebral body.

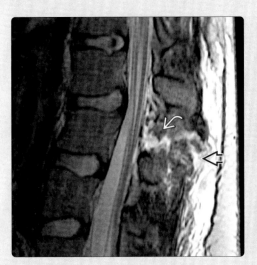
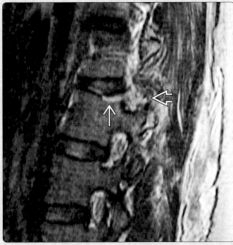

(Left) Sagittal T2WI MR in the same patient shows rupture of the interspinous ➡ and supraspinous ➡ ligaments. The anterior longitudinal ligament and posterior longitudinal ligament appear intact. (Right) Sagittal T2WI MR in the same patient shows a vertebral body fracture ➡ and facet joint disruption ➡. The combination of fracture and ligamentous injury is variable in Chance injury but all types show evidence of anterior compression and posterior distraction without an anterior to posterior vector force.

Anterior Compression Fracture

TERMINOLOGY

- Vertebral body fracture compressing anterior cortex, sparing middle/posterior columns

IMAGING

- Vertebral body shorter anteriorly than posteriorly
  - < 40-50% loss of height in patients with normal bone density
- ± vertebral body endplate abnormality
- ± anterior cortical irregularity
- Normal middle and posterior vertebral columns
- Most common in middle and lower thoracic spine

TOP DIFFERENTIAL DIAGNOSES

- Burst fracture
- Compression-distraction injury (Chance fracture)
- Pathologic fracture due to tumor
- Schmorl node
- Scheuermann kyphosis
- Physiologic vertebral wedging
- Limbus vertebra

CLINICAL ISSUES

- Most common type of thoracic spine fracture due to blunt trauma
  - Young patient (due to significant fall)
  - Osteoporotic patients: Insufficiency fracture
- American Academy of Orthopaedic Surgeons (AAOS) practice guidelines (2011)
  - Against vertebroplasty for osteoporotic spinal compression fracture in patients who are neurologically intact (kyphoplasty is option)
- AAOS guidelines recommend calcitonin for 4 weeks
  - Ibandronate and strontium ranelate are options to prevent additional symptomatic fractures

DIAGNOSTIC CHECKLIST

- Patients often have additional compression, burst, Chance, or shear fractures at other spinal levels

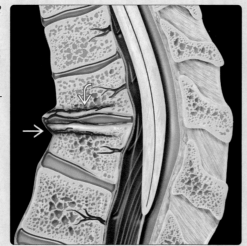

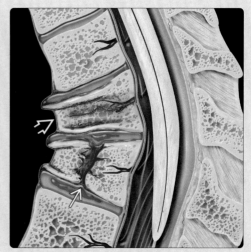

(Left) Sagittal graphic shows 2 types of compression fractures. The most common type is compression of the superior endplate ➡. Isolated compression of the inferior endplate ➡ is rare. Note that in these cases, there is angular deformity of the anterior cortex without focal endplate angulation. (Right) Sagittal graphic shows 2 additional types of compression fractures. The fracture involving both endplates ➡ is common, while the coronally oriented fracture through the vertebral body with wedge deformity ➡ is rare.

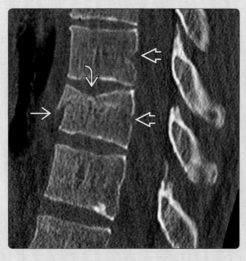

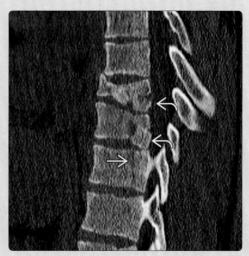

(Left) Sagittal bone CT shows a compression fracture causing angular deformity of the vertebral endplate ➡ and cortical step-off ➡ anteriorly. The normal vascular groove posteriorly ➡ should not be confused with a fracture. (Right) Sagittal bone CT shows multilevel injuries. The T12 compression fracture ➡ has a coronal split. T10 and T11 fractures are not compression fractures but burst fractures, since there is retropulsion of the posterior vertebral body cortex ➡.

Sacral Insufficiency Fracture

TERMINOLOGY

- Sacral fracture resulting from normal physiological stress on weakened (e.g., osteoporotic) bone

IMAGING

- Vertical fracture(s) through sacral alae
  - Either unilateral or bilateral
  - Located lateral to sacral foramina (zone I), roughly parallel to sacroiliac joint
- ± transverse fracture of sacral body
- Subtle ventral cortical disruption of sacral alae
- Sclerotic bands or irregular zones in sacral alae during healing phase
- Sacral marrow edema on MR
  - Hypointense on T1, hyperintense on T2
  - Greatest conspicuity on STIR or T2WI FS
  - May be overlooked on MR of lumbar spine obtained for generalized back pain

- Variable presence of classic H-shaped pattern of radiotracer uptake on bone scan: 19-62%
- Frequency of extrasacral tracer uptake 70% in 1 series
  - Multiple sites of tracer uptake may falsely raise concern for metastatic disease

PATHOLOGY

- Associated abnormalities
  - Vertebral compression fractures
  - Other pelvic insufficiency fractures (pubic rami, iliac wing)
  - Intertrochanteric femur fracture

CLINICAL ISSUES

- In 1 series, only 43% with unilateral fractures and 0% with bilateral fractures regained preinjury levels of mobility
- CT-guided percutaneous sacroplasty is effective procedure to treat painful sacral insufficiency fractures

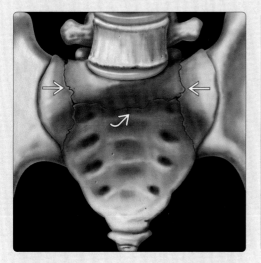

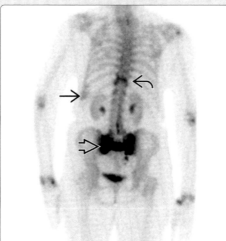

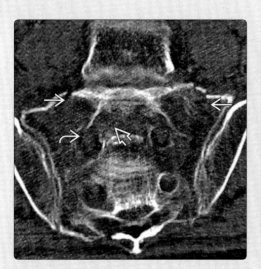

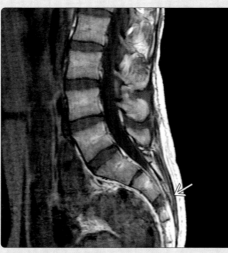

(Left) Sagittal graphic depicts bilateral vertical sacral alar fractures ➡ located lateral to the sacral foramina and a transverse fracture ➡ through the sacral body resulting in the classic H-shaped insufficiency fracture. (Right) Posterior bone scan shows increased sacral uptake in the classic "H" distribution ➡ due to insufficiency fracture. There is also uptake in a T12 compression fracture ➡ and in a pair of lower left rib fractures ➡.

(Left) Coronal reformatted CT shows diffuse osteopenia and bilateral sacral alae cortical defects ➡ due to sacral insufficiency fracture. The right-sided fracture extends into the right S1 neural foramen ➡. There is also a transverse fracture ➡ of the sacral body. (Right) Sagittal T1WI MR shows a small focus of low marrow signal involving the S3 body in the midline ➡ in this patient with insufficiency fracture. This location is important to evaluate in every lumbar spine MR.

IMAGING

- Fusiform intramedullary hyperintensity tracking CSF signal
  - Myelomalacia precedes overt syrinx formation = presyrinx state
- Cystic expansile cord lesion
  - May appear to be expansile lesion, relative finding in presence of cord atrophy
- Consider cine PC CSF flow study if suspected obstruction to CSF flow (e.g., arachnoid adhesions)

TOP DIFFERENTIAL DIAGNOSES

- Gibbs artifact
- Nontraumatic syrinx
- Myelitis
- Myelomalacia

PATHOLOGY

- Current treatment assumes syrinx is related to posttraumatic arachnoid scarring and CSF flow obstruction at trauma level

CLINICAL ISSUES

- Symptoms include spasticity, hyperhidrosis, pain, sensory loss, automotive hyperreflexia
- Classic presentation: Severe pain unrelieved by analgesics; ascending disassociated sensory loss
- Surgery reserved from patients with progressive neurological symptoms
  - 1st-line treatment has moved away from shunting of syrinx to restoring normal CSF flow patterns at traumatic site
    - Untethering of cord
    - Duraplasty
    - Spine realignment or fusion may be added if angulation or stability is problematic

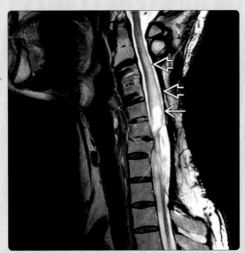

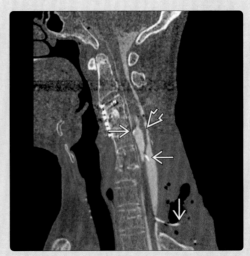

(Left) Sagittal images show extension of the syrinx over time into regions of presyrinx edema. This initial T2 MR after C3-C4 fusion and prior flexion injury at C5-C6 shows the well-defined syrinx cavity at the C5-C6 level with cord expansion ➡. T2 hyperintense signal within the cord extends cephalad from the syrinx to the C2 level due to cord edema ➡. (Right) Sagittal CT myelogram following placement of a syringoperitoneal shunt shows the shunt catheter ➡ within the syrinx cavity, which has decreased in size ➡.

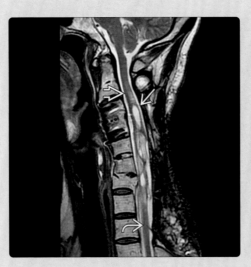

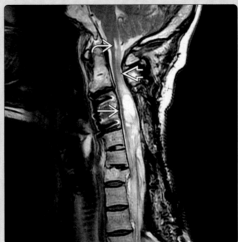

(Left) Follow-up sagittal T2 MR 3 months later shows extension of the syrinx to the C3 level ➡ with slight edema ➡ cephalad to this site. Note the presence of a shunt catheter ➡, which has not stopped the syrinx progression. (Right) Sagittal T2 MR 6 months later shows expansion of the syrinx at the C3 level ➡ and marked, increased presyrinx edema extending cephalad to the medulla ➡ with a small focus of syringobulbia ➡.

Presyrinx Edema

TERMINOLOGY

- Potentially reversible state of spinal cord edema caused by obstruction or alteration of normal CSF flow pathways

IMAGING

- Increased T2 signal within central aspect of cord with slightly decreased and ill-defined T1 signal and cord expansion in setting of pathology that alters CSF flow dynamics

TOP DIFFERENTIAL DIAGNOSES

- Posttraumatic syringomyelia
- Nontraumatic syringomyelia
  - Chiari 1 malformation
  - Tumor associated (ependymoma, astrocytoma, hemangioblastoma)
  - Idiopathic
- Myelitis
  - Demyelinating disease
  - Viral infection
  - Vasculitis (SLE)
- Infarction
- Myelomalacia
- Type I dural arteriovenous fistula
- Radiation myelopathy/necrosis

CLINICAL ISSUES

- Surgical removal of CSF flow obstruction will quickly eliminate cord edema
- Extensive arachnoid scarring gives poor prognosis with high incidence of recurrence

DIAGNOSTIC CHECKLIST

- Presyrinx edema likely represents point on continuum to development of syringomyelia
- May be misinterpreted as syringomyelia on MR studies
- May be related to progressive posttraumatic myelomalacic myelopathy

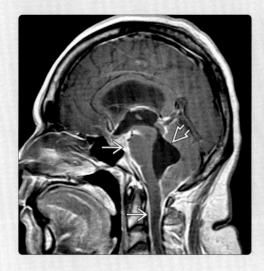

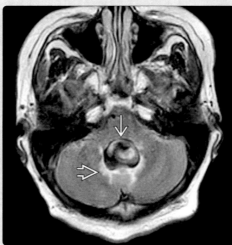

(Left) Sagittal T1WI C+ MR of the brain shows severe hydrocephalus ➡ from diffuse coccidioidomycosis basilar meningitis with diffuse leptomeningeal enhancement ➡. (Right) Axial FLAIR MR through the posterior fossa in this case of coccidioidomycosis meningitis shows transependymal edema ➡ surrounding the markedly dilated 4th ventricle ➡.

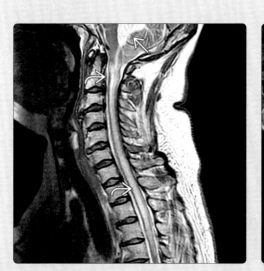

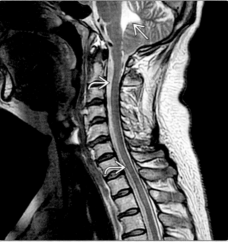

(Left) Sagittal T2 MR shows extensive cervical cord presyrinx edema ➡ that is due to coccidioidomycosis meningitis causing marked hydrocephalus ➡. The cervical subarachnoid space and 4th ventricular outflow obstruction causes abnormal fluid shift into the cord. (Right) For extensive cervical cord edema (presyrinx) resolution following ventricular shunting, a follow-up MR study 7 days after lateral ventricular shunt placement shows resolved cervical cord edema ➡ and diminished 4th ventricular size ➡.

Spinal Cord Contusion-Hematoma

TERMINOLOGY

- Spinal cord injury (SCI)
- Traumatic axonal injury, cord edema, &/or hemorrhage

IMAGING

- Abnormal cord signal on MR in setting of trauma
- Most common level of adult SCI is C4-C6
- Commonly associated fracture or subluxation in younger adults (16-45 years)
- Underlying degenerative change (canal stenosis) predisposes to cord injury in older population
- SCI without radiographic abnormality is common in pediatric population (< 8 years)
- Cord injury typically occult on CT

PATHOLOGY

- Overall incidence of SCI in trauma estimated at 3.7%
- High-velocity mechanisms more common in youth and young adults

- If > 45 years, more likely due to fall; short falls (< 1 m) may result in significant injury in elderly

CLINICAL ISSUES

- Edema without hemorrhage: Good prognosis for recovery
- Hematoma: Poor prognosis, often without recovery
  - Extent of intramedullary hemorrhage and cord swelling are key predictors of neurologic recovery after traumatic cervical cord injury
- 30-60 new cases per million per year in USA

DIAGNOSTIC CHECKLIST

- Sagittal STIR is key sequence
  - Sensitive to cord edema
  - Ligamentous/muscular injury
  - Marrow edema
- Sagittal and axial gradient-echo images for cord hemorrhage

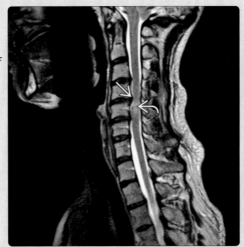

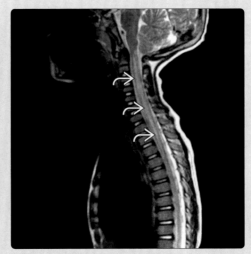

(Left) Sagittal T2 MR of a patient days after a motor vehicle accident with upper > lower extremity weakness shows congenital narrowing of the canal with multiple disc bulges & levels of canal stenosis, worst at C4-C5 ➡. Caudally, mild, patchy T2 hyperintensity shows nonhemorrhagic cord contusion ➡. (Right) Sagittal T2 MR in a child shows diffuse contusion ➡ in the cord from C1 through the upper thoracic cord. This patient presented with 4 extremity neurologic deficits after fall. Plain films would be normal (SCIWORA).

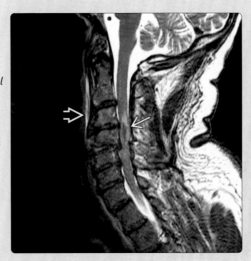

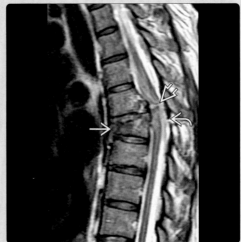

(Left) Sagittal T2 MR in a trauma patient shows low signal intensity cord hemorrhage at C4 ➡ with surrounding edema in the setting of severe cervical canal stenosis. Prevertebral edema is present ➡. (Right) Sagittal T2WI MR shows a midthoracic burst fracture ➡ and disruption of ligamentum flavum ➡. There is complete transection of the spinal cord ➡, demonstrated by a CSF-filled cleft with adjacent edema.

Idiopathic Spinal Cord Herniation

TERMINOLOGY

- Ventral cord herniation
- Herniation of spinal cord through defect in dura of ventral canal

IMAGING

- Best diagnostic clue: Focal anterior displacement of cord with expansion of dorsal subarachnoid space
- Location: Typically in midthoracic spine
  - T2-T8 level
- Focal cord deformity
- Cord displaced anteriorly against posterior edge of vertebral body
- Increased dorsal subarachnoid sac
- May see secondary collection of contrast in extradural sac
- Best imaging tool: CT postmyelography

TOP DIFFERENTIAL DIAGNOSES

- Arachnoid cyst

- Epidermoid cyst
  - Restricted diffusion
- Adhesions
- Cystic schwannoma
  - Peripheral or nodular enhancement
- Epidural hematoma
- Epidural empyema

PATHOLOGY

- Defect or diverticulum in ventral dural sheet into which cord herniates
- Several proposed mechanisms
  - Congenital weakening of ventral dural fibers
  - Damage to ventral dura by disc herniation or other mechanism
  - Abnormal adhesion of cord to anterior dural sleeve progressively wears down dura, leading to herniation

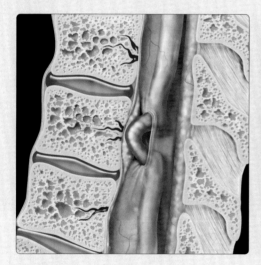
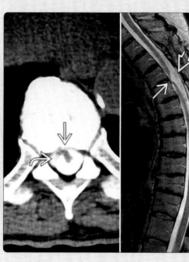

(Left) Sagittal graphic shows a focal dural defect in the thoracic spine allowing cord herniation. Note the distinctive and focal cord kink. (Right) Axial CECT myelogram (L) and sagittal T2WI MR (R) show ventral cord distortion and anterior displacement into the extradural cavity ➡ with focal enlargement of dorsal CSF ➡. Note the extradural CSF collection with slightly less density from delayed leakage of contrast ➡.

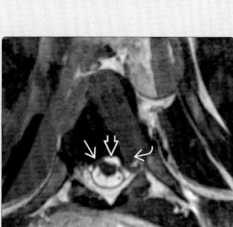
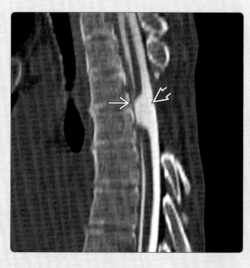

(Left) Axial heavily T2-weighted CISS MR shows the site of cord herniation through the dura ➡ as well as an adjacent extradural fluid collection along the ventral thecal sac ➡. Note the associated disc herniation ➡. (Right) Sagittal CECT (postmyelography) shows a focal kink of the thoracic cord ➡ and anterior adhesion to the back of the vertebral body. The expanded dorsal thecal sac mimics an arachnoid cyst ➡.

KEY FACTS

TERMINOLOGY

- Spinal epidural hematoma
- Posttraumatic accumulation of blood into spinal epidural space

IMAGING

- May be located at any spinal level
  - Typically extends over multiple levels
  - Fusiform, oval, or tubular
- Extends more freely in dorsal epidural space; ventral spread limited by dural attachment to posterior longitudinal ligament, anulus
- "Capping" of hematoma by epidural fat on sagittal imaging
  - Confirms epidural (rather than subdural) location
- MR signal intensity depends on age of hematoma

TOP DIFFERENTIAL DIAGNOSES

- Epidural abscess (or phlegmon)
- Epidural lipomatosis
- Epidural tumor
- Extramedullary hematopoiesis
- Ossification of posterior longitudinal ligament
- Sequestered disc fragment

PATHOLOGY

- Clot characteristics depend on compartment, age of collection
- Venous source more common than arterial

CLINICAL ISSUES

- May be associated with significant compression of spinal cord or cauda equina
- Surgical evacuation/decompression may be necessary to alleviate compression of spinal cord, cauda equina

DIAGNOSTIC CHECKLIST

- IV gadolinium-based contrast and fat saturation for complete characterization
- CT may help identify hemorrhage when MR confusing

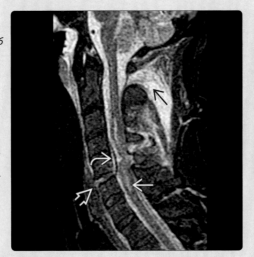

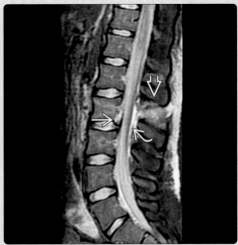

(Left) Sagittal STIR MR shows disruption of the anterior longitudinal ligament at C5-C6 ➡ and a small ventral epidural hematoma ➡. There is contusion of the cervical cord ➡. Injury to the paraspinous musculature is shown by hyperintense signal ➡. (Right) Sagittal STIR MR shows a small dorsal epidural hemorrhage ➡ in this patient with a L2 Chance fracture. This image shows a portion of the fracture extending through the posterior vertebral body ➡ and disruption of the interspinous ligaments at L1-L2 ➡.

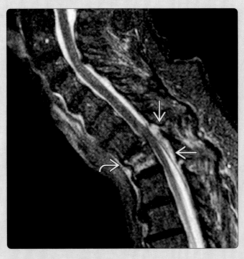

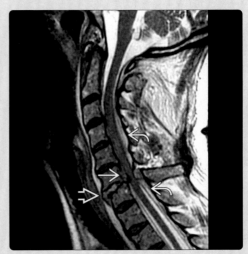

(Left) Sagittal STIR MR shows a compression deformity of T1 ➡ and dorsal epidural hematoma spanning C7 to T2-T3 ➡, which effaces the thecal sac and compresses the cervicothoracic cord. Note how STIR MR shows the complex signal of the hematoma distinct from the homogeneous CSF and the fat-suppressed epidural fat. (Right) Sagittal T2WI MR shows disruption of the anterior longitudinal ligament ➡ and posttraumatic herniation at C6-C7 ➡. There is dorsal epidural hematoma ➡ with cord compression.

Traumatic Subdural Hematoma

TERMINOLOGY

- Accumulation of blood between dura and arachnoid layers of spine

IMAGING

- Lobulated subdural mass with smooth margins
  - May be located at any level of spine
  - Tends to have biconvex or lentiform appearance on both sagittal and axial imaging
- MR signal depends on age of hematoma
  - MR most useful to assess size/extent and to evaluate impact on neurologic structures
- Variable degree of compression of spinal cord or nerve roots

TOP DIFFERENTIAL DIAGNOSES

- Epidural hematoma, traumatic
- Abscess, subdural
- Arachnoid cyst

- Meningioma

CLINICAL ISSUES

- Overall incidence of traumatic subdural hematoma is rare, as subdural space is relatively avascular
  - tSSDH is particularly rare
  - Nontraumatic etiologies are more common
    - Coagulopathy, arteriovenous malformation, or vascular tumor
- May be associated with significant compression of spinal cord or cauda equina
  - Surgical decompression or percutaneous drainage may be performed to alleviate compression of spinal cord or cauda equina
  - Conservative management may be considered
    - Usually resorbs within weeks or several months, depending on size
- Retroclival subdural hematoma requires evaluation for possible atlantooccipital dislocation

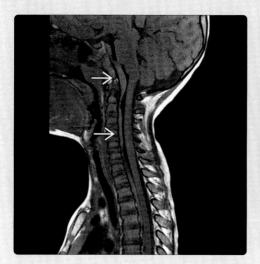
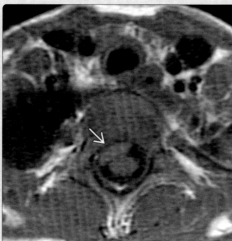

(Left) Sagittal T1WI MR shows a typical case of early subacute clival and subdural hematoma ➡ demonstrating the typical lobulated margin of the arachnoid effacing the ventral thecal sac. (Right) Axial T1WI MR through the lower cervical spine shows early subacute subdural hematoma ➡ demonstrating the typical lobulated margin of the arachnoid effacing the ventral thecal sac and impinging on the anterolateral cervical cord.

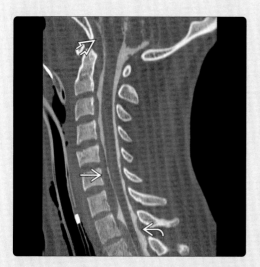
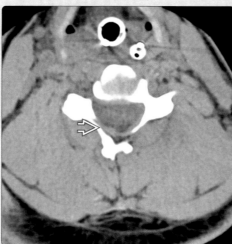

(Left) Sagittal CECT myelogram shows extensive posttraumatic spinal subdural hematoma with contiguous intracranial extension ➡. Note the larger ventral ➡ and smaller dorsal components of the hematoma ➡. (Right) Axial NECT shows posttraumatic spinal subdural hematoma with a small, circumferential subdural hematoma at the level of the midcervical spine ➡.

SECTION 6
Degenerative Diseases and Arthritides

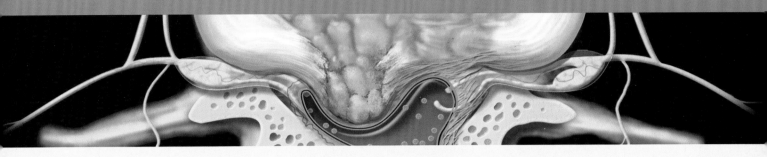

Degenerative Disease

Inflammatory, Crystalline, and Miscellaneous Arthritides

Disc Degeneration

Overview

Describing morphology alterations seen in degenerative disc disease requires common terminology to standardize communication. A series of pathoanatomic terms and definitions proposed by an interdisciplinary committee and endorsed by multiple societies is summarized here. These general terms are descriptive and independent of imaging modality.

It cannot be overemphasized that the specific terms described below do not imply knowledge of etiology, symptoms, prognosis, or need for treatment.

MR Signal Intensity

Any or all of the following can occur with **disc degeneration**: Real or apparent desiccation, fibrosis, narrowed intervertebral disc space, bulging, fissuring/mucinous degeneration of the anulus, osteophytes of the vertebral apophyses, and endplate/adjacent marrow changes.

Severely degenerated discs with markedly decreased signal intensity may demonstrate linear areas of high signal intensity on T2-weighted images that may represent free fluid within cracks or fissures of the degenerated complex. Signal intensity changes in the intervertebral disc on T1-weighted images, while much less common than the loss of signal noted on T2-weighted images, can also be seen with degeneration.

Regions of decreased or absent signal within **heavily calcified discs** may occur. Signal loss has been attributed to a low mobile proton density as well as, in the case of gradient-echo imaging, its sensitivity to the heterogeneous magnetic susceptibility found in calcified tissue.

Focal or diffuse areas of hyperintensity on T1-weighted spin-echo sequences may also be encountered in densely calcified intervertebral discs. These changes are related to T1 relaxation times secondary to a surface relaxation mechanism. These regions of high signal intensity on T1 are unaffected by fat suppression, suggesting that it is a T1-shortening effect rather than the presence of lipid. Hyperintensities within severely degenerated intervertebral discs that suppress on fat-saturation techniques presumably relate to areas of fatty marrow.

Separation between, or avulsion of, anular fibers from their vertebral body insertions, or breaks through fibers that extend transversely in a radial fashion or concentrically through layers of the anular lamellae, are referred to as **anular fissures**. On MR, these changes are seen on T2-weighted images as high signal intensity within the outer anulus/posterior longitudinal ligament complex (the so-called "high intensity zone"). These regions will also sometimes enhance following the administration of paramagnetic contrast, an effect thought to be secondary to reactive reparative tissue. The term "anular tear" should be avoided.

The role of anular disruption as the principle causal agent of disc degeneration has not been proven. In light of the continuing controversy surrounding the concept of "internal disc disruption," it is probably unwarranted to imply that radial tears are more than a manifestation of advanced degeneration. While no data clearly support an unequivocal causal relationship between these degeneration changes and symptoms, anular disruption is important to consider because of a controversial concept of "discogenic pain" and its implications concerning the usefulness of discography for

diagnosis. Back pain is thought to occur in some patients without morphological abnormalities, such as herniation or stenosis, which are thought to be related to leakage of nuclear material through the disrupted anulus into the epidural space.

Facet and ligament degenerative changes can occur with or without accompanying disc degeneration and can be readily identified on imaging studies. These changes are best described level by level, along with the presence of foraminal and canal narrowing, facet fluid, cysts, and other abnormalities.

Bulge vs. Herniation

The term **bulge** is used to describe a generalized extension > 25% of the circumference of the disc tissues, extending a short distance (< 3 mm) beyond the edges of the adjacent apophyses. A bulge is not a herniation, although 1 portion of the disc may be bulging and another portion of the disc may herniate.

A bulge is often a normal variant, particularly in children in whom all normal discs appear to extend slightly beyond the vertebral body margin. A bulge may also be associated with disc degeneration or may occur as a response to axial loading or angular motion with ligamentous laxity. Occasionally, a bulge in 1 plane is really a central subligamentous disc herniation in another plane. Asymmetric bulging of disc tissue > 25% of the disc circumference may be seen as an adaptation to adjacent deformity and is not considered a form of herniation.

Herniations are a localized displacement of disc material beyond the limits of the intervertebral disc space in any direction. The disc space is defined in the craniocaudad direction by the vertebral body endplates and peripherally by the outer edges of the vertebral ring apophyses, exclusive of any osteophytes. Herniations occupy < 25% of the disc circumference. They may be referred to as **focal or localized or broad based**. These descriptors regarding focal and broad-based morphologies have been eliminated in the latest version of the nomenclature.

Protrusions are herniations in which the greatest distance in any plane between the edges of disc material beyond the disc space is less than the distance between the edges of the base in the same plane. In practical terms, this looks like a triangle on sagittal images, with the base of the triangle at the disc margin and the apex of the triangle within the epidural space.

Extrusions are herniations in which, in at least 1 plane, any 1 distance between the edges of the disc material beyond the disc space is greater than the distance between the edges of the base in the same plane, or when no continuity exists between the disc material beyond the disc space and that material within the disc space. In practical terms, this looks like the toothpaste sign on the sagittal image with the larger component of the herniation within the epidural space and a smaller pedicle connecting to the intervertebral disc.

If extruded disc material is not contiguous to the disc space, it is referred to as a **sequestration** (or **"free fragment"**). The extrusion is referred to as "migrated" if it has been displaced from the site of extrusion, regardless of whether or not it is sequestrated. The signal intensity of the extruded portion may be increased or decreased on T2-weighted images. All disc herniations, small or large, can be associated with enhancement, and this enhancement may constitute a large portion of the extradural mass. Acute disc herniations may also cause focal epidural hemorrhage.

Sequestrated fragments can lie anterior to the posterior longitudinal ligament, especially if they have migrated behind the vertebral bodies where the posterior longitudinal ligament is not in direct opposition. Fragments may also lie posterior to the ligament. Sequestrated fragments within the lateral recess and the neural foramen have been shown to produce eroded cortical bone and expansion of those spaces and thus should be considered in the differential diagnosis of a mass arising and expanding the neural foramen and lateral recess.

In rare instances, disc herniation may extend through the dura and arachnoid. The mechanism of **intradural disc herniation** is thought to be the development of chronic inflammation leading to adhesions between the dura and the posterior longitudinal ligament. Nevertheless, there is almost invariably penetration through the posterior longitudinal ligament posteriorly, where it is fused with the anulus, or superiorly or inferiorly, where it fuses with the vertebral body margin. Intradural disc herniations may enhance and mimic neoplasm.

The characterization of a disc herniation is not always clear cut, and it may appear as a protrusion in 1 plane and an extrusion in another. If there is displacement away from the disc space in any plane, it should be referred to as an extrusion. Containment refers to the integrity of the outer anulus covering the disc herniation.

One may view the continuum of herniated disc disease as starting with anular disruption, proceeding on to small focal herniation (which is not broken completely through the anulus-ligamentous complex) to frank herniation (extrusion). The extrusion has dissected through the anulus and posterior ligamentous complex completely. These extrusions may show variable degrees of containment, and a line of decreased signal intensity has been reported around sequestrated fragments and large extruded discs where there has clearly been disruption of the anulus and ligament. This is thought to be secondary to anular and ligamentous fibers that are carried away with the disc herniation.

The anulus fibrosus and posterior longitudinal ligament are so intertwined at the level of the disc that a distinction between the 2 structures may be impossible or, for that matter, irrelevant. Technical limitations of CT and MR usually preclude the distinction of a contained from an uncontained disc herniation. In the transverse plane, the disc abnormality is usually described as **central**, **right** or **left central**, **subarticular**, **foraminal**, or **extraforaminal** (far lateral). In the sagittal plane, **discal**, **infrapedicular**, **suprapedicular**, and **pedicular** are most commonly employed.

Several nonstandard terms should be avoided. These include "disc material beyond the interspace" (DEBIT), which has been superseded by protrusion and extrusion categorization. "Herniated nucleus pulposus" is an old favorite but is not accurate because much of what herniates is not nucleus pulposus (cartilage, fibrous tissue). "Ruptured" disc has no role in a report because this implies a specific knowledge of a traumatic etiology, which is nearly always lacking. Finally, "prolapse" is synonymous with the standard term "protrusion."

Degenerative Endplate Changes

The relationship among the vertebral body, endplate, and disc has been studied by using both degenerated and chymopapain-treated discs as models. A common observation in MR is signal intensity changes in the vertebral body marrow adjacent to endplates of a degenerative disc. These changes appear to take 3 main forms.

Type I changes demonstrate a decreased signal intensity on T1-weighted images and an increased signal intensity on T2-weighted images, and these changes have been identified in ~ 4% of patients scanned for lumbar disease. Type I changes are also seen in ~ 30% of chymopapain-treated discs, which may be viewed as a model of acute disc degeneration.

Type II changes are represented by increased signal intensity on T1-weighted images and an isointense or slightly hyperintense signal on T2-weighted images. These changes are seen in ~ 16% of cases. In both types I and II, there is evidence of associated degenerative disc disease at the level of involvement. Mild enhancement of type I vertebral body marrow changes is seen with Gd-DTPA, which at times can extend to involve the disc itself. This enhancement is presumably related to vascularized fibrous tissue within adjacent marrow.

Histopathological sections of a disc with type I changes demonstrate disruption and fissuring of the endplate and vascularized fibrous tissues within the adjacent marrow, producing prolongation of T1 and T2. Discs with type II changes also show evidence of endplate disruption with yellow marrow replacement in the adjacent vertebral body, resulting in a shorter T1. There appears to be a relationship between the different endplate types, as type I changes have been observed to convert to type II with time, and type II changes seem to remain stable.

Type III changes are represented by decreased signal intensity on both T1- and T2-weighted images. These findings seem to correlate with the presence of extensive bony sclerosis.

Although the signal intensity changes of type I may be similar to those seen in vertebral osteomyelitis, the distinguishing factor (at least in the adult population) is the involvement of the intervertebral disc, which shows abnormal high signal intensity and abnormal configuration on T2-weighted images with infection. Increased signal from the disc may suggest an active inflammatory process. Disc narrowing, sclerosis, and vertebral endplate irregularity suggestive of osteomyelitis have also been demonstrated in long-term hemodialysis and calcium pyrophosphate disease. Classically, in the patient with hemodialysis spondyloarthropathy, the intervertebral disc maintains low signal intensity on both T1- and T2-weighted sequences. Crystal disorders should show increased signal intensity on long TE/TR sequences.

Selected References

1. Fardon DF et al: Lumbar disc nomenclature: version 2.0: recommendations of the combined task forces of the North American Spine Society, the American Society of Spine Radiology and the American Society of Neuroradiology.. Spine J. 14(11):2525-45, 2014
2. Fardon DF et al: Nomenclature and classification of lumbar disc pathology. Recommendations of the Combined task Forces of the North American Spine Society, American Society of Spine Radiology, and American Society of Neuroradiology. Spine (Phila Pa 1976). 26(5):E93-E113, 2001
3. Milette PC: The proper terminology for reporting lumbar intervertebral disk disorders. AJNR Am J Neuroradiol. 18(10):1859-66, 1997

(Left) *Sagittal graphic of a disc bulge shows generalized extension of the disc margin beyond the vertebral body* ➡️*. An axial view must show generalized extension > 90° of the disc margin to be a bulge; < 90° would be a protrusion.* (Right) *Sagittal graphic of a disc protrusion shows extension of disc material beyond the interspace margin where the base of the herniation is wider than the portion in the epidural space* ➡️*.*

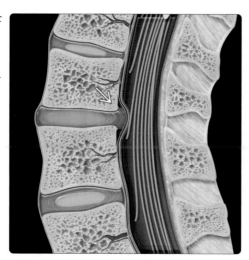
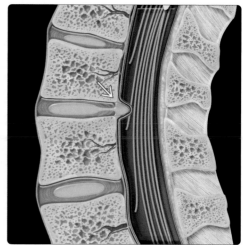

(Left) *Sagittal graphic of a disc extrusion shows extension of disc material beyond the interspace where the base of the herniated material is smaller than the component in the epidural space* ➡️*.* (Right) *Sagittal graphic shows a disc extrusion with free fragment. Extruded disc demonstrates extension of disc material beyond the interspace with the base narrower than the portion in the epidural space* ➡️*. A 2nd component* ➡️ *has separated from the parent disc and is a free fragment or sequestered disc.*

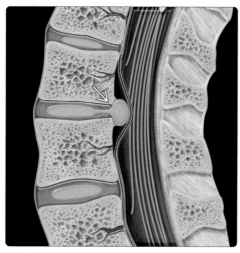
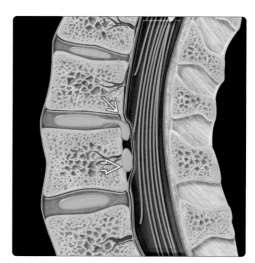

(Left) *Sagittal T1WI MR shows severe disc degeneration at L5-S1 with disc extrusion where the base of herniation is narrower than the portion extending into epidural space* ➡️*. There is inferior migration of herniation consistent with free fragment.* (Right) *Sagittal T1WI MR shows a large L3-L4 far lateral disc extrusion, which is located within the neural foramen (foraminal herniation)* ➡️ *and obscures the exiting L3 nerve root. Note the normal exiting root at the level below for comparison* ➡️*.*

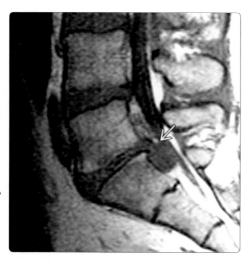
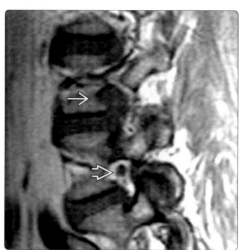

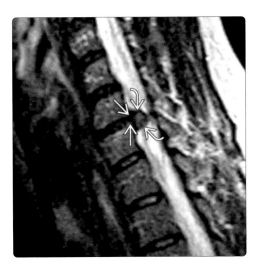

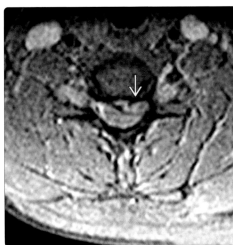

(Left) Sagittal T2WI MR shows C5-C6 disc extrusion where the base of the herniation ➡ is smaller than the rest of the epidural component ➡. (Right) Axial T2* GRE MR shows a large left central disc extrusion with moderate compression of the thecal sac and cord ➡.

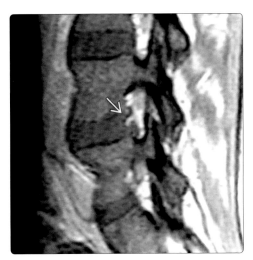

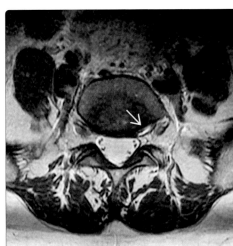

(Left) Sagittal T1 C+ MR shows an anular fissure as focal enhancement within the posterolateral anulus fibrosus ➡. There is no disc herniation, and the foramen is normal in size. The term "anular tear" is to be avoided. (Right) Axial T2WI shows an anular fissure along the posterior lateral margin of the disc defined as linear hyperintensity without focal contour abnormality ➡.

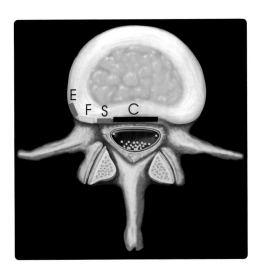

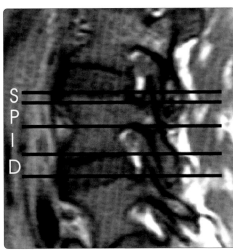

(Left) Axial graphic of a lumbar intervertebral disc shows right-left location nomenclature classification for disc disease: C (central), S (subarticular), F (foraminal), and E (extraforaminal or far-lateral). (Right) Sagittal T1W1 MR through the neural foramen of the lumbar spine shows the level of classification and nomenclature: S (suprapedicular), P (pedicular), I (infrapedicular), and D (disc).

KEY FACTS

TERMINOLOGY

- Generalized and multifactorial process affecting discovertebral unit, leading to biomechanical/morphologic alterations
- Asymptomatic or associated with back/neck pain ± radiculopathy

IMAGING

- Loss of disc space height, vacuum phenomenon seen as low signal within disc
- Degenerative endplate changes I → III
- T2 shows loss of signal from nucleus, loss of horizontal nuclear cleft
- Disc may show linear enhancement with degenerative disc disease, enhancement within Schmorl nodes

TOP DIFFERENTIAL DIAGNOSES

- Disc space infection
- Hemodialysis spondyloarthropathy

- Seronegative spondyloarthropathy

PATHOLOGY

- Etiology of disc degeneration multifactorial
- Individuals involved in manual materials handling, with repeated heavy lifting, at increased risk
- Some studies show strong familial predisposition to discogenic back pain

CLINICAL ISSUES

- Lifetime incidence of back pain in United States 50-80%
- Prevalence among adults ranges from 15-30%
- Back pain most common cause of disability in persons younger than 45 years
- Low back pain (LBP) has benign natural history
  - LBP symptoms self-limited and resolve spontaneously (< 2 weeks)

(Left) *Sagittal graphic shows degeneration of L4-L5 and L5-S1 intervertebral discs with loss of disc height, associated type II fatty endplate change, and osteophyte formation.* (Right) *Sagittal NECT reformat shows multilevel severe loss of disc height and vacuum phenomenon. Endplate eburnation is present at L3-L4 and L4-L5. Osteophyte is present at several levels.*

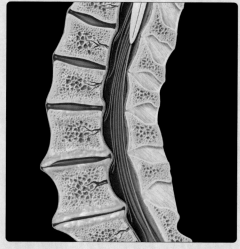
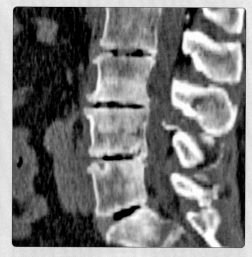

(Left) *Sagittal T2WI MR shows a degenerated disc as low signal at L4-L5, L5-S1 compared with normal disc signal intensity at L3-L4. Degenerative disc disease is also seen as loss of disc height at L4-L5, disc herniation at L5-S1 ➡, and anular tear at L4-L5 ➡.* (Right) *Axial T2WI MR shows protrusion ➡ compressing the exiting root. A degenerated disc shows low signal centrally with disrupted internal disc contents pointing toward the herniation ➡.*

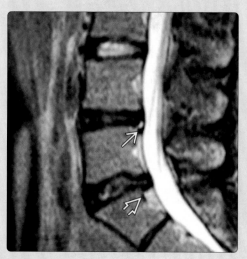
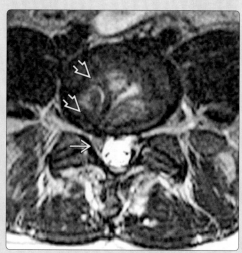

TERMINOLOGY

Synonyms

- Degenerative disc disease (DDD), disc degeneration, spondylosis

Definitions

- Generalized and multifactorial process affecting discovertebral unit, leading to biomechanical/morphologic alterations

IMAGING

General Features

- Best diagnostic clue
  - Decreased signal of intervertebral disc on T2WI
- Location
  - Intervertebral disc, adjacent endplates

Radiographic Findings

- Radiography
  - Late disease shows loss of disc space height, osteophyte formation, bony endplate eburnation "discogenic sclerosis," vacuum phenomenon

CT Findings

- NECT
  - Useful for assessment of bulge, focal disc herniation, osteophyte formation with facet arthropathy, central stenosis

MR Findings

- T1WI
  - Loss of disc space height, vacuum phenomenon seen as low signal within disc
- T2WI
  - T2 shows loss of signal from nucleus, loss of horizontal nuclear cleft
- T1WI C+
  - Disc may show linear enhancement with DDD, enhancement within Schmorl nodes

Nonvascular Interventions

- Myelography
  - Nonspecific extradural defects associated with central stenosis, osteophyte formation, herniation

Nuclear Medicine Findings

- Bone scan
  - Diffuse increased uptake with DDD, osteophyte formation, and facet degenerative arthropathy

DIFFERENTIAL DIAGNOSIS

Disc Space Infection

- Endplate destruction

Hemodialysis Spondyloarthropathy

- Low signal on T1WI, may be indistinguishable from pyogenic infection

Seronegative Spondyloarthropathy

- Inflammatory endplate changes may mimic type I degenerative endplate changes

PATHOLOGY

General Features

- Genetics
  - 2 collagen IX alleles associated with sciatica and disc herniation
  - Disc degeneration associated with aggrecan gene polymorphism, matrix metalloproteinase 3 and 7 gene alleles
  - Some studies show strong familial predisposition to discogenic back pain
- Etiology of symptomatic DDD not fully known

Microscopic Features

- Nucleus becomes progressively disorganized and fibrous, cracks and fissures throughout nucleus
- Endplate fragmentation and disruption with new bone formation, granulation tissue
- Marrow conversion from hematopoietic to fat or fibrous (type II, type I endplate change, respectively)

CLINICAL ISSUES

Presentation

- Most common signs/symptoms
  - Commonly asymptomatic with normal neurologic exam
  - Low back pain (LBP) or neck pain
    - ± radiculopathy
  - Other signs/symptoms
    - Range of motion restricted

Demographics

- Age
  - Back pain peak 45-65 years
- Gender
  - M = F
- Epidemiology
  - Overall incidence of back pain ~ 45 per 1,000 person-years
  - Lifetime incidence of back pain in United States 50-80%
  - Prevalence among adults ranges from 15-30%
  - 2-5% of population receives medical care every year for back pain

Natural History & Prognosis

- LBP has benign natural history
- LBP symptoms self-limited and resolve spontaneously (< 2 weeks)
- 7% of patients with acute symptoms develop chronic pain

Treatment

- Nonoperative treatment with bedrest, exercise, drug therapy, manipulation, epidural steroid injection
- Operative treatment
  - Surgical treatment for axial pain from DDD most commonly involves fusion

DIAGNOSTIC CHECKLIST

Consider

- 30% of normal individuals have abnormal signal in lumbar discs

(Left) H&E-stained section of normal discovertebral junction shows a normal endplate with nucleus ➡, smooth cartilage junction ➡, thin bony trabeculae, and normal hematopoietic marrow ➡. **(Right)** Sagittal T2WI MR shows multiple aspects of DDD, including Schmorl node involving inferior endplates of L3 and T12 ➡, diffuse disc degeneration with loss of height at multiple levels, severe multilevel central canal stenosis with bulging discs effacing the thecal sac, and multilevel ligamentous hypertrophy ➡.

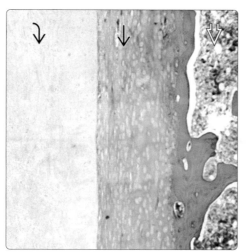

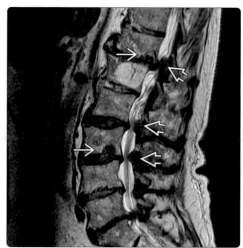

(Left) Micropathology, low-power H&E of severely degenerated discovertebral junction shows a degenerated endplate with disruption of cartilage, fissures in the nucleus ➡, granulation tissue ➡, and cartilage endplate herniation ➡. **(Right)** Axial discogram CT shows contrast extension from the central nucleus pulposus into a midline anular tear ➡ extending to the epidural space.

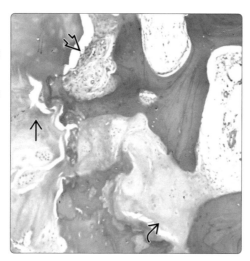

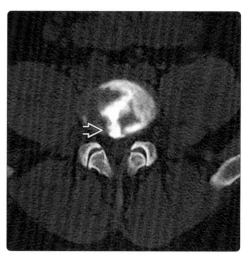

(Left) Sagittal T1WI MR shows prominent type II endplate change at L4-L5 (fatty marrow) ➡ with marked loss of disc space height. The adjacent level L3-L4 shows type I change as low signal marrow ➡ with slight spondylolisthesis. **(Right)** Sagittal STIR MR level shows L3-L4 pronounced type I degenerative endplate change. There is a slight anterolisthesis of L3 on L4 and multilevel disc degeneration.

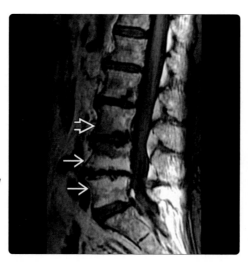

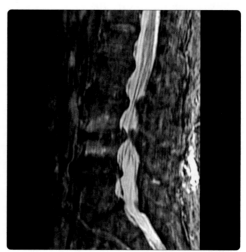

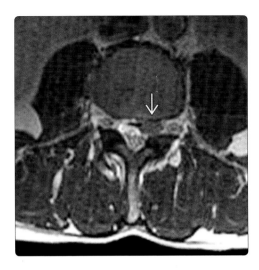

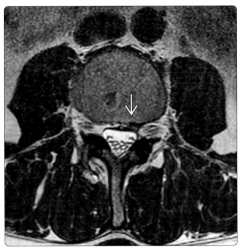

(Left) *Axial T2WI MR at presentation shows a large left-sided disc extrusion with thecal sac compression* ➡ *in this case of natural involution of large disc extrusion.* (Right) *Follow-up axial T2WI MR after conservative therapy shows a markedly decreased size of the previously large disc extrusion* ➡ *seen on the previous image.*

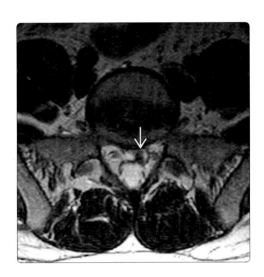

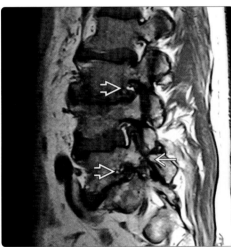

(Left) *Axial T2WI MR study 7 months after the initial diagnosis of typical disc extrusion shows well-defined fluid signal intensity that has replaced the disc herniation, consistent with a "discal cyst"* ➡. *This may reflect involution of a prior hemorrhage with the disc herniation.* (Right) *Sagittal T1WI MR shows chronic L5 spondylolysis* ➡ *with severe multilevel foraminal stenosis with extension of the disc bulge and osteophyte into the inferior neural foramina* ➡.

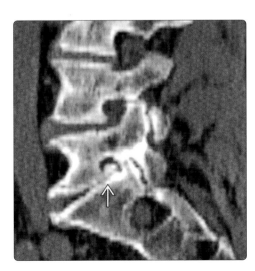

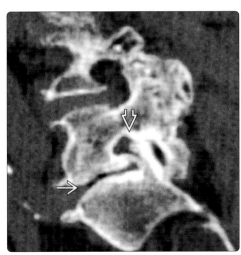

(Left) *Sagittal NECT shows loss of disc height at L5-S1 with resultant rostrocaudal subluxation of facets and foraminal stenosis. Osteophyte causes further stenosis extending into the foramen* ➡. (Right) *Sagittal NECT reformat shows loss of disc space height at L5-S1 with vacuum phenomenon* ➡. *Marked facet hypertrophic degenerative arthropathy* ➡ *gives severe foraminal stenosis.*

KEY FACTS

TERMINOLOGY

- Vertebral endplate change, Modic changes
  - Type I, II, III endplate change
- MR signal abnormalities involving vertebral body endplates related to degenerative disc disease
  - Type I: Hypointense on T1, hyperintense on T2
  - Type II: Hyperintense on T1, isointense on T2
  - Type III: Hypointense on T1 and T2

TOP DIFFERENTIAL DIAGNOSES

- Disc space infection
- Pseudoarthrosis/nonunion
- Seronegative spondyloarthropathy
- Metastatic disease

PATHOLOGY

- Type I: Replacement with fibrovascular marrow
- Type II: Replacement by fatty marrow
- Type III: Replacement by bony sclerosis with little residual marrow

CLINICAL ISSUES

- Type I: Present in 4% of patients undergoing MR for disc disease
- Type II: Present in 16% of patients undergoing MR for disc disease
  - Commonly present after successful segmental fusion
- Type III: Least common (~ 1%)
- Relationship of type I endplate changes to low back pain (discogenic pain) controversial
  - Some studies suggest type I, II changes have high specificity (> 90%) but low sensitivity (20-30%) for painful lumbar disc
  - Type I change shows high positive predictive value with discography

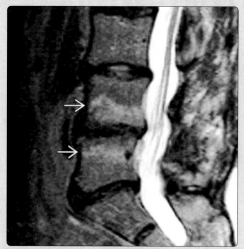
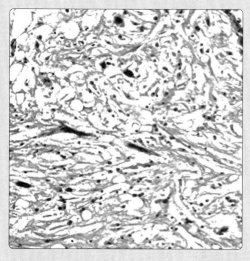

(Left) Sagittal T2WI MR shows increased signal intensity from L4-L5 endplates ➡. The disc at L4-L5 is low signal, reflecting disc degeneration with a slight retrolisthesis. No prevertebral or epidural soft tissue is present to suggest infection. (Right) Micropathology, low-power H&E shows type I change with fibrovascular replacement of hematopoietic marrow. There are prominent interstitial spaces and scattered capillaries among spindle-shaped cells.

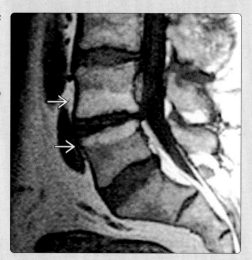
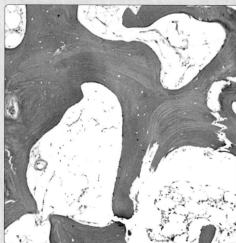

(Left) Sagittal T1WI MR shows classic type II endplate changes ➡ due to fatty marrow replacement at L4-L5 disc level. There is degeneration of L4-L5 with a loss of disc height and vacuum phenomenon. (Right) Micropathology, low-power H&E shows type II changes with fatty replacement of normal hematopoietic marrow. Note the thickened trabeculae with new woven bone formation.

Degenerative Endplate Changes

TERMINOLOGY

Synonyms

- Vertebral endplate change, Modic changes
- Type I, II, III endplate change

Definitions

- MR signal abnormalities involving vertebral body endplates related to degenerative disc disease
  - Type I: Hypointense on T1WI, hyperintense on T2WI
  - Type II: Hyperintense on T1WI, isointense on T2WI
  - Type III: Hypointense on T1WI and T2WI

IMAGING

General Features

- Best diagnostic clue
  - Parallel signal alteration of vertebral endplates, associated with evidence of disc degeneration
- Location
  - Most common in lumbar spine, may occur in any vertebral body
  - L4-L5, L5-S1 most common

MR Findings

- T1WI
  - Type I: Hypointense horizontal bands involving endplates
  - Type II: Hyperintense bands
  - Type III: Hypointense bands
- T2WI
  - Type I: Hyperintense horizontal bands involving endplates
  - Type II: Isointense to slightly hyperintense bands
    - Signal tracks fat on all pulse sequences
  - Type III: Hypointense bands involving endplates
- T1WI C+
  - Type I: May show prominent enhancement
  - Commonly associated with linear intervertebral disc enhancement

DIFFERENTIAL DIAGNOSIS

Disc Space Infection

- Low signal involving endplates similar to type I change
- Endplate destruction
- Hyperintense intervertebral disc on T2WI

Pseudoarthrosis/Nonunion

- Low signal involving endplates similar to type I change

Hemodialysis Spondyloarthropathy

- May be indistinguishable from pyogenic disc space infection

Seronegative Spondyloarthropathy

- Inflammatory endplate changes (Anderson lesions) may mimic type I degenerative endplates

Metastatic Disease

- Focal low signal on T1WI with bone destruction ± epidural extension

PATHOLOGY

General Features

- Etiology
  - Unknown
    - Type I: Probably reflects sequelae of acute disc degeneration
    - Type II: Probably reflects sequelae of chronic disc degeneration
    - Type III: Probably reflects sequelae of chronic disc degeneration
- Genetics
  - Interleukin 1 gene locus polymorphisms reported

Gross Pathologic & Surgical Features

- Disc degeneration with desiccation of disc, bony endplate eburnation

Microscopic Features

- Type I: Spindle cells, capillaries (vascularized fibrous tissue) with prominent interstitial space, thickened trabeculae with new bone production
- Type II: Adipose cells, prominent trabeculae with new bone production (woven bone)
- Type III: Dense woven bone

CLINICAL ISSUES

Presentation

- Most common signs/symptoms
  - Role of endplate changes in back pain is controversial
  - Relationship of type I endplate changes to low back pain (discogenic pain) controversial
    - No significant correlation between concordant pain at discography and presence of endplate changes in some studies
    - Some studies suggest type I, type II changes have high specificity (> 90%) but low sensitivity (20-30%) for painful lumbar disc
    - Some studies show type I correlation with pain (> 70%) but low with type II (10%)
    - Type I change shows high positive predictive value with discography
- Clinical profile
  - Low back pain without major radicular component

Demographics

- Epidemiology
  - Adult with disc degeneration
  - Type I: Present in 4% of patients undergoing MR for disc disease
  - Type II: Present in 16% of patients undergoing MR for disc disease
  - Type III: Least common (~ 1%)
    - Mixed lesions are possible (I/II and II/III)

Natural History & Prognosis

- Natural history variable
  - Type I change may convert to type II over course of months to years
  - Type II more stable change
    - Up to 14% of type II may convert over 3-year follow-up

Disc Bulge

TERMINOLOGY

- Anular bulge
- Generalized extension of disc beyond edges of vertebral ring apophyses

IMAGING

- Circumferential disc "expansion" beyond confines of vertebral endplates
  - Short radius of extension: ≤ 3 mm
  - > 25% of disc circumference
  - If morphologic abnormality is < 25% of disc circumference, then it is herniation and not bulge
- Smooth ventral extradural defect in contrast column, with indentation on anterior thecal sac
  - Central canal and subarticular recesses usually not compromised unless associated with ligamentous hypertrophy
- T1WI and T2WI MR with sagittal and axial planes
- Discography may help identify symptomatic disc

TOP DIFFERENTIAL DIAGNOSES

- Disc protrusion (< 25% of disc circumference)
- Ossification of posterior longitudinal ligament
  - Most common in cervical spine (70%)
- Vertebral endplate bony spur
  - Continuous with vertebral endplate

PATHOLOGY

- Bulge less important as separate entity but associated with disc degeneration and anular fissures → "discogenic" pain

CLINICAL ISSUES

- Low back pain
- Up to 39% of asymptomatic adults have bulging discs
- > 80-90% success rate with conservative treatment

(Left) *Axial T2WI FS MR demonstrates the broad-based appearance of the bulging disc* ⇩ *with predominately low signal intensity. Associated anular fissure would show focal high signal.* (Right) *Sagittal T2WI MR through the lumbar spine shows L4-L5 disc degeneration with loss of signal and a bulging disc touching the ventral thecal sac without significant deformity. An associated hyperintense annular fissure is present* ➡.

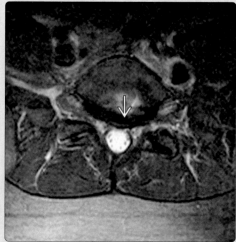
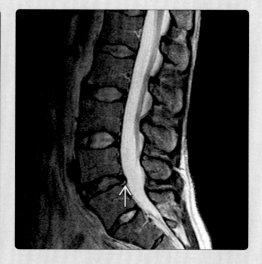

(Left) *Axial NECT after discography shows multiple circumferential annular tears* ➡. *These coalesce into a large dorsal annular defect, allowing contrast extending beyond annulus* ➡. *Note the generalized extension of the posterior disc margin into the epidural space.* (Right) *Sagittal T2WI MR shows grade II spondylolisthesis at L5-S1 with type I degenerative endplate changes* ➡. *There is extensive "uncovering" of L4 and L5 discs, which should not be confused with annular bulge* ➡. *Note the annular fissures at L2-L3 and L3-L4* ➡.

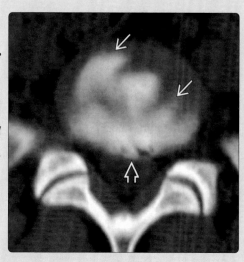
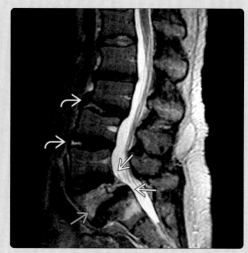

TERMINOLOGY

- Anular defect; high-intensity zone (HIZ) in posterior anulus
- Disruption of concentric collagenous fibers comprising anulus fibrosus
- Term "tear" is nonstandard and may inaccurately imply acute traumatic etiology

IMAGING

- Focal HIZ in anulus on T2WI with low signal of parent disc
- Contrast enhancement on T1WI
- Focally enhancing nidus in posterior disc margin
- Discography is more provocative test (symptom simulation) rather than diagnostic imaging modality

TOP DIFFERENTIAL DIAGNOSES

- Disc space infection
- Focal disc protrusion
- Focal fat or ossification of disc with fatty marrow

CLINICAL ISSUES

- Most anular tears are asymptomatic
  - Autopsy demonstrates high prevalence of fissures
  - MR shows anular fissures in majority of asymptomatic individuals
- Utility of discography remains controversial
- Direct association with disc degeneration
  - Recurrent meningeal nerve and ventral ramus of somatic spinal nerve are sources of innervation
  - Anular disruption may allow inflammatory substances to leak from nucleus

DIAGNOSTIC CHECKLIST

- Consider other sources of low back pain or disc pathology (e.g., disc infection)
- Incidental HIZ of otherwise normal disc is essentially normal finding

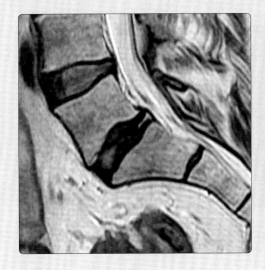

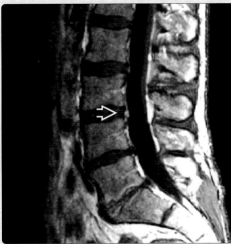

(Left) Sagittal PD FSE MR demonstrates linear hyperintensity within the posterior aspect of the anulus fibrosus at L5-S1, reflecting the anular disruption of an anular fissure. There is mild bulging of the anulus at this level as well. (Right) Sagittal T1WI C+ MR shows focal enhancement within posterior anulus ➡. This is a typical pattern for focal enhancement within anular fissure. There is also enhancement within the posterior anulus at L2-L3 and severe degenerative disc disease at L5-S1.

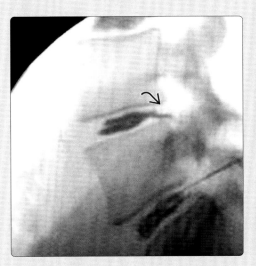

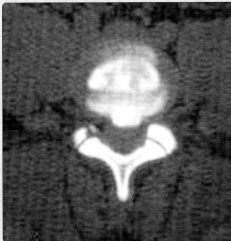

(Left) Lateral radiograph during discography shows leakage of intradiscal contrast at L4-L5 ➘ and fissured and degenerated L4-L5 and L5-S1 discs. Symptoms were reproduced with injection of L5-S1 disc, not at L4-L5. (Right) Axial bone CT in the same patient following the discogram shows the leakage of contrast into the ventral epidural space at L4-L5, verifying the presence of the anular defect.

KEY FACTS

TERMINOLOGY

- Protruded disc, extruded disc, free fragment, sequestered disc
- Localized (< 50% of disc circumference) displacement of disc material beyond edges of vertebral ring apophyses

IMAGING

- Small mass in ventral spinal canal, contiguous with intervertebral disc
- Protrusion is herniated disc with broad base at parent disc
- Extrusion is herniated disc with narrow or no base at parent disc
- Sequestered or free fragment: Extruded disc without contiguity to parent disc
- Migrated: Disc material displaced away from site of herniation, regardless of continuity to parent disc

TOP DIFFERENTIAL DIAGNOSES

- OPLL

- Osteophyte
- Tumor
- Hemorrhage
- Abscess

CLINICAL ISSUES

- 10% of people under age 40 have cervical herniation
- Acute radiculopathy usually self-limited disorder with full recovery expected
  - Neck pain (90%)
  - Radicular pain (65%)
  - Paresthesia (89%)
- Treatment
  - Conservative treatment
  - Multiple surgical approaches without clear consensus

DIAGNOSTIC CHECKLIST

- Use fast STIR for cord disease
- Axial GRE, T2* GRE for disc definition

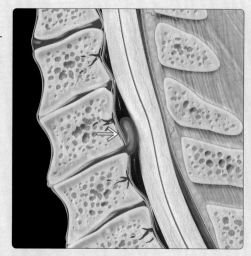

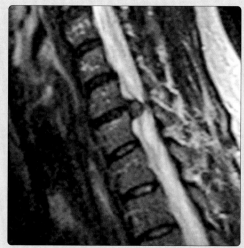

(Left) Sagittal graphic shows disc extrusion ➡ with the base of the herniation smaller than the epidural component, effacing the thecal sac and causing cord compression. (Right) Sagittal T2WI MR shows C5-C6 disc extrusion with the base of herniation smaller than the component extending into the epidural space.

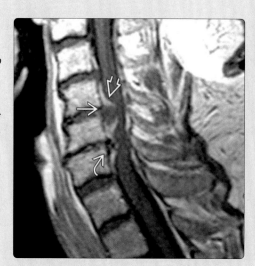

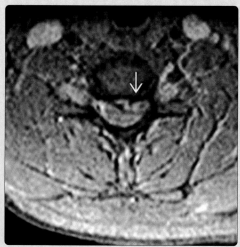

(Left) Sagittal T1WI C+ MR shows C4-C5 extrusion ➡ impinging upon the cord. Smaller C5-C6 protrusion also compresses the ventral cord ➡. Peripheral enhancement ➡ is related to epidural plexus and granulation tissue. (Right) Axial T2* GRE MR shows left-sided extrusion ➡ effacing the left side of the thecal sac and compressing the cord, extending toward the left neural foramen.

KEY FACTS

IMAGING

- Small mass in spinal canal contiguous with intervertebral disc
  - Ventral epidural
  - Rare in upper thoracic spine (T1-T3)
- May enhance peripherally after intravenous contrast material due to granulation tissue or dilated epidural plexus
  - Peripheral enhancement may give "lifted band" or "tent" configuration

TOP DIFFERENTIAL DIAGNOSES

- Osteophyte
  - Sharp margins not arising directly from intervertebral disc level
- Tumor
  - Homogeneous enhancement
- Hemorrhage
  - Elongated within epidural space, tends to be posterior
- Abscess

- May mimic large herniation with peripheral enhancement

CLINICAL ISSUES

- 5th decade
- Uncommon entity
- Thoracic disc surgery uncommon, represents 1-2% of all disc surgery
- History of Scheuermann

DIAGNOSTIC CHECKLIST

- Calcification (65%)
- Multiple herniation (14%)
- T2WI critical since herniation may not be visible on T1WI due to calcification
- **Check and recheck herniation level, counting from C2 and L5 levels**
  - Preoperative placement of gold fiducial markers overlying posterior elements can aid intraoperative level localization

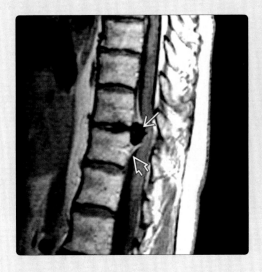
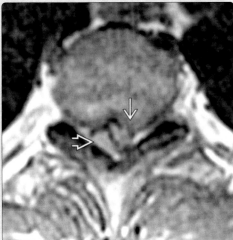

(Left) *Sagittal T1WI MR with contrast shows a large low signal intensity mass contiguous with disc space reflecting a large calcified disc extrusion ➡. Prominent distended epidural veins "tent" around herniation ➡. (Right) Axial T1WI MR demonstrates the large left-sided extrusion ➡ severely compressing the left side of the cord ➡.*

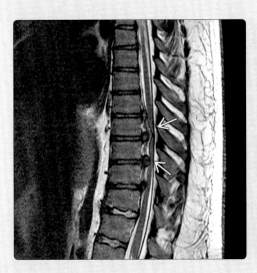
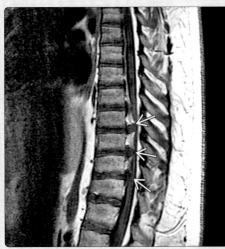

(Left) *Sagittal T2WI MR shows multiple large lower thoracic disc herniations, which severely compress the cord ➡ at multiple levels. Thoracic herniations are most common from T7-T12. (Right) Sagittal T1WI C+ MR shows pronounced peripheral enhancement surrounding the nonenhancing large herniations ➡. The enhancement relates to "tented" and distended epidural plexus and herniation-associated granulation tissue.*

KEY FACTS

TERMINOLOGY

- Localized (< 25% of disc circumference) displacement of disc material beyond confines of disc space
- Protrusion
  - Herniated disc with broad base at parent disc
- Extrusion
  - Herniated disc with narrow or no base at parent disc
- Sequestered: Free fragment
- Migrated: Disc material displaced away from site of herniation

IMAGING

- Anterior extradural mass contiguous with disc space extending into spinal canal
- Axial: Central, subarticular (lateral recess), foraminal, or extraforaminal (far lateral)
- Sagittal: Disc level, infrapedicle, pedicle, suprapedicle

TOP DIFFERENTIAL DIAGNOSES

- Peridural fibrosis
- Epidural abscess
- Epidural metastasis
- Nerve sheath tumor

CLINICAL ISSUES

- Low back pain
- Radiculopathy: Posterolateral radiating pain down lower extremity
  - Positive straight-leg raising test (Lasègue sign)
  - Cauda equina syndrome
- Back pain ± radiculopathy resolves within 6-8 weeks
- Treatments
  - Conservative
  - Minimally invasive techniques (many variations)
  - Standard open techniques, such as laminotomy/discectomy
    - ≥ 90% success rate

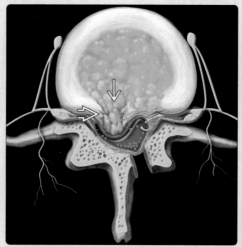
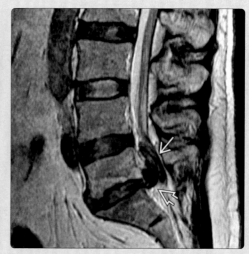

(Left) Graphic of large recurrent disc herniation shows displacement of the nuclear material ➡ through a large defect in the posterior annular fibers ➡ with effacement of the ventral thecal sac and displacement of the intrathecal nerve roots. (Right) Sagittal T2 TSE shows a large extrusion ➡ of the intervertebral disc at the L5-S1 level with a sequestered component (free fragment) ➡ that is migrated superiorly. There is severe thecal sac compression.

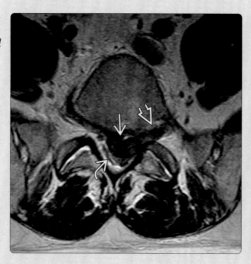
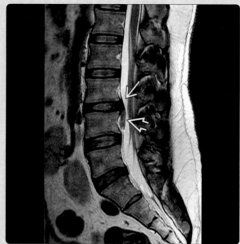

(Left) Axial T2WI MR shows a large central and left extrusion of the intervertebral disc ➡ with severe effacement of the thecal sac ➡. The herniation extends into the left neural foramen ➡. (Right) Sagittal T2WI MR shows a large disc extrusion ➡ with relatively low signal intensity that is migrated inferiorly ➡. There is severe effacement of the ventral thecal sac by the herniation.

KEY FACTS

TERMINOLOGY

- Extruded disc material within neural foramen
- Far lateral is disc material lateral to neural foramen

IMAGING

- Obliterated perineural fat in neural foramen on sagittal images
- Soft tissue mass contiguous with parent disc
- T1WI isointense to parent disc
- T2WI iso-, hypo-, or hyperintense to parent disc
- May enhance peripherally
- Often missed on myelography

TOP DIFFERENTIAL DIAGNOSES

- Schwannoma
- Spinal nerve root diverticulum
- Large facet osteophyte

CLINICAL ISSUES

- May stabilize or resolve spontaneously
- Severe radicular pain
- Mass effect on exiting nerve root in narrow confines of neural foramen
- 5-10% of all disc herniations
- Surgery
  - Failed conservative therapy after 6-8 weeks; progressive deficits
  - Interlaminal approach with partial medial facetectomy
  - Endoscopic lateral approaches more commonly used but no change in outcome relative to open procedures

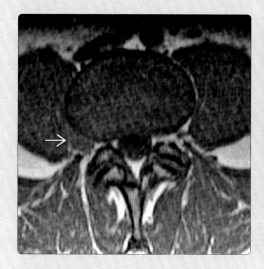

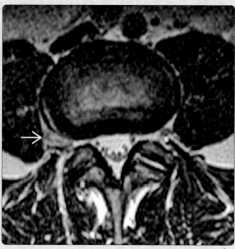

(Left) Axial T1WI MR shows large right lateral and intraforaminal disc herniation at L4-L5 ➡. The disc herniation involves the lateral aspect of the neural foramen and extends to the root ganglion level. (Right) Axial T2WI MR shows the large right lateral and intraforaminal disc herniation ➡ at L4-L5 as near isointense signal to adjacent paravertebral soft tissue. There is slight lateral displacement of the psoas muscle.

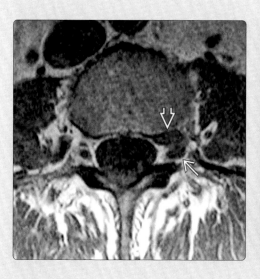

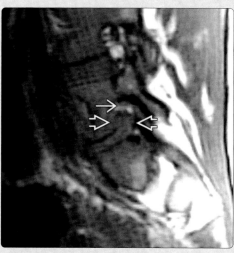

(Left) Axial T1WI MR shows a left L4-L5 foraminal disc extrusion ➡, contacting the exiting left L4 nerve root ➡ at the level of the nerve root ganglion. (Right) Sagittal T1WI MR shows L5-S1 foraminal disc extrusion ➡ displacing the exiting L5 nerve root ➡ superiorly within the foramen.

KEY FACTS

TERMINOLOGY

- Facet arthrosis, degenerative facet disease, degenerative joint disease

IMAGING

- Osseous facet overgrowth impinging on neural foramina in conjunction with articular joint space narrowing
- Facet joint osteophytes producing foraminal narrowing
- Mushroom cap facet appearance
- Joint space narrowing with sclerosis and bone eburnation
- Intraarticular gas (vacuum phenomenon)
- Enhancing inflammatory soft tissue changes surrounding facet joint are common
- Joint space narrowing, thinning of articular cartilage
- Facet effusions as linear hyperintensity

TOP DIFFERENTIAL DIAGNOSES

- Septic facet
- Healing facet fracture

- Inflammatory arthritides
- Paget disease
- Myositis ossificans
- Metastasis

CLINICAL ISSUES

- Clinical pain aggravated by rest and alleviated by movement
- Poor correlation between duration/severity of pain and extent of facet degeneration

DIAGNOSTIC CHECKLIST

- Best detail with thin-section CT
- T2* images overemphasize degree of foraminal or central narrowing

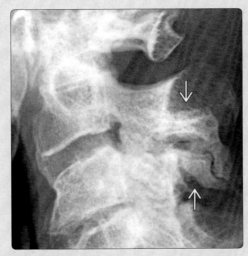
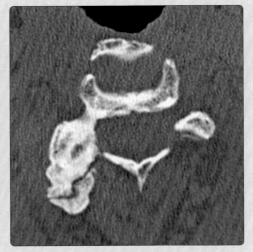

(Left) Lateral radiograph shows severe facet hypertrophic degenerative arthropathy at C2-C3 ➡ with marked hypertrophy of the facets. *(Right)* Axial NECT shows severe, exuberant right facet degenerative arthropathy.

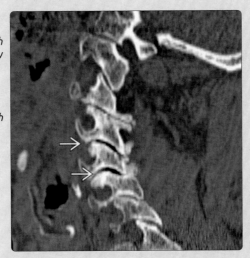
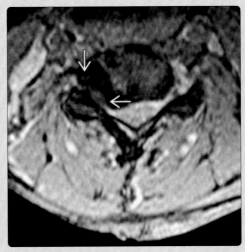

(Left) Sagittal NECT shows multilevel hypertrophic facet degenerative arthropathy with vacuum phenomenon ➡, bony eburnation, and osteophyte formation. *(Right)* Axial T2* GRE MR shows severe right uncovertebral hypertrophic degenerative arthropathy with severe foraminal stenosis ➡ with a facet degenerative change.

Lumbar Facet Arthropathy

KEY FACTS

TERMINOLOGY

- Facet arthrosis, degenerative facet disease, degenerative joint disease, facet hypertrophy
- Osteoarthritis of synovially lined lumbar apophyseal joints

IMAGING

- Osseous overgrowth impinging on foramina in conjunction with articular joint space narrowing
  - Mushroom cap facet appearance
  - Joint space narrowing with sclerosis/bone eburnation, ligamentum flavum hypertrophy
  - Intraarticular gas, effusion
  - Spondylolisthesis not uncommon
- CT more sensitive than plain films for detecting presence and degree of arthrosis
  - Facet hypertrophic degenerative arthropathy, particularly superior articular facet
- MR best demonstrates degenerative facet compression of thecal sac and fat-filled neural foramina
  - Enhancing inflammatory soft tissue changes surrounding facet joint not uncommon
- Consider CT myelography if MR contraindications or MR does not demonstrate facet relationship to neural foramina

TOP DIFFERENTIAL DIAGNOSES

- Septic facet
- Inflammatory arthritides
- Paget disease
- Tumor
  - Metastasis
  - Lymphoma

CLINICAL ISSUES

- Symptoms aggravated by rest and alleviated by movement
- Poor correlation between duration and severity of pain and extent of degeneration

DIAGNOSTIC CHECKLIST

- Look for associated **synovial cysts**

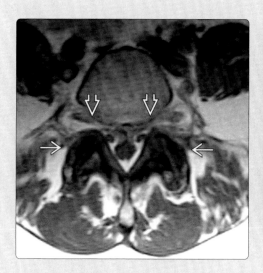

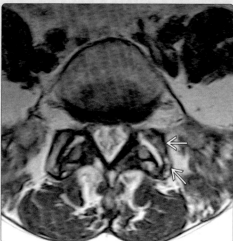

(Left) Axial T1WI MR shows marked facet hypertrophic degenerative arthropathy with enlarged facets ➡ producing moderately severe foraminal stenosis ➡. (Right) Axial T2WI MR shows bilateral facet hypertrophy and small bilateral facet effusions ➡. There is mild deformity of the posterior margin of the thecal sac but no significant central stenosis.

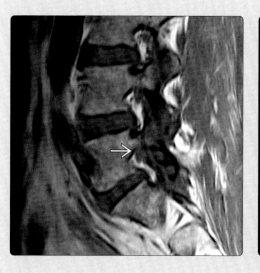

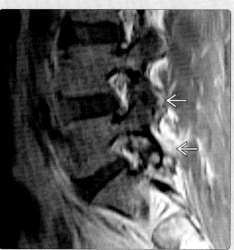

(Left) Sagittal T1WI MR shows L4-L5, L5-S1 facet degenerative arthropathy with bony hypertrophy and low signal involving the facets from bony sclerosis. There is narrowing of the L5-S1 foramen primarily by the hypertrophied superior articular facet of S1 ➡. (Right) Sagittal T1WI C+ MR shows enhancement of the L4-L5 and L5-S1 facets ➡ due to degenerative arthropathy.

KEY FACTS

TERMINOLOGY

- Juxtaarticular cyst
- Facet joint ganglion cyst
- Synovial cyst formed from degenerative facet joint

IMAGING

- Posterolateral extradural cystic mass communicating with facet joint
- Posterolateral to thecal sac
- Adjacent to facet joint
- Lumbar spine: 90%
  - Cervical and thoracic spine uncommon

TOP DIFFERENTIAL DIAGNOSES

- Extruded disc fragment
- Nerve sheath tumor
- Septic facet arthritis/epidural abscess
- Asymmetric ligamentum flavum hypertrophy

PATHOLOGY

- Facet osteoarthropathy
- Facet instability and hypermobility
- Greatest mobility at L4-L5
- Degenerative spondylolisthesis

CLINICAL ISSUES

- Chronic low back pain, radicular symptoms
- May spontaneously regress
- High postsurgical success rate in symptomatic patients
- Myelopathy if cervical or thoracic location
- Treatment
  - Conservative
  - Laminectomy with cyst excision
  - Percutaneous cyst aspiration/steroid injection
- High surgical success rate in symptomatic patients

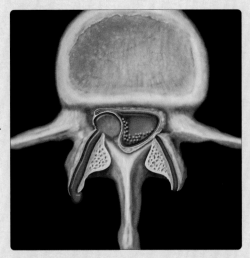

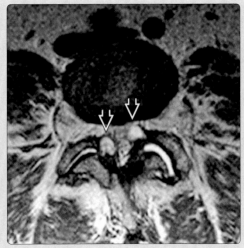

(Left) Axial graphic depicts a right facet joint synovial cyst. Fluid expands the right facet joint, extending into a subarticular recess in a loculated collection. There is mass effect on the thecal sac. (Right) Axial T2WI MR shows bilateral subarticular hyperintense masses ➡ at L4-L5, consistent with bilateral facet synovial cysts. There is bilateral facet degeneration with facet effusions.

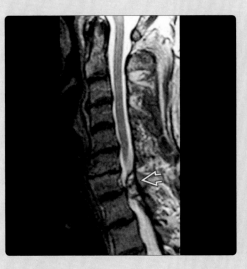

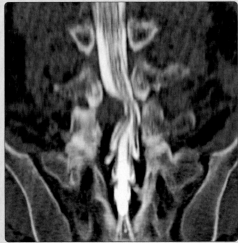

(Left) Sagittal T2WI MR shows peripheral low signal and central heterogeneous hyperintensity ➡ within a dorsal extradural mass at C7-T1 due to a juxtaarticular cyst. (Right) Axial bone CT after myelography with coronal reformation shows an extradural mass abutting the right L4-L5 facet joint, severely distorting the thecal sac.

Baastrup Disease

KEY FACTS

TERMINOLOGY

- Close approximation and contact of adjacent spinous processes with enlargement, flattening, and sclerosis of apposing interspinous surfaces
- Putative source of back pain exacerbated by extension, relieved with flexion

IMAGING

- Plain films/CT: Contact of adjacent spinous processes with sclerosis ("kissing" spinous processes)
- T1WI: Apposing surfaces of spinous processes may show low signal with bony sclerosis or marrow edema
- T2WI: Increased signal from interspinous ligament cystic degeneration and bursa formation

TOP DIFFERENTIAL DIAGNOSES

- Ligamentum flavum hypertrophy
- Osteomyelitis, pyogenic
- Metastases, lytic osseous

- Juxtaarticular cyst
- Tumoral calcinosis

CLINICAL ISSUES

- Interspinous bursitis appearance seen in 8% of subjects undergoing MR of lumbar spine for back or leg pain
- Associations with Baastrup
  - Increasing age
  - Central canal stenosis
  - Anterolisthesis
  - Facet degenerative change with facet effusions
- Treatment
  - Conservative therapy with NSAIDs
  - Direct steroid injection into bursa
  - X-Stop or other interspinous spacing device for treatment of canal stenosis (less common)
  - Resection of offending spinous processes

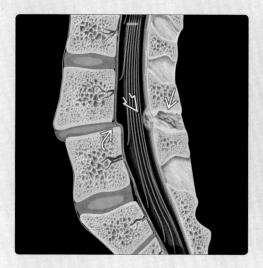

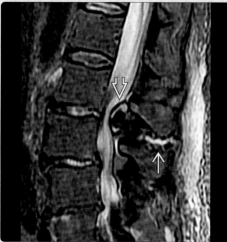

(Left) Sagittal graphic shows degeneration of the L4-L5 interspinous ligament ➡ with spinous process flattening and sclerosis of apposing interspinous surfaces. There is associated ligamentum flavum hypertrophy ➡ and spondylolisthesis ➡. (Right) Sagittal STIR MR shows Baastrup disease as irregular hyperintensity at the L2-L3 interspinous ligament level ➡. There is an associated protein containing a synovial (juxtaarticular) cyst with central low signal within the dorsal epidural space causing severe canal stenosis ➡.

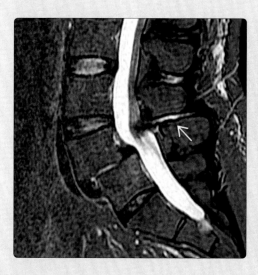

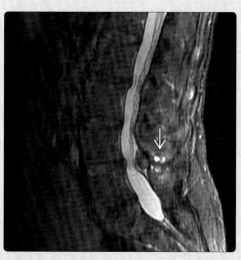

(Left) Sagittal STIR MR shows bursa formation of the interspinous ligament at the L4-L5 level ➡ seen as linear hyperintensity. No adjacent marrow signal abnormality is seen. Note the grade II spondylolisthesis at L4-L5. (Right) Sagittal STIR MR shows irregularity of apposed margins of L4-L5 spinous processes with ligamentum flavum and interspinous process hypertrophy ➡. Cystic degeneration is shown as focal high signal.

KEY FACTS

TERMINOLOGY

- Back pain related to unilateral or bilateral enlargement of transverse process of most caudal lumbar vertebra, which may articulate or fuse with sacrum or ilium

IMAGING

- Partial sacralization of caudal segment of lumbar body on plain films, CT, or MR

TOP DIFFERENTIAL DIAGNOSES

- Normal variant
- Osteochondroma
- Posttraumatic ossification
- Sacroiliac joint degenerative change
- Facet joint arthropathy

PATHOLOGY

- 4-6% of normal patients show transitional segment
  - Hypothesized mechanism is reduced and asymmetrical motion at lumbosacral junction

- Type I: Unilateral (Ia) or bilateral (Ib) dysplastic transverse process measuring at least 19 mm craniocaudal
- Type II: Unilateral (IIa) or bilateral (IIb) lumbarization/sacralization with enlarged transverse process with diarthrodial joint with sacrum
- Type III: Unilateral (IIIa) or bilateral (IIIb) lumbarization/sacralization with complete osseous fusion of transverse process to sacrum
- Type IV: Unilateral type II transition with type III on contralateral side

CLINICAL ISSUES

- Causal relationship to low back pain controversial
- Conservative treatment with NSAIDs, physical therapy
- Steroid and local anesthetic infiltration into anomalous lumbosacral articulation
- Resection of accessory joint
- Posterolateral fusion of transitional segment

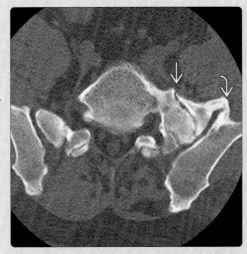

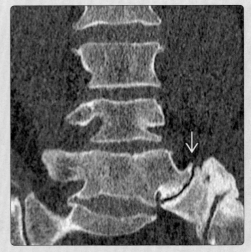

(Left) Axial NECT shows large bridging pseudoarticulation ➡ of the caudal lumbar segment with the sacrum and ilium ➡ on the left, contrasted with the normal right-sided anatomy. (Right) Coronal NECT shows the large neoarticulation of the caudal lumbar body with the sacrum with articular irregularity and vacuum phenomenon ➡.

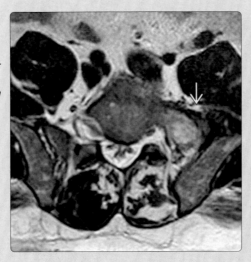

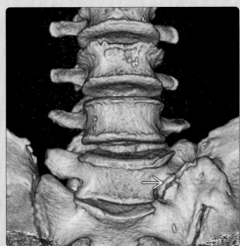

(Left) Axial T2WI MR shows the transitional anatomy at the caudal lumbar segment with partial sacralization on the left ➡. (Right) Coronal CT reconstruction shows the anomalous pseudoarticulation ➡ at the caudal lumbar level on the left between the body, sacrum, and ilium.

Schmorl Node

KEY FACTS

TERMINOLOGY

- Definition: Node within vertebral body due to vertical disc extension (intravertebral disc herniation) through vertebral endplate

IMAGING

- Focal invagination of endplate by disc material surrounded by sclerotic (old) or edematous (acute) bone
- Plain films
  - Contour defect within endplate, extending from disc space into vertebral body spongiosa with well-corticated margins
- CT
  - Island of low density surrounded by condensed bone on axial slice through vertebral body
- MR
  - Focal defect in endplate filled by disc ± adjacent marrow edema, fatty marrow conversion

TOP DIFFERENTIAL DIAGNOSES

- Acute compression fracture
- Degenerative endplate change
- Discitis
  - Both endplates show defect
- Limbus vertebrae
  - Seen at vertebral body corners
- Bone island
  - Sclerotic nodule
- Focal metastasis
  - No contiguity with parent disc

CLINICAL ISSUES

- Seen in up to 75% of all normal spines
- Conservative management

DIAGNOSTIC CHECKLIST

- Schmorl node is always contiguous with parent disc

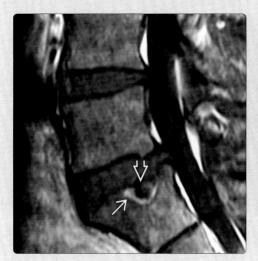

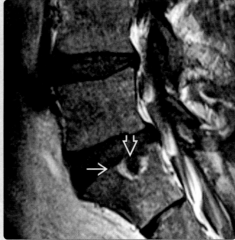

(Left) Sagittal T1WI MR shows a well-defined focus of low signal ⮕ involving the superior endplate of S1 due to endplate herniation. There is a thin rind of fatty marrow conversion adjacent to the Schmorl node ➡. (Right) Sagittal T2WI MR in the same patient demonstrates the typical pattern of fatty marrow ➡ outlining low signal intensity chronic endplate herniation ⮕.

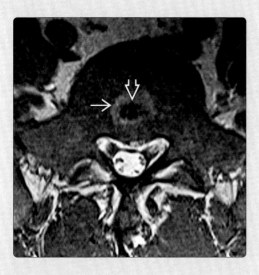

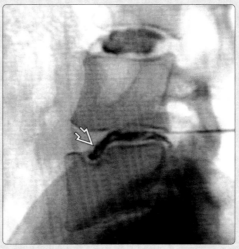

(Left) Axial T2WI MR in the same patient shows a well-defined focus of low signal ⮕ in the superior S1 endplate representing a Schmorl node. There is a thin concentric rind of fatty marrow conversion ➡ surrounding the Schmorl node. (Right) Lateral fluoroscopy image in a different patient during discography reveals a superior endplate Schmorl node ⮕. Contrast injected into the contiguous intervertebral disc fills the herniated disc within the vertebral defect.

KEY FACTS

TERMINOLOGY

- Juvenile kyphosis, Scheuermann kyphosis
- Kyphosis secondary to multiple Schmorl nodes → vertebral body wedging

IMAGING

- Wedged-shaped thoracic vertebrae with irregular endplates
  - ≥ 3 contiguous vertebrae, each showing ≥ 5° of kyphosis
  - Undulation of endplates secondary to extensive disc invaginations
  - Disc spaces narrowed with greatest narrowing anteriorly
  - Well-defined Schmorl nodes

TOP DIFFERENTIAL DIAGNOSES

- Postural kyphosis
- Wedge compression fractures
- Congenital kyphosis
- Tuberculosis

- Osteogenesis imperfecta
- Neuromuscular disease

PATHOLOGY

- Disc extrusions through weakened regions of vertebral endplates
- Weightlifting, gymnastics, and other spine-loading sports may contribute

CLINICAL ISSUES

- Thoracic spine pain worsened by activity
- Kyphosis develops in adolescence, may present later in life
- Peak incidence: 13-17 years
- Initial treatment includes observation, bracing
- Surgical treatment for > 75° kyphosis in skeletally immature person

DIAGNOSTIC CHECKLIST

- Schmorl nodes without anterior wedging are not indicative of Scheuermann disease

(Left) Sagittal graphic demonstrates anterior vertebral wedging and herniation of disc material through the vertebral endplates, creating focal subcortical bone defects in conjunction with thoracic kyphotic deformity. Undulation of endplates reflects sequelae of the osseous reparative process. (Right) Lateral radiography reveals anterior wedging deformity and undulation of vertebral endplates with multiple Schmorl nodes at each level ⊟.

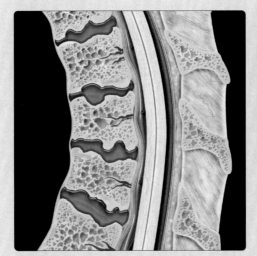
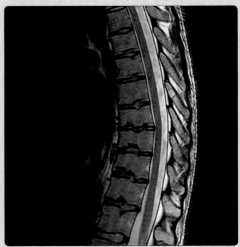

(Left) Sagittal bone CT shows loss of anterior vertebral height and endplate irregularity involving multiple thoracic discs. There are multiple (> 3) contiguous levels of endplate irregularities (Schmorl node) and increased thoracic kyphosis. (Right) Sagittal T2WI MR (same patient) confirms loss of disc height and signal intensity at multiple thoracic levels. The thoracic spinal cord is normal and there are no associated thoracic disc herniations into the spinal canal.

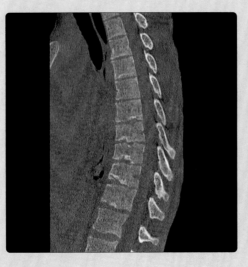
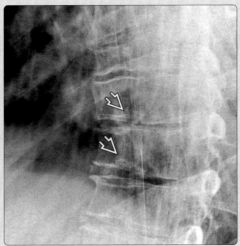

Acquired Lumbar Central Stenosis

KEY FACTS

TERMINOLOGY

- Spinal canal narrowing secondary to multifactorial degenerative changes; is progressive and dynamic process

IMAGING

- Trefoil appearance of lumbar spinal canal on axial imaging
- Sagittal diameter of bony lumbar canal < 12 mm relative stenosis
- Sagittal diameter of bony lumbar canal < 10 mm absolute stenosis
- Hourglass appearance of central canal on sagittal T2WI

TOP DIFFERENTIAL DIAGNOSES

- Disc herniation
- Metastatic disease
- Paget disease
- Epidural hemorrhage

CLINICAL ISSUES

- Chronic low back pain
- Neurogenic claudication
  - Leg pain (80%)
  - Bilateral lower extremity pain, paresthesia, and weakness
  - Relief of pain by squatting or sitting (flexion) in 80%
- Bladder dysfunction and sexual difficulty (10%)
- Radicular pain (10%)
- Operative treatment includes surgical decompression (common) or X-Stop interspinous implant-like devices (less common)
- Natural history: Majority of symptomatic patients stable over months to years (40-70%)
  - 1/3 improve with nonoperative treatment
  - 1/3 deteriorate

DIAGNOSTIC CHECKLIST

- Axial T2WI mandatory for stenosis identification

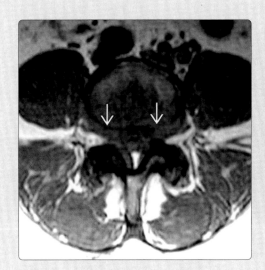

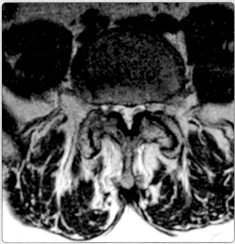

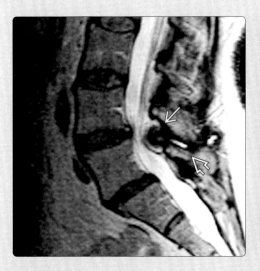

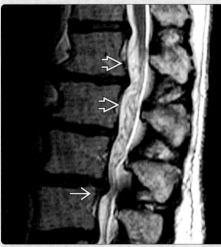

(Left) Axial T1WI MR shows severe central canal stenosis due to a diffusely bulging anulus ➡ anteriorly and posterior facet hypertrophic degenerative arthropathy, which combine to compress the thecal sac. (Right) Axial T2WI MR demonstrates severe central canal stenosis with marked facet degenerative arthropathy. The thecal sac has assumed a trefoil appearance.

(Left) Sagittal T2WI MR shows severe central stenosis at L4-L5 due to marked posterior ligamentum flavum thickening ➡. Hyperintensity within the interspinous ligament denotes degeneration ➡, which is also called Baastrup disease or interspinous bursitis. (Right) Sagittal T2WI MR shows canal stenosis at L3-L4 with a bulging disc and ligamentous thickening ➡. Note serpentine areas of low signal within the cephalad thecal sac due to redundant nerve roots ➡.

Degenerative Diseases and Arthritides

TERMINOLOGY

- Reduced AP canal diameter secondary to short, squat pedicles and laterally directed laminae

IMAGING

- Central canal diameter is smaller than normal
  - Cervical spine: Absolute AP diameter < 14 mm
  - Spinal stenosis present if AP canal diameter at L1 < 20 mm, L2 < 19 mm, L3 < 19 mm, L4 < 17 mm, L5 < 16 mm, S1 < 16 mm
    - Lumbar spine: Critical stenosis at L4 < 14 mm, L5 < 14 mm, S1 < 12 mm
- Short, thick pedicles
- Trefoil-shaped lateral recesses
- Laterally directed laminae

TOP DIFFERENTIAL DIAGNOSES

- Acquired spinal stenosis
- Inherited spinal stenosis
  - Achondroplasia
  - Mucopolysaccharidoses

PATHOLOGY

- Torg ratio (AP canal diameter/AP vertebral body diameter) < 0.8
- Idiopathic

CLINICAL ISSUES

- Symptomatic cervical or lumbar stenosis symptoms at younger age than typical of degenerative stenosis
  - These patients typically lack complicating medical problems (diabetes or vascular insufficiency)
- Athletes present with temporary neurological deficit following physical contact that subsequently resolves
- Lumbar: Decompressive laminectomy, posterior foraminotomy at involved levels
- Cervical: Posterior cervical laminectomy or laminoplasty

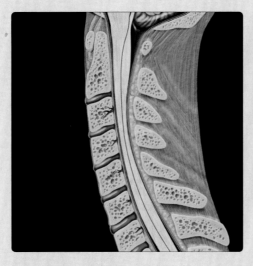
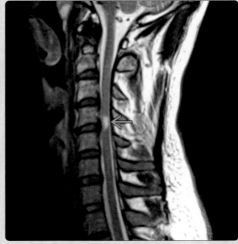

(Left) Sagittal graphic shows marked congenital anteroposterior narrowing of the central spinal canal. (Right) Sagittal T2WI MR reveals moderate congenital AP canal narrowing exacerbated by C4-C5 disc herniation. The protrusion produces spinal cord T2 hyperintensity ➡ corresponding to clinical myelopathy.

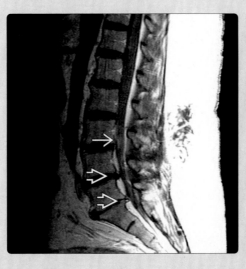
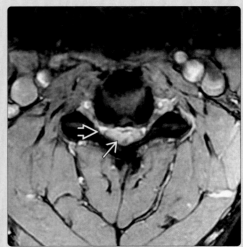

(Left) Sagittal T1 C+ MR shows diffuse congenital central canal stenosis with superimposed acquired stenosis at L4-L5 and L5-S1 levels ➡ with disc bulges. Note the root enhancement at L3-L4 secondary to the stenosis ➡. (Right) Axial GRE study at C3-C4 shows diffuse high signal throughout the substance of the cord ➡, which is a typical pattern for chronic traumatic myelomalacia related to disc disease. Note the small AP diameter of the bony canal due to congenital stenosis ➡.

Cervical Spondylosis

KEY FACTS

TERMINOLOGY

- Spinal canal and neural foraminal narrowing in cervical spine 2° to multifactorial degenerative changes

IMAGING

- Cervical spine, ventral epidural, centered at disc levels
- Sagittal diameter of cervical canal < 13 mm
- Disc osteophyte complex protruding into canal and compressing thecal sac and cord
- Completely effaced subarachnoid space at disc levels in cervical spine → "washboard spine"
- Variable degrees of cord compression

TOP DIFFERENTIAL DIAGNOSES

- Ossification of posterior longitudinal ligament
- DDx of abnormal cord signal
  - Cord tumor
  - Syrinx
  - Multiple sclerosis

- Motor neuron disease

PATHOLOGY

- Multilevel disc degeneration with decreased disc hydration and fissures
- Disc herniation, bulge with associated broad osteophytes
- Uncovertebral joint osteoarthritic change with foraminal stenosis

CLINICAL ISSUES

- Acquired cervical spinal canal stenosis has no pathognomic symptoms or signs
  - Spastic paraparesis commonly seen
  - Upper extremity numbness, weakness ("myelopathic hand")
- Natural history of insidious onset, periods of static disability, and episodic worsening
- Most common cause of spinal cord dysfunction worldwide

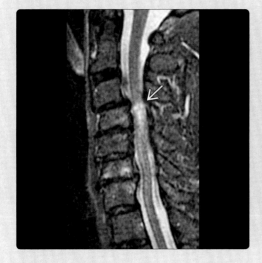
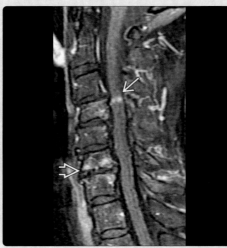

(Left) Sagittal T2WI MR shows multilevel degenerative disc disease and disc osteophyte complexes with canal stenosis spanning C3-C4 through C6-C7. T2 hyperintensity present within the cord centered at C3-C4 ➡ reflects myelomalacia. (Right) Sagittal T1WI C+ FS MR shows horizontal linear enhancement within the cervical cord ➡ at C3-C4 due to chronic myelomalacia. There is also enhancement of type I degenerative endplate changes at C6-C7 ➡.

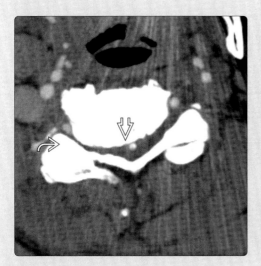
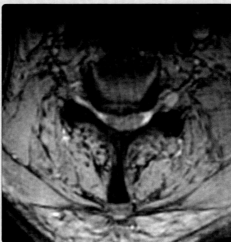

(Left) Axial CT angiogram shows severe central canal stenosis ➡ from ventral disc-osteophyte complex with marked cord compression. There is severe right foraminal stenosis ➡ with uncovertebral joint hypertrophy. (Right) Axial GRE MR shows severe central canal stenosis from ventral disc-osteophyte complex with underlying congenital central stenosis.

Degenerative Diseases and Arthritides

TERMINOLOGY

- Diffuse idiopathic skeletal hyperostosis (DISH)
- Forestier disease, senile ankylosing hyperostosis, asymmetrical skeletal hyperostosis

IMAGING

- Flowing anterior vertebral ossification with minimal degenerative disc disease, facet arthropathy, absent facet ankylosis
- Thoracic spine (100%) > cervical (65-80%), lumbar spine (68-90%); R > L
- Lateral radiography inexpensive, reliable
- Reserve MR to evaluate for coexistent OPLL or spondylosis-related cord compression

TOP DIFFERENTIAL DIAGNOSES

- Spondylosis
- Ankylosing spondylitis
- Psoriatic or reactive (Reiter) arthritis

PATHOLOGY

- Exact cause for exaggerated new bone formation stimuli unknown
  - Exuberant entheseal reaction at tendon, ligament, and joint capsule insertions
  - Associated with OPLL
  - Dysphagia related to DISH multifactorial
- Primary diagnostic criteria for DISH
  - Flowing anterior ossification extending over at least 4 contiguous vertebral bodies
  - No apophyseal or sacroiliac joint ankylosis
  - Mild degenerative disc changes, no facet ankylosis

CLINICAL ISSUES

- Majority of cases incidental
- Osteophyte resection if severe symptoms
- Increased risk of extension-type fractures with high morbidity

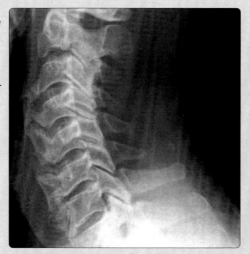
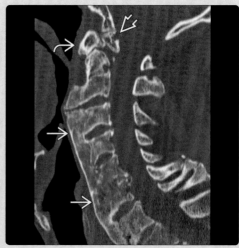

(Left) Lateral radiograph shows a large anterior ossified mass that is discontinuous at several disc spaces, a variation implying some degree of continued cervical spine mobility. (Right) Sagittal NECT shows large flowing ventral osteophytes from C2 through the upper thoracic spine ➡. There is no bony fusion at C2-C3, allowing limited motion at this segment. Note the blunted odontoid with a hypertrophic anterior C1 arch ➡ and os odontoideum articulating with the basion ➡.

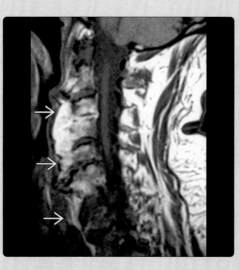
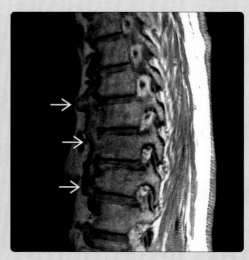

(Left) Sagittal T1WI MR shows bulky anterior flowing ossification ➡ consistent with diffuse idiopathic skeletal hyperostosis (DISH). Fatty marrow is responsible for high T1 signal intensity within the anterior ossification. (Right) Sagittal T1WI MR right parasagittal slice shows bulky flowing anterior longitudinal ligament ossification ➡ spanning more than 4 vertebral levels but minimal disc abnormality that is typical of DISH.

KEY FACTS

TERMINOLOGY

- Ossification of posterior longitudinal ligament (OPLL)

IMAGING

- Flowing multilevel ossification posterior to vertebral bodies with relatively minimal degenerative disc disease, absent facet ankylosis
  - Midcervical (C3-C5) > midthoracic (T4-T7)
  - PLL ossification narrows AP spinal canal dimension → spinal stenosis, cord compression
- Characteristic "upside-down T" or "bowtie" PLL configuration on axial images
  - CT with sagittal reformats to confirm MR diagnosis, clarify extent of ossification for surgical planning
  - Sagittal T1WI, T2WI to evaluate spinal cord compression, extent of ligamentous ossification

TOP DIFFERENTIAL DIAGNOSES

- Spondylosis

- Calcified herniated disc
- Meningioma

PATHOLOGY

- Continuous → ossified mass over several vertebral segments
- Segmental → fragmented ossified lesions behind each vertebral body
- Mixed → combination of continuous and segmental
- Other → ossification confined to disc level
- Diffuse idiopathic skeletal hyperostosi seen in 25% of patients with OPLL
- OPLL present in 16-20% of cases of ossification of ligamentum flavum

CLINICAL ISSUES

- Spastic paresis → paralysis (17-22%)
- ↑ risk for developing progressive myelopathy if > 60% canal stenosis, ↑ cervical range of motion

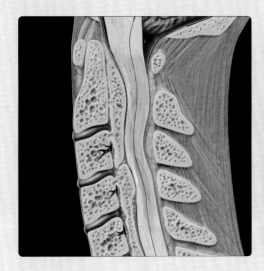

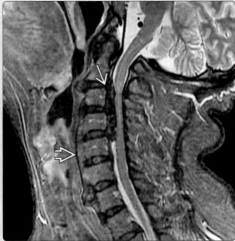

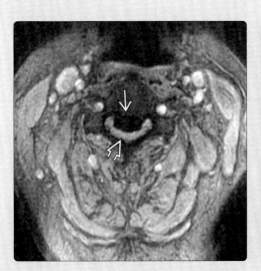

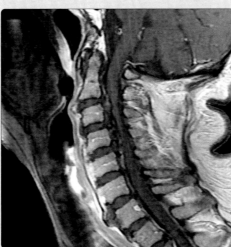

(Left) Sagittal graphic shows flowing multilevel ossification of the posterior longitudinal ligament (OPLL), producing canal narrowing and cord compression. (Right) Sagittal STIR MR shows the typical pattern of continuous-type OPLL seen as low signal ventral to the cord ➡ with severe cord compression. Note the associated diffuse idiopathic skeletal hyperostosis with multilevel fusion ➡.

(Left) Axial GRE MR shows a rectangular focus of markedly low signal ventral to the cord, consistent with OPLL ➡. There is severe cord compression ➡. (Right) Sagittal T1 C+ MR shows a slightly heterogeneous mass ventral to the cervical cord with severe cord compression. OPLL may show low or heterogeneous increased signal on T1WI due to marrow content with fat elements.

KEY FACTS

TERMINOLOGY

- Ossification of ligamentum flavum, ossification of vertebral arch ligaments, ligamentum flavum "pseudogout"
- Calcification/ossification of ligamentum flavum

IMAGING

- Linear thickening of ligamentum flavum with imaging characteristics similar to adjacent vertebral marrow ossification
- Curvilinear hyperdense thickening of ligamentum flavum
- Hypointense linear "mass" within ligamentum flavum ± cord myelomalacia, ↑ signal intensity 2° to compression
- CT imaging best modality for primary diagnosis, "lesion conspicuity"

TOP DIFFERENTIAL DIAGNOSES

- Facet arthrosis
- Meningioma

PATHOLOGY

- Ectopic bone formation within ligamentum flavum
- In majority of patients (idiopathic presentation) mechanism is unclear
  - Some cases clearly associated with metabolic or endocrine disease
- Variably coexists with DISH, OPLL

CLINICAL ISSUES

- Often incidental observation on imaging study ordered for other reasons
- May be associated with cord compression and chronic thoracic myelopathy
  - Ambulation difficulty, weakness, back pain, and lower extremity paresthesias
  - 4th → 6th decade
  - Symptomatic presentation more common in Japanese, North African descent > > Caucasian > African American

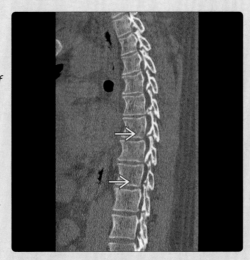

(Left) Sagittal NECT shows that, at essentially every thoracic level, there are various patterns of ligamentum flavum ossification ➡. These areas of ossification merge with the facets along their ventral margins. (Right) Axial NECT shows typical thoracic ligamentum flavum ossification as clumped and linear calcifications ventral and medial to the facets ➡. They may have variable mass effect upon the thecal sac but can be a source of thoracic myelopathy.

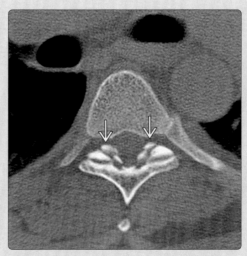

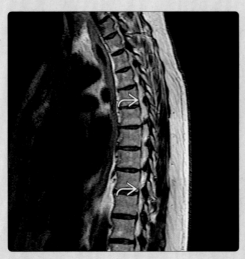

(Left) Sagittal T2WI MR shows ossified ligamentum flava as low signal ➡ at every thoracic level, merging with the low signal of the cortex of the facet joints. (Right) Axial T2* GRE MR demonstrates the ossified ligaments as low signal ➡ with compression of the dorsal thecal sac producing central canal stenosis. This should be distinguished from congenital stenosis with shortened pedicles.

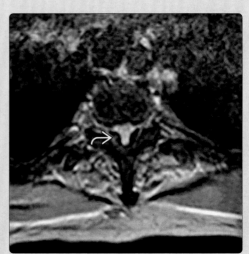

TERMINOLOGY

- Calcium pyrophosphate dihydrate deposition disease (CPPD); articular chondrocalcinosis
- Crowned dens syndrome: Fever with cervicooccipital junction pain, stiffness with associated calcification of transverse ligament and nonenhancing retroodontoid soft tissue; associated with CPPD or hydroxyapatite deposition
- Pseudogout: Arthritis caused by CPPD crystal inflammation with symptoms like gout

IMAGING

- Calcification of transverse ligament on CT
- T1WI: Iso- to low-signal mass posterior to odontoid
- T2WI: Low-signal mass posterior to odontoid
- T1WI C+: May show peripheral enhancement

TOP DIFFERENTIAL DIAGNOSES

- Rheumatoid arthritis
- Osteoarthritis

- OPLL
- Osteomyelitis
- Meningioma
- Metastatic disease
- Longus colli calcific tendinitis

PATHOLOGY

- Nodular deposits of birefringent, rhomboid crystals

CLINICAL ISSUES

- Age 60 or older, prevalence of CPPD deposition = 34%
- Crowned dens: Inflammatory indicators + (fever, CRP, elevated WBC count)
- Conservative treatment including NSAIDs, steroids, or both; physical therapy

DIAGNOSTIC CHECKLIST

- Calcification of transverse ligament common in elderly but symptomatic CPPD very uncommon

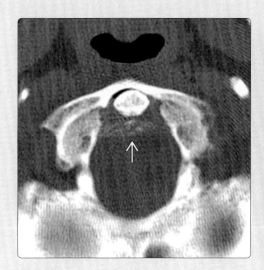

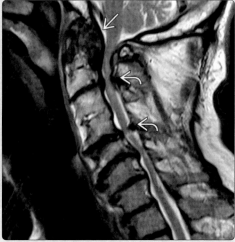

(Left) Axial NECT shows amorphous calcification within the transverse ligament at the C1-C2 junction ➡. There is also osteoarthritic degenerative change at the anterior C1-C2 joint with vacuum phenomenon. (Right) Sagittal T2WI MR shows a low-signal pseudotumor posterior to the odontoid process ➡ with moderate mass effect upon the cervical cord. A low-signal mass extends over the superior margin of the odontoid. Note the associated calcification of ligamentum flavum ➡.

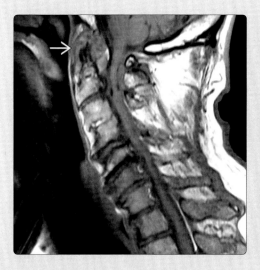

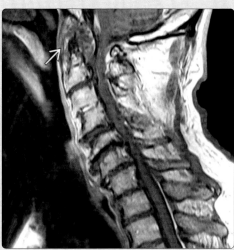

(Left) Sagittal T1WI MR shows prominent soft tissue surrounding the odontoid process ➡ with mass effect upon ventral thecal sac and cord at C1 level. There is severe multilevel disc degeneration and canal stenosis. (Right) Sagittal T1WI C+ MR shows mild peripheral enhancement of the calcium pyrophosphate dihydrate deposition pseudotumor involving the periodontal soft tissues ➡. Low T2 signal and peripheral enhancement are typical of this soft tissue.

KEY FACTS

TERMINOLOGY

- Defects in pars interarticularis thought to result from repetitive stress injury
  - Pars is junction of pedicle, lamina, and facet

IMAGING

- Most common at L5: 80-90%
- Discontinuity in neck of "Scotty dog" on oblique plain films
- Elongation of spinal canal at level of pars defects on axial imaging
- Incomplete ring sign on axial imaging

TOP DIFFERENTIAL DIAGNOSES

- Acute traumatic fracture of posterior elements
- Facet arthropathy with marrow edema
- Septic facet with marrow edema
- Bone tumor with marrow edema
- Pedicle stress fracture
- Congenital defect with pars cleft

PATHOLOGY

- Repeated microfractures of pars interarticularis lead to fatigue fracture

CLINICAL ISSUES

- 6-8% in general population, 10-20 years old
- Symptoms of chronic low back pain
- Conservative measures in grade 1-2 spondylolisthesis
- Wide variety of practice patterns for treatment
  - Epidural or pars steroid injection
  - Surgical intervention
    - Fail conservative treatment
    - Have worsening slippage
  - No consensus on optimum surgical strategy
    - Laminectomy/fusion
    - Transforaminal lumbar interbody fusion/posterior lumbar intervertebral fusion
    - Anterior lumbar interbody fusion with posterior instrumentation

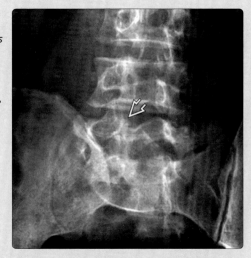
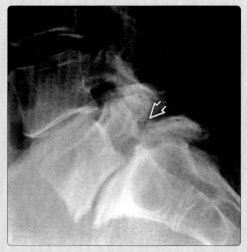

(Left) Coronal oblique radiograph shows a thin lucency ➡ in the right L5 pars interarticularis with adjacent bony sclerosis. (Right) Lateral radiography shows a defect and mild angulation in the L5 pars interarticularis ➡. There is disc height loss at L5-S1 with associated sclerotic endplate changes.

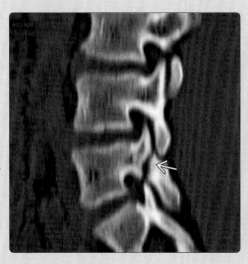
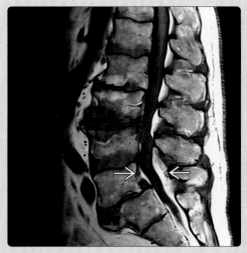

(Left) Sagittal bone CT reformation shows a chronic-appearing L5 pars defect with smooth corticated margins without anterolisthesis ➡. (Right) Sagittal T1WI MR shows grade I anterolisthesis of L5 on S1 with severe disc degeneration and loss of disc height. There is a widened canal sign with increased distance between the posterior margin of L5 and the spinous process ➡, indicating bilateral spondylolysis. Note the degenerative endplate changes at L2-L3 and L3-L4.

IMAGING

General Features

- Best diagnostic clue
  - Bony defect or cortical discontinuity in pars interarticularis (PI)
- Location
  - Most common at L5: 80-90%
  - L4 2nd most common
- Morphology
  - Horizontal orientation on axial imaging

Radiographic Findings

- Radiography
  - Radiolucent band in PI on oblique views of lumbar spine (discontinuity in neck of "Scotty dog")
  - Oblique lucency at base of laminae on lateral view
  - Contralateral pedicle and lamina hypertrophy and sclerosis
    - Unilateral spondylolysis; best seen on frontal lumbar spine
  - Variable degree of spondylolisthesis
  - Disc height loss at level below spondylolysis
  - Secondary degenerative sclerotic endplate changes and spurring

CT Findings

- Bone CT
  - Incomplete ring sign on axial imaging
    - Disruption of ring formed by vertebral body and arch
  - May simulate facet joints
    - Extrafacet sign; horizontal vs. oblique orientation; irregular vs. smooth bony cortex
  - Pars defects well seen on oblique reformation
  - Variable spondylolisthesis and foraminal narrowing on sagittal reformation
    - Disc space loss; degenerative endplate changes
  - Canal may be widened even without spondylolisthesis

MR Findings

- T1WI
  - Focally decreased signal in PI on sagittal and axial imaging; similar appearance on T2WI
- T2WI
  - Hyperintensity may be present within pars defects and adjacent marrow of pedicle
- STIR
  - Marrow edema adjacent to pars defects and pedicle
- Elongation of spinal canal
- MR sensitivity: 57-86%; MR specificity: 81-82%

Nonvascular Interventions

- Myelography
  - Neural foraminal narrowing with anterolisthesis and disc height loss

Nuclear Medicine Findings

- Bone scan
  - Foci of increased radiotracer uptake in posterior elements; suggests bone healing; SPECT is better but still relatively high false-positives and false-negatives

Imaging Recommendations

- Best imaging tool
  - Axial thin-section CT with bone algorithm (sagittal and oblique reformation)

DIFFERENTIAL DIAGNOSIS

Acute Traumatic Fracture of Posterior Elements

- History of acute trauma

Facet Arthropathy With Marrow Edema

- Hypertrophied facet and ligamentum flavum

Septic Facet With Marrow Edema

- Clinical findings of fever, elevated WBC, and sedimentation rate

Bone Tumor With Marrow Edema

- Osteoid osteoma typical
- Metastatic disease

Pedicle Stress Fracture

- Stress reaction may show adjacent marrow edema

Congenital Defect With Pars Cleft

- Hypoplasia of spinal accessory process

CLINICAL ISSUES

Presentation

- Most common signs/symptoms
  - Commonly asymptomatic; chronic low back pain, particularly in children and adolescents
  - Other symptoms: Back spasm; hamstring tightness; radiculopathy and cauda equina syndrome; gait disturbance

Treatment

- Conservative measures in patients with grade 1 and 2 spondylolisthesis
  - Antiinflammatory medications; epidural steroid injection; brace/physical therapy
- Surgical intervention: Fail conservative treatment; have worsening slippage; preserve neural function and prevent instability
- Wide variety of practice patterns for treatment; 50% of surgeons agreed on surgical treatment in 1 study
- No consensus on optimum surgical strategy
  - Laminectomy/fusion; transforaminal lumbar interbody fusion/posterior lumbar intervertebral fusion; anterior lumbar interbody fusion (ALIF) with posterior instrumentation

DIAGNOSTIC CHECKLIST

Consider

- L5-S1 isthmic spondylolysis stand-alone ALIF failure has been reported; unique axial load and shear stresses; supplementary posterior fixation recommended

Image Interpretation Pearls

- Look for integrity of PI on sagittal MR

IMAGING

- Erosions of dens, uncovertebral joints, facet joints
- Atlantoaxial instability in 20-86% patients with rheumatoid arthritis (RA)
- Atlantoaxial subluxation in 5% of cervical RA
- Cranial settling occurs in 5-8% of RA patients
- Lower cervical spine: Facet and uncovertebral joint erosions, instability
- Neutral, flexion, and extension lateral radiographs performed for evaluation of instability
  - Normal: 2 mm between inner margin anterior ring of C1 and dens
  - High correlation to neurologic symptoms with distance ≥ 9 mm
- Pannus is mass-like and surrounds and erodes dens, facet joints, uncovertebral joints
  - Low signal on T1WI
  - Heterogeneous signal on T2WI, STIR
  - Enhances avidly with gadolinium

TOP DIFFERENTIAL DIAGNOSES

- Seronegative spondyloarthropathy
- Calcium pyrophosphate dihydrate deposition (CPPD) disease
- Juvenile chronic arthritis
- Osteoarthritis
- Degenerative disc disease

CLINICAL ISSUES

- 50-60% of RA patients have involvement of cervical spine
- Never involves spine before hands &/or feet
- May develop radiculopathy, myelopathy
- Instability → significant morbidity, mortality

DIAGNOSTIC CHECKLIST

- Calcifying mass with odontoid erosions is **not** RA
  - Indicates crystalline arthropathy, usually CPPD

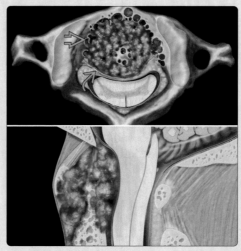

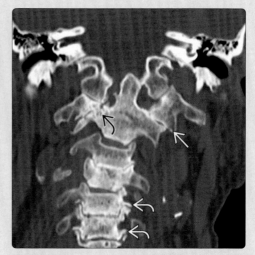

(Left) Axial and sagittal graphics show erosion of dens by hypertrophied synovial tissue ⇨ (pannus). The pannus has eroded the transverse ligament of the dens ⤳, resulting in instability. The spinal cord is compressed. (Right) Coronal CT reconstruction illustrates erosive changes at the right C1-C2 joint ⤳ and lateral subluxation of C1 with respect to C2 ➡. Inflammatory synovial proliferation and destruction of surrounding bone also affect the uncovertebral joints in the subaxial spine ⤳.

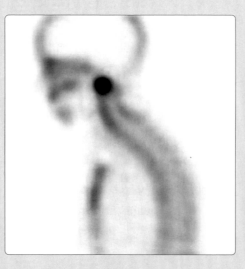

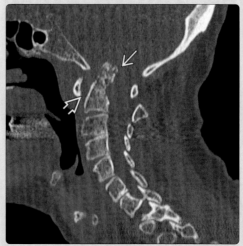

(Left) Lateral view from a bone scan shows focal marked uptake at the C1-C2 junction in this patient with rheumatoid arthritis (RA). (Right) Sagittal NECT scan shows upward translocation of the odontoid ➡ and widened atlantodental interval ➡. The skull and C1 have remained together with the ligamentous laxity and disruption at C1-C2 (coupled with the C1 lateral mass collapse), allowing C2 to migrate cephalad into the foramen magnum with brainstem compression (not shown).

TERMINOLOGY

Abbreviations

- Rheumatoid arthritis (RA)

IMAGING

General Features

- Location
  - Cervical spine: ~ 50-60% of RA patients
    - C1-odontoid articulations, occipital condyles, facets

Radiographic Findings

- Radiography
  - Erosions of dens, uncovertebral joints, and facet joints
  - Neutral, flexion, and extension lateral radiographs to evaluate for instability
  - C1-C2 instability
    - Normal: < 2 mm between anterior ring of C1 and dens
      □ Neurologic symptoms present if distance ≥ 9 mm
    - Atlantoaxial instability in 20-86% of patients
  - Basilar impression: Decreased distance occiput to C2
    - Used synonymously with cranial settling
    - Bony erosions of occipital condyles/C1 lateral masses where cranium moves downward relative to dens
      □ Dens may protrude through foramen magnum
  - Instability may also be present at lower levels of cervical spine

CT Findings

- Bone CT
  - Odontoid erosions
  - Pannus around dens may be seen; **never** calcifies

MR Findings

- Pannus
  - Low signal intensity on T1WI
  - Contrast-enhanced T1WI MR may be able to discriminate between joint effusion and various forms of pannus
- Subluxations may lead to spinal stenosis
  - Myelopathic changes are common

Imaging Recommendations

- Best imaging tool
  - Cervical spine radiographs in flexion/extension
  - Plain radiographs of hands &/or feet
  - Thin-section bone algorithm CT
  - MR imaging in patients with cord symptoms

DIFFERENTIAL DIAGNOSIS

Seronegative Spondyloarthropathy

- Corner erosions of anterior cortex vertebral bodies

Calcium Pyrophosphate Dihydrate Deposition Disease

- Inflammatory mass around odontoid with calcification

Juvenile Idiopathic Arthritis

- Fusion of vertebral bodies, facet joints, erosions

Osteoarthritis

- Osteophytes and joint narrowing

- May cause "pseudopannus" at dens

Gout

- Rare in spine

PATHOLOGY

General Features

- Laboratory findings
  - ESR, C-reactive protein (CRP) elevated
  - Autoantibodies, such as rheumatoid factor (RF) and anticitrullinated protein antibody (ACPA)

Staging, Grading, & Classification

- 2010 American College of Rheumatology/European League Against Rheumatism criteria
  - Target population: Patients with at least 1 joint with clinical synovitis not explained by other disease
  - Joint involvement
  - Serology
    - Presence of RF, ACPA
  - Acute-phase reactants
    - CRP, ESR
  - Duration of symptoms

CLINICAL ISSUES

Presentation

- Most common signs/symptoms
  - Morning pain and stiffness
  - Radiculopathy

Demographics

- Gender
  - 3x more common in women

Natural History & Prognosis

- Increased morbidity and mortality with CVJ instability
- Neurologic symptoms poor prognostic sign as mortality rate increases dramatically

Treatment

- Medical treatment
  - Corticosteroids
  - Disease-modifying agents slow disease progression
    - Tumor necrosis factor inhibitors, methotrexate (MTX), cyclosporine
    - Biological treatment, such as infliximab, for failure of initial MTX treatment
- Surgical indications for atlantoaxial instability
  - Pain, myelopathy, cord compression, symptomatic vertebral artery compromise
  - Atlantodental interval > 8-10 mm
  - C1-C2 transarticular surgical fusion for atlantoaxial subluxation
- Surgical indications for basilar impression
  - Lower cranial neuropathy (C9-C12)
  - Myelopathy, pain, symptomatic vertebral artery compromise, deformity
  - Severe compression of cervicomedullary junction
- Transoral odontoidectomy for cord compression

(Left) *Sagittal CT demonstrates superior migration of the dens ➡. Cranial settling may lead to compression of the brainstem by the dens with compression of the autonomic centers with labile blood pressures, arrhythmias, or sudden death.* **(Right)** *Sagittal NECT shows cranial settling with upward translocation of the odontoid process ➡ relative to the foramen magnum. There are also odontoid erosions ➡ and increased atlantodental interval ➡.*

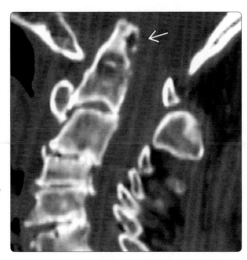
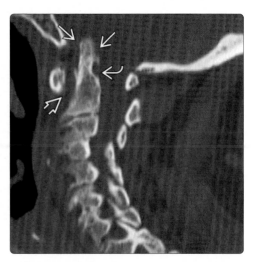

(Left) *Sagittal CT reconstruction exhibits erosions along the posterior margin of the dens ➡ and widening of the anterior atlantodental interval (AADI) ➡.* **(Right)** *Sagittal T1WI MR depicts widening of the AADI ➡ related to the inflammatory pannus and erosive changes of the posterior dens ➡, consistent with known RA.*

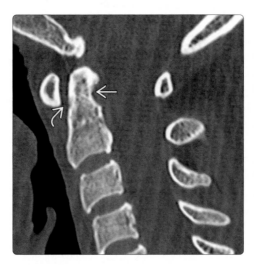
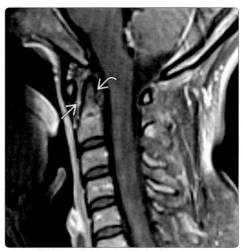

(Left) *Sagittal NECT (bone window) shows extensive erosive changes of the anterior arch of C1 ➡ and odontoid process ➡. The odontoid is malpositioned and touching the clivus.* **(Right)** *Sagittal T1WI MR shows a large amount of the pannus both ventral and dorsal to the odontoid ➡ with effacement of the thecal sac and posterior displacement of cord ➡.*

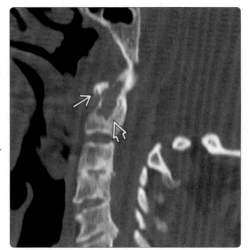
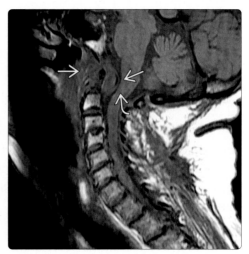

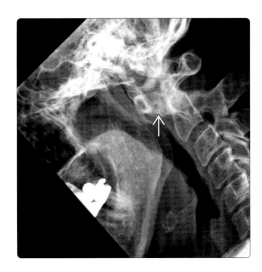

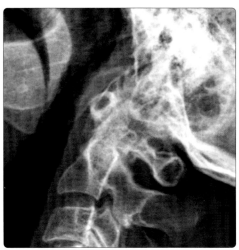

(Left) *Sagittal radiograph in the flexed position illustrates marked widening of the AADI ➡. Inflammatory destruction via synovitis of the atlantal transverse ligament leads to anteroposterior instability of the atlantoaxial joint.* **(Right)** *Sagittal radiograph in the same patient shows a decrease in the AADI with the neck extended. However, posterior atlantodental interval (PADI) has been shown to be a more reliable predictor of whether neurologic symptoms will develop. MR is recommended when PADI is ≤ 14 mm.*

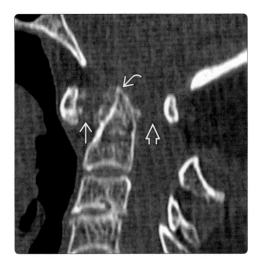

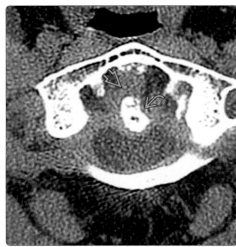

(Left) *Sagittal CT demonstrates marked erosive change of the dens ➡. Erosion of the odontoid process frequently coincides with the development of anterior atlantoaxial subluxation. Widening of the AADI is also noted ➡. There is narrowing of the PADI ➡ and the space for the cord is markedly narrowed.* **(Right)** *Axial NECT displays abnormal soft tissue widening the predental space ➡. There are erosive changes along the margin of the dens ➡. The pannus is the main cause of bone destruction.*

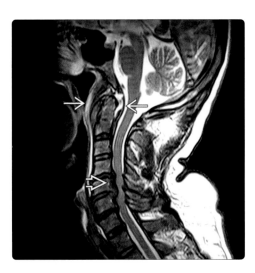

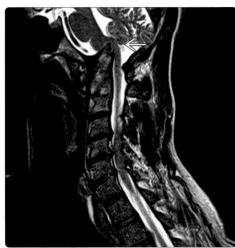

(Left) *Initial MR shows rapid development cranial settling & severe inflammatory response surrounding C1-C2 articulation with a ventral and dorsal soft tissue mass ➡ but a relatively preserved relationship of C2 with the foramen magnum. Large disc extrusion is seen at C5 ➡.* **(Right)** *Follow-up MR 6 months later (a further example of rapid development cranial settling) shows rapid progression of cranial settling with upward translocation of the odontoid process through the foramen magnum with severe cervicomedullary cord compression ➡.*

Juvenile Idiopathic Arthritis

TERMINOLOGY

- Spectrum of idiopathic inflammatory arthropathies occurring in childhood

IMAGING

- Cervical spine subluxations, fusions, and growth disturbance
- Bony overgrowth due to hyperemia may also be seen
- Cranial settling and basilar invagination are common
- Involves discs, facets, and uncovertebral, costovertebral and costotransverse joints
- Progresses to ankylosis
  - Fused vertebrae are small in anteroposterior dimension if fused early in childhood
- Pannus on MR: Rounded, periarticular mass
  - ↓ signal on T1WI; intermediate, heterogeneous signal on T2WI, STIR
- Synovitis: Effusions in facets and sacroiliac joints

TOP DIFFERENTIAL DIAGNOSES

- Congenital spinal fusion
- Physiologic cervical spine subluxations
- Down syndrome
- Osteogenesis imperfecta
- C1-C2 osteomyelitis

PATHOLOGY

- Rheumatoid factor is negative

CLINICAL ISSUES

- Vague, pauciarticular pain
- Limited neck movement

DIAGNOSTIC CHECKLIST

- Diagnosis is often delayed due to subtle imaging findings and nonspecific symptoms
- Sacroiliac joints normally wide in children; diagnose juvenile ankylosing spondylitis only if inflammatory changes seen

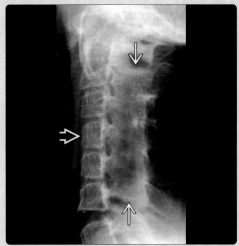
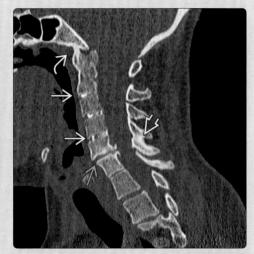

(Left) *Lateral radiograph shows fusion of the posterior elements and vertebral bodies from C2-C6 ➡. Fusion occurred at a young age and the vertebral bodies across the fused section ceased to grow, resulting in small body size in the fused portion ➡. (Right) Sagittal NECT of the cervical spine shows multiple fused vertebral bodies ➡ that also involve the posterior elements ➡. The fusion extends to the craniocervical junction ➡. There is severe disc degeneration below the fusion site ➡.*

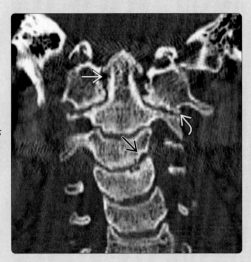
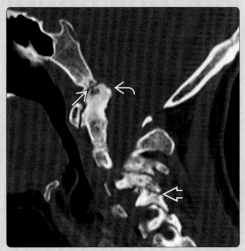

(Left) *Coronal CT shows erosions along the dens ➡, C1-C2 facet joint ➡, and C3-C4 uncovertebral joint ➡. Joint space narrowing and growth disturbances are key radiologic manifestations of juvenile idiopathic arthritis. (Right) Sagittal CT shows superior migration of the dens into the foramen magnum ➡. Erosive changes of the dens, clivus ➡, and subaxial facet joints ➡ are seen.*

Neurogenic (Charcot) Arthropathy

KEY FACTS

TERMINOLOGY

- Destructive arthropathy occurring when pain and proprioception are impaired while joint mobility is maintained

IMAGING

- Almost always in lumbar spine
- Vertebral endplate destruction
- Facet joint destructive arthropathy
- Preserved bone density
- Nonunited fractures
- Bony debris around vertebrae
- Vertebral subluxations
- Soft tissue mass, which may be large
- Heterogeneous enhancement
  - Both of affected vertebrae and soft tissue mass

TOP DIFFERENTIAL DIAGNOSES

- Pyogenic infection

- Atypical infection: Tuberculosis, fungi
- Soft tissue sarcoma
- Bone tumor
- Degenerative disc disease with instability

CLINICAL ISSUES

- Instability of spine
- Spine deformity
- Treated with rigid internal fixation and fusion of affected spinal levels
- Treatment
  - Rigid internal fixation and fusion of affected spinal level
  - Can also be treated with bracing but success limited

DIAGNOSTIC CHECKLIST

- Distinction between neuropathic joint and infection is 1 of most difficult problems radiographically
- Only 2 processes can destroy joint in 1 month: Infection and neurogenic arthropathy

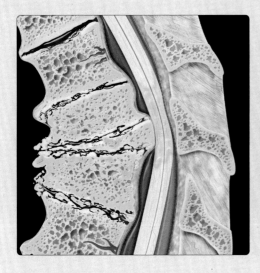

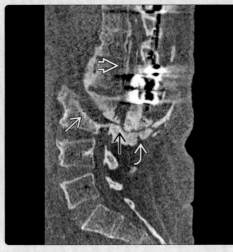

(Left) Sagittal graphic shows arthropathy centered at 3 adjacent discs with endplate erosions, bony debris, and deformity. (Right) Sagittal NECT shows a Charcot joint with pseudoarthrosis at L2-L3 ➡ and remodeling of adjacent vertebral bodies with extensive hypertrophic bone production about the posterior elements ➡. Note the posterior retrolisthesis of the spinal canal at the L2-L3 level ➡. Note also the linear calcification involving the dura in the lower thoracic spine from arachnoiditis ➡.

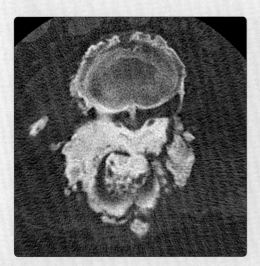

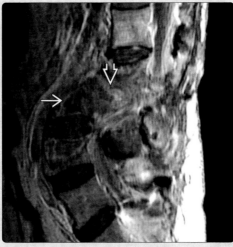

(Left) Axial NECT shows the typical massive bone production associated with neuropathic pseudoarthrosis. (Right) Sagittal T1 C+ MR in a paraplegic with cord transection shows heterogeneous enhancement and destructive arthropathy at L2-L3 ➡ with posterior subluxation, with central fluid-filled areas ➡ surrounded by enhancing reparative tissues. L3-L4 is affected to a lesser extent. The striking soft tissue abnormalities seen on MR of Charcot arthropathy often raise concern for infection or sarcoma.

KEY FACTS

TERMINOLOGY

- Destructive spondyloarthropathy
- Discocentric destructive arthritis in patient on long-term hemodialysis

IMAGING

- Vertebral and endplate destruction in patient on long-term hemodialysis, ± vertebral collapse
  - Cervical, thoracic, or lumbar spine
  - Often involves multiple levels
- Endplate destruction with sharply marginated erosions
- Amorphous material in disc, spinal canal, &/or prevertebral soft tissues
  - Usually lower signal intensity than infection on T2WI, STIR

TOP DIFFERENTIAL DIAGNOSES

- Infection
- Neuropathic joint

- Gout
- Calcium pyrophosphate deposition disease

PATHOLOGY

- 2 types of arthropathy associated with hemodialysis
  - Amyloid deposition: β-2 microglobulin
  - Crystal deposition: Hydroxyapatite

CLINICAL ISSUES

- Indolent
- May result in spinal instability
- Back pain, radiculopathy, cord compression
- Fusion for stabilization

DIAGNOSTIC CHECKLIST

- Specimen must be sent for crystal analysis in saline or ethanol; formalin dissolves crystals
- History is key to making diagnosis

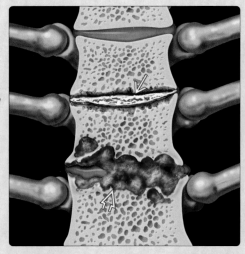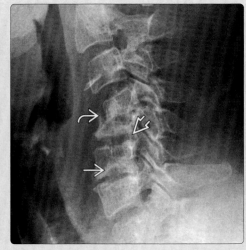

(Left) Coronal graphic shows 2 types of hemodialysis arthropathy: Crystal deposition ➡ and amyloid deposition ⇒, both of which may cause endplate erosions. (Right) Lateral radiograph shows severe bone destruction ➡ centered at the C4-C5 disc ➡ with smaller, punched-out erosions at C5-C6 ⇒ and C6-C7. This patient was on hemodialysis and had chronic, worsening neck pain and findings consistent with cord compression.

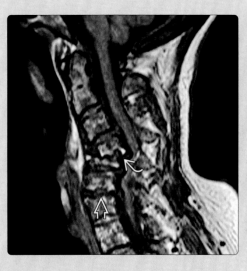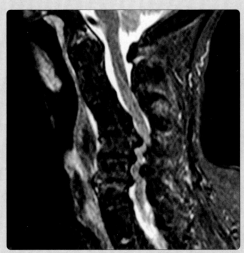

(Left) Sagittal T1WI MR shows severe bone destruction centered at the C4-C5 disc ➡ with smaller, punched-out erosions at C5-C6 ⇒ and C6-C7. This patient was on hemodialysis and had chronic, worsening neck pain and findings consistent with cord compression. Soft tissue posteriorly could represent discs or crystal deposition. (Right) Sagittal STIR MR of the same patient shows severe cord compression. Of note, discs and masses remain very low signal intensity, unlike pyogenic infection.

TERMINOLOGY

Synonyms
- Destructive spondyloarthropathy (DSA)

Definitions
- Discocentric destructive arthritis in patient on long-term hemodialysis

IMAGING

General Features
- Best diagnostic clue
  - Vertebral and endplate destruction in patient on long-term hemodialysis, ± vertebral collapse
- Location
  - Cervical, thoracic, or lumbar spine
  - Often involves multiple levels

Radiographic Findings
- Radiography
  - Endplate destruction
  - Soft tissue mass
    - May contain amyloid
    - May contain crystals with visible calcification

CT Findings
- Sharply marginated endplate erosions
- Soft tissue mass
  - ± calcifications
  - Vertebral body collapse

MR Findings
- Vertebral endplate destruction
- Abnormal signal intensity in vertebral bodies
  - High signal intensity on T2WI, STIR mimics infection
- Amorphous material in disc, spinal canal, &/or prevertebral soft tissues
  - Usually lower signal intensity than infection on T2WI, STIR

Nuclear Medicine Findings
- Bone scan
  - Positive 3-phase bone scan

Imaging Recommendations
- Best imaging tool
  - MR
  - Differentiation from active infection may require biopsy

DIFFERENTIAL DIAGNOSIS

Infection
- Endplate destruction, adjacent soft tissue abscess
- High signal intensity in disc on T2WI, STIR
- Calcifications absent

Neuropathic Joint
- Lumbar spine
- Bone debris, subluxations prominent

Gout
- Imaging appearance may be identical

Calcium Pyrophosphate Deposition Disease
- Disc, ligamentum flavum linear calcifications
- Endplate destruction, erosions

PATHOLOGY

General Features
- Etiology
  - 2 types of arthropathy associated with hemodialysis
    - Amyloid deposition: β-2 microglobulin
      - Less common today due to advances in hemodialysis
    - Crystal deposition: Hydroxyapatite
- Associated abnormalities
  - Adynamic bone disease
    - Absolute or partial parathyroid hormone deficit associated with low or absent bone remodeling
    - Patients often present with bone fractures and collapse, myopathy

CLINICAL ISSUES

Presentation
- Most common signs/symptoms
  - Asymptomatic unless severe
  - Other signs/symptoms
    - Back pain, radiculopathy, cord compression

Demographics
- Epidemiology
  - Uncommon, incidence increases with length of time on dialysis

Natural History & Prognosis
- Indolent, may result in instability

Treatment
- Options, risks, complications
  - Fusion for stabilization

DIAGNOSTIC CHECKLIST

Consider
- Specimen must be sent for crystal analysis in saline or ethanol; formalin dissolves crystals

Image Interpretation Pearls
- History is key to making diagnosis

SELECTED REFERENCES

1. Rizzo MA et al: Neurological complications of hemodialysis: state of the art. J Nephrol. 25(2):170-82, 2012
2. Spinos P et al: Surgical management of cervical spondyloarthropathy in hemodialysis patients. Open Orthop J. 4:39-43, 2010
3. Yamamoto S et al: Recent progress in understanding dialysis-related amyloidosis. Bone. 45 Suppl 1:S39-42, 2009
4. Sarraf P et al: Non-crystalline and crystalline rheumatic disorders in chronic kidney disease. Curr Rheumatol Rep. 10(3):235-48, 2008
5. Theodorou DJ et al: Imaging in dialysis spondyloarthropathy. Semin Dial. 15(4):290-6, 2002
6. Leone A et al: Destructive spondyloarthropathy of the cervical spine in long-term hemodialyzed patients: a five-year clinical radiological prospective study. Skeletal Radiol. 30(8):431-41, 2001

KEY FACTS

IMAGING

- Location
  - Discs and synovial joints of spine
  - Joints of axial skeleton, less commonly peripheral joints
  - Tendon and ligament attachments (entheses)
- Sacroiliac joints: Bilaterally symmetric erosive arthropathy → fusion
- Facet, uncovertebral joints: Erosions → fusion
- Squaring of vertebral bodies → corner erosions → shiny corner (corner sclerosis) → ankylosis
- Erosions, new bone formation at tendon and ligament attachments
- Trauma
  - Often hyperextension injury involving all 3 columns of spine
  - Fracture may occur through fused regions
  - MR should be considered to exclude occult fracture as these may be subtle secondary to osteopenia

TOP DIFFERENTIAL DIAGNOSES

- DISH
- Psoriatic arthritis and reactive arthropathy
- Rheumatoid arthritis
- Osteitis condensans ilii

PATHOLOGY

- Associated findings
  - Pulmonary interstitial fibrosis, decreased chest excursion, uveitis, aortitis, aortic valve insufficiency
- 90% of patients HLA-B27 positive

CLINICAL ISSUES

- Complications: Kyphotic deformity, fractures of fused spine
- Pain centered over sacroiliac joints, back stiffness

DIAGNOSTIC CHECKLIST

- Normal sacroiliac joints preclude imaging diagnosis of ankylosing spondylitis

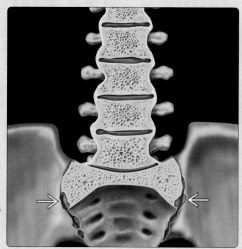

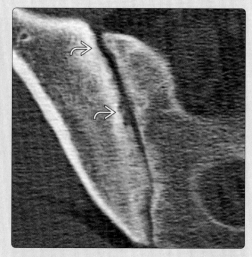

(Left) *Graphic shows sacroiliac joint erosions ➡. Erosions are best seen in the inferior 1/3 of the joint, which is primarily synovial. More superiorly, the articulation is primarily ligamentous with only a small synovial portion and erosions are difficult to see. (Right) Axial bone CT shows the classic appearance of sacroiliac joint inflammatory arthropathy: Small erosions ➡, blurring of the subchondral bone plate, and adjacent sclerosis. Findings are more severe on the iliac side of the joint.*

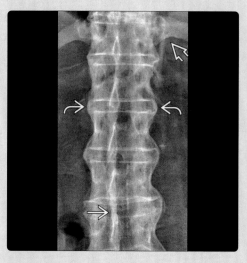

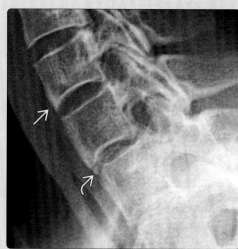

(Left) *Anteroposterior radiograph shows the bamboo spine that is typical of advanced ankylosing spondylitis (AS) where ossification of the outer fibers of the annulus fibrosus ➡ mimics the joints of the bamboo plant. Fusion of the costotransverse joints ➡ and between the spinous processes ➡ is also visible. (Right) Lateral radiograph shows the shiny corner sign ➡. Bone resorption beneath the anterior longitudinal ligament creates a squared vertebral body contour. A single, thin syndesmophyte ➡ is visible.*

TERMINOLOGY

Definitions

- Syndesmophyte: Paraspinous ligamentous or disc ossification bridging 2 adjacent vertebral bodies

IMAGING

General Features

- Location
  - Intervertebral discs
  - Synovial joints of spine: Facet, uncovertebral, costotransverse, costovertebral
  - Joints of axial skeleton
  - Tendon and ligament attachments (entheses)
    - Plantar fascia origin erosions common

Radiographic Findings

- Sacroiliac joints: Sacroiliitis
  - Bilaterally symmetric erosive arthropathy
  - Findings seen on iliac side of joint before sacral side
  - Early: Loss of definition of subchondral bone plate
  - Later: Erosions, widened joint space
    - Erosions often small, indistinct
  - Later: Sclerosis surrounding joint
  - End stage: Fusion of joint
- Vertebral bodies
  - Earliest: Squaring of vertebral bodies → corner erosions → shiny corner (corner sclerosis)
  - Later: Thin syndesmophytes bridge vertebrae
  - End stage: Widespread ankylosis (bamboo spine)
- Facet, uncovertebral joints
  - Erosions → fusion
- Enthesopathy
  - Erosions, periosteal new bone formation at tendon and ligament attachments
- Osteopenia

CT Findings

- Same findings as radiograph, but ↑ sensitivity

MR Findings

- Bone marrow edema: Low-signal T1, high-signal T2, and STIR
  - Sacroiliac joints
  - Corners of vertebral bodies, facet joints
- Joint effusions
- Erosions: Loss of subchondral bone plate, irregular margins of joint
- Squaring of vertebral bodies
- Ankylosis not striking MR finding
  - Syndesmophytes are thin, low signal intensity on all sequences

Imaging Recommendations

- Best imaging tool
  - MR and CT have good sensitivity for sacroiliitis

Imaging of Trauma in Ankylosing Spondylitis

- C2, cervicothoracic junction, thoracolumbar junction
  - Often hyperextension injury involving all 3 columns of spine
  - Fracture may be through vertebral body or fused disc space
  - MR should be considered to exclude occult fracture as these may be subtle secondary to osteopenia

DIFFERENTIAL DIAGNOSIS

DISH

- Bulky ossification of paraspinous ligaments
- Symmetric sacroiliac joint usually normal, rarely fused by bulky osteophytes

Rheumatoid Arthritis

- Ankylosis not feature
- Involves synovial joints, spares discs
- Primarily in cervical spine

Psoriatic Arthritis and Reactive Arthropathy

- Bulky ossification of paraspinous ligaments
- Sacroiliac joint involvement often asymmetric

Osteitis Condensans Ilii

- Sclerosis adjacent to sacroiliac joint
- Subchondral bone plate preserved, no erosions
- Joint space normal or narrow

Infection

- Unilateral sacroiliitis

PATHOLOGY

General Features

- Associated abnormalities
  - Pulmonary interstitial fibrosis, decreased chest excursion, uveitis, aortitis, aortic regurgitation
  - 90% of patients HLA-B27 positive

CLINICAL ISSUES

Presentation

- Most common signs/symptoms
  - Pain centered over sacroiliac joints, back stiffness
- Other signs/symptoms
  - Kyphotic deformity, fracture

Treatment

- Corticosteroids
- Disease modifying agents: Tumor necrosis factor inhibitors, sulfasalazine, methotrexate
  - Early initiation of treatment helps prevent ankylosis

DIAGNOSTIC CHECKLIST

Image Interpretation Pearls

- Normal sacroiliac joints preclude imaging diagnosis of ankylosing spondylitis

SELECTED REFERENCES

1. Navallas M et al: Sacroiliitis associated with axial spondyloarthropathy: new concepts and latest trends. Radiographics. 33(4):933-56, 2013
2. Campagna R et al: Fractures of the ankylosed spine: MDCT and MRI with emphasis on individual anatomic spinal structures. AJR Am J Roentgenol. 192(4):987-95, 2009
3. Braun J et al: Ankylosing spondylitis. Lancet. 369(9570):1379-90, 2007

(Left) *Coronal bone CT shows erosions and sclerosis at the C1-C2 facet joints ➡. There is extensive periosteal reaction (enthesopathy) surrounding the dens ➡. Occiput-C1 joints are fused ➡. (Right) Sagittal bone CT shows fractures at C2 ➡ and C7 ➡ in a patient with AS. Fractures in this population are often multilevel and difficult to see on CT because of osteopenia. Fracture of the C7 spinous process alerts the radiologist to look for a fracture of the anterior column.*

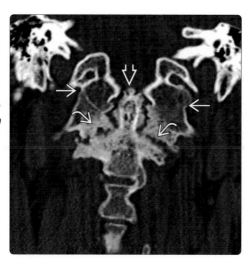
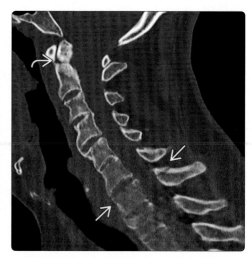

(Left) *Sagittal T1WI MR shows the characteristically unimpressive MR appearance of syndesmophytes ➡. At C3-C4 the entire disc has ossified ➡. (Right) Sagittal T2WI MR in a different patient shows ligamentous ossification extending from the clivus to the thoracic spine ➡. Note the upper thoracic kyphosis. Spinal deformity in patients with AS may preclude use of a cervical MR coil; flexible surface coils are often a better option.*

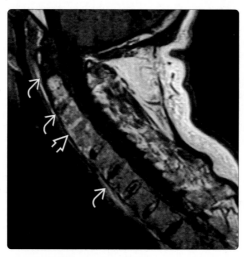
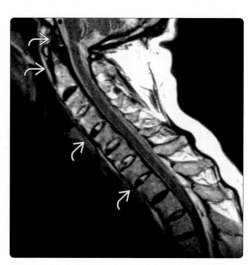

(Left) *Lateral radiograph in a 46-year-old woman shows fixed deformity from AS. Vertebral bodies and facet joints are fused with loss of cervical lordosis. Thoracic kyphosis is severe and the patient's chin was on her chest. Spinal deformity of AS can be debilitating. This patient also had limited chest expansion due to ankylosis of rib articulations. (Right) Sagittal bone CT shows the same patient after extension osteotomy and posterior fusion. A focal lordosis has been created at C6-C7 ➡.*

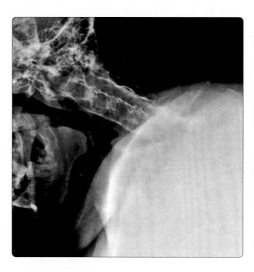
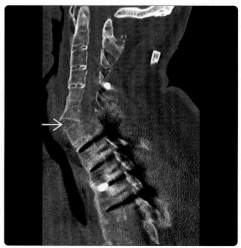

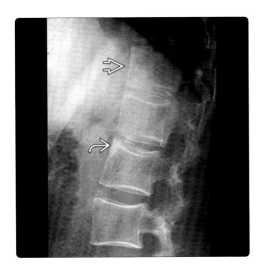

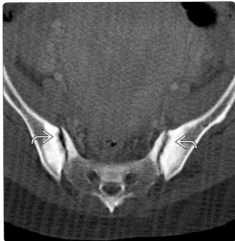

(Left) *Lateral radiograph shows the shiny corner sign* ➡️ *at L1 and L2. There is squaring of the vertebral body contour* ⇨ *of T12-L3. AS initially involves the sacroiliac joints, then typically skips to the thoracolumbar junction.* (Right) *Axial bone CT shows bilaterally symmetric sacroiliitis. Small erosions* ➡️ *are seen with widening of the joint and reactive sclerosis. Osteitis condensans ilii, in contrast, shows bone sclerosis without erosions or joint space widening.*

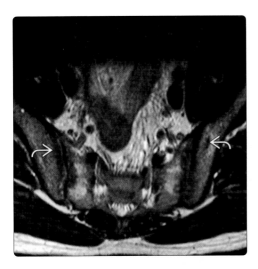

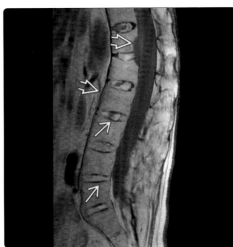

(Left) *Axial T2WI MR shows bilateral sacroiliac joint erosions* ➡️. *Bone marrow edema is slightly more prominent on the left. As is typical, the erosions are more severe on the iliac side of the joint.* (Right) *Sagittal T1W MR shows the typical changes of longstanding AS with ossified discs with fatty marrow replacement* ➡️, *syndesmophytes, and a ventral dural diverticulum* ⇨ *(which can be associated with cauda equina syndrome).*

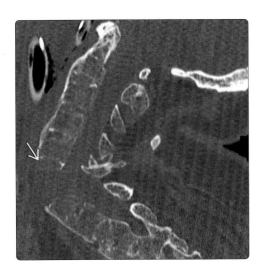

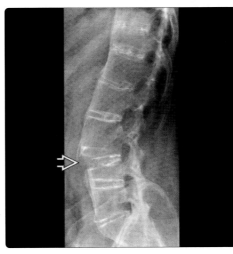

(Left) *Sagittal bone CT shows a severe extension fracture through the C5-C6 ossified disc space* ➡️ *in this patient with longstanding AS.* (Right) *Lateral radiograph in the same patient shows hyperextension-type fracture* ⇨ *of L4. The rigidity of the ankylosed spine renders it vulnerable to fracture. Fractures may occur through syndesmophytes or, as in this case, through the vertebral body or ossified disc space.*

TERMINOLOGY

- Calcium pyrophosphate dihydrate deposition (CPPD) disease
- Crowned dens syndrome: Pain due to CPPD deposition around dens
- Pseudogout: Acute painful episode due to CPPD

IMAGING

- Soft tissue calcifications
  - Usually linear, occasionally globular
  - Seen in ligaments, discs, facet joint capsules, hyaline cartilage
  - Horseshoe-shaped calcification around dens
- Erosions of odontoid process, vertebral endplates
  - Usually sharply demarcated, often corticated
- MR findings nonspecific
  - Calcium usually not visible, low signal intensity on all sequences
  - Soft tissue mass surrounding dens
  - Erosions of dens, vertebral endplates

TOP DIFFERENTIAL DIAGNOSES

- Degenerative disc disease
- Rheumatoid arthritis, adult
- Osteomyelitis, pyogenic
- Seronegative spondyloarthropathy
- Hemodialysis arthropathy
- Hyperparathyroidism
- Gout

CLINICAL ISSUES

- Chronic back pain
- Acute attack of pain ± fever ± radiculopathy
- Myelopathy due to cord compression

DIAGNOSTIC CHECKLIST

- CT useful in distinguishing from rheumatoid arthritis, which does not calcify

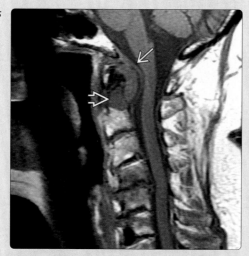
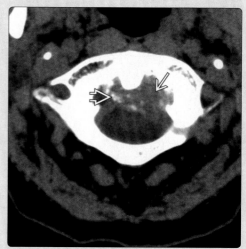

(Left) Sagittal T1WI MR shows a large pseudopannus posterior to the odontoid process ➡ with moderately severe effacement of the ventral thecal sac and mild mass effect upon the cervicomedullary junction. A large degenerative cyst is present in the odontoid process ➡. (Right) Axial bone CT shows marked thickening of the retroodontoid soft tissues ➡ with scattered calcifications ➡ that are consistent with a diagnosis of CPPD.

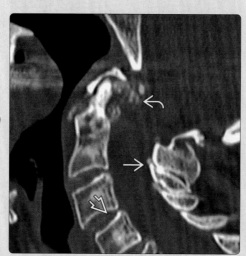
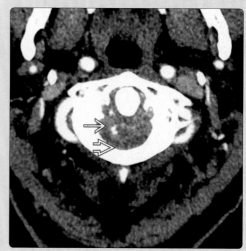

(Left) Sagittal bone CT shows severe CPPD at the craniocervical junction. There is a large calcified mass posterior to the dens ➡ and severe odontoid erosion. Calcification is seen in the ligamentum flavum ➡ and intervertebral discs ➡. (Right) Axial CTA study shows multiple punctate foci of calcification ➡ within a large soft tissue mass posterior to the odontoid process, which causes cord compression ➡.

Gout

KEY FACTS

TERMINOLOGY

- Arthropathy secondary to urate crystal deposition

IMAGING

- Generally involves only 1-2 levels
- Disc or facet joints, sacroiliac joint
- Most common in lumbar spine
- Typically have peripheral joint disease
- Endplate, facet erosions
  - Usually sharply demarcated (punched out)
- Preserved bone density
- Tophi
  - Mass in disc space, facet joint, paravertebral, spinal canal
  - May compress cord or nerve roots
  - May contain faint, amorphous calcifications on CT
  - Low signal intensity on T1WI
  - Low to intermediate signal intensity on T2WI, STIR
  - Variable enhancement with gadolinium
  - ± bone marrow edema adjacent to tophi

TOP DIFFERENTIAL DIAGNOSES

- Osteomyelitis
- Hemodialysis arthropathy
- Calcium pyrophosphate deposition
- Neuropathic arthropathy
- Seronegative spondyloarthropathy
- Rheumatoid arthritis

PATHOLOGY

- Uric acid crystal deposition in soft tissues
- May be secondary to chronic diseases

CLINICAL ISSUES

- Treatment
  - Colchicine
  - Uric acid production inhibitors (e.g., allopurinol)
  - Uricosuric medications (e.g., probenecid)

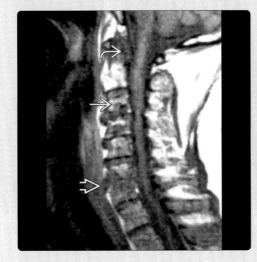
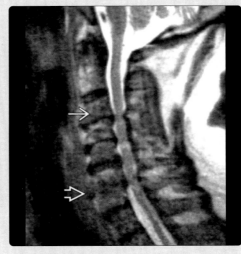

(Left) Sagittal PD/intermediate MR shows punched-out vertebral body erosions at multiple levels. There is near-complete endplate destruction at C6-C7 ➡. Tophus is present posterior to C2 ➡ and there are multiple intraosseous tophi ➡. (Right) Sagittal T2 MR in the same patient shows endplate destruction at C6-C7 ➡. Intraosseous tophus ➡ has low signal intensity and is almost indistinguishable from the surrounding marrow.

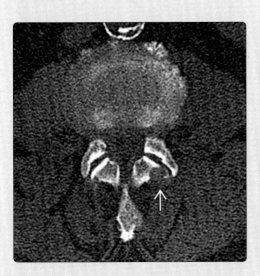
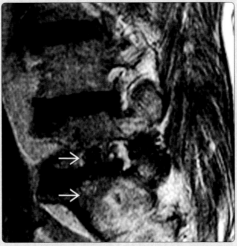

(Left) Axial NECT shows a focal punched-out lesion of soft tissue density in the left facet ➡ not directly contiguous with the joint space. Metastatic disease was the primary consideration but gout was diagnosed by biopsy. (Courtesy N. Farhataziz, MD.) (Right) Sagittal T2 MR shows focal erosions ➡ of L5 and S1 in a patient with uncontrolled peripheral gout and a flare-up of back pain. There was minimal enhancement with gadolinium.

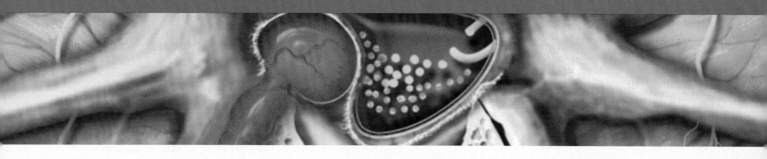

SECTION 7
Infection and Inflammatory Disorders

Infection

Inflammatory and Autoimmune

Anatomy-Based Imaging Issues

Spread of infection may occur along one of many different tracts, including **direct extension**, **lymphatic spread**, **hematogenous spread**, and along the **cerebrospinal fluid pathways**. **Direct extension**, as its name implies, occurs when bone or soft tissue comes into contact with a directly adjacent infection leading to a soft tissue abscess or osteomyelitis. For the spine, this route is typically seen adjacent to a decubitus ulcer where there is adjacent osteomyelitis. An infection of the disc space can extend into the adjacent paravertebral soft tissues and produce psoas muscle abscesses. Direct extension is also the mechanism for epidural abscess involvement cranial or caudal to the site of disc space infection. This route can also be seen for an intramedullary spinal cord abscess where the infection occurs through congenital dysraphism or a dermal sinus tract. Lymphatic spread is of limited importance in the spine relative to the much more commonly seen direct extension and hematogenous spread. **Lymphatic spread** may be seen in cases of retroperitoneal node enlargement from pelvic or abdominal primary neoplasms.

Hematogenous Spread

Hematogenous spread is the major pathway of infection spread to the axial skeleton; which route is more important (arterial or venous) is controversial. The arterial route is classically more important for spread of spinal infection. Vertebral bodies have areas that function physiologically in a similar manner to long bone metaphyses. The metaphyseal equivalent bone occurs near the anterior longitudinal ligament and has an end-arteriole network making it susceptible to bacterial seeding. These areas have distal nonanastomosing vessels that have slow flow, and occlusion of these vessels will lead to avascular necrosis. In the vertebral bodies, segmental arteries usually supply 2 adjacent vertebral bodies and the intervening disc, giving the typical disc space infection patterns. The venous route is classically through the Batson plexus, which is a longitudinal network of valveless veins running parallel to the spinal column. These veins lie outside of the thoracoabdominal cavity. These veins communicate with multiple aspects of the venous system, including the vena cava, portal venous system, azygos system, intercostal veins, and pulmonary and renal veins. Flow direction within the plexus is variable due to the variable intrathoracic and intraabdominal pressures. The pharyngovertebral plexus serves the same physiologic purpose. The contiguity of the cerebrospinal fluid spaces between the intracranial vault and the thecal sac allows for direct communication of the neoplasm and infection. Intracranial neoplasms may seed throughout the cervical, thoracic, or lumbar thecal sac. Likewise, even distal neoplasms involving the caudal thecal sac may propagate cephalad and extend into the intracranial cerebrospinal fluid space.

Pathologic Issues

Types of spinal infection can be divided into disc space infection/vertebral osteomyelitis, subdural empyema, meningitis, intramedullary cord abscess, and septic arthritis/facet joint involvement. Disc space infection shows the typical pattern of low signal intensity on T1-weighted images involving the disc space proper and extending to the adjacent endplates. Endplate irregularity is a typical feature. T2 hyperintensity is generally present within the intervertebral disc in a nonanatomic pattern with adjacent T2 hyperintensity extending to the vertebral bodies. Contrast enhancement tends to be irregular when it involves the intervertebral disc with diffuse enhancement extending to the involved vertebral bodies. Extension into the paravertebral soft tissues is an important aspect of disc space infections and should be evaluated via either fat-suppressed, postcontrast T1-weighted images looking for enhancement of the paravertebral and psoas musculature or on T2-weighted images looking for T2 hyperintensity. It is important to comment not only on the level of involvement but also on any instability or malalignment that may be present and whether there is extension into the paravertebral regions, epidural space, and psoas musculature.

Epidural Abscess and Meningitis

Isolated epidural abscesses can occur without concomitant disc space infections, but they can be associated with indwelling spinal catheters or prior spinal instrumentation. Uncommonly, these may occur as a result of hematogenous spread. Meningitis typically manifests on postcontrast T1-weighted images as linear enhancement along the pial surface of the cord or the roots of the cauda equina. With fungal infection, a more nodular enhancement pattern can be seen, which mimics the appearance of neoplastic spread. Spinal subdural empyemas are an uncommon manifestation of infection but may be seen in the setting of a severe disc space infection with adjacent extension into the epidural space. Presumably, this is the result of direct extension through the dura and infection of the subdural space.

Intramedullary spinal cord abscesses are uncommon but can occur via both the hematogenous route and by direct extension. In adults, direct extension is the more typical mechanism. In children, the typical mechanism is direct extension through a dermal sinus. Septic arthritis/facet joint involvement may occur via hematogenous extension or by direct extension. Early infection may only be identified by slight T2 hyperintensity involving the bone of the facets, which is associated with facet effusion.

Adult vs. Pediatric

The routes of pyogenic infection will differ between adults and children due to developmental differences. In adults, the vertebral endplates become infected first, spreading to adjacent disc space and subsequently to the adjacent vertebral body, paravertebral tissues, and epidural space. In children, vascular channels are present across the growth plate, allowing primary infection of the intervertebral disc with subsequent secondary infection of the vertebral body. Disc space infections occur most commonly in the lumbar spine, followed by thoracic and cervical regions. Risk factors are many but include over 50 years of age, diabetes, rheumatoid arthritis, AIDS, steroid administration, urinary tract instrumentation, prior spinal fracture, and paraplegia. *Staphylococcus aureus* is the most common organism. Pseudomonas may occur in the setting of drug abuse. *Salmonella* is the classic infection seen in sickle cell patients; however, *S. aureus* is still the most common overall in this population.

Classification

The Cierny and Mader classification of bone infection divides the pathology into 4 anatomic disease types and 3 host categories, yielding 12 clinical stages. The 4 anatomic disease types are: (1) Early hematogenous or medullary osteomyelitis, (2) superficial osteomyelitis (contiguous spread), (3) localized or full thickness sequestration, and (4) diffuse osteomyelitis. The 3 host classifications are: (A) Normal physiologic response,

(B) locally or systemically compromised response, and (C) treatment of the osteomyelitis would be worse than the infection itself.

The spinal tuberculosis classification of Mehta (2001) divides the disease into 4 groups: (1) Stable anterior lesions without kyphotic deformity are treated with anterior debridement and strut grafting, (2) global lesions with kyphosis and instability are treated with posterior instrumentation and anterior strut grafting, (3) patients who are at high risk if treated by transthoracic surgery are treated with posterior decompression and instrumentation, and (4) isolated posterior lesions can be treated with posterior decompression.

Clinical Implications

Spinal involvement with infection represents 2-5% of all osteomyelitis sites. Axial spine pain is the most common presentation. This is progressive, although it can have a fairly insidious onset, producing pain without relief from rest. Fever is variable and may be present in < 50% of cases. High-grade fever is present in < 5% and motor and sensory deficits occur in 10-15% of patients. Rarely, intramedullary abscess can present with motor or sensory neurological deficits. Delay in diagnosing spinal infection is common. Intramedullary abscesses are fatal in 8% with persistent neurological deficits in over 70%. Erythrocyte sedimentation rate is positive in more than 90%. C-reactive protein is also elevated. Blood cultures are positive with spinal osteomyelitis in 25-60% of cases.

Operative debridement with fusion may be necessary for a variety of reasons, including the necessity to obtain a specific microorganism, abscess drainage, persistent neurological deficit, presence of spine instability and deformity, and failure of medical treatment. Long-term intravenous antibiotics remain the 1st-line of therapy if there is no acute or evolving neurological deficit. A 6-week course of intravenous antibiotics is typical, which may also include an additional oral antibiotic regimen at the completion of the intravenous phase. External spine immobilization and bracing may be used. Recurrent bacteremia, paravertebral abscesses, and chronically draining sinuses are associated with relapse. Chronic autofusion of the infected level with successful nonoperative treatment is a common outcome.

Differential Diagnosis

The primary diagnostic modality in the evaluation of epidural abscess is MR, which is as sensitive as CT myelography for epidural infection but also allows the exclusion of other diagnostic choices, such as herniation, syrinx, tumor, and cord infarction. MR imaging of epidural abscess demonstrates a soft tissue mass in the epidural space with tapered edges and an associated mass effect on the thecal sac and cord. The epidural masses are usually isointense to the cord on T1-weighted images and of increased signal on T2-weighted images. Contrast-enhanced MR is necessary for full elucidation of the abscess. The patterns of MR contrast enhancement of epidural abscess include: (1) Diffuse and homogeneous, (2) heterogeneous, and (3) thin peripheral. Enhancement is a very useful adjunct for identifying the extent of a lesion when the plain MR scan is equivocal, demonstrating activity of an infection, and directing needle biopsy and follow-up treatment. Successful therapy should cause a progressive decrease in enhancement of the paraspinal soft tissues, disc, and vertebral bodies. In the initial stages of vertebral osteomyelitis, when the disc space is not yet involved, it may be difficult to exclude neoplastic disease, type I degenerative endplate changes, or compression fracture from the differential diagnosis using only MR. Follow-up studies are usually necessary to further define the nature of the lesion.

Boden et al. suggested that in the postoperative spine, the triad of intervertebral disc space enhancement, annular enhancement, and vertebral body enhancement leads to the diagnosis of disc space infection, with the appropriate laboratory findings, such as an elevated sedimentation rate. However, there is a group of normal postoperative patients with annulus enhancement (at the surgical curette site), intervertebral disc enhancement, and vertebral endplate enhancement without evidence of disc space infection. In postoperative normal enhancement, the intervertebral disc enhancement is typically seen as thin bands paralleling the adjacent endplates, and the vertebral body enhancement is enhancement associated with type I degenerative endplate changes. This pattern should be distinguished from the amorphous enhancement seen within the intervertebral disc with disc space infection.

Selected References

1. Floccari LV et al: Surgical site infections after pediatric spine surgery. Orthop Clin North Am. 47(2):387-94, 2016
2. Boody BS et al: Vertebral osteomyelitis and spinal epidural abscess: an evidence-based review. J Spinal Disord Tech. 28(6):E316-27, 2015
3. Duarte RM et al: Spinal infection: state of the art and management algorithm. Eur Spine J. 22(12):2787-99, 2013
4. Malghem J et al: Necrotizing fasciitis: Contribution and limitations of diagnostic imaging. Joint Bone Spine. 80(2):146-54, 2013
5. Go JL et al: Spine infections. Neuroimaging Clin N Am. 22(4):755-72, 2012
6. DeSanto J et al: Spine infection/inflammation. Radiol Clin North Am. 49(1):105-27, 2011
7. Celik AD et al: Spondylodiscitis due to an emergent fungal pathogen: Blastoschizomyces capitatus, a case report and review of the literature. Rheumatol Int. 29(10):1237-41, 2009
8. Hong SH et al: MR imaging assessment of the spine: infection or an imitation? Radiographics. 29(2):599-612, 2009
9. Karikari IO et al: Management of a spontaneous spinal epidural abscess: a single-center 10-year experience. Neurosurgery. 65(5):919-23; discussion 923-4, 2009
10. Mylona E et al: Pyogenic vertebral osteomyelitis: a systematic review of clinical characteristics. Semin Arthritis Rheum. 39(1):10-7, 2009
11. Petruzzi N et al: Recent trends in soft-tissue infection imaging. Semin Nucl Med. 39(2):115-23, 2009
12. Posacioglu H et al: Rupture of a nonaneurysmal abdominal aorta due to spondylitis. Tex Heart Inst J. 36(1):65-8, 2009
13. Sobottke R et al: Treatment of spondylodiscitis in human immunodeficiency virus-infected patients: a comparison of conservative and operative therapy. Spine (Phila Pa 1976). 34(13):E452-8, 2009
14. Thwaites G et al: British Infection Society guidelines for the diagnosis and treatment of tuberculosis of the central nervous system in adults and children. J Infect. 59(3):167-87, 2009
15. Dai LY et al: Anterior instrumentation for the treatment of pyogenic vertebral osteomyelitis of thoracic and lumbar spine. Eur Spine J. 17(8):1027-34, 2008
16. Mehta JS et al: Tuberculosis of the thoracic spine. A classification based on the selection of surgical strategies. J Bone Joint Surg Br. 83(6):859-63, 2001
17. Mader JT et al: Staging and staging application in osteomyelitis. Clin Infect Dis. 25(6):1303-9, 1997
18. Boden SD et al: Postoperative diskitis: distinguishing early MR imaging findings from normal postoperative disk space changes. Radiology. 184(3):765-71, 1992

(Left) *Sagittal graphic shows lumbar disc space infection with vertebral body osteomyelitis with endplate destruction and marrow edema. There are ventral and dorsal abscess collections.* **(Right)** *Sagittal T1WI C+ FS MR in this case of disc space infection shows enhancement of L5 and S1 bodies* ➡ *and an intervertebral disc with prevertebral and epidural phlegmon* ➡ *extension.*

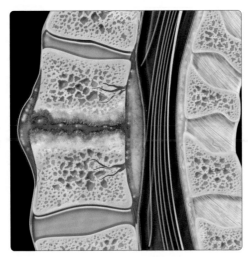
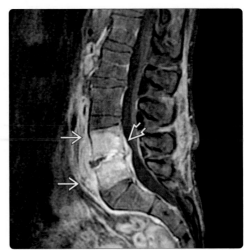

(Left) *Axial T1WI C+ MR of a disc space infection shows inflammatory extension into the prevertebral space, psoas muscles, and dorsal spinal muscles. Phlegmon extends into the ventral epidural space with thecal sac compression* ➡. **(Right)** *Axial T2WI FS MR shows inflammatory extension into the prevertebral space, psoas muscles* ➡, *and dorsal spinal muscles* ➡.

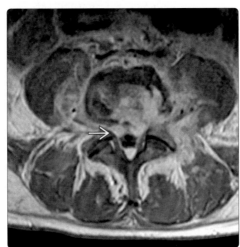
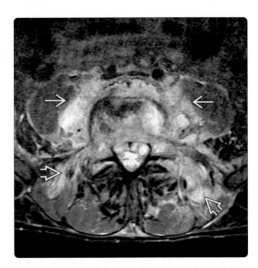

(Left) *Axial T1WI C+ MR shows disseminated coccidioidomycosis with diffuse bone and soft tissue involvement and adjacent paraspinal extension and extension into lung.* **(Right)** *Axial T2WI MR in coccidioidomycosis shows huge paraspinal abscesses* ➡. *There is effacement of the normal thecal sac within the spinal canal due to disc space infection and osteomyelitis.*

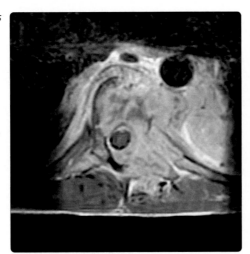
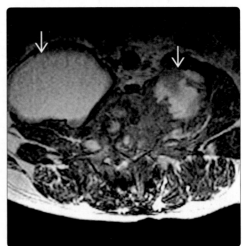

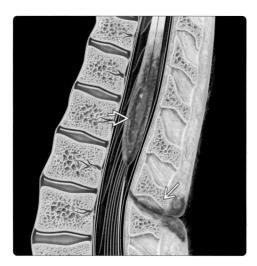

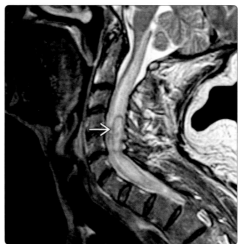

(Left) Sagittal graphic shows the dermal sinus ⇶ extending from the skin surface to the conus, with conus abscess ⇶ and extensive cord edema. (Right) Sagittal T2WI MR in a patient with a cervical cord abscess and streptococcal endocarditis shows diffuse cord expansion with a ring-shaped area of low T2 signal (abscess capsule) within the cord from C4 to C5-C6 ⇶.

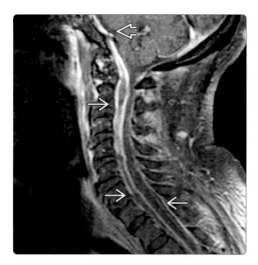

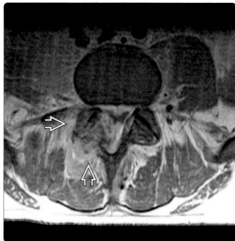

(Left) Sagittal T1WI C+ MR with fat suppression shows extensive subdural empyema with peripheral enhancement ⇶ throughout the cervical spine and extending along clivus ⇶. (Right) A septic facet joint is shown. Axial T1WI C+ MR at L4-L5 shows extension of the infection to the right facet joint with diffuse facet bone enhancement and juxta facet soft tissue involvement ⇶.

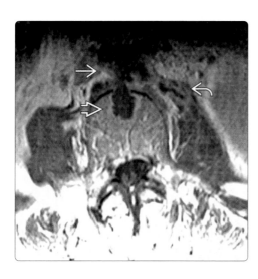

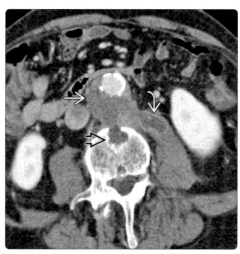

(Left) Axial T1WI C+ MR shows direct extension of infection from a mycotic aortic aneurysm ⇶ into the ventral vertebral body, producing bone destruction and osteomyelitis ⇶. There is also direct extension of infection into psoas muscle ⇶. (Right) Axial CECT shows direct extension of infection from a mycotic aortic aneurysm ⇶ into the vertebral body ⇶ and left psoas muscle ⇶.

Infection and Inflammatory Disorders

KEY FACTS

TERMINOLOGY

- Definition: Bacterial suppurative infection of vertebrae and intervertebral disc
- Synonyms: Pyogenic spondylodiscitis, disc space infection

IMAGING

- Ill-defined hypointense T1 vertebral marrow with loss of endplate definition on both sides of disc
- Loss of disc height and abnormal disc signal
- Destruction of vertebral endplate cortex
- Vertebral collapse
- Paraspinal ± epidural infiltrative soft tissue ± loculated fluid collection
- Follow-up MR
  - Should focus on soft tissue findings
  - No single MR imaging parameter is associated with clinical status

TOP DIFFERENTIAL DIAGNOSES

- Degenerative endplate changes
- Tuberculous vertebral osteomyelitis
- Spinal neuropathic arthropathy

PATHOLOGY

- Predisposing factors
  - Intravenous drug use
  - Immunocompromised state
  - Chronic medical illnesses (renal failure, cirrhosis, cancer, diabetes)
- *Staphylococcus aureus* is most common pathogen

CLINICAL ISSUES

- Acute or chronic back pain
- Focal spinal tenderness
- Fever
- ↑ ESR, ↑ CRP, ↑ WBC

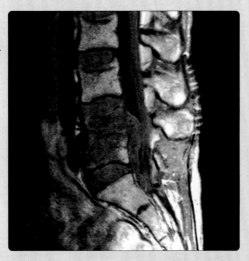
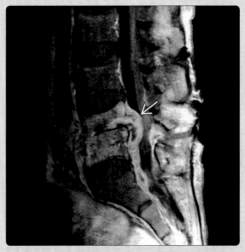

(Left) *Sagittal T1WI MR in a patient with a history of lumbar surgery shows findings of disc space infection at L4-L5 with hypointense marrow, vertebral collapse, endplate erosion, disc space loss, and epidural phlegmon.* (Right) *Sagittal T1WI C+ MR demonstrates enhancing vertebral bodies and intervening disc. There is an epidural abscess ➡ extending from L4-L5 to S1, consistent with pyogenic vertebral osteomyelitis. Severe central canal narrowing is present at L4-L5.*

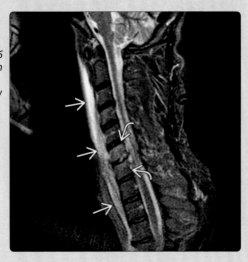
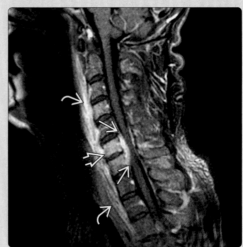

(Left) *Sagittal STIR MR shows increased fluid in the retropharyngeal/prevertebral space ➡. Marrow edema in C6 and C7 vertebral bodies is seen ➡. There is fluid signal within the disc space with irregularity along the endplate cortical margins.* (Right) *Sagittal T1WI C+ FS MR shows homogeneously enhancing epidural phlegmon at the C6-C7 level ➡ causing mass effect on the cord. C6 & C7 vertebral bodies exhibit avid homogeneous enhancement ➡. Note the prevertebral, enhancing soft tissues ➡ representing phlegmon.*

TERMINOLOGY

Synonyms

- Pyogenic spondylodiscitis, disc space infection

Definitions

- Bacterial suppurative infection of vertebrae and intervertebral disc

IMAGING

General Features

- Best diagnostic clue
  - Ill-defined hypointense vertebral marrow on T1WI with loss of endplate definition on both sides of disc
- Morphology
  - Loss of disc height, abnormal signal
  - Destruction of vertebral endplate cortex
  - Paraspinal ± epidural infiltrative soft tissue ± loculated fluid collection

CT Findings

- NECT
  - Endplate osteolytic/osteosclerotic changes
  - Increase in paraspinal soft tissue

MR Findings

- Disc space
  - Hypointense on T1WI, hyperintense on T2WI
  - Diffuse or rim enhancement with gadolinium
- Vertebral marrow signal abnormality abutting disc
- Paraspinal and epidural phlegmon or abscess
- Cord compression

Nuclear Medicine Findings

- Bone scan
  - 3-phase technetium-99m diphosphonate scan shows increased activity in all phases
- Gallium scan
  - Increased uptake of gallium citrate (Ga-67)
- WBC scan
  - Often false-negative in patients with chronic vertebral osteomyelitis

Imaging Recommendations

- Best imaging tool
  - Sagittal and axial T2WI and T1WI MR
    - Sensitivity (96%), specificity (92%), accuracy (94%)
  - SPECT Ga-67 scan good alternative
    - Sensitivity and specificity in low 90%

DIFFERENTIAL DIAGNOSIS

Degenerative Endplate Changes

- Most common mimic
- Disc desiccation
- Vertebral endplates preserved

Tuberculous Vertebral Osteomyelitis

- Vertebral collapse, gibbus deformity
- Large dissecting paraspinal abscesses out of proportion to vertebral involvement

Spinal Neuropathic Arthropathy

- Sequela of spinal cord injury
- Disc space loss/T2 hyperintensity, endplate erosion/sclerosis, osteophytosis, soft tissue mass

Chronic Hemodialysis Spondyloarthropathy

- Disc space loss, endplate erosion, vertebral destruction

Spinal Metastases

- Discrete or ill-defined vertebral lesions
  - Postgadolinium enhancement
- Disc space preserved

PATHOLOGY

General Features

- Etiology
  - Predisposing factors
    - Intravenous drug use
    - Immunocompromised state
    - Chronic medical illnesses (renal failure, cirrhosis, cancer, diabetes)
  - *Staphylococcus aureus* is most common pathogen
    - *Escherichia coli* most common of gram-negative bacilli
    - *Salmonella* common in patients with sickle cell disease
  - Bacteremia from extraspinal primary source
  - Direct inoculation from penetrating trauma, surgical intervention, or diagnostic procedures
  - Extension from adjacent infection
    - Diverticulitis, appendicitis, inflammatory bowl disease

CLINICAL ISSUES

Presentation

- Most common signs/symptoms
  - Back pain, tenderness, fever
- Other signs/symptoms
  - Myelopathy if cord compromised
  - Elevated erythrocyte sedimentation rate, C-reactive protein, white cell count

Natural History & Prognosis

- Mortality rate: 2-12%
- Favorable outcome; resolution of symptoms if prompt diagnosis & treatment
- Recurrence due to incomplete treatment (2-8%)
- Irreversible neurological deficits
  - Delay in diagnosis & neurologic impairment at diagnosis significant predictors of neurologic deficit at follow-up
- Improvement in imaging findings may lag behind clinical improvement

Treatment

- CT-guided or open biopsy yields causative organism > blood cultures (77% vs. 58%)
  - Previous antibiotic treatment lowers yield (23% vs. 60%)
- Early empiric antibiotics, broad spectrum coverage until causative pathogen isolated
- Spinal immobilization with bracing for 6-12 weeks
- Surgical treatment
  - Laminectomy, debridement, ± stabilization
  - Intervention if epidural abscess, instability present

Infection and Inflammatory Disorders

(Left) *Sagittal STIR MR illustrates marrow edema related to discitis-osteomyelitis at the T12-L1 level ⇨. Intervertebral fluid extends into the paraspinal soft tissues ⇨. Cortical irregularity along the adjacent endplate margins is observed.* **(Right)** *Sagittal T1WI C+ MR shows peripheral enhancement of the T12/L1 disc ⇨ and paraspinal enhancing phlegmon ⇨. Follow-up MR images often depict less paraspinal inflammation and less epidural enhancement compared with baseline images.*

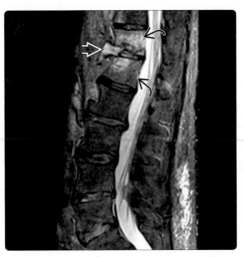
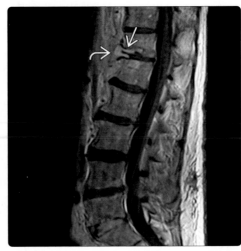

(Left) *Sagittal STIR MR depicts marrow edema in the L5 and S1 vertebral bodies ⇨. A presacral fluid-intensity collection ⇨ is observed. The anterior cortical margin is obscured. On follow-up MR vertebral body disc space enhancement and bone marrow edema may be equivocal or appear worse compared with the baseline.* **(Right)** *Axial CT reconstruction exhibits an irregular cortical break along the anterior superior margin of the S1 body ⇨, subtle sclerosis ⇨, and a presacral soft tissue component ⇨.*

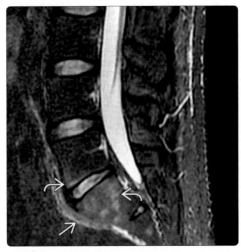
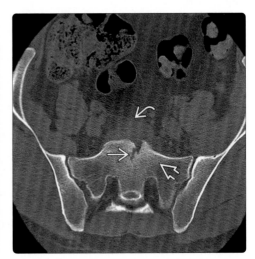

(Left) *Abnormal T1 hypointensity ⇨ is seen in the marrow of 2 adjacent midthoracic vertebral bodies. Thin syndesmophytes ⇨ are compatible with ankylosing spondylitis (AS).* **(Right)** *Sagittal T1 C+ MR shows enhancement of the adjacent irregular endplates ⇨. Aseptic spondylodiscitis can complicate AS. Proliferative epidural tissue without inflammatory infiltrates and new bone reaction, suggesting the contribution of mechanical factors, may cause neurological complications.*

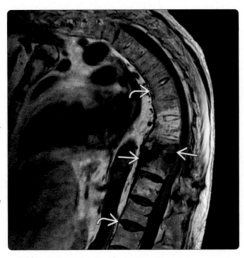
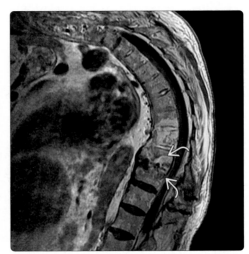

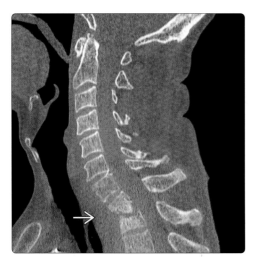

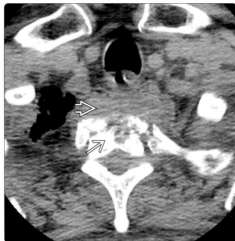

(Left) *Sagittal NECT (bone window) of upper thoracic disc space infection shows destruction of the T1 and T2 bodies centered about the collapsed disc space* ➡ *with marked endplate irregularity and kyphotic deformity.* (Right) *Axial NECT shows destruction of the T1 and T2 bodies with marked endplate irregularity* ➡ *and a large ventral paravertebral soft tissue mass (abscess)* ➡.

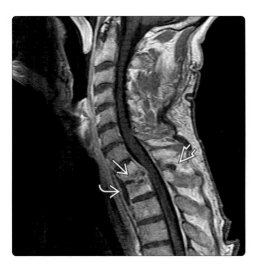

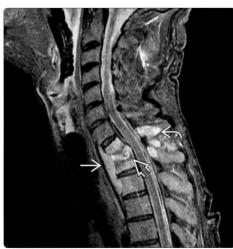

(Left) *Sagittal C+ MR shows multiple compartments involved by infection with destruction and collapse of the adjacent vertebral endplates* ➡, *a large ventral abscess* ➡, *and extension to involve the posterior elements* ➡. (Right) *Sagittal STIR MR shows T1 and T2 collapse with endplate destruction* ➡ *and a large ventral abscess that displaces the anterior longitudinal ligament* ➡. *There is extension that involves the posterior elements* ➡.

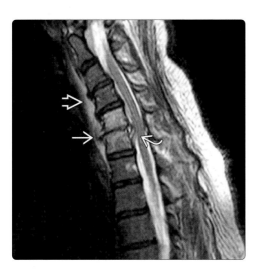

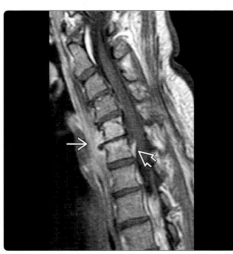

(Left) *Sagittal T2 MR shows C5-C6 disc space infection* ➡ *with increased signal from the contiguous bodies and extensive prevertebral edema* ➡. *There is a small epidural abscess that mildly effaces the cord* ➡. (Right) *Sagittal T1 C+ MR shows enhancement of the C5 and C6 bodies with mild disc irregularity and diffuse prevertebral soft tissue enhancement* ➡. *A small ventral epidural abscess is also present* ➡.

Infection and Inflammatory Disorders

TERMINOLOGY

- Tuberculous spondylitis (TS)
- Granulomatous infection of spine and adjacent soft tissue secondary to tuberculosis

IMAGING

- Gibbus vertebrae with relatively intact intervertebral discs, large paraspinal abscesses
- Midthoracic or thoracolumbar > lumbar, cervical
- Isolated posterior element involvement possible
- Sagittal STIR or FSE T2 with fat saturation most sensitive for bone marrow edema, epidural involvement
  - MR best modality to evaluate extent of disease, assess response to treatment

TOP DIFFERENTIAL DIAGNOSES

- Pyogenic spondylitis
  - Initial infection in subchondral bone
  - Intervertebral discs typically affected

- Fungal spondylitis
- Spinal metastases
  - Extraosseous epidural or paraspinal extension
  - Disc space preserved
- Brucellar spondylitis

PATHOLOGY

- Hematogenous or lymphatic spread
- Initial inoculum in anterior vertebral body
- Spread to noncontiguous vertebral bodies beneath longitudinal ligaments

CLINICAL ISSUES

- Chronic back pain, focal tenderness, fever
- Neurologic deficits more common with TS than other granulomatous infections
- Concomitant pulmonary tuberculosis in ~ 10% of patients
- Spinal tuberculosis accounts for 2% of all tuberculosis cases

(Left) Sagittal graphic through the lumbar spine depicts multifocal granulomatous osteomyelitis. Frank abscesses are present at the L3-L4 disc space ➡ and between the spinous process of L2 and L3 ➡. (Right) Sagittal STIR MR in a patient with tuberculosis (TB) infection shows involvement of contiguous vertebral bodies with subligamentous abscess spread and partial disc involvement ➡. Multiple focal bone lesions are present without adjacent disc involvement ➡.

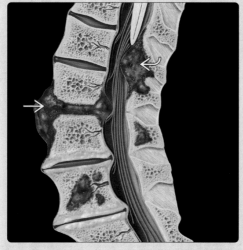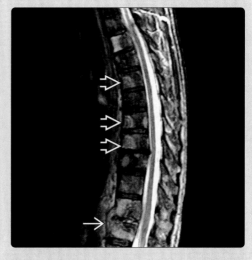

(Left) Sagittal T1WI C+ FS MR demonstrates focal kyphosis at L2-L3, collapse of the disc space, avid vertebral body enhancement ➡, and ventral and dorsal paravertebral abscesses ➡. There are peripherally enhancing abscesses in the paraspinal soft tissues ➡, which exhibit hypointense rims ➡. (Right) Coronal T1WI C+ FS MR shows TB osteomyelitis with L2 vertebra plana ➡. Psoas involvement with swelling and marked enhancement ➡ is present. Inflammatory soft tissue surrounds the disc ➡.

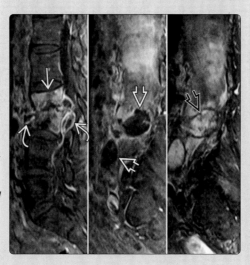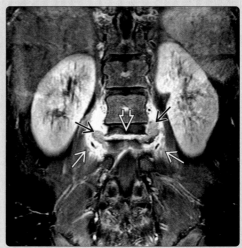

Fungal and Miscellaneous Osteomyelitis

KEY FACTS

TERMINOLOGY

- Noncaseating, acid-fast negative or fungal infections primarily occurring as opportunistic infection in immunocompromised patient
- Involvement of spine and adjacent soft tissue typically secondary to fungal pathogen

IMAGING

- Osseous destruction ± disc, epidural, or paraspinal involvement
  - Mixed lytic and sclerotic foci within vertebral bodies
  - Marrow edema
  - ± paravertebral mass, epidural phlegmon
- Diffuse > focal, lobulated contours
- May produce spinal deformity

TOP DIFFERENTIAL DIAGNOSES

- Pyogenic osteomyelitis
- Granulomatous osteomyelitis

  - Tuberculosis
  - Brucellosis

PATHOLOGY

- Hematogenous spread
- Direct extension from adjacent tissues
  - Direct implantation from trauma, hematogenous, local extension, iatrogenic after lumbar puncture, nucleoplasty

CLINICAL ISSUES

- Neck pain or back pain
- Clinical signs of systemic illness
- Risk factors: Immunosuppression, diabetes, hemodialysis, corticosteroid use, chemotherapy, or malnutrition

DIAGNOSTIC CHECKLIST

- Also consider fungal entities when tuberculosis is in imaging differential diagnosis list

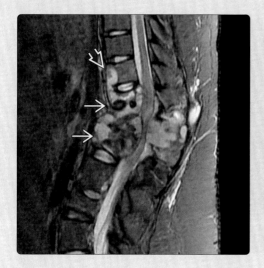
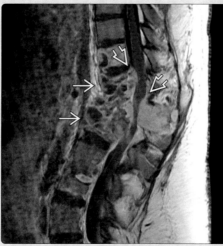

(Left) Sagittal STIR MR (coccidioidomycosis) shows destruction and abnormal signal involving multiple vertebral bodies at the thoracolumbar junction ⇨. There is severe compression of the thecal sac. Note the anterior extension underneath the anterior longitudinal ligament ⇨. (Right) Sagittal T1 C+ MR (coccidioidomycosis) shows extensive, multiple vertebral body irregular enhancement and destruction ⇨ with dorsal and ventral epidural extension and thecal sac compression ⇨.

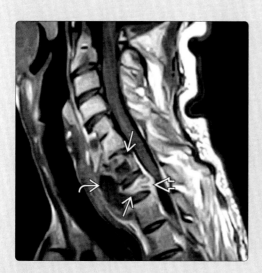
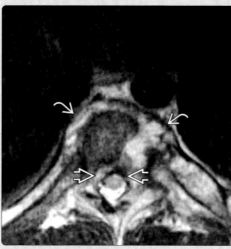

(Left) Sagittal T1 C+ MR (coccidioidomycosis) shows a rim-enhancing prevertebral abscess ⇨ due to chronic infection. There is destruction of C7 and T1 vertebral bodies ⇨, relative sparing of the intervertebral discs, and ventral epidural phlegmon ⇨. (Right) Axial T2WI MR (blastomycosis) illustrates hyperintense paraspinal phlegmon ⇨. A ventral epidural mass ⇨ mildly displaces the cord without cord signal abnormality.

TERMINOLOGY

- Infection of C1-C2 articulation (pyogenic or tuberculous)

IMAGING

- Soft tissue mass within prevertebral space centered at C1-C2
  - Prevertebral increased soft tissue/edema
  - Variable extension into epidural space, dural sac, or cord compression
  - Low T1 signal, increased T2/STIR signal from vertebral bodies, soft tissue mass
- ± bone destruction involving anterior arch of C1, odontoid, and body of C2
- Diffuse enhancement of vertebral bodies, soft tissue mass within prevertebral region/epidural space
  - May show nonenhancing abscess focus
- MRA/CTA: Evaluation of skull base, C1-C2 instability with vertebral artery compromise

TOP DIFFERENTIAL DIAGNOSES

- Rheumatoid arthritis
- Odontoid fracture
- C1-C2 osteoarthritis
- Primary bone tumor/metastases

PATHOLOGY

- Hematogenous seeding to capillary ends/end arterioles in subchondral regions

CLINICAL ISSUES

- Neck pain, limited range of motion, dysphagia
- C1-C2 subluxation, medulla compression, and motor/sensory deficit
- Vertebral artery compression with posterior circulation infarction

DIAGNOSTIC CHECKLIST

- Severe C1-C2 subluxation ± epidural phlegmon/abscess

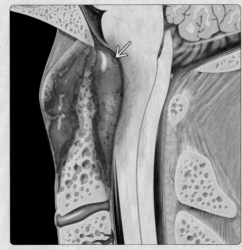
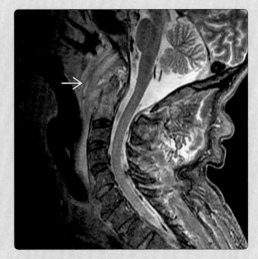

(Left) Sagittal graphic illustrates osteomyelitis involving the odontoid with bone destruction, extension to the anterior arch of C1, and formation of epidural abscess ➡. (Right) Sagittal STIR MR in this patient with a septic C1-C2 joint shows extensive abnormal signal from the odontoid and C2 body with phlegmon extension into the prevertebral soft tissues ➡.

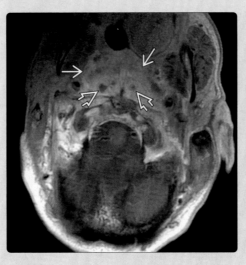
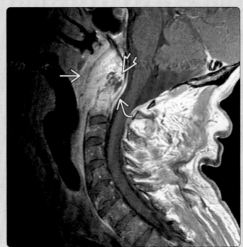

(Left) Axial T1 C+ MR shows a large amount of enhancing phlegmon within the prevertebral soft tissues ➡ with scattered smaller nonenhancing abscesses ➡. (Right) Sagittal T1 C+ MR shows an irregular area of decreased enhancement in the odontoid that is consistent with bone infarction ➡. There is extensive prevertebral enhancing phlegmon ➡. A small amount of epidural phlegmon is also present ➡.

Septic Facet Joint Arthritis

KEY FACTS

TERMINOLOGY

- Suppurative bacterial infection of facet joint, adjacent soft tissue

IMAGING

- Abnormal enhancement within facet joint with associated facet marrow, adjacent soft tissue edema
  - Typically single level, unilateral involvement
  - Facet joint widening
  - Ill-defined facet marrow signal alteration
  - Eroded facet cortex
- Lumbar spine most common
- Protocol advice
  - Sagittal STIR or FSE T2 with fat saturation most sensitive for bone marrow edema and epidural involvement
  - Postgadolinium T1WI with fat saturation better delineates extent of facet, epidural, and paraspinal involvement

TOP DIFFERENTIAL DIAGNOSES

- Facet joint osteoarthritis
  - Bilateral joint space narrowing with vacuum phenomenon
- Facet synovial cyst
  - Juxtaarticular thin-walled, well-defined mass
- Rheumatoid arthritis
  - Widened facets with enhancing synovium
  - Facet joint erosion

PATHOLOGY

- Most common cause: Hematogenous contamination
  - *Staphylococcus aureus* in 86%; *Streptococcus* in 9%
- Direct inoculation from penetrating trauma, surgical intervention, or diagnostic procedures
- Extension from adjacent infection in paraspinal soft tissues
  - Associated findings
    - Spondylodiscitis
    - Epidural paravertebral abscess

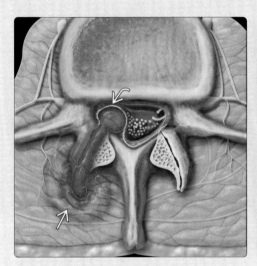
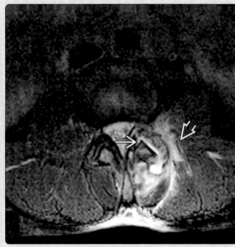

(Left) *Axial graphic at a lumbar vertebral level demonstrates a septic right facet joint with adjacent osteomyelitis and abscess extending into subarticular recess ➡ and posterior paraspinal muscle ➡. (Right) Axial T2WI MR with fat suppression through lumbar vertebra shows fluid in the left facet joint ➡ with posterior extension and loculation. Edema is present in surrounding soft tissue ➡.*

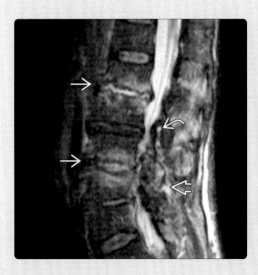
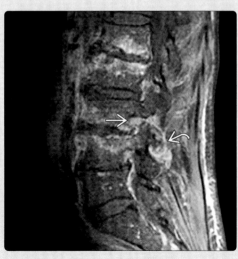

(Left) *Sagittal STIR MR shows multilevel discitis-osteomyelitis ➡ with interdiscal fluid and adjacent endplate erosive changes. There is also infection of the facet joints of 2 adjacent levels. Fluid is seen within the facet joints ➡. There is marrow edema of the articular pillars as well as the surrounding soft tissues ➡. (Right) Sagittal T1WI C+ FS MR depicts the peri facet inflammation associated with septic facet arthritis ➡. Epidural phlegmon extends into the neural foramen ➡.*

Infection and Inflammatory Disorders

KEY FACTS

TERMINOLOGY

- Paraspinal phlegmon surrounding peripherally enhancing fluid collections

IMAGING

- **Pre**vertebral/**para**vertebral space
- Multiple or multiloculated collections along muscle plane
- NECT
  - Amorphous low-density intramuscular collection
  - Calcified psoas abscesses characteristic of tuberculous paraspinal abscess (PA)
  - Endplate destruction
- MR
  - Iso- to hypointense on T1WI
  - Hyperintense fluid collection and surrounding muscle on T2WI and STIR
  - Diffuse enhancement: Phlegmon
  - Peripherally enhancing fluid collection(s): Abscess

TOP DIFFERENTIAL DIAGNOSES

- Neoplasm, primary or metastatic
- Retroperitoneal hematoma
- Extramedullary hematopoiesis

PATHOLOGY

- Most common pathogens
  - *Staphylococcus aureus*
  - *Mycobacterium tuberculosis*
  - *Escherichia coli*

CLINICAL ISSUES

- Fever (50%) at presentation
- Back pain and tenderness
- ↑ ESR, ↑ WBC

DIAGNOSTIC CHECKLIST

- Peripherally enhancing collection in paravertebral soft tissue with associated spondylitis characteristic of PA

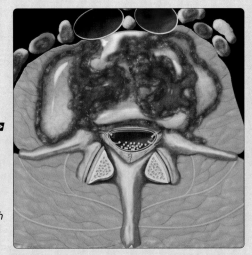

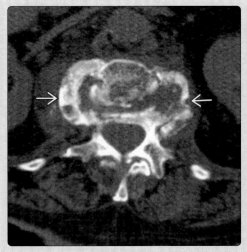

(Left) *Axial graphic through the lumbar disc space demonstrates an extensive abscess infiltrating bilateral psoas muscles and the epidural space. Abnormal retroperitoneal lymph nodes are also present.* **(Right)** *Axial NECT depicts bilateral calcified paraspinal masses ➡ in a patient with tuberculosis spondylodiscitis. The anterior aspect of the vertebral body adjacent to the subchondral plate is affected with spread to adjacent discs. Abscesses may descend down the sheath of the psoas and are typically calcified.*

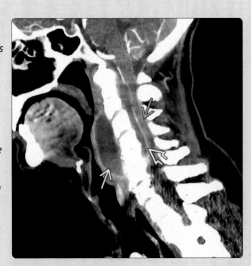

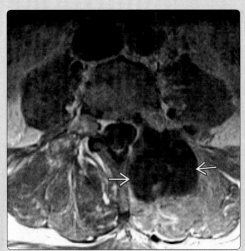

(Left) *Sagittal contrast-enhanced CT shows a large anterior paravertebral abscess ➡ with narrowing of the airway from adjacent disc space infection. Also note the large ventral epidural abscess ➡ with cord compression ➡.* **(Right)** *Axial T1WI C+ MR shows a peripherally enhancing collection ➡ in the left neural foramen operative site in this patient presenting with fever following resection a schwannoma.*

Epidural Abscess

TERMINOLOGY

- Spinal epidural abscess
- Extradural spinal infection with abscess formation

IMAGING

- Lower thoracic and lumbar > upper thoracic and cervical
- CT
  - Enhancing epidural mass narrowing central canal
- MR
  - T1WI: Iso- to hypointense to cord
  - T2WI/STIR: Hyperintense
  - T1WI C+: Homogeneously or heterogeneously enhancing **phlegmon**
  - Peripherally enhancing necrotic **abscess**
- Fat saturation: STIR, T2WI FS, T1WI C+ FS
  - Increases lesion conspicuity by suppressing signal from epidural fat and vertebral marrow
- Signal alteration in spinal cord secondary to compression, ischemia, or direct infection

- Persistent epidural enhancement without mass effect on follow-up MR imaging
  - Probable sterile granulation tissue or fibrosis
  - Correlate with ESR and CRP for disease activity

TOP DIFFERENTIAL DIAGNOSES

- Extradural metastasis
  - Often contiguous with vertebral lesion
- Epidural hematoma
  - ± mild peripheral enhancement

PATHOLOGY

- *Staphylococcus aureus* most common cause; *Mycobacterium tuberculosis* next most frequent

CLINICAL ISSUES

- Fever, acute or subacute spinal pain and tenderness
- Radiculopathy, paraparesis/paralysis, paresthesia, loss of bladder and bowel control

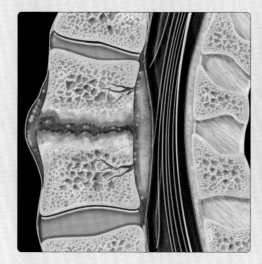

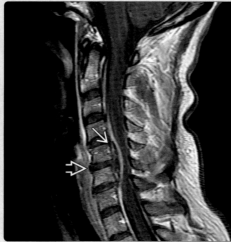

(Left) Sagittal graphic through the lumbar spine demonstrates vertebral osteomyelitis with an intervertebral abscess extending ventrally and dorsally and narrowing the central canal. (Right) Sagittal T1WI C+ MR in an intravenous drug abuser shows a large ventral epidural abscess collection ➡ with peripheral enhancement causing severe mass effect upon the cervical cord. There is relative preservation of the C5-6 endplates ➡ with no disc enhancement.

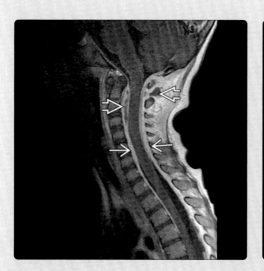

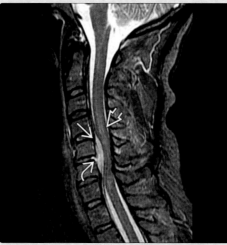

(Left) Sagittal T1 C+ MR shows abnormal circumferential epidural thickening and enhancement in this patient with meningitis complicated by epidural phlegmon ➡ and abscess ➡. (Right) Sagittal STIR MR shows a large ventral epidural abscess ➡ as T2 hyperintensity with severe mass effect upon the cord. Involvement of the posterior C5-6 disc is seen as linear hyperintensity ➡. There is cord hyperintensity in this patient ➡, who was quadriparetic.

KEY FACTS

TERMINOLOGY

- Infection of spinal cord with necrosis
- Very rare, typically associated with dermal sinus in children

IMAGING

- Irregular ring-enhancing mass within cord with appropriate clinical history of inflammation/infection
- Increased T2WI signal from abscess core and surrounding edema; cord expansion
- Capsule may show low signal as in brain abscess
- May show positive diffusion (reduced apparent diffusion coefficient) similar to brain abscess

TOP DIFFERENTIAL DIAGNOSES

- Hypervascular cord primary neoplasms
- Metastasis
- Acute transverse/viral myelitis
- Acute multiple sclerosis
- Cavernous malformation

PATHOLOGY

- 2 major etiologies
  - Adult intramedullary abscess either hematogenous seeding from cardiopulmonary source or idiopathic
  - Children often have congenital cause allowing direct extension of infection
    - Dermal sinus tract or spinal dysraphism

CLINICAL ISSUES

- Often presents with signs/symptoms of structural cord lesion rather than infection
- Mixed neurologic deficits including fever, pain, motor deficit, sensory disturbance, and sphincter dysfunction
- Mortality of 8% in antibiotic era (1977-1997)

DIAGNOSTIC CHECKLIST

- Brain MR to exclude concomitant brain abscess
- Serial WBC count, ESR, enhanced MR important for postoperative follow-up, detection of recurrence

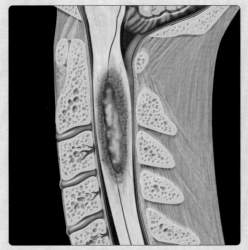
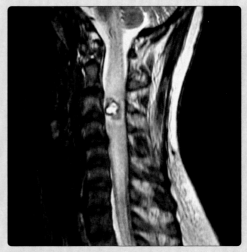

(Left) Sagittal graphic shows an irregular abscess cavity in the cervical cord with cord expansion and edema. (Right) Sagittal T2WI MR shows high signal intensity centrally with a dark rim, which is often seen in inflammatory lesions and extensive edema, tracking rostrally into the medulla and caudally into the thoracic spinal cord. This appearance is not specific for abscess and primary or secondary cord neoplasm would have to be considered as well.

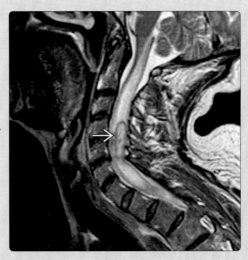
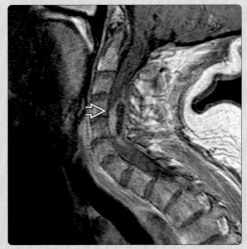

(Left) Sagittal T2WI MR in a patient with streptococcal endocarditis shows diffuse cord expansion with a ring-shaped area of low T2 signal (abscess capsule) within the cord from C4 to C5-6 ➡. (Right) Sagittal T1WI C+ MR in a patient with streptococcal endocarditis demonstrates the abscess capsule region shows ring enhancement ➡.

KEY FACTS

TERMINOLOGY

- Noncompressive myelopathy
- Etiologies include inflammatory causes [acute transverse myelitis (ATM)] + vascular disease + radiation + paraneoplastic + idiopathic (unknown)
  - ATM is broad generic term encompassing heterogeneous group of disorders causing cord dysfunction
    - Is more specific term for cord dysfunction that is inflammatory in etiology
    - Inflammation defined by CSF findings and MR enhancement

IMAGING

- Hyperintense lesion on T2WI with mild cord expansion ± enhancement
- Longitudinally extensive T2 signal abnormality = neuromyelitis optica, acute disseminated encephalomyelitis, viral infection

TOP DIFFERENTIAL DIAGNOSES

- Inflammatory etiologies
  - Acquired demyelinating
    - Multiple sclerosis
    - Neuromyelitis optica
    - Acute disseminated encephalomyelitis
  - Parainfectious
  - Systemic autoimmune
  - Paraneoplastic (antineuronal immune disorder associated with cancer)
- Noninflammatory mimics
  - Radiation
  - Metabolic
  - Tumor and cysts
  - Vascular
    - Cord infarction
    - Dural fistula (type I AVF)
- Idiopathic ATM

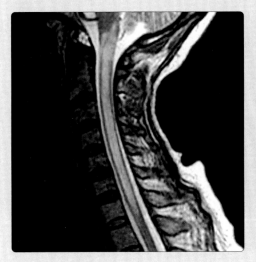
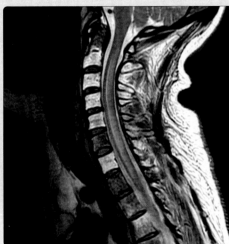

(Left) *Sagittal T2WI MR shows longitudinally extensive T2 hyperintensity throughout the cervical cord and lower medulla. Differential diagnoses include neuromyelitis optica, acute disseminated encephalomyelitis, and parainfectious and systemic autoimmune disorders.* (Right) *Sagittal T2 FS MR in this patient with multiple bone metastases and prior radiation therapy shows diffuse increased signal in the cord. Primary considerations would be radiation myelopathy vs. paraneoplastic myelopathy.*

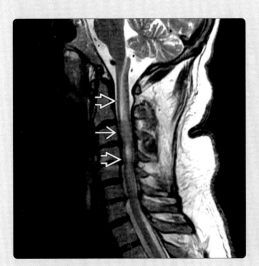
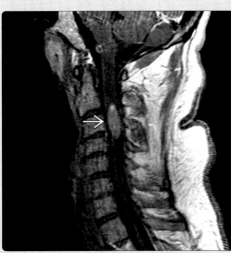

(Left) *Sagittal T2 TSE MR in this patient with lung cancer shows a focal mass at the C3 level ➡ with adjacent cord edema ⇒ from a focal cord parenchymal metastasis.* (Right) *Sagittal T1 C+ MR shows enhancement of focal cord metastasis ➡ in this patient with lung carcinoma and worsening myelopathy.*

KEY FACTS

TERMINOLOGY

- Primary demyelinating disease of CNS with multiple lesions disseminated over time and space
  - Concomitant intracranial lesions in periventricular, subcallosal, brain stem, or cerebellar white matter

IMAGING

- Isolated spinal cord disease (10-20%)
- Cervical segment is most commonly affected
  - Dorsolateral aspect of cord
  - < 1/2 of cross-sectional area of spinal cord
  - < 2 vertebral segments in length
- Sagittal and axial T1WI & T2WI sequences with gadolinium
  - Lesions typically oval, peripheral, and asymmetric
  - Discrete vs. vague hyperintense lesions
  - Enhancement lasts 1-2 months but does not reflect disease progression

TOP DIFFERENTIAL DIAGNOSES

- Intramedullary neoplasm
- Idiopathic transverse myelitis
- Neuromyelitis optica

PATHOLOGY

- Autoimmune, inflammatory process focused on CNS myelin

CLINICAL ISSUES

- Peak onset: 20-40 years
- Relapsing-remitting: Distinct periods of new or worsening symptoms alternating with complete or partial recovery
- Secondary progressive: From relapsing-remitting multiple sclerosis, worsening deficits
- Primary progressive: Steady progression of symptoms
- Progressive relapsing: Includes distinct periods of exacerbation but without recovery

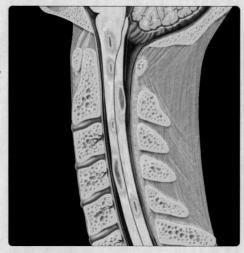
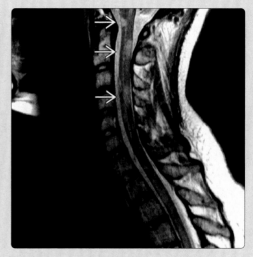

(Left) Sagittal graphic depicts multiple demyelinating plaques within the cervical spinal cord. (Right) Sagittal T2WI MR of the cervical spinal cord demonstrates multiple T2 hyperintense foci ➡, some well defined and others ill defined. The multiplicity of lesions & lack of edema or significant cord expansion is typical for demyelinating disease.

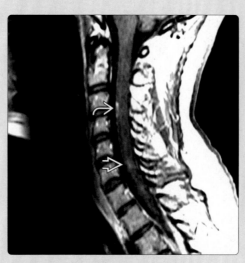
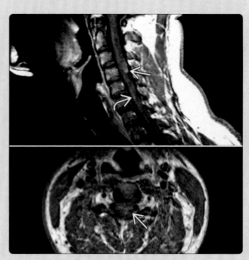

(Left) Sagittal T1WI C+ MR shows multiple enhancing demyelinating lesions within the cervical spinal cord. Enhancement varies from focal ➡ to ill defined ➡. The enhancement pattern changes with evolution of inflammation. (Right) T1WI C+ MR (sagittal on top, axial on bottom) images illustrate an incomplete rim-enhancing lesion ➡ in the dorsal cervical cord at the C3-4 level. A 2nd small enhancing focus is noted in the ventral cord at the C6 level ➡.

Neuromyelitis Optica

TERMINOLOGY

- Synonyms: Devic disease, optic-spinal multiple sclerosis
- Autoimmune inflammatory disorder involving myelin of neurons of optic nerves and spinal cord with limited brain parenchymal involvement

IMAGING

- Longitudinally extensive (> 3 vertebral segments) T2 hyperintensity within cord + enhancement of optic nerves (85% of cases)
- T2 abnormality tends to involve entire cross section of cord, unlike more focal involvement of multiple sclerosis

TOP DIFFERENTIAL DIAGNOSES

- Inflammatory etiologies
  - Multiple sclerosis
  - Acute disseminated encephalomyelitis (ADEM)
  - Parainfectious myelitis (viral, bacterial)
- Systemic autoimmune disease

- Noninflammatory mimics
  - Dural fistula
  - Tumor
- Idiopathic acute transverse myelitis

PATHOLOGY

- Autoimmune disease targeting water channel proteins (aquaporin-4)

CLINICAL ISSUES

- **Revised diagnostic criteria (2006)**
  - Optic neuritis, myelitis, and at least 2 of 3 supportive criteria
    - Contiguous cord lesion 3 or more segments in length, initial brain MR nondiagnostic for multiple sclerosis, or neuromyelitis optica (NMO)-IgG seropositivity

DIAGNOSTIC CHECKLIST

- Simultaneous optic neuritis and myelitis → NMO cannot be distinguished from ADEM at 1st attack

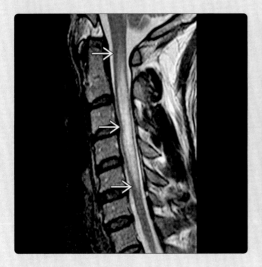
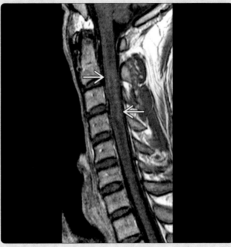

(Left) Sagittal T2WI MR shows a long segment of cord enlargement with T2 hyperintensity ➡. (Right) Sagittal T1WI C+ MR shows cord enlargement and ill-defined enhancement ➡. Neuromyelitis optica (NMO) is an autoimmune disease possibly targeting the aquaporin-4 transmembrane water channel. The vasculocentric distribution of NMO-IgG antigen correlates with the sites of immunoglobulin and complement deposition seen in spinal cord lesions of patients with NMO.

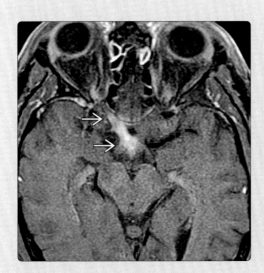
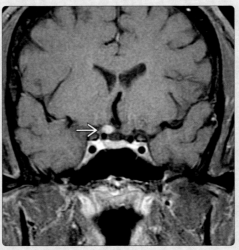

(Left) Axial T1WI C+ FS MR reveals intense enhancement and mild enlargement of the intracanalicular and prechiasmatic segments of the right optic nerve ➡. (Right) Coronal T1WI C+ FS MR reveals intense enhancement and mild enlargement of the intracanalicular and prechiasmatic segments of the right optic nerve ➡. This is the classic appearance of Devic disease involving the optic nerves and spinal cord with no brain parenchymal abnormalities.

KEY FACTS

TERMINOLOGY

- Para-/postinfectious immune-mediated inflammatory disorder of white matter
  - Antibodies to pathogens exhibit cross immunoreactivity with myelin basic protein

IMAGING

- Multifocal white matter lesions with relatively little mass effect or vasogenic edema
  - Flame-shaped lesions with slight cord swelling
  - Dorsal white matter more voluminous
  - May see gray matter involvement
  - Variable enhancement depending on stage of disease
  - May see nerve enhancement
- Brain almost always involved

TOP DIFFERENTIAL DIAGNOSES

- Inflammatory etiologies
  - Acquired demyelinating
    - Multiple sclerosis
    - Neuromyelitis optica
  - Parainfectious myelitis
  - Systemic autoimmune (vasculitis)
- Noninflammatory mimics
  - Vascular malformation
  - Infarction, spinal cord
  - Tumor and cysts
- Idiopathic acute transverse myelitis

CLINICAL ISSUES

- Typically monophasic illness lasting 2-4 weeks
  - Encephalopathy, paresis
- Typically in childhood or young adult

DIAGNOSTIC CHECKLIST

- Rescanning if initially negative
  - Typically delay between clinical onset and appearance of imaging findings

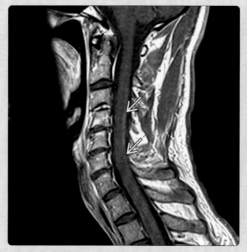

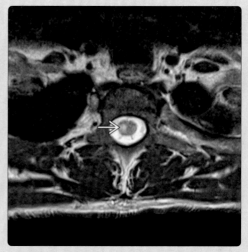

(Left) Sagittal T1WI C+ MR shows linear enhancement along the dorsal surface of the midcervical cord ➡. Acutely, there is perivenous edema, demyelination, and infiltration with macrophages and lymphocytes with relative axonal sparing. The late course of the disease is characterized by perivascular gliosis. (Right) Axial T2WI MR depicts a hyperintense focus in the right hemicord ➡ with minimal cord enlargement. ADEM is a postinfectious disease mediated by autoreactive cells or molecules.

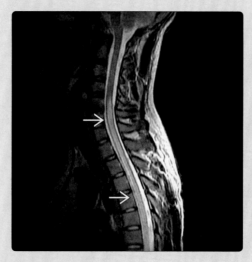

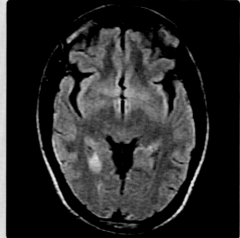

(Left) Sagittal T2 MR in this patient with postvaccination ADEM shows diffuse lower cervical and thoracic cord expansion and T2 hyperintensity ➡. (Right) Axial FLAIR MR shows focal demyelination involving right posterior temporal white matter in this patient with postvaccination demyelination.

Sarcoidosis

TERMINOLOGY

- Neurosarcoidosis
- Noncaseating granulomatous disease

IMAGING

- Intramedullary
  - Fusiform cord enlargement
  - Enhancing intramedullary masses
  - Focal or diffuse T2-hyperintense lesions
- Intradural extramedullary
  - Leptomeningeal enhancement
  - Dural masses
- Extradural
  - CT/radiographs: Sclerotic or mixed lytic and sclerotic lesions
- Combination of leptomeningeal and peripheral intramedullary mass-like enhancement suggestive of spinal sarcoidosis

TOP DIFFERENTIAL DIAGNOSES

- Intramedullary neoplasm
- Idiopathic transverse myelitis
- Lymphoma
- Intradural metastases
- Multiple sclerosis

CLINICAL ISSUES

- Clinical CNS involvement in patients with sarcoidosis (5%)
  - Spinal intramedullary sarcoidosis (< 1%)
- Lower extremity weakness, paresthesia
- Bladder and bowel dysfunction
- Protean imaging manifestations
  - Mimicking multiple spinal pathologies
  - Typically, systemic disease present; rarely, intramedullary sarcoid as initial presentation
- Treatment: Intravenous ± oral corticosteroids
  - Immunosuppressive therapy

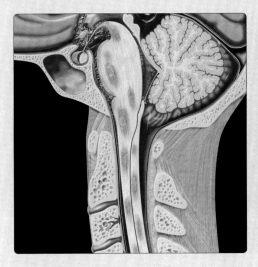

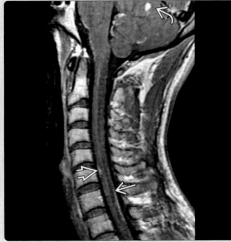

(Left) Graphic depicts multiple intramedullary sarcoid granulomas in brainstem & upper cervical cord. The intramedullary, intradural extramedullary, & extradural regions can be involved. Rare findings, such as calcifications & cyst formation, have also been described. (Right) Sagittal T1WI C+ MR demonstrates diffuse linear leptomeningeal enhancement ➡ with areas of nodularity ➡. There is intracranial involvement with sarcoidosis ➡. Bulky leptomeningeal disease is unusual with neurosarcoidosis.

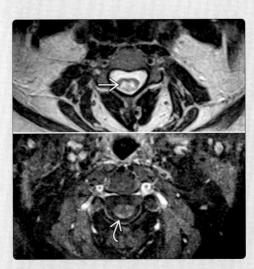

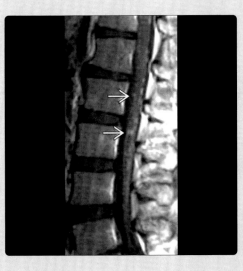

(Left) Axial T2WI MR (top) shows intramedullary hyperintensity ➡. Axial T2WI MR (bottom) reveals irregular leptomeningeal enhancement along the cord ➡. (Right) Sagittal T1WI C+ MR exhibits multiple enhancing subarachnoid nodules interspersed among the cauda equina ➡. Intradural extramedullary lesions are usually represented by leptomeningeal sarcoidosis infiltration, present in up to 60% of spinal cord lesions.

KEY FACTS

TERMINOLOGY

- Atlantoaxial rotary subluxation accompanying respiratory infection or otolaryngologic surgery

IMAGING

- Fixed, rotated head occurring in child soon after upper respiratory infection or otolaryngologic surgery
- Difficult to obtain adequate films 2° to head position
- Open-mouth odontoid: Asymmetric C1 lateral masses
  - Anteriorly rotated side wider and closer to odontoid
  - Opposite side smaller and farther from odontoid
- Lateral view: ± widened atlantodental interval
- Dynamic CT: Should include occiput C1-C2
  - Initial scan: Maintain position of comfort
  - 2nd scan: Rotate head to contralateral side
  - Interpretation: C1-C2 relationship fixed or C1 unable to rotate past neutral to contralateral side
- MR may replace CT to eliminate radiation dose

TOP DIFFERENTIAL DIAGNOSES

- Torticollis
  - Resolves within few days to weeks
- Septic C1-C2 joint

PATHOLOGY

- Multiple theories: Common theme tracking of inflammatory mediators from upper airway

CLINICAL ISSUES

- Pain, head tilt, restricted neck movement
- Cock-robin position: Head rotated and tilted to 1 side with chin lifted to opposite side
- Associated with otitis media, pharyngitis, retropharyngeal abscess, upper respiratory infection, otolaryngologic surgery
- 68% < 12 years old; 90% < 21 years old
- Leads to permanently fixed deformity if left untreated
- Reduction and immobilization are key

(Left) Lateral radiograph shows typical retropharyngeal effusion due to strep pharyngitis ➡. Grisel syndrome may occur with any stage of infection, from effusion to extensive abscess. (Right) Axial CECT shows retropharyngeal space abscess ➡ due to left palatine tonsillitis ➡. Although the C1-C2 articulation is not affected, one can appreciate how easily inflammatory changes can track to that articulation.

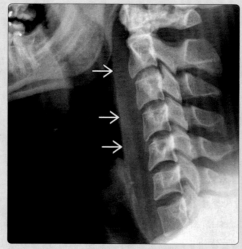
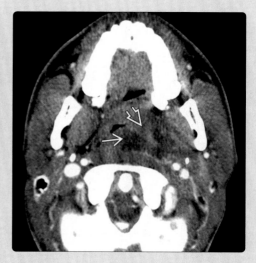

(Left) Sagittal STIR MR in a florid case of craniovertebral junction bacterial infection shows marked increased signal involving prevertebral space ➡, odontoid, and loss of anterior C1 arch margin. This is to be contrasted with the less aggressive appearance of Grisel syndrome. (Right) Axial T1 C+ MR shows infection involving the craniovertebral junction with multiple small abscesses within the posterior nasopharyngeal tissue ➡. Note the close anatomic relationship, which would allow for C1-C2 joint involvement.

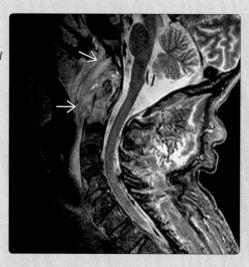
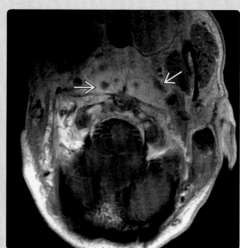

IgG4-Related Disease/Hypertrophic Pachymeningitis

KEY FACTS

TERMINOLOGY

- Idiopathic hypertrophic pachymeningitis
- IgG4-related hypertrophic pachymeningitis (IgG4-RHP)
- Multiorgan immune-mediated condition, which mimics multiple malignant, infectious, and inflammatory disorders
  - Chronic progressive diffuse inflammatory fibrosis of dura of brain or spine

IMAGING

- Linear low-signal mass involving dura with variable mass effect upon cord
- Low-signal linear mass effacing CSF and cord
- Peripheral enhancement related to peripheral zone of active inflammation vs. chronic central fibrosis

TOP DIFFERENTIAL DIAGNOSES

- Meningioma
- Lymphoma
- Tuberculosis

- Sarcoidosis
- Dural metastases
- Venous engorgement (CSF leak)

PATHOLOGY

- Autoreactive IgG4 antibodies observed in IgG4-related disease
  - No evidence they are directly pathogenic
- Central pathology features
  - Lymphoplasmacytic infiltration
  - Obliterative phlebitis
  - Storiform fibrosis
  - Mild to moderate tissue eosinophilia

CLINICAL ISSUES

- Spinal presentation as mass with myelopathy or radiculopathy
- Histopathology remains cornerstone of diagnosis

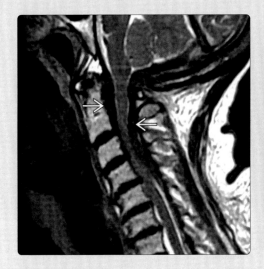

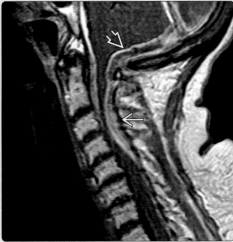

(Left) *Sagittal T2WI MR shows extensive low signal intensity thickening of the dura involving the posterior fossa and extending to involve the upper cervical dura to the C4 level ➡. There is severe cord compression with loss of normal CSF signal from the C1-3 level.* (Right) *Sagittal T1WI C+ MR shows diffuse enhancement of dural thickening of the posterior fossa and upper cervical dura. Note the variable enhancement with areas that homogeneously enhance ➡ and other areas with more peripheral enhancement ⇛.*

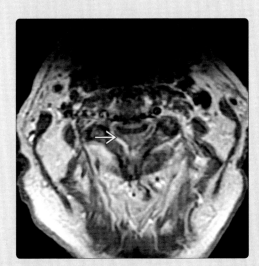

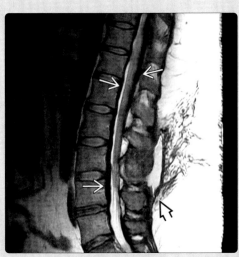

(Left) *Axial T1WI C+ MR shows diffuse enhancement of the markedly thickened dura circumferentially surrounding the cord ➡.* (Right) *Sagittal T2WI MR shows extensive linear low signal ➡ involving the dura throughout both the ventral and dorsal aspects of the lumbar spine. This patient has undergone dural biopsy ➡.*

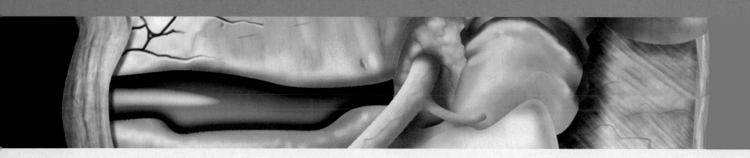

SECTION 8
Neoplasms, Cysts, and Other Masses

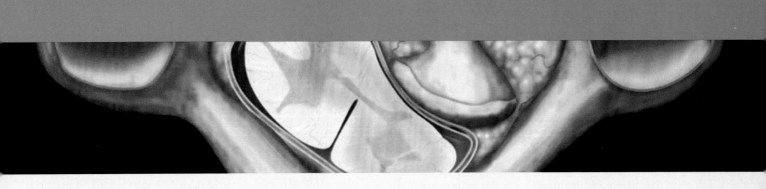

Nonneoplastic Cysts and Tumor Mimics

Anatomy-Based Imaging Issues

Neoplasms affecting the spine may spread by direct extension via the lymphatic system, the hematogenous route, or along the cerebrospinal fluid pathways. There can also be combinations of these pathways involved with the most typical being hematogenous metastatic dissemination to vertebral bodies with subsequent direct extension into the epidural space.

Primary tumors located in soft tissues may extend into the vertebral column by direct extension. An example would include lung carcinoma extending into the chest wall and subsequently the paravertebral region and into the spinal column and epidural space. Prostate, bladder, or bowel carcinoma may extend into the presacral space and subsequently into the vertebral column and epidural space. Nasopharyngeal carcinoma extends into the clivus and skull base and may track along the cranial nerves. In rare cases, there may be direct extension of a CNS tumor along the biopsy or surgical tract. There are also rare cases of CNS tumors extending through access via indwelling shunt tubing to give systemic metastases. Findings of direct extension of a neoplasm in the spine consist of a soft tissue mass with adjacent bone destruction and variable neural compromise. Direct extension of a neoplasm into the epidural space is more likely from the vertebral body through the posterior longitudinal ligament. The anterior longitudinal ligament and disc are relatively resistant to tumor invasion. The anterior longitudinal ligament is stronger than the posterior longitudinal ligament and has fewer perforating vessels. Once the tumor has access into the epidural space, it comes against the tough dura, which is an effective barrier to tumor penetration. These barriers result in the distinguishing features between a disc space infection with adjacent vertebral osteomyelitis (with the epicenter at the level of the disc space) and neoplastic involvement (with the epicenter involving the vertebral bodies with sparing of the disc space). Direct extension of tumor may also be seen with a primary cord tumor within the cervical spine, with extension into the infratentorial space. Rarely, brainstem or cerebellar neoplasms may extend into the upper cervical cord.

Lymphatic spread is of limited importance in spine imaging relative to the more ubiquitous hematogenous spread. Local spread of pelvic tumors within the lumbar spine without pulmonary metastases would suggest a venous or lymphatic route of extension.

Hematogenous spread is the major pathway of extension of malignant tumors to the axial skeleton. The Batson plexus is a longitudinal network of valveless veins running parallel to the spinal column. These veins lie outside of the thoracoabdominal cavity and communicate with multiple aspects of the venous system, including the vena cava, spinal, portal, azygos, intercostal, pulmonary, and renal veins. Flow direction in the Batson plexus is variable due to the variable intrathoracic and intraabdominal pressures. Tumors in multiple anatomic sites could cause metastatic lesions along the course of the venous plexus without lung or liver involvement. Prostate carcinoma cells could seed vertebral bodies via the Batson plexus and not necessarily extend into the vena cava. Breast carcinoma might also seed the vertebral bodies via the azygos system into the Batson plexus. There is only 5-10% of portal blood flow that might shunt to the Batson plexus, explaining the relatively low frequency of spinal metastatic lesions with GI and GU primaries. For the vast majority of spinal metastases, there may be no clear answer to the precise route to the end target. Homing properties of the tumor cells and receptive properties of the implantation site may be more important than any particular vascular route.

Spread along the CSF pathways is an important route for primary intracranial tumors. Tumor emboli gain access to the CSF via fragmentation, as well as being shed during surgical manipulation. CNS tumor types showing subarachnoid spread include medulloblastoma, ependymoma, pineal tumors, astrocytoma, lymphoma and leukemia, choroid plexus carcinoma, and retinoblastoma (poor prognosis with MYCN gene amplification). Spread along the CSF pathways can also occur following initial hematogenous dissemination of tumor. For example, this pattern of spread would be present in cord and leptomeningeal metastatic disease following the initial hematogenous dissemination in lung and breast metastatic disease.

Pathologic Issues

Forty percent of patients with cancer will develop visceral or bony metastases during their illness. The spinal column is the most common site of osseous metastases. Men are more frequently affected with vertebral metastases, with a male to female ratio of 3:2. Prostate, lung, and breast carcinomas account for the vast majority of spinal metastases. Locations are primarily thoracic (70%) > lumbar (20%) > cervical.

Primary tumors are generally composed of a variety of biologically different cells in regard to ultimate metastatic potential. Cells continually shed from the primary tumor and gain access to the circulatory system. Less than 0.01-0.1% of tumor cells survive to reach a distant site. Successful tumor spread requires completion of a complex pathway, including tumor separation from the primary source, access to blood, CSF or lymphatic system, survival within the transport process, attachment to the endothelium of a distant vessel as well as exiting that vessel into the interstitial space, and finally developing the vascular supply at a distant site. The distant host environment site is a complex milieu. Multiple anatomic pathways may be involved with varying flow patterns within the veins and arteries.

Mechanisms of Tumorigenesis

Tumorigenesis in humans appears to be a multistep process. These steps reflect genetic alterations that drive progressive transformation of normal human cells into highly malignant versions. Cancers in humans have been shown to have an age-dependent incidence, which implicates 4-7 rate limiting, stochastic events. Tumor development proceeds via a succession of genetic changes, each conferring one or another type of growth advantage, which leads to the progressive conversion of normal human cells into cancer cells. By definition, cancer cells will have defects in regulatory circuits that govern cell proliferation and homeostasis. These defects have been categorized into 6 types of alterations in cell physiology: (1) Self-sufficiency in growth signals, (2) insensitivity to growth inhibitory signals, (3) evasion of programmed cell death (apoptosis), (4) limitless replicative potential, (5) sustained angiogenesis, and (6) tissue invasion and metastasis. Each of these 6 physiologic changes reflects the successful breaching of an anticancer defense mechanism that is hardwired into cells and tissues.

Normal cells require growth signals before they can move into an active proliferative state. The signals are transmitted to the cell via transmembrane receptors that bind a variety of signaling molecules, such as diffusible growth factors, extracellular matrix components, and cell-to-cell adhesion molecules (CAMs). Many cancer cells acquire the ability to synthesize growth factors to which they are responsive, which creates an abnormal positive feedback loop. Examples would be the production of platelet-derived growth factor (PDGF) by glioblastoma and tumor growth factor alpha (TGF) by sarcomas. Epidermal growth factor receptor (EGF-R) is upregulated in brain tumors.

Normal tissues have a variety of mechanisms that limit proliferation. Signals include both growth inhibitors and inhibitors within the extracellular matrix on the surface of adjacent cells. Many antiproliferative signals are channeled through the retinoblastoma tumor suppressor protein (pRb) and its variations. Disruption of the retinoblastoma protein pathway will allow cell proliferation by rendering the cells insensitive to antigrowth factors by repressing the E2F transcription factors.

Evasion of programmed cell death (apoptosis) commonly occurs through mutations involving the *p53* tumor suppressor gene. The inactivation of this *p53* protein is seen in over 50% of human cancers.

The limitless replicative potential of cancer tumors is seen in cultures of tumor cells that have become immortalized. Normal human cell types in culture have a capacity for no more than 60-70 doublings. The ends of the chromosomes appear to be involved in this process, which are called the telomeres. The erosion of the telomeres occurs through successive cycles of normal cell replication causing them to lose their ability to protect the ends of the chromosome DNA. This leads to eventual cell crisis and cell death. In contrast, telomere maintenance is evident in all types of malignant cells. In cancer, telomeres are maintained at a length above some critical threshold, which allows unlimited cell multiplication.

Abnormal angiogenesis is perhaps one of the more recognized aspects of abnormal cell physiology in cancer. Angiogenesis promoting signals are classically seen with vascular endothelial growth factor (VEGF) and fibroblast growth factors (FGF). More than 2 dozen angiogenic-inducing factors are known, with a similar number of inhibiting-type proteins.

Metastatic Disease and Cell Motion

Tumor metastases are the cause of 90% of human cancer deaths. Tumor invasion and tumor metastases are very complex processes, with multiple genetic and biochemical factors. These can be described as tumor invasion, tumor cell dissemination through the blood stream or lymphatic system, colonization of distant organs, and outgrowth of the metastasis. Several classes of proteins are involved in tethering cells to their surroundings and are altered in invasion and metastases. CAMs and integrins are involved in this cell-to-cell regulatory signaling. The basement membrane is the 1st barrier tumor cells must breech. Receptors on the surface of cells recognize the glycoprotein of the basement membrane to which they attach. Attachment is followed by proteolysis of type IV collagen of the basement membrane by tumor-specific collagenase. Locomotion follows basement membrane lysis, with cells crossing that defective basement membrane with access to the interstitial space, lymphatics, and blood vessels. Chemoattractants can activate cell migration and invasion through activation of specific

receptors and downstream intracellular signaling pathways. This appears to ultimately reorganize the actin cytoskeleton. Rho/Rac GTPases are well-known regulators of cytoskeletal organization. Rac activation induces membrane ruffles, adhesion complexes, and lamellipodia formation.

Tumor dissemination and cell motility occurs along 3 different pathways, including epithelial-to-mesenchymal transition (EMT), amoeboid transcription, and collective migration. In EMT, the cell elongates and degrades the local matrix by enzymes and migrates with pseudopodia-like projections. In amoeboid transcription the cells become spherical and pass through gaps in the extracellular matrix. In collective migration, sheets or clusters of tumor cells migrate. EMT includes the downregulation of epithelial markers in tight junctions and cytokeratin filament network and upregulation of mesenchymal markers, like N-cadherin, vimentin, integrins, tenascin C, and fibronectin, fibroblast- specific protein 1. N-cadherin seems to be the most important of this group of markers. EMT can be controlled by intrinsic oncogenic activation like *KRAS* mutation or Her2 overexpression. In some cancers, such as lung, the central role of EMT regulator belongs to TGFβ. TGFβ ultimately promotes EMT by regulating genes that control cell proliferation, apoptosis, differentiation, motility and migration.

Clinical Implications

Spine metastatic involvement presents with unrelenting back pain. Objective signs are uncommon, or occur late in the disease (such as palpable mass and deformity). Back pain and weakness is a sign of epidural tumor extension. Due to spinothalamic tract crossing pattern, sensory levels may be 1-2 segments below the site of compression. Sensory abnormalities are an uncommon presenting sign of metastatic disease in the spine.

Selected References

1. Balic M et al: Circulating tumor cells: from bench to bedside. Annu Rev Med. 64:31-44, 2013
2. Perlikos F et al: Key molecular mechanisms in lung cancer invasion and metastasis: a comprehensive review. Crit Rev Oncol Hematol. 87(1):1-11, 2013
3. Ianari A et al: Cell death or survival: The complex choice of the retinoblastoma tumor suppressor protein. Cell Cycle. 9(1):23-4, 2010
4. Chen HZ et al: Emerging roles of E2Fs in cancer: an exit from cell cycle control. Nat Rev Cancer. 9(11):785-97, 2009
5. Fiorentino FP et al: Senescence and p130/Rbl2: a new beginning to the end. Cell Res. 19(9):1044-51, 2009
6. Mazel C et al: Cervical and thoracic spine tumor management: surgical indications, techniques, and outcomes. Orthop Clin North Am. 40(1):75-92, vi-vii, 2009
7. Sciubba DM et al: Solitary vertebral metastasis. Orthop Clin North Am. 40(1):145-54, viii, 2009
8. Fokas E et al: Metastasis: the seed and soil theory gains identity. Cancer Metastasis Rev. 26(3-4):705-15, 2007
9. Guillevin R et al: Spine metastasis imaging: review of the literature. J Neuroradiol. 34(5):311-21, 2007
10. Christofori G: New signals from the invasive front. Nature. 441(7092):444-50, 2006
11. Demopoulos A: Leptomeningeal metastases. Curr Neurol Neurosci Rep. 4(3):196-204, 2004
12. Batson OV: The function of the vertebral veins and their role in the spread of metastases. Ann Surg. 112(1):138-49, 1940

(Left) *Axial graphic shows a hematogenously disseminated lytic metastatic lesion to the thoracic vertebral body and pedicle with subsequent direct epidural tumor extension and cord compression.* **(Right)** *Axial T1WI C+ MR shows a large, hematogenously disseminated metastatic paravertebral mass lesion involving thoracic body with direct tumor extension to the posterior elements, chest wall, and epidural space with cord compression ⮞.*

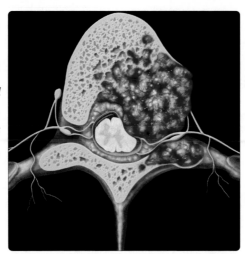
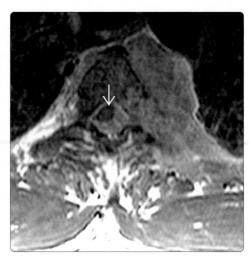

(Left) *AP bone scan in a case of extensive blastic prostate carcinoma shows multiple foci of increased radiotracer uptake that is consistent with diffuse bone metastasis.* **(Right)** *Sagittal T1WI C+ MR in a patient with extensive blastic prostate carcinoma shows diffuse abnormal decreased signal from all vertebral bodies and posterior elements with multiple foci of ventral epidural tumor extension ⮞ causing mild cord compression.*

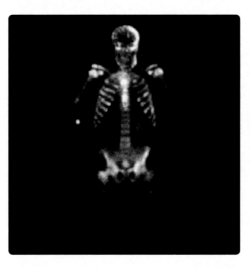
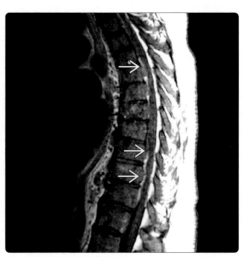

(Left) *Sagittal T2WI MR in a patient with multiple myeloma shows 2 levels of bony tumor involvement and slight spinous process expansion. There is severe cord compression at both levels.* **(Right)** *Sagittal T1 C+ FS MR of multiple myeloma shows 2 levels of focal tumor involvement with enhancement and slight spinous process expansion. Cord compression is present at both levels.*

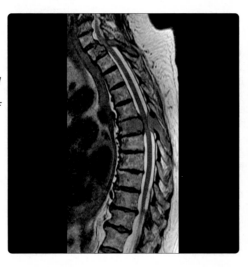
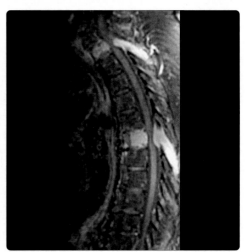

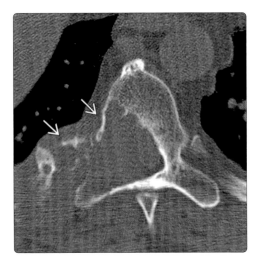

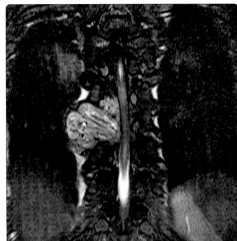

(Left) *Axial NECT in a patient with renal cell metastasis shows a mass destroying the right side of T7-T8 bodies, extending into posterior elements and crossing to involve right ribs and costovertebral joint. There is bony expansion with a thin rim soap bubble pattern* ➡. **(Right)** *Coronal T2WI FS MR in a patient with renal cell metastasis shows a mass involving the ribs and right side of T7-T8 bodies with epidural extension and cord compression. Multiple flow voids are present within the mass.*

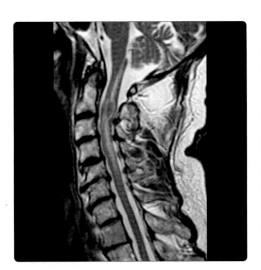

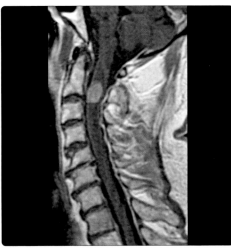

(Left) *Unenhanced T2WI MR in a patient with a large cervical cord metastatic lesion from lung carcinoma shows diffuse cord edema from the cervicomedullary junction inferiorly to C5. More focal signal abnormality is present at the C2-C3 level.* **(Right)** *Sagittal T1WI C+ MR in a patient with large cervical cord metastatic lesion from lung carcinoma via hematogenous dissemination shows enhancement of a large intramedullary metastatic lesion at the C2-C3 level.*

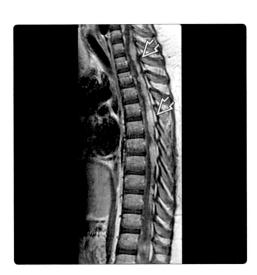

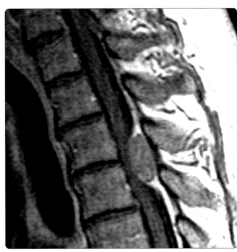

(Left) *Sagittal T1 C+ MR in a patient with extensive nodular leptomeningeal metastatic disease from high-grade brain oligodendroglioma shows a massive nodular-enhancing leptomeningeal tumor following contrast administration* ➡. *This child had rapid onset of flaccid paraplegia suggesting cord infarction from tumor compression.* **(Right)** *Sagittal T1 C+ MR shows a focal epidural mass with cord compression from metastatic melanoma. The route of dissemination is presumed hematogenous.*

KEY FACTS

TERMINOLOGY

- Extension of primary tumor to spine where bone production exceeds bone destruction

IMAGING

- Multiple osteoblastic lesions in spine
  - May coexist with areas of osteolytic tumor, soft tissue mass
- MR signal typically diminished on T1, T2WI in areas of osteoblastic metastases
- Sclerotic metastases usually tracer avid on bone scan

TOP DIFFERENTIAL DIAGNOSES

- Treated metastases
- Discogenic sclerosis
- Hemangioma
- Paget disease
- Osteosarcoma

PATHOLOGY

- Marrow infiltration, tumor stimulates osteoblastic response
  - New bone deposition on trabeculae, within intertrabecular spaces
- Primary tumor, adults: Prostate, breast, carcinoid, lung, GI, bladder, nasopharynx, pancreas
- Primary tumor, children: Medulloblastoma, neuroblastoma

CLINICAL ISSUES

- Pain: Progressive axial, referred, or radicular
- Epidural tumor, if present, may cause neurologic dysfunction
- 90% of prostate metastases involve spine, with lumbar 3x more often than cervical

DIAGNOSTIC CHECKLIST

- Defining response to therapy difficult since osteolytic conversion (tumor progression) and fading (good response) may look identical

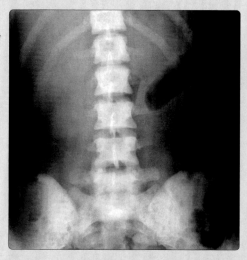
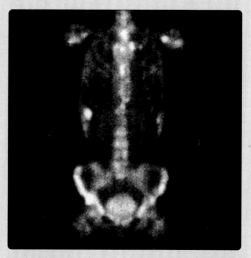

(Left) *Anteroposterior plain film shows diffuse extensive bone sclerosis of the spine and pelvis due to diffuse osseous metastases from breast carcinoma.* (Right) *Anteroposterior bone scan shows diffuse, patchy tracer uptake in the thoracolumbar spine, pelvis, sternum, and multiple ribs due to diffuse osseous metastases from breast carcinoma.*

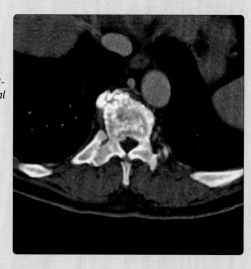
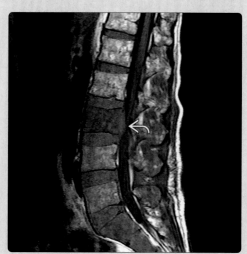

(Left) *Axial NECT through the lower thoracic spine shows patchy sclerosis of the vertebral body due to blastic metastases from prostate carcinoma.* (Right) *Sagittal T1-weighted MR shows low signal involving the L3 body and sacrum, reflecting diffuse metastatic disease. Extraosseous extension into the epidural space is seen at L3 ⤹. There is no specific signal change on the MR to define the blastic nature of these metastatic lesions.*

Lytic Osseous Metastases

KEY FACTS

TERMINOLOGY

- Spread of primary tumor to spine where bone destruction exceeds bone production

IMAGING

- Multiple osteolytic lesions in spine
- Compression fracture with bowing of posterior cortex, osteolysis extending into neural arch, extraosseous soft tissue
- Lesion distribution proportional to red marrow (lumbar > thoracic > cervical)
- Radiography requires 50-70% bone destruction and tumor size > 1 cm for detection
- Bone scan can give false-negatives with aggressively lytic tumor or with very small lesions

TOP DIFFERENTIAL DIAGNOSES

- Hematopoietic malignancy
- Benign (osteoporotic) compression fracture

- Schmorl node
- Normal heterogeneous marrow
- Spondylodiscitis

PATHOLOGY

- Spine is most common site of osseous metastases
- Common primaries causing osteolytic metastases
  - Renal, lung, breast, thyroid, GI tract, urothelial, ovarian, melanoma, chordoma, paraganglioma

CLINICAL ISSUES

- Pain: Progressive axial, referred, or radicular
- Epidural tumor extension may cause neurologic dysfunction
- Compression fracture
- Cord compression in 5% of adults with systemic cancers (70% solitary, 30% multiple sites)
- Spine metastases found in 5-10% of cancer patients

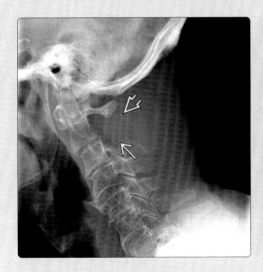

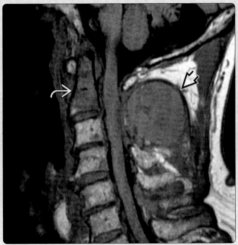

(Left) Lateral radiograph shows osteolysis of the C2 neural arch ⤳ and superior margin of the C3 arch ➡. (Right) Sagittal T1WI MR in the same patient shows a large soft tissue mass replacing the C2 arch ➡. There is also replacement of marrow in the C2 body and dens ➡. Subsequent work-up disclosed non-small cell lung carcinoma in the right upper lobe.

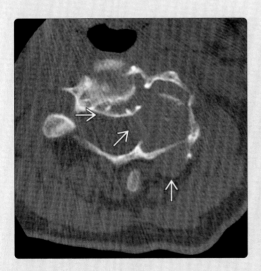

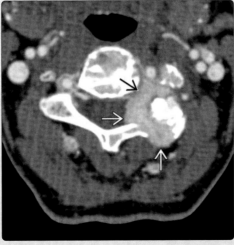

(Left) Axial NECT shows large thyroid carcinoma metastasis to the vertebral body and left facet/lamina of C3. There is a thin rim of expanded bone partially surrounding the lesion. The extraosseous soft tissue mass is not clearly seen ➡. (Right) Axial contrast-enhanced CT shows enhancement of the mass ➡ that is typical of hypervascular tumors like thyroid carcinoma. The medial margin of the mass is in the spinal canal, effacing the thecal sac and contacting the cervical cord. There is extension into the foramen ➡.

KEY FACTS

TERMINOLOGY

- Common benign venous malformation within vertebrae
- Usually intraosseous, may have epidural component
- Typically incidental lesion identified on imaging performed for unrelated reasons

IMAGING

- CT: Well-circumscribed, hypodense lesion with coarse vertical trabeculae (white polka dot appearance on axial CT)
- MR: Circumscribed lesion, hyperintense on both T1 and T2WI with hypointense vertical striations
  - Atypical hemangiomas may have reduced T1 signal due to paucity of fat
- Often multiple (20-30%)

PATHOLOGY

- 11% of adult population
- Complications in < 1%
  - Pathologic compression fracture

- Epidural hemangioma component with cord compression
- Histology
  - Thin-walled sinusoidal channels lined by vascular endothelium
  - Interspersed bony trabeculae with fat
- Majority confined to vertebral body proper
  - Uncommon in posterior elements/pedicles (10-15%)

CLINICAL ISSUES

- Bone CT may supplement MR evaluation in atypical hemangioma to look for typical osseous findings
- No follow-up typically necessary with pathognomonic imaging with small lesions and no extraosseous extension
- Aggressive hemangiomas
  - Vertebroplasty in conjunction with embolization may be considered if concern for pathologic fracture
  - Surgical resection (corpectomy) or radiation therapy

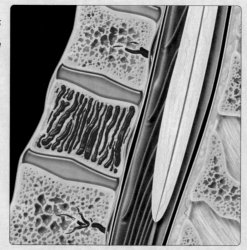
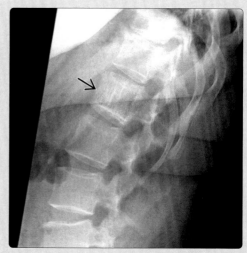

(Left) Sagittal graphic of the thoracolumbar junction shows the typical striated pattern of a hemangioma with thickened bony trabeculae. There is neither extraosseous extension nor thecal sac compromise. (Right) Lateral radiograph shows vertical striations within the L1 vertebral body ➡, the so-called "corduroy vertebra," due to vertebral hemangioma.

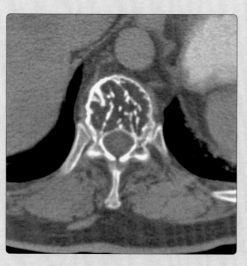
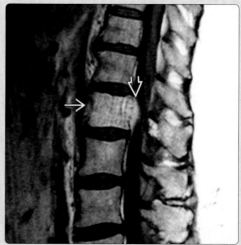

(Left) Axial CECT shows fatty attenuation within the lower thoracic vertebral body with multiple punctate thickened trabeculae. (Right) Sagittal T1 C+ MR shows prominent vertical striations within the vertebral body consistent with a hemangioma ➡. There is extraosseous extension of the tumor into the ventral epidural space ➡.

Osteoid Osteoma

KEY FACTS

TERMINOLOGY

- Benign osteoid-producing tumor < 1.5 cm in size
- Tumor often called nidus to distinguish it from surrounding reactive zone due to host response

IMAGING

- 10% occur in spine, in neural arch
- Focal scoliosis, concave on side of tumor
- Central nidus
  - Variable amount of ossification
- Reactive zone
  - Dense sclerosis, edema around nidus
  - Involves much larger area than tumor
  - Periosteal reaction variably present
  - Soft tissue mass or pleural thickening/effusion
  - Low signal on T1WI, high signal on T2WI, STIR
  - Enhances with gadolinium, iodinated contrast

TOP DIFFERENTIAL DIAGNOSES

- Osteoblastoma
- Stress fracture of pedicle or lamina
- Unilateral spondylolysis
- Unilateral absent pedicle or pars interarticularis
- Sclerotic metastasis
- Lymphoma
- Osteomyelitis
- Ewing sarcoma

CLINICAL ISSUES

- Night pain relieved by aspirin, NSAIDs
- 70% have scoliosis related to muscle spasm, concave on side of tumor

DIAGNOSTIC CHECKLIST

- Thin-section CT most accurate in visualizing nidus
- Edema on MR mimics infection, malignancy

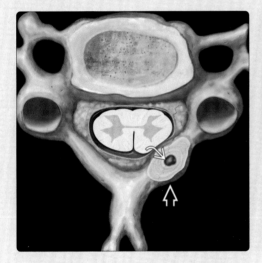

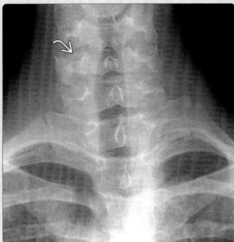

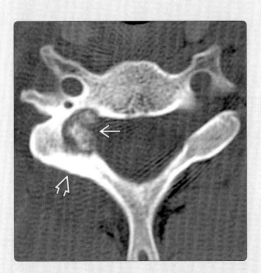

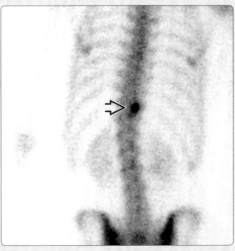

(Left) Axial graphic shows a small, highly vascular tumor nidus ➡ of osteoid osteoma in the left lamina, surrounded by dense reactive bone ➡. (Right) Anteroposterior radiograph shows focal, short-curve levoscoliosis in a young man with neck pain and no trauma history. Painful scoliosis raises concern for a tumor or infection. Sclerosis ➡ at C6 on the right suggested a possible diagnosis of osteoid osteoma.

(Left) Axial bone CT in the same patient shows a sclerotic C6 osteoid osteoma nidus ➡. Nidus may range from purely radiolucent to completely sclerotic. The lesion is sharply demarcated and surrounded by reactive sclerosis ➡. The lesion was missed on a prior routine cervical spine MR. (Right) Posteroanterior bone scan (3-hour image) shows scoliosis and intense, focal uptake on the right at a T11 osteoid osteoma ➡. Scoliosis due to osteoid osteoma is always concave on the side of the tumor.

Neoplasms, Cysts, and Other Masses

TERMINOLOGY

- Benign tumor that forms osteoid
- Differentiated grossly from osteoid osteoma by larger size (> 1.5 cm)

IMAGING

- 40% of osteoblastomas occur in spine
- Well-circumscribed, expansile lesion of neural arch
  - Frequent extension into vertebral body
  - Narrow zone of transition, sclerotic rim
- Periosteal inflammatory response of adjacent ribs, pleural thickening, effusion
- Peritumoral edema (flare phenomenon)
  - On MR, edema enhances, obscures tumor margins, and mimics malignancy

TOP DIFFERENTIAL DIAGNOSES

- Osteoid osteoma
- Aneurysmal bone cyst
- Metastasis
- Osteogenic sarcoma
- Chordoma
- Infection

PATHOLOGY

- Tumor prostaglandins release causes extensive peritumoral edema

CLINICAL ISSUES

- 90% in 2nd-3rd decades of life
- Dull, localized pain
- Painful scoliosis
- Neurologic symptoms due to compression of cord, nerve roots

DIAGNOSTIC CHECKLIST

- May be occult on radiographs; consider MR in young patients with painful scoliosis

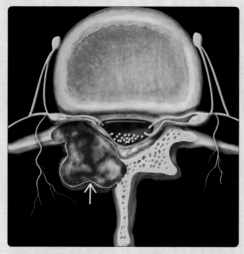
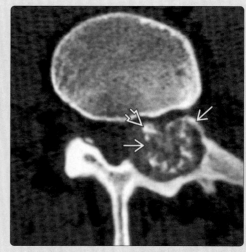

(Left) Axial graphic shows expansile, highly vascular osteoblastoma (OB) ➡ arising in the right lamina and impinging on the exiting nerve root. (Right) Axial bone CT in the same patient shows an expansile mass ➡ containing thin, irregular bone trabeculae ➡ that is characteristic of OB. Although cortical breakthrough is present, the zone of transition to adjacent bone is narrow and sclerotic.

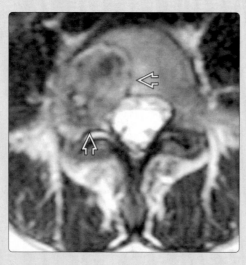
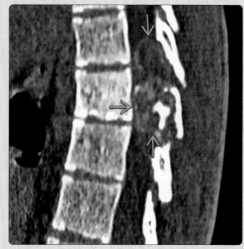

(Left) Axial T2WI MR shows an osteoblastoma ➡ of L5 with characteristic heterogeneous signal intensity. The bony matrix is low signal. There is edema in the adjacent vertebral body. (Right) Sagittal bone CT shows expansile lower thoracic OB ➡ extending from the lamina into the spinal canal. The lesion is sharply circumscribed and bilobed, involving 2 adjacent levels.

Aneurysmal Bone Cyst

KEY FACTS

IMAGING

- 10-30% of aneurysmal bone cysts (ABCs) occur in spine and sacrum
- Centered in neural arch, extends into vertebral body
- Balloon-like expansile remodeling of bone
  - Thinned, "eggshell" cortex
  - Focal cortical destruction common
- Absent pedicle sign: Expansion of pedicle results in loss of pedicle contour on AP radiographs
- Contains multiple round cysts with fluid-fluid levels
  - Caused by hemorrhage, blood product sedimentation
- Blood-filled cysts separated by septa of varying thickness
  - Periphery and septa enhance
  - Solid ABC variant enhances diffusely
- Calcified tumor matrix absent
- Narrow, nonsclerotic zone of transition with adjacent bone
- CT best to differentiate from telangiectatic osteogenic sarcoma
  - Narrow zone of transition in ABC
  - Absence of infiltration into surrounding soft tissues
- MR shows epidural extent, cord compromise

TOP DIFFERENTIAL DIAGNOSES

- Osteoblastoma
- Telangiectatic osteogenic sarcoma
- Metastases
- Giant cell tumor
- Tarlov cyst

PATHOLOGY

- Now considered true neoplasm since cytogenetic abnormalities found in > 50%
- Translocation between chromosomes 16 and 17

CLINICAL ISSUES

- Young patient with back pain of insidious onset

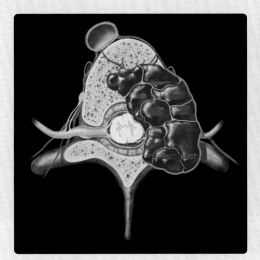

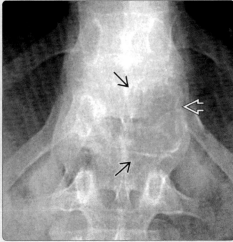

(Left) Axial graphic shows an aneurysmal bone cyst with an expansile, multicystic mass in the posterior vertebral body and pedicle extending into the epidural space. Fluid-fluid levels are characteristic. (Right) Anteroposterior radiograph shows an aneurysmal bone cyst of T12 with an absent pedicle sign ➡. The superior and inferior extent of tumor is shown by bone destruction ➡, which involved the vertebral body as well as the neural arch.

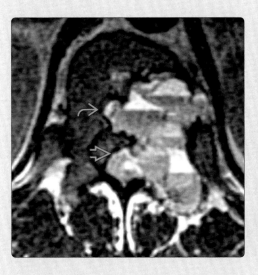

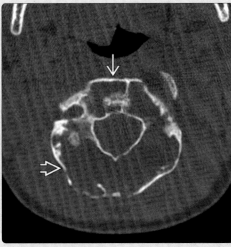

(Left) Axial T2WI MR shows an aneurysmal bone cyst of T12 with multiple fluid-fluid levels due to layering blood products. The zone of transition ➡ to normal bone is narrow and sclerotic. There is cortical breakthrough as well as extension into the spinal canal ➡ compressing the spinal cord. (Right) Axial NECT shows an extensive aneurysmal bone cyst involving the entire C2 body with body ➡ and posterior element ➡ expansion. The bony expansion is the typical soap bubble type with intact cortical margins.

Giant Cell Tumor

KEY FACTS

TERMINOLOGY

- Giant cell tumor (GCT)
- Locally aggressive neoplasm composed of osteoclast-like giant cells

IMAGING

- 3% of all GCTs occur in spine
- 4% of all GCTs occur in sacrum
- Lytic, expansile lesion of vertebral body or sacrum
- Narrow zone of transition, margin not sclerotic
- Matrix absent but may have residual bone trabeculae
- May have cortical breakthrough
- Heterogeneous contrast enhancement
- Nonenhancing areas of necrosis often present
- May be associated with aneurysmal bone cyst component

TOP DIFFERENTIAL DIAGNOSES

- Metastasis
- Myeloma
- Chordoma
- Osteogenic sarcoma

CLINICAL ISSUES

- Back pain of insidious onset, greatest at night
- Locally aggressive: 12-50% recurrence rate
- Curettage alone associated with high rate of recurrence
  - Curettage defect filled with methylmethacrylate or bone graft
  - Denosumab: Human monoclonal antibody to RANKL
    - In one study, 86% of patients had tumor response

DIAGNOSTIC CHECKLIST

- Most likely causes of solitary sacral mass in adult patient are GCTs, chordoma, and plasmacytoma
- Malignant GCTs rare, difficult to distinguish from typical GCT
  - Zone of transition usually less well defined

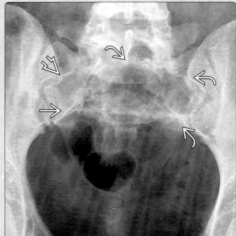

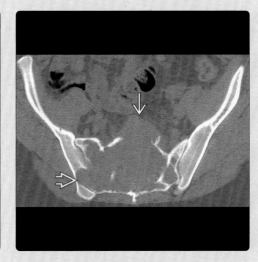

(Left) AP radiograph shows a giant cell tumor (GCT) ➡ of the sacrum. Lytic lesions in this region are difficult to see on radiographs and may be mistaken for bowel gas. Arcuate lines are a useful landmark. In this case, the S1 ➡ & S2 ➡ arcuate lines are visible on the normal right side but destroyed on the left. (Right) Axial NECT shows a nearly complete cortical rim around a large sacral mass. There is a small region of cortical breakthrough ➡ & extension of tumor from the sacrum into right iliac wing across the sacroiliac joint ➡.

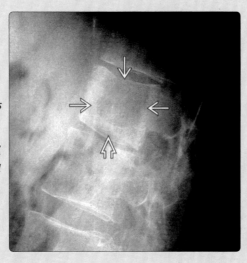

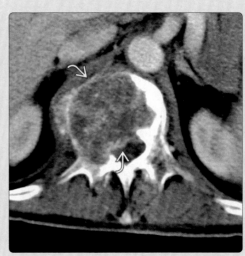

(Left) Lateral radiograph shows a lytic lesion ➡ of L1. The lesion is sharply demarcated with a nonsclerotic margin. There is probable cortical breakthrough inferiorly ➡. This constellation of findings is consistent with GCT and other intermediate aggressivity lesions, such as plasmacytoma, chordoma (rare at this site), or some metastases. (Right) Axial CECT in the same patient shows a heterogeneously enhancing mass with cortical breakthrough ➡.

Osteochondroma

KEY FACTS

TERMINOLOGY

- Osteochondroma (OC)
- Osteocartilaginous exostosis, exostosis
- Cartilage-capped osseous growth contiguous with parent bone

IMAGING

- Sessile or pedunculated osseous cauliflower-like lesion
- Continuity of bony cortex and medullary space between lesion and underlying bone
- May see chondroid calcifications in cartilage cap
- Center follows normal marrow signal on MR
- Cartilage cap of similar intensity to cord on T1WI, hyperintense on T2WI

TOP DIFFERENTIAL DIAGNOSES

- Chondrosarcoma
- Osteoblastoma
- Aneurysmal bone cyst

- Tumoral calcinosis
- Enthesopathy

PATHOLOGY

- Idiopathic, trauma, perichondrial ring deficiency
- Radiation-induced OC
- Syndromic: Hereditary multiple exostoses (HME)
- Vertebral OC rare; 1-5% of sporadic OC, 1-9% OC in HME

CLINICAL ISSUES

- Often asymptomatic; incidental diagnosis on radiography
- Palpable mass
- Mechanical impingement of joint, muscle
- Cord compression, radiculopathy unusual
- Peak age = 10-30 years

DIAGNOSTIC CHECKLIST

- Multiplicity → consider HME
- Cartilage cap > 1.5 cm in adults raises concern for malignant transformation (chondrosarcoma)

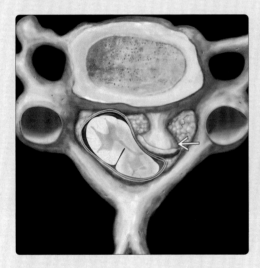

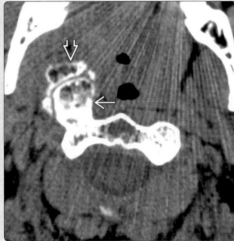

(Left) Axial graphic of the cervical spine demonstrates a typical osteochondroma (exostosis) ➡ protruding into the spinal canal causing canal stenosis and cord compression. (Right) Axial NECT shows a large osseous excrescence projecting ventrally from the right lateral mass of C2 ➡. There is ossification of the cartilaginous cap ➡.

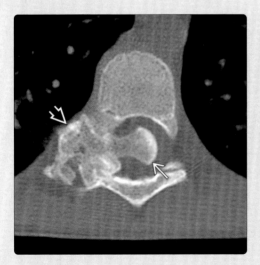

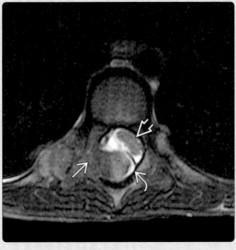

(Left) Axial bone CT shows a pedunculated osseous lesion ➡ extending into the canal from the right pedicle with cortical and medullary continuity. There is resulting canal stenosis. The right pedicle and superior facet are irregularly enlarged ➡ due to the sessile component of the osteochondroma. (Right) Axial T2WI FS MR in the same patient shows the medullary continuity of the osseous mass with the right pedicle ➡ and a hyperintense cartilaginous cap ➡. The spinal cord ➡ is displaced and compressed.

KEY FACTS

TERMINOLOGY

- Malignant tumor of connective tissue characterized by formation of cartilage matrix by tumor cells

IMAGING

- Lytic mass with chondroid matrix
  - Higher grade lesions tend to have larger areas without calcifications
- Lobular morphology often seen
- Enhancing periphery and internal septa
- May penetrate cortex with epidural or paravertebral extension
- Thoracic most commonly involved spine segment
  - Both posterior elements and body (45%)
  - Posterior elements (40%)
- Variable size, typically large at presentation

TOP DIFFERENTIAL DIAGNOSES

- Metastases

- Plasmacytoma
- Lymphoma
- Osteosarcoma
- Malignant fibrous histiocytoma

PATHOLOGY

- Lobulated tumor composed of translucent hyaline nodules (resemble normal cartilage)
- May be primary or secondary

CLINICAL ISSUES

- Palpable mass
- Localized pain, typically long duration of symptoms
- Neurologic symptoms in 45% of vertebral chondrosarcoma
  - Weakness, paresthesias, paralysis
- Age at presentation: 20-90 years; peak: 40-60 years

DIAGNOSTIC CHECKLIST

- Enlarging or painful enchondroma or osteochondroma suspicious for sarcomatous transformation

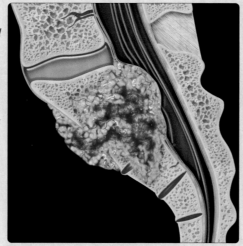

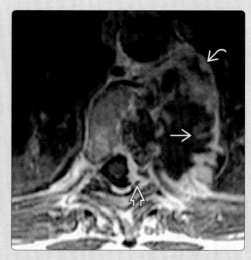

(Left) Sagittal graphic of the lumbosacral junction shows a large soft tissue mass centered within the sacrum. This tumor produces bone destruction with presacral and epidural extension. (Right) Axial T1WI C+ MR shows a large vertebral mass with paraspinal ➡ and epidural ➡ extension. There is irregular peripheral enhancement with some faintly enhancing central septations ➡.

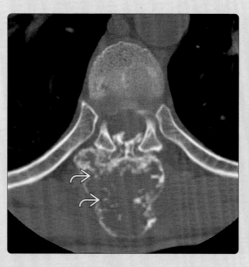

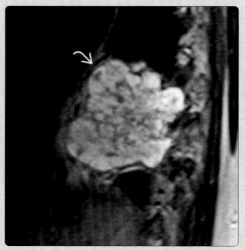

(Left) Axial unenhanced bone CT shows a large mass arising from the neural arch, containing ringed and stippled calcifications ➡, the typical appearance of a chondroid tumor matrix. (Right) Left paravertebral sagittal T2WI in the same patient shows a large, lobulated mass ➡ and a predominately hyperintense signal with thin, hypointense signal around the periphery of the lobules due to calcification. This is the typical MR appearance of a chondroid neoplasm.

Osteosarcoma

KEY FACTS

TERMINOLOGY

- Sarcoma containing osteoid matrix produced directly by malignant cells

IMAGING

- Permeative or moth-eaten appearance
- Cortical breakthrough
- Bone sclerosis due to production of immature bone
- Wide zone of transition
- Discontinuous periosteal reaction, usually multilaminar
- Soft tissue mass [fluid-fluid levels seen in telangiectatic osteogenic sarcoma (OGS)]

TOP DIFFERENTIAL DIAGNOSES

- Sclerotic metastasis
- Osteoblastoma
- Aneurysmal bone cyst
- Chordoma
- Osteomyelitis

- Ewing sarcoma
- Chondrosarcoma
- Lymphoma
- Malignant giant cell tumor

PATHOLOGY

- 4% of all primary OGS occurs in spine and sacrum
- Majority of OGS are of unknown etiology = primary OGS
- Association with retinoblastoma (*Rb* gene mutation)

CLINICAL ISSUES

- Insidious onset of back pain, greatest at night
- Neurologic symptoms including radicular pain, weakness
- 3% of 10-year survivors of all OGS develop 2nd malignancy

DIAGNOSTIC CHECKLIST

- CT scan best method for evaluation of tumor matrix, zone of transition
- All telangiectatic OGS are lytic on radiographs and CT but not all lytic OGS are telangiectatic

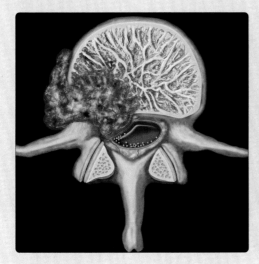

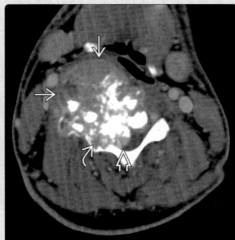

(Left) *Axial graphic shows secondary osteosarcoma arising in a Pagetic vertebral body, destroying the cortex and invading adjacent soft tissues. The soft tissue mass in osteosarcoma usually contains ossification.* (Right) *Axial CECT shows a very aggressive-appearing soft tissue mass ➡ that both produces a bony matrix and has areas of bone destruction ➡. There is a large epidural soft tissue component with cord compression ➡.*

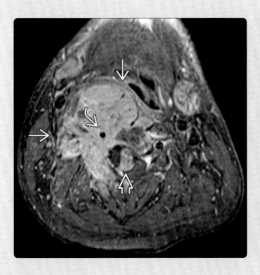

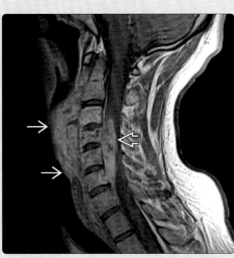

(Left) *Axial T2 FS MR shows a large soft tissue mass ➡, which has a relatively low T2 signal that is consistent with a highly cellular tumor. The mass has epidural extension with the cord displaced to the left ➡. The right vertebral artery is encased by tumor ➡.* (Right) *Postcontrast T1W MR shows diffuse enhancement of the mass with prevertebral ➡ and paravertebral extension as well as extensive epidural extension ➡ and cord compression.*

Chordoma

TERMINOLOGY

- Malignant tumor arising from notochord remnants

IMAGING

- Sacrococcygeal > sphenooccipital > mobile spine
- Osseous destruction with disproportionately large soft tissue mass
- Circumscribed, scalloped, or sclerotic bony margins
- Amorphous intratumoral calcifications
- Hyperintense to disc on T2WI with multiple septa
- May extend into disc space, involve 2 or more adjacent vertebrae

TOP DIFFERENTIAL DIAGNOSES

- Chondrosarcoma
- Giant cell tumor
- Metastases
- Plasmacytoma

PATHOLOGY

- Lobulated, soft, grayish gelatinous (myxoid) mass
- Areas of calcification and hemorrhage

CLINICAL ISSUES

- Skull base
  - Diplopia (CNV2 palsy, most common)
  - Headaches
  - Facial pain
- Mobile spine: Cord compression, radiculopathy (50%)
- Sacral: Altered sacrogluteal sensation
- Symptoms tend to be longstanding (4-24 months)
- Recurrence common
- 5-year survival: 50-68%; 10-year survival: 28-40%

DIAGNOSTIC CHECKLIST

- High signal intensity mass on T2WI with septations, little enhancement is chordoma or chondrosarcoma

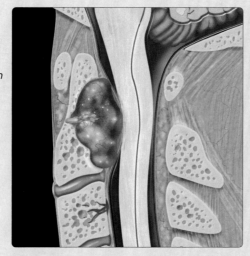

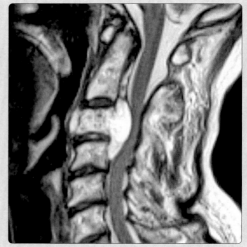

(Left) Sagittal graphic of the cervical spine shows an extradural soft tissue mass with the epicenter in the posterior aspect of the C2 body causing bone destruction and epidural extension with cord compression. (Right) Sagittal T2WI MR shows a hyperintense mass involving the C3 body with extensive epidural extension and cord compression.

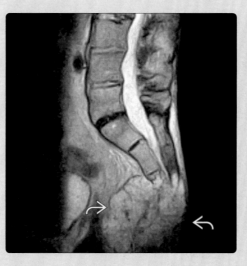

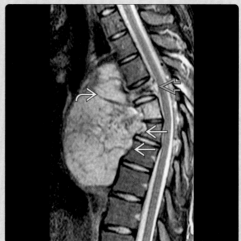

(Left) Sagittal T2WI show a large, well-defined hyperintense soft tissue mass engulfing the distal sacrum and coccyx with extension into the presacral space and dorsal soft tissues ➡. (Right) Sagittal T2WI FS MR shows a posterior mediastinal mass with involvement of 4 adjacent thoracic vertebral bodies. The mass is hyperintense with fine septations ➡. There is a pathologic compression fracture of the top vertebra with ventral epidural tumor ➡. Note the scalloped anterior margins ➡.

Ewing Sarcoma

TERMINOLOGY

- Ewing sarcoma family of tumors
- Aggressive childhood cancer, which includes Ewing sarcoma, Askin tumor, and peripheral primitive neuroectodermal tumor

IMAGING

- Spine: 5% of all Ewing tumors
  o Sacrum most common spinal site
  o Spreads along peripheral nerves
- May originate in epidural or paraspinous soft tissues
- Permeative/moth-eaten bone destruction
  o 5% sclerotic (represents host reaction, not tumor matrix)
  o Areas of central necrosis common
  o "Percolates" through tiny perforations in cortex
- Lower signal intensity than disc or muscle on T1WI
  o May be isointense to red marrow on T2WI
  o Intermediate to high signal intensity on STIR

- MR best shows involvement of adjacent bones and soft tissues, which can be underestimated on CT scan
  o Heterogeneous enhancement with gadolinium
- CT useful to confirm absence of tumor matrix, distinguish from osteogenic sarcoma

TOP DIFFERENTIAL DIAGNOSES

- Primitive neuroectodermal tumor
- Langerhans cell histiocytosis
- Osteosarcoma
- Metastatic neuroblastoma
- Osteomyelitis

CLINICAL ISSUES

- 90% of all Ewing sarcoma patients present before 20 years of age
- Fever, leukocytosis, elevated ESR (simulating osteomyelitis)
- Spine and sacral lesions often present in older patients than peripheral Ewing sarcoma

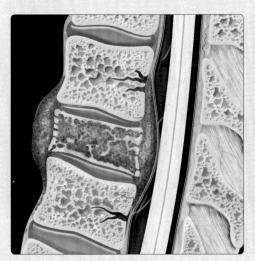
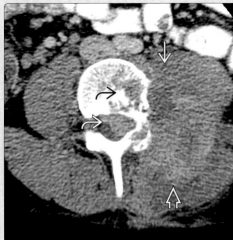

(Left) Sagittal graphic shows a vertebral body replaced by Ewing sarcoma resulting in mild collapse. Tumor extends into adjacent soft tissues through small perforations in the bone cortex. (Right) Axial CECT shows a large paraspinal soft tissue mass of Ewing sarcoma engulfing the left psoas muscle with extension into the dorsal musculature, destruction of left side of lumbar body, and epidural extension.

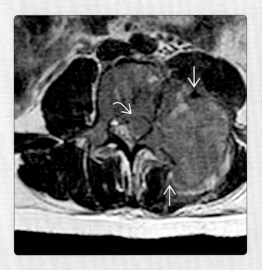
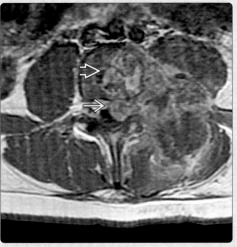

(Left) Axial T2WI MR shows Ewing sarcoma involving the paraspinal muscles and extending into the epidural space, compressing and displacing the thecal sac to the right. Infiltration of the vertebral body is poorly defined on this sequence. (Right) Axial T1WI C+ MR shows diffuse heterogeneous enhancement of the tumor involving the left side of lumbar body, epidural space, and paravertebral and dorsal muscles.

Lymphoma

TERMINOLOGY

- Lymphoreticular neoplasms with myriad of specific diseases and cellular differentiation

IMAGING

- Multiple types with variable imaging manifestations
- Epidural lymphoma: Thoracic > lumbar > cervical
  - Enhancing epidural mass ± vertebral involvement
- Osseous lymphoma: Long bones > spine
  - Bone destruction (ivory vertebra, rare), vertebra plana
- Lymphomatous leptomeningitis
  - Smooth/nodular pial enhancement
- Intramedullary lymphoma: Cervical > thoracic > lumbar
  - Poorly defined, enhancing mass
- Secondary > primary involvement
- Extradural > intradural > intramedullary
- FDG PET useful for staging, monitoring treatment response, predicting treatment outcomes, and risk stratifying lymphoma patients

PATHOLOGY

- Non-Hodgkin lymphoma (NHL) > > Hodgkin disease (HD); 80-90% are B cell
  - CNS lymphoma > 85% NHL (B cell > > T cell)
- CNS lymphoma may be primary or secondary (hematogenous or direct geographic extension)

CLINICAL ISSUES

- Most common presenting symptom = back pain
- Intramedullary = myelopathy (weakness, numbness)
- Cord compression occurs in up to 5-10% of systemic lymphomas
- Generally poor prognosis for CNS lymphoma
- Markedly sensitive to chemotherapy/XRT
- Depressed humoral and cell-mediated immunity leads to opportunistic infections
- Treatment: XRT ± chemotherapy (markedly sensitive to chemotherapy/XRT); ± surgery

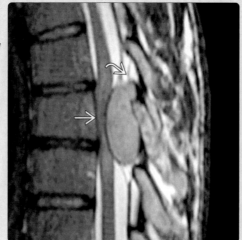

(Left) Sagittal T2WI MR demonstrates a discrete hypointense mass in the posterior epidural space with a cap of epidural fat ➡. The spinal cord is displaced anteriorly ➡. Lymphoma is the most common malignancy of the epidural space. (Right) Sagittal T2WI MR (left) shows an amorphous hypointense tumor mass insinuating along the cauda equina ➡. Sagittal T1WI C+ MR (right) reveals enhancing lymphoma within the leptomeninges surrounding the distal conus and involving the nerve roots diffusely ➡.

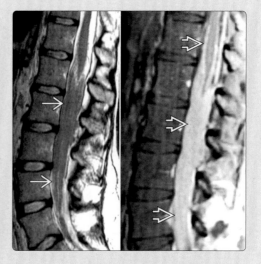

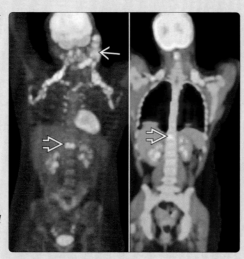

(Left) Coronal PET (left) shows FDG uptake in the left cervical lymph node mass ➡ that was clinically evident. PET/CT fused image (right) shows abnormal activity at T11 ➡. This is an example of osseous metastases from cervical Hodgkin lymphoma primary tumor. (Right) Sagittal CT (left) demonstrates a pathologic compression fracture of a midthoracic vertebral body ➡. Sagittal T1WI C+ MR (right) confirms abnormal marrow enhancement ➡ and a ventral paraspinal mass ➡.

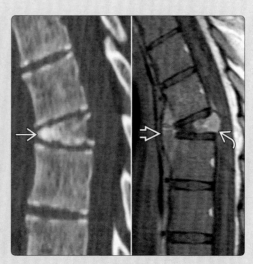

Leukemia

KEY FACTS

TERMINOLOGY

- Acute or chronic myeloid or lymphoid white blood cell neoplasia with spinal involvement as component of systemic disease

IMAGING

- Radiographs/CT
  - Diffuse osteopenia with multiple vertebral fractures ± lytic spine lesions
  - Variable enhancing isodense soft tissue mass with adjacent bone destruction
- MR
  - T1WI: Hypointense marrow and focal tumor masses
  - T2WI: Hyperintense marrow ± focal vertebral mass, cord signal abnormality
  - T1WI C+: Abnormal enhancement of marrow, focal lesion, or leptomeninges

TOP DIFFERENTIAL DIAGNOSES

- Metastases
- Lymphoma
- Ewing sarcoma
- Langerhans cell histiocytosis

CLINICAL ISSUES

- Localized or diffuse bone pain
- Symptomatic patients present with fever, ↑ ESR, hepatosplenomegaly, lymphadenopathy, joint effusions, petechial and retinal hemorrhage, anemia, frequent infections

DIAGNOSTIC CHECKLIST

- Marrow infiltration in child with osteoporosis raises suspicion for leukemia
- Consider leukemia in patient with unexplained compression fractures

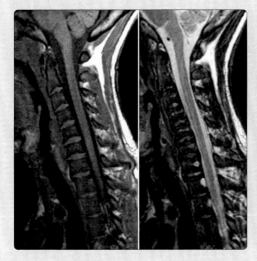
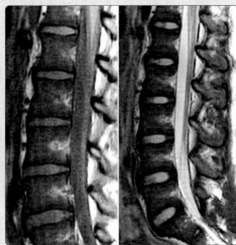

(Left) Sagittal T1WI MR (left) and T2WI MR (right) of the cervical spine demonstrate diffuse abnormal hypointense signal intensity within the vertebra. Signal intensity is lower than the adjacent disc spaces. (Right) Sagittal T1WI MR (left) and T2WI MR (right) of the lumbar spine exhibit diffuse abnormal hypointense signal intensity within the vertebra as compared to the adjacent disc spaces. The signal abnormality may be a combination of tumor marrow infiltration and hyperplastic marrow secondary to anemia.

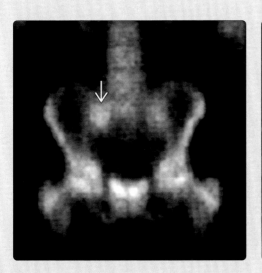
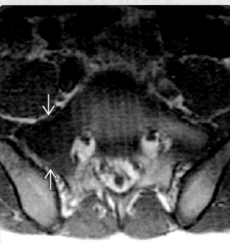

(Left) Coronal planar bone scan of the pelvis reveals abnormal increased uptake within the right sacral ala ➡️ in this case of focal leukemic metastasis to the axial skeleton. Bone scan may underestimate disease extent, especially in absence of significant cortical destruction. (Right) Axial T1WI MR in the same patient clarifies the right sacral alar metastatic lesion ➡️. There is no definite cortical breakthrough.

KEY FACTS

TERMINOLOGY

- Solitary monoclonal plasma cell tumor of bone or soft tissue
- Diagnosis of solitary bone plasmacytoma (SBP) requires
  - Solitary lesion, biopsy showing plasma cells
  - Negative skeletal survey, negative MR spine, pelvis, proximal femora/humeri
  - Negative clonal cells in marrow aspirate
  - No anemia, hypercalcemia, or renal involvement suggesting systemic myeloma

IMAGING

- Axial skeleton > extremities
  - Thoracic vertebral body most common site
- Radiographs/CT
  - Lytic, multicystic-appearing lesion ± vertical dense striations
  - Pathologic compression fracture common

- T1 hypointense, T2/STIR hyperintense marrow with low-signal, curvilinear areas
  - Posterior elements involved in most cases
  - ± associated soft tissue mass (paraspinous or epidural with draped curtain sign)

PATHOLOGY

- SBP may reflect early (stage I) multiple myeloma
- SBPs considered clinical stage I Durie-Salmon lesions

CLINICAL ISSUES

- Most common symptom = pain due to bone destruction
- Epidural extension may cause compression of cord or nerve root
- Mean age = 55 years (younger than age of patients with multiple myeloma)

DIAGNOSTIC CHECKLIST

- Must exclude 2nd unanticipated lesion (33% of cases)

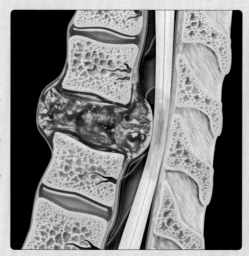
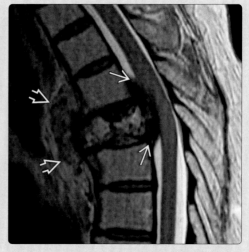

(Left) Sagittal graphic shows collapse of the thoracic vertebral body due to tumor infiltration. There is retropulsion of the anterior and posterior margins. Posterior retropulsion and tumor mass may result in cord compression. (Right) Sagittal T2WI MR demonstrates a heterogeneously hyperintense thoracic vertebral body lesion with hypointense ventral epidural ➡ and paravertebral ➡ soft tissue components producing cord compression.

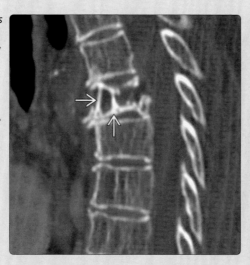
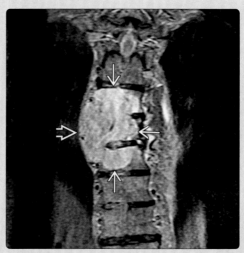

(Left) Sagittal bone CT exhibits the characteristic appearance of thickened cortical struts ➡, a result of stress phenomenon from the lytic process forcing remaining bone to increase thickness as a compensatory response to weakening bone. (Right) Coronal STIR MR of the thoracic spine demonstrates hyperintense lesions involving 3 contiguous vertebral bodies ➡ with an associated soft tissue mass extending in the right paravertebral region ➡.

Multiple Myeloma

KEY FACTS

TERMINOLOGY

- Multifocal malignant proliferation of monoclonal plasma cells within bone marrow

IMAGING

- Skeletal survey is initial diagnostic imaging evaluation
  - Diffuse osteopenia and multiple lytic lesions
- NECT (bone algorithm)
  - Multifocal lytic lesions
  - Vertebral destruction and fractures
- MR patterns
  - Normal
  - Focal marrow involvement
  - Diffuse marrow involvement
  - Variegated pattern (micronodular, salt and pepper appearance)
- Compression fractures with variable central canal narrowing
- FDG PET
  - Identifies active multiple myeloma; useful in monitoring treatment response
- FSE T2 with fat saturation, STIR, or T1WI C+ with fat suppression increase lesion conspicuity

TOP DIFFERENTIAL DIAGNOSES

- Metastases
- Leukemia/lymphoma
- Osteoporosis
- Hyperplastic marrow

CLINICAL ISSUES

- Bone pain: 75%
- Marrow failure: Anemia, infection
- Renal insufficiency/failure
- M protein (monoclonal immunoglobulin): Blood ± urine
- Hypercalcemia
- Treatment: Supportive care, local radiation, chemotherapy, transplants

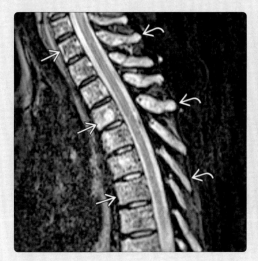

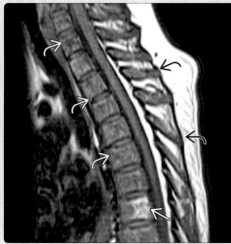

(Left) Sagittal STIR MR illustrates innumerable hyperintense foci in the cervical and thoracic vertebral bodies ➡ and spinous processes ➡. Advanced imaging is recommended in those with normal radiographs and monoclonal gammopathy or a solitary plasmacytoma. (Right) Sagittal T1WI MR demonstrates heterogeneous marrow signal due to countless hypointense lesions in the cervical and thoracic vertebral bodies ➡ and the spinous processes ➡. There is a benign vertebral hemangioma at T8 ➡.

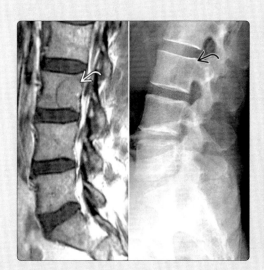

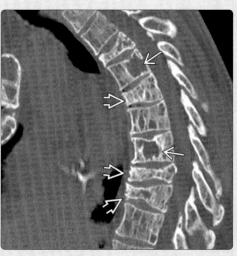

(Left) Sagittal T2WI MR (left) shows marrow heterogeneity with a hypointense L3 vertebral body lesion ➡, barely detectable on lateral MR (right) ➡. Radiographs allow identification of only those lesions with advanced destruction affecting at minimum 30% of trabecular bone. (Right) Sagittal CT shows diffuse osteopenia with multiple vertebral body lytic lesions ➡. Pathologic compression fractures ➡ are seen in multiple midthoracic vertebral bodies. Compression fractures can cause variable central canal narrowing.

KEY FACTS

TERMINOLOGY

- Neuroblastoma (NB), ganglioneuroblastoma (GNB), and ganglioneuroma (GN) are tumors of varying maturity derived from primordial neural crest cells that form sympathetic nervous system

IMAGING

- Abdominal (adrenal, paraspinal ganglia) > thoracic > pelvic > cervical
- Radiographs
  - Widened paraspinal soft tissues ± scoliosis
  - ± stippled abdominal or mediastinal calcifications
- CT
  - Widened neural foramina & intercostal spaces, pedicle erosion, adjacent rib splaying (GN, GNB) or destruction (NB)
- MR for diagnosis, presurgical planning
  - T1WI: Hypo-/isointense paraspinal mass
  - T2WI: Hypo-/hyperintense paraspinal mass
  - ± epidural extension through neural foramina
  - Variable enhancement ± internal hemorrhage, necrosis
- MIBG for NB staging, posttreatment surveillance

TOP DIFFERENTIAL DIAGNOSES

- Ewing sarcoma
- Vertebral metastasis
- Lymphoma

CLINICAL ISSUES

- Abdominal mass/pain, bone pain, fatigue, weight loss, blanching subcutaneous nodules
- Paraparesis/paraplegia (cord compression)
- NB 5-year survival ~ 83% for infants, 55% for children 1-5 years, and 40% for children > 5 years

DIAGNOSTIC CHECKLIST

- Critical to determine whether tumor extends into spinal canal or neural foramina

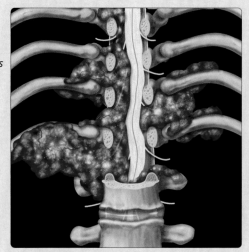
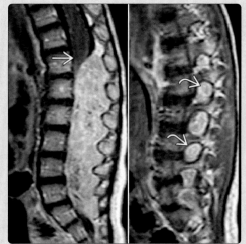

(Left) Coronal graphic depicts a vascular paraspinal neuroblastoma (NB) originating on the right with spread through the contiguous neural foramina across the midline to the left (stage 3). (Right) Sagittal T1 C+ MR illustrate a large mass involving the entire lumbar epidural space with marked compression of the thecal sac and compression of the conus medullaris ➡. This NB mass enhances avidly and homogeneously. The mass extends from the retroperitoneum through multiple lumbar foramina ➡.

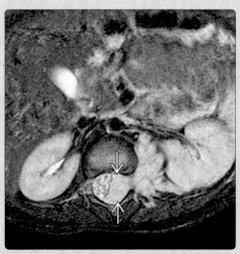
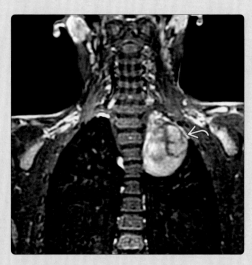

(Left) Axial STIR MR displays a paraspinal NB transgressing across the neural foramen into epidural space ➡ & displacing the thecal sac medially. Report whether the tumor extends into the spinal canal or neural foramina, as epidural extension complicates surgical management. (Right) Sagittal T1 C+ FS MR shows an avidly enhancing posterosuperior mediastinal mass ➡. This ganglioneuroblastoma directly contacts adjacent vertebral bodies & ribs without abnormal marrow enhancement to imply invasion.

Schwannoma

TERMINOLOGY

- Neurinoma, neurilemmoma (outdated terms)
- Neoplasm of nerve sheath (Schwann cells)

IMAGING

- 70-75% intradural extramedullary
  - Most common intradural extramedullary mass
- 15% completely extradural
- 15% transforaminal, dumbbell masses
- Bone remodeling due to large intraspinal or intraforaminal tumor common
- Cystic change common
- Calcifications, hemorrhage are rare
- Uniform, heterogeneous, or peripheral enhancement patterns

TOP DIFFERENTIAL DIAGNOSES

- Neurofibroma (NF)
- Perineural root sleeve cyst

- Myxopapillary ependymoma
- Meningioma
- Leptomeningeal carcinomatosis
- Neuroblastic tumor

PATHOLOGY

- WHO grade I
- NF2: Loss of tumor suppressor (merlin) on chromosome 22
- Sporadic schwannoma more common than NF2
  - Inactivating mutations of merlin gene in ~ 60%

CLINICAL ISSUES

- Pain, weakness, paresthesias most common clinical findings
- Typically solitary unless part of inherited tumor syndrome

DIAGNOSTIC CHECKLIST

- Schwannoma most likely when solitary enhancing dumbbell-shaped spinal lesion present

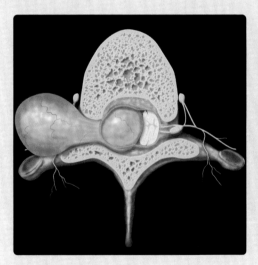

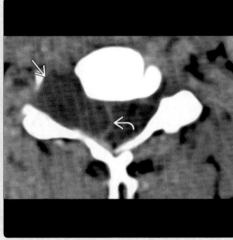

(Left) Axial graphic portrays a right-sided dumbbell-shaped spinal nerve root schwannoma enlarging the neural foramen and compressing the spinal cord. Both intra- and extradural components (dumbbell) are present. (Right) Axial CECT shows a hypodense transforaminal mass ➡ enlarging the right neural foramen. The intraspinal component effaces the thecal sac ➡ and causes canal stenosis.

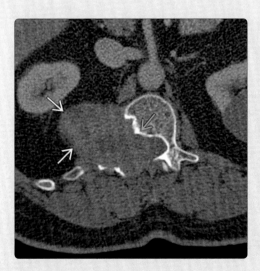

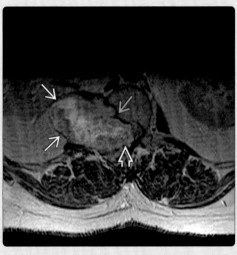

(Left) Axial NECT demonstrates a large soft tissue mass ➡ enlarging the right L1-2 neural foramen. There is conspicuous scalloping of the vertebral body ➡. The full intraspinal component is not seen. (Right) Axial T2WI MR in the same patient reveals heterogeneous mass ➡ signal intensity. Foraminal enlargement and vertebral body scalloping are again seen ➡. The extradural component within the spinal canal is causing significant canal stenosis ➡.

KEY FACTS

IMAGING

- Intradural extramedullary mass
- Thoracic (80%) > cervical (16%) > lumbar (4%)
- Typically round or ovoid (en globe)
  - en plaque variety pancaked or flat along dura
- Broad dural attachment (more often ventral or ventrolateral)
- Strong homogeneous enhancement
- Calcification in 1-5%
- No bony remodeling or hyperostosis in spine

TOP DIFFERENTIAL DIAGNOSES

- Schwannoma
- Ependymoma, myxopapillary
- Lymphoma
- Intradural metastases

PATHOLOGY

- Arise from arachnoid cap cells

- > 95% WHO grade I
- Most solitary, sporadic
  - Almost all have 22q12 abnormalities
- Syndromes
  - Multiple lesions with neurofibromatosis type 2
    - Intradural extramedullary meningiomas and schwannomas
    - Intramedullary ependymomas
  - Familial clear cell meningioma syndrome
  - Multiple meningiomatosis

CLINICAL ISSUES

- Peak incidence: 5th-6th decades
- > 80% female
- 2nd most common intradural extramedullary tumor
- Sensory and motor deficits (84%)
- Gait disturbances (83%)
- Local pain (47%)

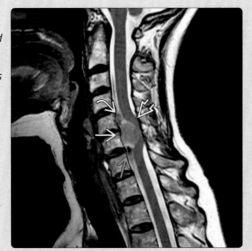
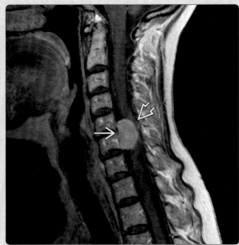

(Left) Sagittal T2 MR shows a ventral, dural-based mass at C5-6 level ➡ compressing and displacing the cervical cord posteriorly ➡. An intradural extramedullary mass displaces the cord with concomitant widening of the CSF spaces adjacent to the mass ➡. This T2 image shows CSF flow dephasing with signal loss adjacent to the mass ➡. (Right) Sagittal T1W C+ MR shows a large intradural extramedullary meningioma with prominent enhancement. Note the broad ventral dural attachment ➡ and severe cord compression ➡.

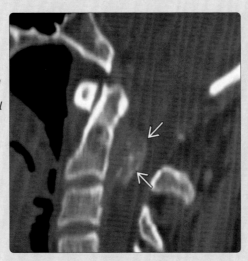
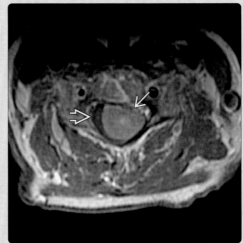

(Left) Sagittal reconstructed bone CT shows a sizable, partially calcified meningioma ➡ arising on the ventral margin of the canal at the level of C2. The mass results in significant canal stenosis and cord compression. (Right) Axial T1 C+ MR shows a large cervical meningioma with a ventral, dural-based attachment at the C5-6 level ➡ severely compressing and displacing the cervical cord posteriorly and to the right ➡.

Solitary Fibrous Tumor/Hemangiopericytoma

KEY FACTS

TERMINOLOGY

- Hemangiopericytoma (HPC)
- Solitary fibrous tumor (SFT)

IMAGING

- HPC may occur in any compartment of spine except intramedullary
- Circumscribed, multilobulated morphology
- Vivid enhancement characteristically seen

TOP DIFFERENTIAL DIAGNOSES

- Meningioma
- Schwannoma
- Chordoma and other primary bone malignancies
- Aggressive hemangioma
- Vascular metastases
- Angiosarcoma

PATHOLOGY

- Hypervascular neoplasm; currently considered mesenchymal tumor of unknown etiology
- Hemangiopericytoma considered part of SFT spectrum ("cellular" or "malignant" SFT)
- Majority of HPC likely classified within cellular end of SFT spectrum

CLINICAL ISSUES

- Natural history
  - Progressive growth
  - Local recurrence
  - Metastases
- Primary treatment is surgical resection
- Radiation therapy as adjuvant to surgery, primary treatment for unresectable tumor
  - Limited benefit of chemotherapy
- Continued radiographic surveillance for late recurrence

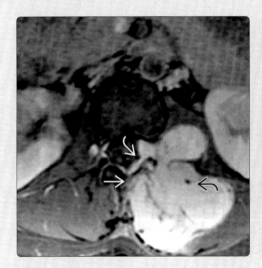
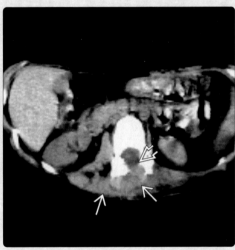

(Left) Axial T1WI C+ MR shows a lobulated, avidly enhancing paraspinous mass with internal flow voids ➡ due to hypervascularity. There is transforaminal extension with an intradural component ➡. Bony invasion of the lamina ➡ is also seen. (Right) Axial NECT shows a dorsal soft tissue mass ➡ destroying the lamina and extending into the dorsal epidural space ➡.

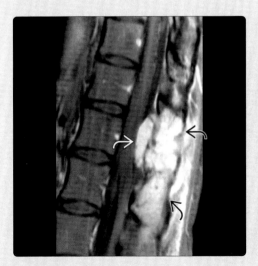
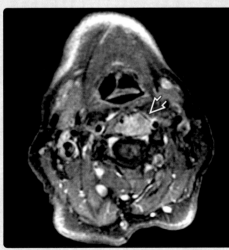

(Left) Sagittal T1WI C+ MR shows an avidly enhancing mass ➡ invading the dorsal elements and adjacent soft tissues at 3 levels of the thoracic spine. An intraspinal component ➡ is not clearly in the epidural or intradural extramedullary compartments. (Right) Axial T1WI C+ MR shows an avidly enhancing osseous metastasis ➡ from an intracranial hemangiopericytoma to the C3 vertebral body.

KEY FACTS

TERMINOLOGY

- Neoplasm containing Schwann cells, fibroblasts, myxoid material, and peripheral nerve fibers

IMAGING

- Locations
  - Extradural/paraspinal; intradural extramedullary
- Variable involvement of spinal root, neural plexus, peripheral nerve, or end organs
- Size varies from small circumscribed mass to large plexiform neurofibromatosis (NF) involving multiple body compartments
- Plexiform neurofibroma pathognomonic for NF1
- Target sign on T2WI suggestive but not pathognomonic for NF
- FDG avidity suggests malignant degeneration

TOP DIFFERENTIAL DIAGNOSES

- Schwannoma
- Spinal meningioma
- Perineural root sleeve cyst
- Chronic interstitial demyelinating polyneuropathy
- Malignant nerve sheath tumors

PATHOLOGY

- Neoplastic Schwann cells + fibroblasts
- Tumor, nerve fascicles intermixed (presence of axons characteristic of NF)
- 90% of neurofibromas are sporadic

CLINICAL ISSUES

- Malignant transformation of plexiform NF to malignant peripheral nerve sheath tumor (MPNST) in 10% of NF1 patients

DIAGNOSTIC CHECKLIST

- Rapidly growing NF or atypical pain concerning for malignant transformation to MPNST
- Solitary spinal lesion more likely schwannoma than NF

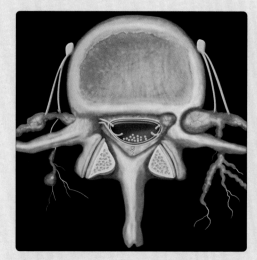

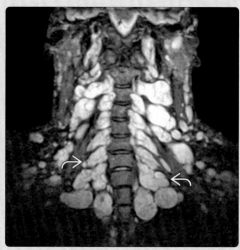

(Left) Axial graphic portrays bilateral lobulated plexiform neurofibromas in neurofibromatosis type 1 (NF1). There is erosion of the left pedicle by the tumor. (Right) Coronal STIR shows extensive, bulky plexiform neurofibromas ➡ involving bilateral cervical nerve roots. This appearance is virtually pathognomonic for NF1.

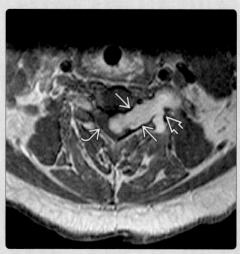

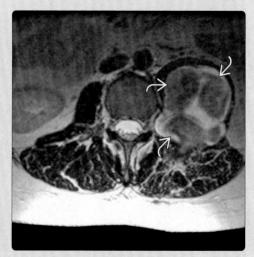

(Left) Axial T1WI C+ MR shows an oblong enhancing mass ➡ extending through the left C4-5 neural foramen. Longstanding remodeling has enlarged the neural foramen ➡. The intraspinal component of the mass causes canal stenosis and cord compression ➡. (Right) Axial T2WI MR in the same patient shows central areas of T2 hypointense signal ➡ with a peripheral rim of hyperintensity. This target sign is not specific but is seen more commonly with neurofibroma than with schwannoma.

Malignant Nerve Sheath Tumors

TERMINOLOGY

- Malignant peripheral nerve sheath tumor (MPNST)
- Soft tissue sarcoma that arises from or differentiates toward cells of peripheral nerve sheath

IMAGING

- CT and MR: Large, infiltrative, often hemorrhagic, soft tissue mass
  - Arise spontaneously or from malignant degeneration within preexisting neurofibroma
  - Heterogeneous areas correspond to hemorrhage, calcifications, and necrosis
  - Bony erosion, destruction
  - Marked enhancement
  - Indistinct margins
- FDG PET diagnoses neurofibromatosis type 1 (NF1)-associated MPNST with sensitivity of 89% and specificity of 95%

- CT significantly less accurate than FDG PET for characterizing tumors as malignant or benign

TOP DIFFERENTIAL DIAGNOSES

- Benign peripheral nerve sheath tumor, other soft tissue sarcoma, hematoma

PATHOLOGY

- Incidence in general population: 0.001%
- 50-60% associated with NF1

CLINICAL ISSUES

- Enlarging soft tissue mass
- Local or radicular pain, sensory disturbance
- Paraparesis
- Sporadic MPNST presents in 4th decade (mean age: 39.7 years)
- If associated with NF1: 26-42 years (mean age: 28.7)
- Local recurrence: 26-65%; metastases: 20-65%
- Worse prognosis with NF1

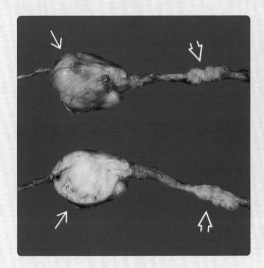

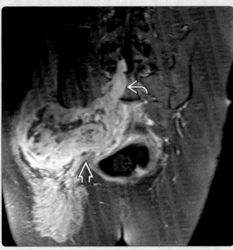

(Left) *Malignant peripheral nerve sheath tumors (MPNSTs) often arise from a major nerve trunk, such as this sciatic nerve tumor forming a fusiform, lobulated, intraneural mass* ➡. *These tumors can extend along a nerve to form satellite nodules* ➡. **(Right)** *Coronal T1 C+ FS MR shows a large heterogeneously enhancing mass in the right pelvis extending through a sacral foramen into the spinal canal* ➡ *and through the sciatic notch* ➡ *into the buttocks.*

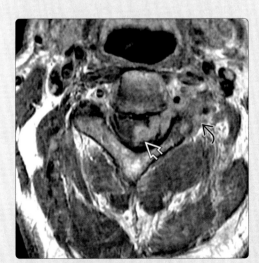

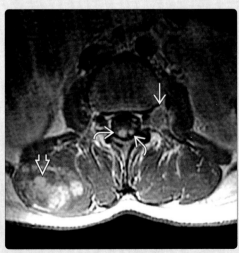

(Left) *Axial T1 C+ MR shows an enhancing dumbbell-shaped mass involving the cervical spine. There is infiltration of the paravertebral soft tissues* ➡. *Tumor invades the cord parenchyma* ➡ *within the spinal canal.* **(Right)** *Axial T1 C+ MR in a patient with neurofibromatosis type 1 shows neurofibromas in the left neural foramen* ➡ *and within the spinal canal* ➡. *The enhancing tumor in the right sacrospinalis muscle* ➡ *has slightly indistinct margins and was pathologically proven to be a MPNST.*

KEY FACTS

TERMINOLOGY

- Spread of malignant tumor through subarachnoid spaces of brain and spinal cord

IMAGING

- Smooth or nodular enhancement along cord, cauda equina
- Located at any point along CSF pathway
- 4 basic patterns
  - Solitary focal mass at bottom of thecal sac or along cord surface
  - Diffuse, thin, sheet-like coating of cord/roots (carcinomatous meningitis)
  - Rope-like thickening of cauda equina
  - Multifocal discrete nodules along cord/roots

TOP DIFFERENTIAL DIAGNOSES

- Multifocal primary tumor
- Pyogenic meningitis
- Granulomatous meningitis

- Chemical meningitis
- Recent lumbar puncture
- Congenital hypertrophic polyradiculoneuropathies
- Thick nerve roots/cauda equina

PATHOLOGY

- Hematogenous dissemination from solid tumors (1-5%)
- Drop metastases from patients with primary CNS tumor (1-2%)
- Leukemia, lymphoma (5-15%)
- False-negative CSF cytology in up to 40%

CLINICAL ISSUES

- Typically seen in advanced cancer cases
- Prevalence increasing as cancer patients are living longer
- Median patient survival of 3-6 months with treatment, 4-6 weeks without

DIAGNOSTIC CHECKLIST

- MR more sensitive than CSF cytology

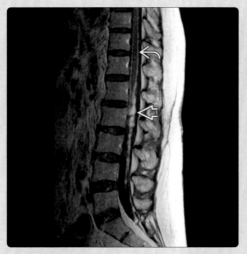
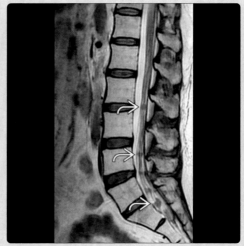

(Left) Sagittal T1WI C+ MR shows a mixed nodular ⤷ and smooth ➡ leptomeningeal tumor along the distal cord and conus medullaris due to drop metastases from glioblastoma multiforme. (Right) Sagittal T2WI MR shows multiple nodular low signal intensity rounded drop metastases ➡ involving roots of the cauda equina, spreading from an intracranial glioblastoma multiforme.

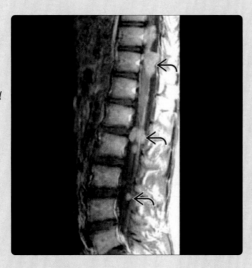
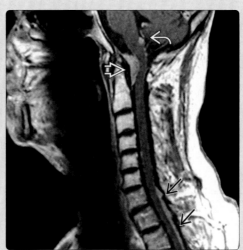

(Left) Sagittal T1WI C+ MR shows bulky nodular drop metastases ➡ from a pineal germinoma along the conus and cauda equina. (Right) Sagittal T1WI C+ MR shows CSF metastasis from small cell lung carcinoma with a bulky enhancing dural mass compressing the cervicomedullary junction ➡ and linear enhancing metastases along the dorsal pial surface of the cord from C7 caudally ➡. An additional enhancing focus is seen in the region of the gracile tubercle ➡.

Paraganglioma

TERMINOLOGY

- Synonyms: Glomus tumor, extraadrenal pheochromocytoma, chemodectoma

IMAGING

- Hypervascular, intensely enhancing intradural extramedullary mass
  - Prominent flow voids due to enlarged draining veins
  - ± cystic areas, hemosiderin from prior hemorrhage
- Large tumors may show osseous remodeling
- Malignant paraganglioma may → osteolytic spinal metastases
- Usually positive on I-123 or I-131 MIBG scan

TOP DIFFERENTIAL DIAGNOSES

- Myxopapillary ependymoma
  - Usually indistinguishable from paraganglioma on imaging studies
- Schwannoma

- Rarely associated with dilated vessels
- Meningioma
- Metastasis
- Hemangioblastoma of filum terminale

PATHOLOGY

- WHO grade I
- Slow-growing, generally benign behavior

CLINICAL ISSUES

- Presents with back pain/radiculopathy (often chronic)
- Prognosis varies with tumor location but generally excellent

DIAGNOSTIC CHECKLIST

- MR imaging features nonspecific
- Ependymoma and schwannoma much more common than paraganglioma

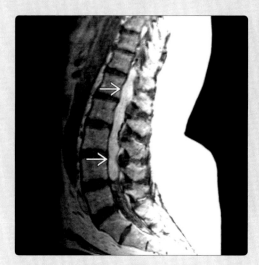

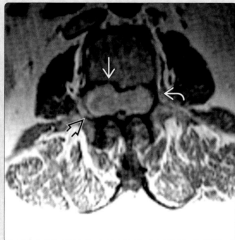

(Left) Sagittal T1WI C+ MR of the lumbar spine demonstrates a large, homogeneously enhancing intradural mass ➡ filling the lumbar canal from T12 through L4. (Right) Axial T1WI C+ MR of the same patient shows posterior vertebral body scalloping ➡, neuroforaminal enlargement ➡, and thinning of the left pedicle ➡ secondary to longstanding osseous remodeling. Recognition of these osseous changes confirms the slow-growing nature of the tumor.

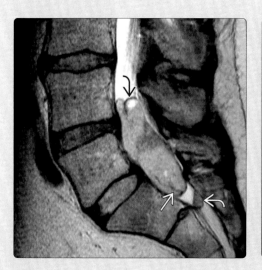

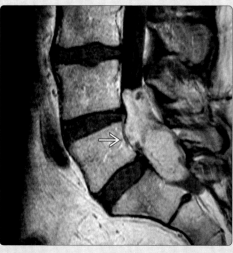

(Left) Sagittal T2WI MR reveals a heterogeneous mass within the caudal thecal sac demonstrating a cystic area superiorly ➡ and a prominent flow void ➡ indicating hypervascularity. A small amount of hemorrhage layers dependently ➡ in the caudal tip of the thecal sac. (Right) Sagittal T1WI C+ MR in the same patient confirms diffuse, mildly heterogeneous enhancement throughout the tumor. Mild scalloping of the posterior L5 vertebral body is also noted, indicating chronic remodeling ➡.

TERMINOLOGY

- Primary neoplasm of astrocytic origin within spinal cord

IMAGING

- Fusiform expansion of cord with enhancing component of variable morphology
  - Almost always enhances
- Cervical > thoracic
- Usually ≤ 4 segments
  - Occasionally multisegmental, even holocord (more common with pilocytic astrocytoma)
- ± cyst/syrinx (fluid slightly T1 hyperintense to CSF)
- Hyperintense on proton density and T2WI MR

TOP DIFFERENTIAL DIAGNOSES

- Ependymoma
- Hemangioblastoma
- Metastasis
- Syringohydromyelia

- Autoimmune or inflammatory myelitis

PATHOLOGY

- 80-90% low grade
- 10-15% high grade

CLINICAL ISSUES

- Slow onset of myelopathy
- May cause painful scoliosis
- Most are slow growing
  - Malignant tumors may cause rapid neurologic deterioration
- Most common intramedullary tumor in children and young adults
- Overall, ependymomas > astrocytomas (2:1)

DIAGNOSTIC CHECKLIST

- Myelopathy should be evaluated with MR

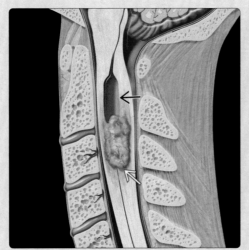
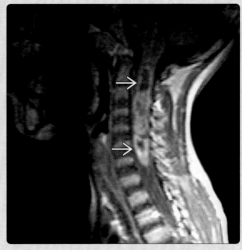

(Left) Sagittal graphic of cervical spine astrocytoma shows a fusiform solid mass ➡ with a rostral cystic cord component ➡. (Right) Sagittal T1WI C+ MR reveals a heterogeneously enhancing cervical cord mass ➡. The tumor subtype and histological grade are the most important prognostic factors. Malignant transformation, while common in recurrent adult low-grade gliomas, is unusual in pediatric low-grade intramedullary spinal cord tumors.

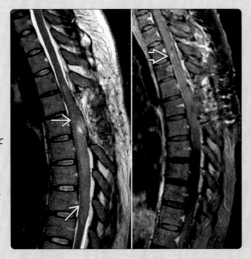
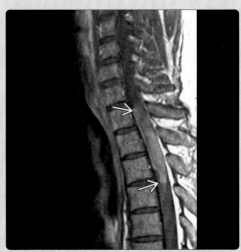

(Left) Sagittal T2WI MR (left) illustrates an anaplastic astrocytoma of the thoracic cord with a long segment of cord expansion and hyperintensity ➡. Sagittal T1WI C+ FS MR (right) reveals minimal enhancement ➡ of the lesion. (Right) Sagittal T1WI C+ MR depicts a large enhancing mass in the thoracic cord with long segment fusiform expansion ➡. Differential diagnoses include astrocytoma vs. ependymoma. Pathology revealed glioblastoma multiforme. High-grade astrocytomas account for ~ 10% of cases.

IMAGING

General Features

- Best diagnostic clue
  - Enhancing infiltrating mass expanding spinal cord (SC)
- Location
  - Cervical > thoracic
- Size
  - Usually ≤ 4 segments
  - May be extensive, especially with pilocytic histology
- Morphology
  - Fusiform spinal expansion with enhancing component of variable morphology
  - Occasionally asymmetric, even exophytic
    - Eccentric > central growth pattern

Radiographic Findings

- Radiography
  - ± scoliosis
  - ± expansion of osseous canal

CT Findings

- NECT
  - Enlarged SC
  - ± expansion, remodeling of osseous canal
- CECT
  - Mild/moderate enhancement

MR Findings

- T1WI
  - Cord expansion
    - Usually < 4 segments; occasionally multisegmental, even holocord (more common with pilocytic astrocytoma)
  - ± cyst/syrinx (fluid slightly hyperintense to CSF)
  - Solid portion hypo-/isointense [minority of cases may have areas of hyperintensity (methemoglobin)]
- T2WI
  - Hyperintense
- T2* GRE
  - Hyperintense; minority of cases may have hypointense areas if hemorrhagic products
- DWI
  - ↓ fractional anisotropy, ↑ ADC
- T1WI C+
  - Usually enhance (partial > total)
  - Mild/moderate > intense enhancement
  - Heterogeneous/infiltrating > homogeneous/sharply delineated

Imaging Recommendations

- Best imaging tool
  - Contrast-enhanced multiplanar MR
- Protocol advice
  - Sagittal and axial T2WI and T1WI C+ MR

DIFFERENTIAL DIAGNOSIS

Ependymoma

- Intense, sharply delineated enhancement
- Central > eccentric growth pattern
- More often seen in low thoracic cord

Other Neoplasms

- Ganglioglioma
  - Mixed T1 signal intensity due to solid, cystic components
  - Homogeneous > heterogeneous T2 hyperintensity
- Lymphoma
  - Intramedullary form presents as poorly defined, enhancing lesion
- Metastasis
  - Intramedullary nidus of enhancement much more focal with extensive edema
  - Pial metastasis can simulate hemangioblastoma
- Hemangioblastoma
  - Focal, enhancing pial/subpial nodule
  - Associated syrinx simulates astrocytoma

Syringohydromyelia

- Cyst fluid similar to CSF; no enhancement

Autoimmune or Inflammatory Myelitis

- Demyelinating disease (± patchy, ill-defined enhancement if acute)
  - Multiple sclerosis
  - Transverse myelitis
  - Infectious myelitis
    - Viral myelitis, granulomatous osteomyelitis, bacterial meningitis
- Spinal cord infarction
  - Abrupt onset
  - Risk factors: Atherosclerosis, hypertension, diabetes
  - Clinical setting: Aortic dissection, abdominal aortic aneurysm, or surgery
- Dural vascular malformation
  - Typically, cord shows mild edema and enlargement
  - Prominent pial vessels

CLINICAL ISSUES

Presentation

- Most common signs/symptoms
  - Slow onset of myelopathy
- Other signs/symptoms
  - Painful scoliosis; radiculopathy; sensory or motor deficits; incontinence

Treatment

- Serial monitoring for asymptomatic individuals; resection reserved for progressive neurologic decline
- Microsurgical resection (low-grade tumors)
- Adjuvant therapy
  - Option for WHO grades III-IV astrocytomas; no evidence that radiation therapy and chemotherapy improve long-term outcome

DIAGNOSTIC CHECKLIST

Consider

- Myelopathy should be evaluated with MR

Image Interpretation Pearls

- Axial and sagittal T1WI enhanced fat-saturated MR to exclude dural or pial lesion inciting syringomyelia

KEY FACTS

TERMINOLOGY

- Neoplasm arising from ependyma lining spinal cord central canal

IMAGING

- Circumscribed, enhancing hemorrhagic cord mass with surrounding edema
- Associated cysts common
- Cervical > thoracic > conus
- T1WI: Isointense or slightly hypointense to spinal cord
- T2WI: Hyperintense relative to spinal cord
- Cap sign: Hemosiderin at cranial or caudal margin
- Most tumors enhance
- Peripheral enhancement of tumoral cysts

TOP DIFFERENTIAL DIAGNOSES

- Astrocytoma
- Hemangioblastoma
- Demyelinating disease

- Idiopathic transverse myelitis

PATHOLOGY

- Arises from ependymal cells of central cord canal
  - Most intramedullary
  - Rarely can be intradural extramedullary
- Most WHO grade II
- Rarely WHO grade III
  - Anaplastic ependymoma
- Association with neurofibromatosis type 2

CLINICAL ISSUES

- Most common presentation
  - Neck or back pain
- Other presentations
  - Progressive paraparesis, paresthesias

DIAGNOSTIC CHECKLIST

- Spinal cord neoplasm with associated peripheral hemorrhage suggestive of cellular ependymoma

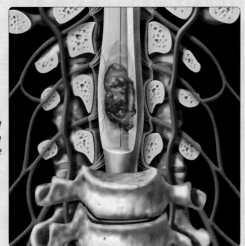
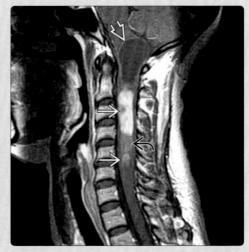

(Left) *Coronal graphic depicts an intramedullary ependymoma mildly expanding the cervical cord. Cranial and rostral cysts, as well as hemorrhagic products, are associated with this mass.* (Right) *Sagittal T1WI C+ MR demonstrates a cervical intramedullary mass with solid and cystic components causing fusiform cord expansion. There are 2 areas of enhancing solid components ➡ and a rostral cyst ➡ extending cephalad into the brainstem. The adjacent solid portion shows little enhancement ➡.*

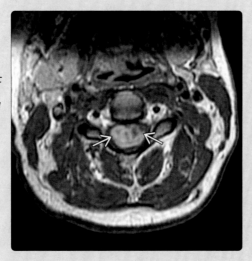
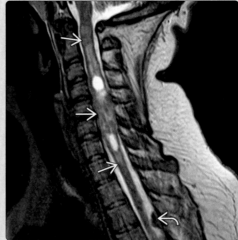

(Left) *Axial T1WI C+ MR reveals an expansile intramedullary ependymoma ➡ with robust enhancement pattern.* (Right) *Sagittal T2WI MR illustrates the mixed cystic and solid appearance of cervical ependymomas ➡ in a patient with neurofibromatosis type 2. In addition, there is a dural-based intradural extramedullary meningioma ➡.*

TERMINOLOGY

Synonyms

- Spinal ependymoma

Definitions

- Neoplasm arising from ependyma lining spinal cord central canal

IMAGING

General Features

- Best diagnostic clue
  - Circumscribed, enhancing hemorrhagic cord mass
- Location
  - Cervical > thoracic > conus
- Size
  - Multisegmental: Typically 3-4 segments
- Morphology
  - Symmetric cord expansion
  - Well circumscribed
  - ± exophytic component

MR Findings

- T1WI
  - Isointense or slightly hypointense to spinal cord
  - Hemorrhage hyperintense
- T2WI
  - Hyperintense relative to spinal cord
  - Focal hypointensity: Hemosiderin
    - Cap sign: Hemosiderin at cranial or caudal margin
  - Surrounding cord edema
- T2* GRE
  - Hypointensity (hemorrhage)
- T1WI C+
  - Tumor enhancement patterns
    - Intense, well-delineated homogeneous enhancement (50%)
    - Nodular, peripheral, or heterogeneous enhancement
    - Minimal or no enhancement (rare)

Imaging Recommendations

- Protocol advice
  - Sagittal, axial T2WI and T1WI MR ± gadolinium

DIFFERENTIAL DIAGNOSIS

Astrocytoma

- May be indistinguishable from ependymoma
  - Often longer, ± holocord
  - More often eccentric, infiltrative with indistinct margins
- Hemorrhage uncommon

Hemangioblastoma

- Cyst with enhancing highly vascular nodule
  - Flow voids often prominent
- Extensive surrounding edema relative to tumor size
- 1/3 with von Hippel-Lindau disease

Demyelinating Disease

- Multiple sclerosis
- Acute disseminated encephalomyelitis

- Ill-defined
- Typically < 2 vertebral segments in length

Idiopathic Transverse Myelitis

- Cord expansion less pronounced than ependymoma
- Centrally located, 3-4 vertebral segments in length
- Variable enhancement

PATHOLOGY

General Features

- Etiology
  - Arises from ependymal cells of central cord canal
- Genetics
  - Ependymoma associated with neurofibromatosis type 2 (NF2)
    - Deletions, translocations of chromosome 22
- Associated abnormalities
  - Superficial siderosis
  - NF2
- 4 subtypes: Cellular, papillary, clear cell, tanycytic
  - Cellular most common intramedullary tumor subtype

Staging, Grading, & Classification

- Most WHO grade II

Gross Pathologic & Surgical Features

- Soft red or grayish-purple mass
- Well circumscribed
- Cystic change common

Microscopic Features

- Immunohistochemistry: Positive for GFAP, S100, vimentin

CLINICAL ISSUES

Presentation

- Most common signs/symptoms
  - Neck or back pain
- Other signs/symptoms
  - Progressive paraparesis

Demographics

- Age
  - 35-45 years
- Epidemiology
  - Ependymomas: 4% of all primary central nervous system neoplasms in adults (30% spinal)
  - Most common primary spinal cord tumor in adults

Natural History & Prognosis

- Metastasis rare
- 5-year survival: 85%

Treatment

- Grade II ependymomas may be observed carefully after imaging confirms complete resection
- Grade III tumors require adjuvant radiation treatment
- Surgical resection
  - Gross total resection in > 85% of cases
- Radiotherapy for subtotal resection or recurrent disease
  - Typical doses of radiation therapy range from 4,000-5,400 cGy

Myxopapillary Ependymoma

TERMINOLOGY

- Slow-growing glioma arising from ependymal cells of conus, filum terminale, cauda equina

IMAGING

- Usually spans 2-4 vertebral segments
  - May fill entire lumbosacral thecal sac
- Ovoid, lobular, sausage-shaped
- CT/radiographs
  - ± osseous canal expansion, thinned pedicles, vertebral scalloping
  - May enlarge, extend through neural foramina
- T1WI: Isointense→ hyperintense to cord
- T2WI: Almost always hyperintense to cord
  - Hypointensity at tumor margin = hemosiderin
- T1WI C+: Intense enhancement

TOP DIFFERENTIAL DIAGNOSES

- Nerve sheath tumor
- Intradural metastases
- Meningioma
- Paraganglioma

PATHOLOGY

- WHO grade I
- May have local seeding or subarachnoid dissemination
- Subarachnoid hemorrhage

CLINICAL ISSUES

- Symptoms mimic disc herniation
- Back pain most common
- Other issues include paraparesis, radiculopathy, or bladder and bowel dysfunction

DIAGNOSTIC CHECKLIST

- Slow tumor growth may delay diagnosis
- Always image conus in patients presenting with back pain

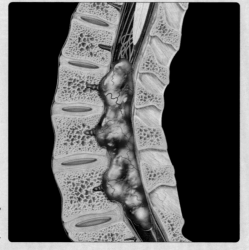
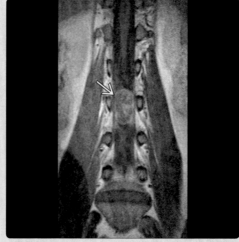

(Left) Sagittal graphic shows a multilevel cauda equina myxopapillary ependymoma. The mass is vascular with old intratumoral hemorrhage & acute subarachnoid hemorrhage along the dorsal conus. Indolent tumor growth has enlarged spinal canal & remodeled posterior vertebral cortex. (Right) Coronal T1WI MR shows a well-delineated, intradural extramedullary mass in the lumbar spine ➡. The lesion is predominantly isointense with cord & nerves. Almost 70% of filum terminale masses are ependymomas, mostly the myxopapillary-type.

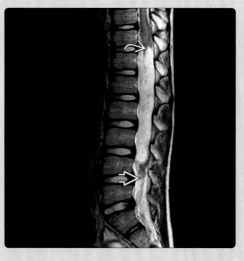
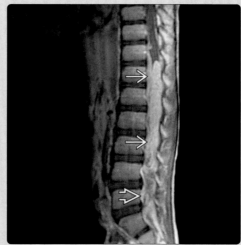

(Left) Sagittal T2WI MR reveals an extensive intradural tumor distorting the conus ➡ and cauda equina ➡. Myxopapillary ependymomas are unique in their intracellular and perivascular accumulation of proteinaceous mucin, which appears T1/T2 hyperintense. (Right) Sagittal T1WI C+ MR exhibits avid homogeneous tumor enhancement ➡. Note diffuse intradural tumor seeding ➡. Smaller tumors tend to displace the cauda equina nerve roots, whereas large tumors often compress or encase them.

Hemangioblastoma

KEY FACTS

TERMINOLOGY

- Low-grade, capillary-rich neoplasms of cerebellum and spinal cord that occur sporadically or in setting of von Hippel-Lindau (VHL) syndrome

IMAGING

- Thoracic > cervical > lumbar, sacral
- Subpial and posterior aspect of spinal cord but can arise in any cord location
- Usually shows intense and uniform contrast enhancement
- Large lesions have vessel flow voids
- Often associated with intraspinal cyst
- Extensive syrinx suggests hemangioblastoma (HB)
- Spinal cord thickening remote from tumor and without syrinx

TOP DIFFERENTIAL DIAGNOSES

- Arteriovenous malformation
- Cavernous malformation

- Hypervascular cord neoplasms
  - o Ependymoma
  - o Astrocytoma
  - o Vascular metastasis
- Intradural extramedullary tumors

PATHOLOGY

- WHO grade I
- No malignant degeneration

CLINICAL ISSUES

- 68% of spinal hemangioblastomas are sporadic (32% VHL-associated)
  - o Multiple HBs indicate VHL syndrome
- Patients with suspected hemangioblastoma and VHL should undergo contrast-enhanced MR imaging of entire neural axis to exclude multiple lesions
- Symptoms: Sensory > motor > pain

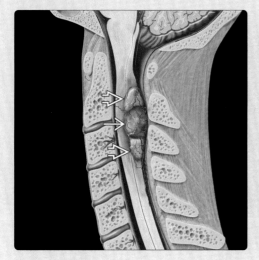

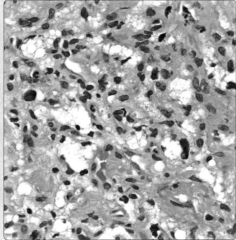

(Left) Sagittal graphic depicts a focal intramedullary mass ➡ in the cervical cord with prominent feeding vessels, adjacent cysts ➡, and cord expansion with edema. (Right) Low-power H&E shows typical stromal cells (neoplastic component of the tumor) with pale vacuolated cytoplasm (clear cells) containing lipid droplets.

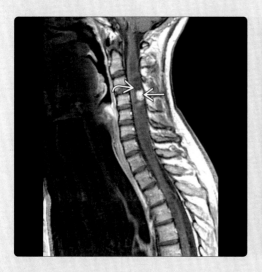

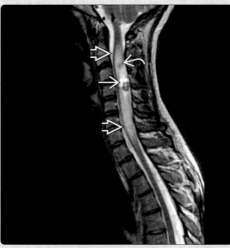

(Left) Sagittal T1WI C+ MR shows a focal enhancing mass in the dorsal cervical cord at the C4 level ➡. Distinct appearances of spinal hemangioblastoma have been described, including associated cyst/syrinx ➡, diffuse cord enlargement, exophytic morphology with minimal spinal cord reaction, and extramedullary location. (Right) T2WI MR displays a peripheral cystic component and focal mass ➡ with edema enlarging the cervical cord ➡. The ring of hypointensity ➡ suggests susceptibility due to prior hemorrhage.

KEY FACTS

TERMINOLOGY

- Metastatic lesion from primary carcinoma in another organ (including brain)

IMAGING

- Focal, enhancing cord lesion(s) with extensive edema
- Typically small (< 1.5 cm)
- T1WI: Enlarged cord
- T2WI/PD/STIR: Focal high signal represents diffuse edema
  - Rarely syrinx
- T1W C+: Focal enhancement
  - Rim sign: Intense, thin rim of peripheral enhancement around enhancing lesion
  - Flame sign: Ill-defined, flame-shaped region of enhancement at superior/inferior margins
- T2* GRE: Hypointensity due to hemorrhagic components

TOP DIFFERENTIAL DIAGNOSES

- Demyelinating disease
  - Multiple sclerosis
  - Acute disseminated encephalomyelitis
- Primary cord tumor
- Inflammatory granuloma
  - Tuberculosis
  - Sarcoidosis
- Inflammatory myelitis

CLINICAL ISSUES

- Brown-Séquard syndrome
- Rapidly progressive flaccid paraparesis
- Intramedullary spinal cord metastatic heralds poor prognosis
- Pain

DIAGNOSTIC CHECKLIST

- Full craniospinal imaging when focal cord lesion found
- Edema out of proportion to focal small cord lesion suggests metastasis, even if solitary

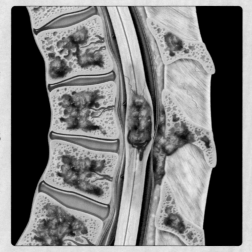
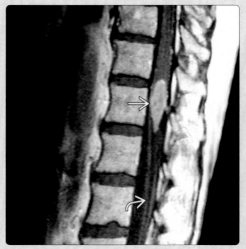

(Left) Metastases to skeleton, epidural space, & cord is shown. Hemorrhagic intramedullary metastasis expands cord. Rapid onset of symptoms is characteristic for intramedullary spinal cord metastatic (ISCM) disease. Asymmetric dysfunction of spinal cord mimicking Brown-Séquard is reported in 30-40% of ISCM disease but is exceptional in epidural spinal cord compression patients. (Right) Sagittal T1WI C+ MR shows enhancing non-small cell metastasis to the conus ➡. Note slight enhancement of cauda equina roots ➡.

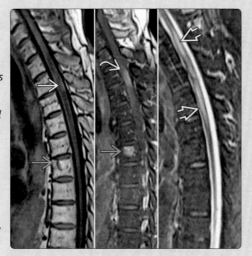
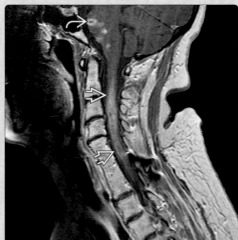

(Left) Sagittal MR shows a T1-hyperintense intramedullary lesion ➡. This ill-defined enhancing lesion ➡ on T1WI C+ FS MR was found to be a melanoma metastasis. There is extensive intramedullary edema ➡. Note the vertebral metastasis ➡. (Right) Sagittal T1WI C+ MR reveals direct extension of glioma ➡ from the brainstem inferiorly into the cervical cord. There are multiple foci of abnormal enhancement within the brainstem ➡. Spinal metastases of glioblastoma multiforme usually occurs late in the course of the disease.

KEY FACTS

TERMINOLOGY

- Uncommon neoplasms derived from normal leptomeningeal melanocytes
- Morphologic spectrum from low-grade melanocytoma to melanocytic tumor of intermediate differentiation to malignant melanoma
  - Distinct from other melanotic lesions, such as meningioma, schwannoma, melanoma

IMAGING

- Most common presentation is intradural enhancing mass showing T1 hyperintensity, not fat suppressing
  - Rarely intramedullary
- MR
  - T1WI: Isointense to hyperintense intradural lesion
    - Signal relates to paramagnetic free radicals in melanin, with shortening of T1, T2
  - T2WI: Isointense to hypointense to normal cord

- T2* GRE: May show blooming of low signal related to melanin susceptibility effect
- T1WI C+: Heterogeneous enhancement

TOP DIFFERENTIAL DIAGNOSES

- Hemorrhagic cord neoplasm
- Cavernous malformation
- Arteriovenous malformation
- Pigmented intradural extramedullary tumors
  - Malignant melanoma, meningioma, schwannoma

CLINICAL ISSUES

- Progressive back pain, extremity numbness, weakness
- Progressive, low-grade lesions curable by resection
- Can be locally invasive
- Treatment
  - Total tumor resection is optimal to prevent recurrence
  - Adjuvant radiotherapy after incomplete resection

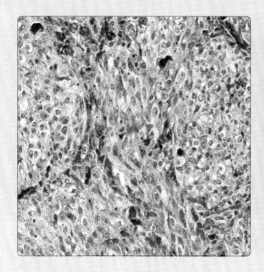
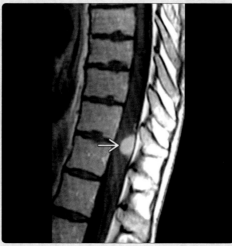

(Left) Tight nests of bland, slightly spindled cells are key features of melanocytoma. Sparsely pigmented or amelanotic tumors may be misinterpreted as meningioma. (Right) Sagittal T1 C+ MR shows there is homogeneous, marked enhancement of a T1 hyperintense intramedullary lesion ➡ in the conus medullaris.

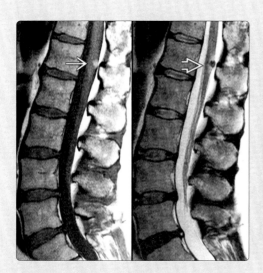
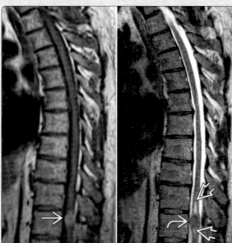

(Left) Sagittal nonenhanced T1 MR (left) shows a primary intramedullary melanocytoma of the cord with intrinsic T1 shortening ➡ that is characteristic of melanin. Sagittal T2 MR (right) shows focal low signal ➡. (Courtesy P. Hildenbrand, MD.) (Right) Sagittal T1 MR shows a well-delineated intramedullary mass in the lower thoracic cord that demonstrates high T1 ➡ (left) and low T2 signal ➡ (right). There is surrounding cord edema ➡.

KEY FACTS

TERMINOLOGY

- CSF flow-related phenomenon due to time of flight (TOF) effects and turbulent flow

IMAGING

- Location: Intrathecal, subarachnoid space
  - Most prominent in cervical and thoracic spine
- Low or high signal intensity
- Ill-defined margins

TOP DIFFERENTIAL DIAGNOSES

- Vascular malformation, type I dural arteriovenous fistula
- Vascular malformation, type IV arteriovenous fistula
- CSF drop metastases

CLINICAL ISSUES

- TOF effects
  - Dark CSF signal

- Positive relationship between CSF velocity and TOF losses
- Typically occurs in spin-echo or fast spin-echo imaging
- Flow-related enhancement produces bright CSF signal
- Turbulent flow
  - Abnormally dark signal intensity
- Ghosting artifact motion
  - Periodic motion, such as CSF pulsation, cardiac motion, and respiratory motion

DIAGNOSTIC CHECKLIST

- Flow artifacts frequently have bizarre nonanatomic appearance
- Cross-reference other imaging planes and compare with faster imaging sequences (GRE, true FISP) that reduce superimposed flow phenomenon
- Ghosting artifacts in phase-encoding direction often accompany TOF- and FRE-related signal changes, help point out true nature of those changes

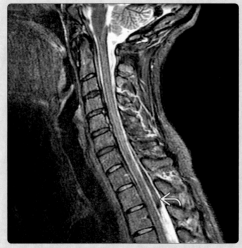

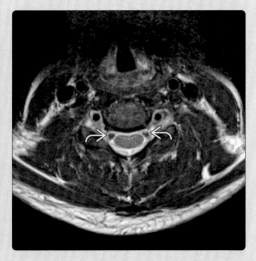

(Left) Sagittal STIR MR shows an ill-defined signal void in the dorsal subarachnoid space of the thoracic spine ➾. This artifact is due to a combination of respiratory- and cardiac-related pulsatile CSF flow superimposed on cranially directed bulk CSF flow. There is also contribution from turbulent CSF flow moving from the ventral to dorsal subarachnoid space. This complex CSF motion results in phase incoherence leading to signal loss. (Right) Axial T2WI MR confirms the CSF flow artifact ➾.

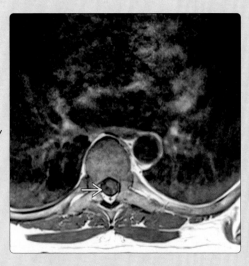

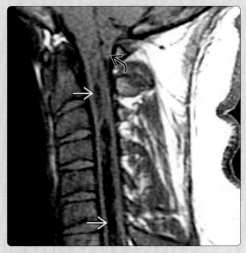

(Left) Axial T1WI MR depicts isointense CSF flow artifact dorsal to the thoracic cord in the subarachnoid space ➾. (Right) Sagittal T1WI MR exhibits syringomyelia in the cervical cord ➾. CSF flow dynamics are altered because of the cerebellar tonsillar ectopia ➾. The turbulent flow results in a broader spectrum of proton velocities, which result in more rapid dephasing and signal loss. There is also a positive relationship between CSF velocity and time of flight losses.

TERMINOLOGY

Definitions

- CSF flow-related phenomenon due to time-of-flight (TOF) effects, turbulent flow

IMAGING

General Features

- Location
  - Intrathecal, subarachnoid space
  - More prominent in cervical and thoracic spine

Imaging Recommendations

- Protocol advice
  - Turbulence dephasing ↓ by shorter TE sequences and smaller voxel volume (decreased slice thickness or higher matrix)
  - Flow-related enhancement (FRE) ↓ by applying saturation bands or by using ultrafast techniques, such as true FISP
  - BLADE shown to be superior to turbo spin-echo sequences
  - ↓ ghosting artifact by ↑ number of excitations
  - T1 FLAIR at 3T and 1.5T shows superior CSF nulling, better conspicuity of normal anatomic structures and degenerative and metastatic lesions, and improved image contrast

MR Findings

- T1WI
  - Hyperintense relative to CSF
- T2WI
  - Hypointense relative to CSF
  - Ill-defined margins
- FLAIR
  - CSF flow artifacts at 3T > 1.5T
    - Crosstalk between each inversion pulse
- T2* GRE
  - Resistant to TOF loss because of short TE
- **T1 FLAIR**
  - Relatively short TI/TR pair to produce effective nulling of CSF signal, achieve heavy T1 weighting, and optimize contrast between abnormal tissues and cord/bone marrow

DIFFERENTIAL DIAGNOSIS

Vascular Malformation, Type I Dural Arteriovenous Fistula

- Dilated pial veins cover abnormally enlarged, hyperintense distal cord

Vascular Malformation, Type IV Arteriovenous Fistula

- Intradural extra-/perimedullary arteriovenous fistula with multiple well-defined serpentine flow voids on ventral or dorsal surface of cord

CSF Drop Metastases

- Administer intravenous contrast, image in multiple planes if necessary

PATHOLOGY

General Features

- Etiology
  - Pulsatile to-and-fro movement of CSF due to expansion and contraction of brain produced by expansion and contraction of intracranial vessels associated with cardiac cycle
    - Results in significant motion-related effects that can alter visualized signal of CSF

CLINICAL ISSUES

Demographics

- Age
  - More prominent in pediatric patients

Natural History & Prognosis

- TOF effects
  - Dark CSF signal
    - More pronounced with faster proton velocity, thinner slices, longer TE, and imaging plane perpendicular to flow
    - Typically occurs in spin-echo or fast spin-echo imaging
  - Single-shot fast spin-echo (SS FSE): TOF loss during systole without TOF loss in diastole
  - Relationship between CSF velocity and TOF losses
  - Laminar flow: Peripherally located protons move at slower velocity → reduction in TOF losses
- FRE produces bright CSF signal
  - Bright signal from unsaturated protons flowing into slice replace outflowing, partially saturated protons during TR
  - Seen on more slices with single slice acquisition techniques in which every slice is entry slice
- Turbulent flow
  - Abnormal dark signal intensity
  - Varied flow velocities and directions → more rapid dephasing and signal loss, intravoxel dephasing
- Ghosting artifact motion
  - Periodic motion, such as CSF pulsation, cardiac motion, and respiratory motion
  - Phase-encoding direction
  - Bright if in phase or dark if out of phase with background signal

DIAGNOSTIC CHECKLIST

Image Interpretation Pearls

- Flow artifacts frequently have bizarre nonanatomic appearance

SELECTED REFERENCES

1. Lavdas E et al: Reduction of motion, truncation and flow artifacts using BLADE sequences in cervical spine MR imaging. Magn Reson Imaging. 33(2):194-200, 2015
2. Kwon JW et al: Three-dimensional isotropic T2-weighted cervical MRI at 3T: comparison with two-dimensional T2-weighted sequences. Clin Radiol. 67(2):106-13, 2012
3. Lisanti C et al: Normal MRI appearance and motion-related phenomena of CSF. AJR Am J Roentgenol. 188(3):716-25, 2007

KEY FACTS

TERMINOLOGY

- Intraspinal extramedullary loculated CSF collection

IMAGING

- Nonenhancing extramedullary loculated CSF intensity collection displacing cord or nerve roots
  - Solitary, multiple, or multiloculated
- Extradural or intradural extramedullary location
  - Extradural meningeal cyst (MC) may extend through enlarged neural foramina
  - Presence of intradural MC suggested by mass effect on spinal cord
- CSF intensity on T1WI, T2WI, STIR
- Cyst wall may be imperceptible
  - No enhancement
- Cap sign: Extradural MC outlined by rostral and caudal epidural fat

TOP DIFFERENTIAL DIAGNOSES

- Idiopathic spinal cord herniation
  - Focal cord atrophy and ventral deviation
- Dural ectasia
  - Spinal cord not distorted
- Spinal nerve root avulsion
  - Contiguous with subarachnoid space

PATHOLOGY

- Nabors classification of spinal MC
  - Type I: Extradural MC without spinal nerve root fibers
  - Type II: Extradural MC with spinal nerve root fibers
  - Type III: Intradural MC

CLINICAL ISSUES

- Most patients asymptomatic
- Other signs/symptoms
  - Pain, paraparesis, paresthesia
- Worsening neurologic deficits with enlarging cyst

(Left) Sagittal graphic demonstrates a type III intradural meningeal cyst in the mild dorsal thoracic canal with moderate mass effect on the spinal cord. (Right) Sagittal T2WI MR depicts an intradural dorsal meningeal cyst causing mild spinal cord compression. The cyst margins can be visualized ➡ adjacent to areas of turbulent CSF flow. This is a typical case of an intradural meningeal cyst presenting with myelopathy. The cyst was treated with surgical fenestration.

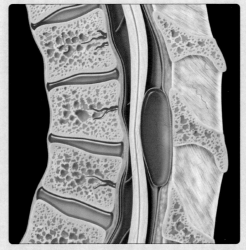
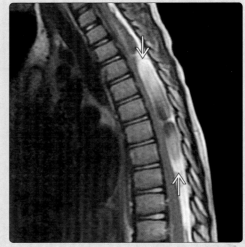

(Left) Sagittal T2 TSE MR shows a giant extradural meningeal cyst ➡ with high signal, extensive bony remodeling, and intracystic septation ➡. (Right) Axial T2WI MR shows bilateral extension of a giant extradural meningeal cyst out along both neural foramina ➡ with bony expansion and remodeling. There is ventral cord displacement and compression ➡.

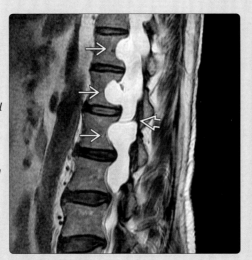
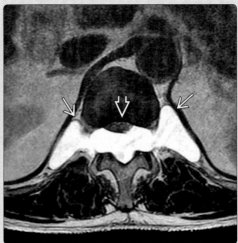

Perineural Root Sleeve Cyst

TERMINOLOGY

- Dilatation of arachnoid and dura of spinal posterior nerve root sheath containing nerve fibers

IMAGING

- Occurs anywhere along spine
  - Most common in lower lumbar spine and sacrum
  - S2 and S3 nerve roots most commonly involved
- Thin-walled cyst mass
  - Contents follow CSF density/signal intensity
  - No enhancement
- ± neural foraminal widening (bone remodeling)

TOP DIFFERENTIAL DIAGNOSES

- Facet synovial cyst
- Nerve sheath tumor
- Spinal nerve root avulsion
- Metastases
- Meningocele

PATHOLOGY

- Nabors classification of spinal meningeal cyst (MC)
  - Type I: Extradural MC without spinal nerve root fibers
    - IA: Extradural MC
    - IB: Occult sacral meningocele (outdated term)
  - Type II: Extradural MC with spinal nerve root fibers
  - Type III: Intradural MC

CLINICAL ISSUES

- Majority asymptomatic: > 80%
- Symptoms may worsen with postural changes, Valsalva maneuvers
- Cyst rupture → spontaneous intracranial hypotension
- Symptoms simulate disc herniation and spinal stenosis

DIAGNOSTIC CHECKLIST

- CSF intensity mass enlarging neural foramen or sacral canal characteristic of perineural root sleeve cyst

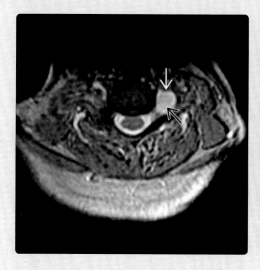

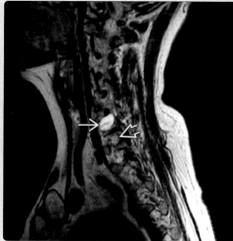

(Left) Axial T2WI MR demonstrates a focal, well-circumscribed, hyperintense perineural cyst ➡ within the left C6-C7 foramen. Subtle linear low signal ➡ within the cyst represents the exiting nerve within it. (Right) Sagittal T2WI MR confirms focal expansion of the left C6-C7 foramen by a large perineural root sleeve cyst ➡. Note the hyperintense cyst signal compared to the normal dorsal root ganglia ➡ within the adjacent level neural foramina.

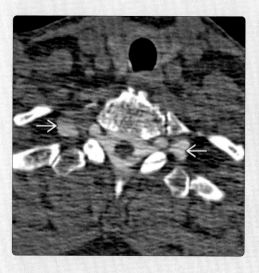

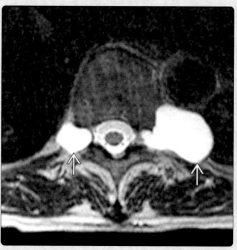

(Left) Axial CT myelography shows multiloculated bilateral T1 nerve root contrast-filled cysts ➡, confirming contiguity with the contrast-filled dural sac. Only part of the right cyst contains contrast. (Right) Axial T2WI MR of the thoracic spine demonstrates bilateral, well-circumscribed CSF intensity perineural cysts ➡ extending through the neural foramina. There is enlargement of the right neural foramen by the cyst.

Syringomyelia

KEY FACTS

TERMINOLOGY

- Hydromyelia = cystic central canal dilatation
- Syringomyelia = cystic spinal cord cavity not contiguous with central cord canal
- Syringobulbia = brainstem syrinx extension

IMAGING

- Expanded spinal cord due to dilated, beaded, or sacculated cystic cavity

TOP DIFFERENTIAL DIAGNOSES

- Ventriculus terminalis
- Cystic spinal cord tumor
- Myelomalacia

PATHOLOGY

- Hydrocephalus, Chiari 1 or 2 malformation, myelomeningocele or other spinal dysraphism, tethered cord, congenital scoliosis, spinal cord injury

CLINICAL ISSUES

- Cloak-like pain and temperature/sensory loss with preservation of position sense, proprioception, light touch
- Distal upper extremity weakness, gait instability
- Cranial neuropathy (2° to syringobulbia)
- Etiologies
  - Primary syrinx usually in young patients
    - ↑ prevalence with basilar invagination, Chiari 1 or 2 malformation
  - Secondary syrinx at any age
    - 25% of spinal cord injury patients develop syrinx

DIAGNOSTIC CHECKLIST

- Despite septated appearance, large syrinx cavities usually contiguous
- Contrast administration essential to exclude tumor in complicated cavitary lesions

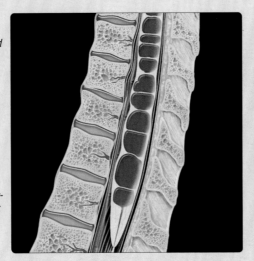

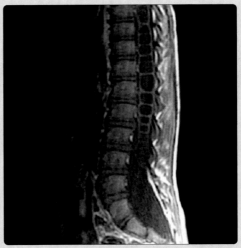

(Left) Sagittal graphic demonstrates a large, sacculated, beaded spinal cord syrinx extending to the conus. Despite the loculated appearance of large syringes, the individual fluid spaces are contiguous and drainable using a single shunt catheter. (Right) Sagittal T1WI MR (Chiari 2 malformation, not shown) depicts a large sacculated spinal cord syrinx that extends the entire length of the spinal cord into the low-lying terminal spinal cord that inserts into the dural closure at L4.

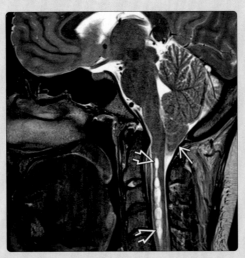

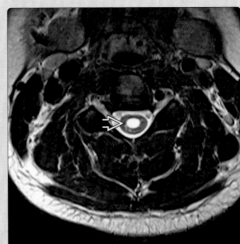

(Left) Sagittal T2WI FS MR (Chiari 1 malformation) shows inferior displacement of pointed ectopic cerebellar tonsils ➡ below the foramen magnum. Note associated cervical syringohydromyelia ⇒. (Right) Axial T2WI MR (Chiari 1 malformation, not shown) reveals typical cervical spinal cord syringohydromyelia ➡ characterized by smooth dilation of the central spinal cord canal and absence of nodularity, eccentric cavitation, or myelomalacia.

Fibrous Dysplasia

TERMINOLOGY

- McCune-Albright syndrome: Polyostotic fibrous dysplasia (FD), precocious puberty, café au lait skin lesions

IMAGING

- Most spine lesions occur with polyostotic disease
- Often causes scoliosis
- Neural arch > vertebral body
- Fusiform expansion of bone
- Cortical thinning
- Commonly ground-glass matrix
  - However, matrix may range from purely lytic to purely sclerotic lesion
- Narrow zone of transition ± sclerotic margin
- Low to intermediate signal intensity on T1WI, heterogeneous on T2WI and STIR with variable enhancement
- Mild to marked increase in radionuclide uptake

TOP DIFFERENTIAL DIAGNOSES

- Aneurysmal bone cyst
- Paget disease
- Osteoblastoma
- Osteosarcoma
- Tuberous sclerosis

PATHOLOGY

- Sporadic mutation in *GNAS* gene

CLINICAL ISSUES

- Growth disturbance, pathologic fracture
- Rarely undergoes sarcomatous transformation

DIAGNOSTIC CHECKLIST

- Do not confuse with Paget disease on imaging
  - Paget disease thickens cortex and trabeculae
  - FD thins cortex and replaces trabeculae

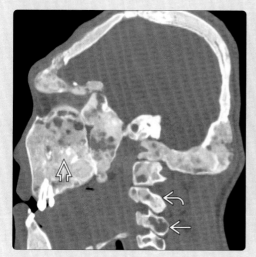

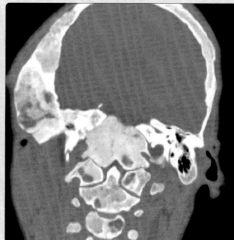

(Left) Sagittal bone CT shows severe polyostotic fibrous dysplasia (FD) involving the skull, facial bones, and cervical spine. Some areas are ground glass ➚, others are purely lytic ➔, and there are a few foci of calcified cartilage ⇒. (Right) Coronal bone CT in the same patient shows loss of normal trabeculae in the majority of the included bones replaced by FD matrix. Thinning of tables of skull is a characteristic finding.

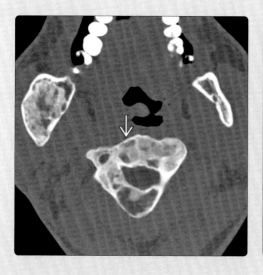

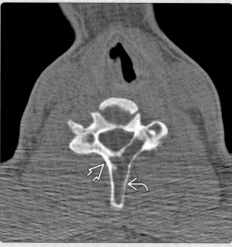

(Left) Axial bone CT shows variation in density ➔ in a single vertebra with nearly complete marrow replacement. This variability is common and should not raise suspicion for malignant degeneration. (Right) Axial bone CT shows lytic FD ➚ in the posterior elements. The narrow zone of transition ➔ (sometimes sclerotic) helps to distinguish FD from more aggressive processes. Vertebral bodies tend to be less severely involved than the posterior elements.

KEY FACTS

TERMINOLOGY

- Posttraumatic avascular necrosis of vertebral body

IMAGING

- Radiographs, CT
  - Loss of height, sclerosis of vertebral body
  - Narrow, horizontally oriented band of gas in vertebral body
  - Filling cleft in vertebral body due to fracture nonunion
- MR
  - Vertebral body collapse
  - Gas-filled cleft is low signal intensity on all sequences (unless fluid-filled)
  - Fracture line may or may not be visible
  - Less well seen than on CT scan

TOP DIFFERENTIAL DIAGNOSES

- Infection
- Nontraumatic bone infarction

- Gas within degenerated intervertebral discs
- Calcium pyrophosphate dihydrate deposition

PATHOLOGY

- Radiographically occult vertebral body clefts common in patients with fracture
- Nonunited vertebral body fracture cleft undergoes 2° necrosis, collapse
- Nitrogen accumulates in fracture cleft

CLINICAL ISSUES

- Presents with pain, kyphosis
- Usually occurs in elderly, osteoporotic patients
- Progressive vertebral body collapse if untreated

DIAGNOSTIC CHECKLIST

- Kümmell disease may be rarely associated with pathologic fracture

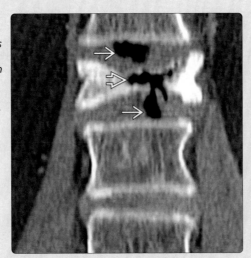 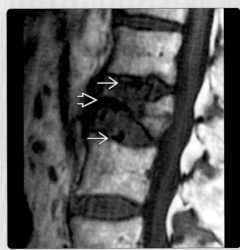

(Left) Coronal bone CT shows gas ➡ within a collapsed, sclerotic vertebral body. Gas is also present in the adjacent disc spaces ➡. The gas seen in Kümmell disease probably migrates into the vertebral body from a degenerated disc. (Right) Sagittal T1WI MR shows gas ➡ in an osteoporotic burst fracture and adjacent discs ➡. Gas could easily be mistaken for calcification on the MR.

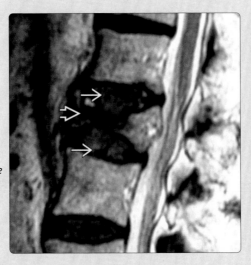 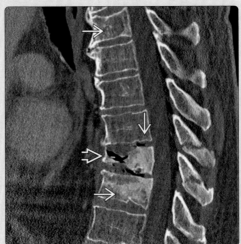

(Left) Sagittal T2WI MR reveals band-like gas in the vertebral body ➡ and gas in the intervertebral discs ➡. The findings are less conspicuous and less specific than demonstrated with bone CT. (Right) Sagittal bone CT shows gas ➡ in a collapsed vertebral body. This unusual case has occurred in a patient with metastatic disease ➡. Kümmell disease should not be presumed to always indicate a benign compression fracture. This patient had blastic metastases from prostate carcinoma.

TERMINOLOGY

Definitions

- Posttraumatic avascular necrosis of vertebral body

IMAGING

General Features

- Best diagnostic clue
  - Gas-filled cleft in flattened vertebral body
- Location
  - Thoracic or lumbar vertebral body

Radiographic Findings

- Radiography
  - Loss of height, sclerosis of vertebral body
  - Narrow, horizontally oriented band of gas in vertebral body
  - Filling cleft in vertebral body due to fracture nonunion

CT Findings

- Bone CT
  - Horizontal band of gas-filling cleft in vertebral body
  - Gas often in adjacent disc space

MR Findings

- Vertebral body collapse
- Fracture line may or may not be visible
  - Horizontal low signal intensity line on T1WI
  - Band-like high signal intensity on T2WI, STIR
- Gas-filled cleft
  - Low signal intensity on all sequences
    - May occasionally be fluid-filled, follow fluid signal intensity
  - Less well seen than on CT scan

Nuclear Medicine Findings

- Bone scan
  - Positive 3-phase bone scan

Imaging Recommendations

- Best imaging tool
  - CT scan
- Protocol advice
  - MDCT with sagittal, coronal reformations

DIFFERENTIAL DIAGNOSIS

Infection

- Small bubbles of gas sometimes present, but not cleft
- Endplate destruction
- Heterogeneous enhancement of disc and vertebral body
- Fluid collections in paraspinous soft tissues

Nontraumatic Bone Infarction

- Serpentine contour of infarction with peripheral enhancement
- Associated with steroids, sickle cell disease, pancreatitis, vasculitis, emboli, and caisson disease

Gas Within Degenerated Intervertebral Discs

- Gas forms in degenerated discs, may enter Schmorl nodes

Calcium Pyrophosphate Dihydrate Deposition (CPPD)

- Calcifications appear similar to gas on MR

PATHOLOGY

General Features

- Etiology
  - Kyphoplasty data suggests radiographically occult vertebral body clefts are common in patients with fracture
  - Nonunited vertebral body fracture undergoes secondary necrosis and collapse
  - Nitrogen accumulates in fracture cleft

CLINICAL ISSUES

Presentation

- Most common signs/symptoms
  - Pain, kyphosis

Demographics

- Age
  - Usually elderly, osteoporotic patients
- Epidemiology
  - Uncommon

Natural History & Prognosis

- Progressive vertebral body collapse if untreated

Treatment

- Options, risks, complications
  - Vertebroplasty or kyphoplasty relieves pain

DIAGNOSTIC CHECKLIST

Image Interpretation Pearls

- Kümmell disease rarely can occur in pathologic fracture due to tumor
- Gas may be seen in infection
  - Usually small bubbles, not linear cleft

SELECTED REFERENCES

1. Wang Q et al: Pathomechanism of intravertebral clefts in osteoporotic compression fractures of the spine: basivertebral foramen collapse might cause intravertebral avascular necrosis. Spine J. 14(6):1090-1, 2014
2. Lin CL et al: MRI fluid sign is reliable in correlation with osteonecrosis after vertebral fractures: a histopathologic study. Eur Spine J. 22(7):1617-23, 2013
3. Voulgari PV et al: Avascular necrosis in a patient with systemic lupus erythematosus. Joint Bone Spine. 80(6):665, 2013
4. Wu AM et al: Vertebral compression fracture with intravertebral vacuum cleft sign: pathogenesis, image, and surgical intervention. Asian Spine J. 7(2):148-55, 2013
5. van der Schaaf I et al: Percutaneous vertebroplasty as treatment for Kummell's disease. JBR-BTR. 92(2):83-5, 2009
6. Swartz K et al: Kümmell's disease: a case report and literature review. Spine (Phila Pa 1976). 33(5):E152-5, 2008
7. Jang JS et al: Efficacy of percutaneous vertebroplasty in the treatment of intravertebral pseudarthrosis associated with noninfected avascular necrosis of the vertebral body. Spine. 28(14):1588-92, 2003
8. Lane JI et al: Intravertebral clefts opacified during vertebroplasty: pathogenesis, technical implications, and prognostic significance. AJNR Am J Neuroradiol. 23(10):1642-6, 2002
9. Young WF et al: Delayed post-traumatic osteonecrosis of a vertebral body (Kümmell's disease). Acta Orthop Belg. 68(1):13-9, 2002
10. Chou LH et al: Idiopathic avascular necrosis of a vertebral body. Case report and literature review. Spine. 22(16):1928-32, 1997

KEY FACTS

TERMINOLOGY

- Synonyms: Hirayama flexion myelopathy, juvenile spinal muscular atrophy, monomelic amyotrophy, juvenile asymmetric segmental spinal muscular atrophy
- Definition: Cervical myelopathy related to anterior displacement of posterior cervical dura with flexion

IMAGING

- Asymmetric cord atrophy
- Flexion study shows increased posterior epidural space with ventral dural displacement, cord compression
- T1WI C+ shows enhancing enlarged posterior epidural space with flexion

TOP DIFFERENTIAL DIAGNOSES

- Motor neuron disease
- Chronic radiculopathy

PATHOLOGY

- Tight dural canal during flexion related to disproportionate length between vertebral column and dural canal
- Generally sporadic but familial cases have been reported
- Anterior horn cells of spinal cord levels C5-T1 show shrinkage, degeneration, and necrosis with mild gliosis

CLINICAL ISSUES

- Nonprogressive muscular atrophy confined to hand and forearm (2nd-3rd decades)
- Usually unilateral but can be bilateral
- Avoidance of neck flexion can stop progression
- May treat with posterior decompression/duraplasty

DIAGNOSTIC CHECKLIST

- Asymmetric atrophy of lower cervical cord on routine MR in patient with distal upper limb weakness is highly suspicious for Hirayama
  - Flexion cervical MR recommended

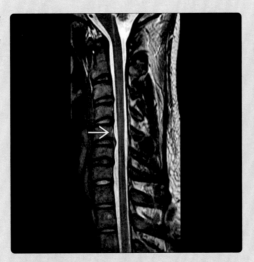
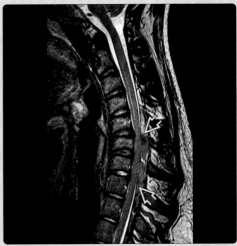

(Left) Sagittal T2WI MR shows the classic appearance of Hirayama disease. The neutral position of the MR shows mild cord atrophy at the C5-C6 level ➡ but is otherwise normal. (Right) Flexion T2WI MR shows marked ventral displacement of the posterior dural margin with cord compression ➡. A hypointense T2 signal filling the dorsal epidural space is a distended venous plexus, which will homogeneously enhance with contrast (not shown).

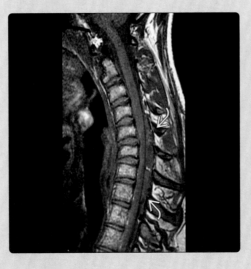
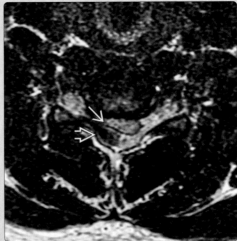

(Left) Flexion T1WI MR shows marked ventral displacement of the posterior dural margin with a long segment of cord compression. A slightly heterogeneous signal filling the dorsal epidural space reflects a distended venous plexus ➡. (Right) Axial T2WI MR in flexion shows a markedly distended posterior epidural plexus ➡. There is ventral displacement of the posterior dura with asymmetrical cord compression, worse on the right ➡.

TERMINOLOGY

Synonyms

- Hirayama flexion myelopathy, juvenile spinal muscular atrophy, monomelic amyotrophy, juvenile asymmetric segmental spinal muscular atrophy

Definitions

- Cervical myelopathy related to anterior displacement of posterior cervical dura with flexion

IMAGING

General Features

- Best diagnostic clue
  - Anterior displacement of posterior cervical dura on MR
- Location
  - Cervical
- Size
  - Variable
- Morphology
  - Anterior displacement of linear posterior dura

CT Findings

- Myelography shows unilateral cord atrophy
- Flexion studies difficult due to contrast movement

MR Findings

- T1WI
  - Asymmetric cord atrophy
  - Flexion study shows increased posterior epidural space with ventral dural displacement, cord compression
- T2WI
  - Asymmetric cord atrophy, cord hyperintensity at atrophic area
  - Flexion study shows increased posterior epidural space with ventral dural displacement, cord compression
- T1WI C+
  - Enhancing enlarged posterior epidural space with flexion

Imaging Recommendations

- Best imaging tool
  - Flexion MR

DIFFERENTIAL DIAGNOSIS

Motor Neuron Disease

- Diagnosis of exclusion without spinal imaging findings

Chronic Radiculopathy

- Disc disease

PATHOLOGY

General Features

- Etiology
  - Controversial
  - Dynamic spinal cord compression with neck flexion
  - Tight dural canal during flexion related to disproportionate length between vertebral column and dural canal
    - Length of cervical canal increases with flexion

- Dural sac compensates for this lengthening in normal subjects
- Imbalance of growth of vertebrae and dura in Hirayama causes tight dural canal with flexion with anterior shift
- Genetics
  - Generally sporadic but familial cases have been reported

Gross Pathologic & Surgical Features

- Anterior horn cells of spinal cord levels C5-T1 showed shrinkage, degeneration, and necrosis with mild gliosis
  - Suggested circulatory insufficiency in these areas related to chronic trauma of cord compression
- Abnormal posterior dura with few elastic fibers

CLINICAL ISSUES

Presentation

- Most common signs/symptoms
  - Muscular atrophy confined to hand and forearm
  - Usually unilateral but can be bilateral
  - Disease onset insidious
  - No sensory or pyramidal tract involvement

Demographics

- Age
  - 2nd to 3rd decades
- Gender
  - M > F

Natural History & Prognosis

- Clinical course characterized by steady progression with eventual stabilization

Treatment

- Avoidance of neck flexion can stop progression
  - Cervical collar for 3-4 years
- Selected patients treated with posterior decompression with duraplasty, rarely anterior fusion

DIAGNOSTIC CHECKLIST

Image Interpretation Pearls

- Asymmetric atrophy of lower cervical cord on routine MR in patient with distal upper limb weakness suspicious for Hirayama
  - Flexion MR recommended

SELECTED REFERENCES

1. Paredes I et al: A severe case of Hirayama disease successfully treated by anterior cervical fusion. J Neurosurg Spine. 20(2):191-5, 2014
2. Lehman VT et al: Cervical spine MR imaging findings of patients with Hirayama disease in North America: a multisite study. AJNR Am J Neuroradiol. 34(2):451-6, 2013
3. Patel TR et al: Lack of epidural pressure change with neck flexion in a patient with Hirayama disease: case report. Neurosurgery. 64(6):E1196-7; discussion E1197, 2009
4. Zhou B et al: Clinical features of Hirayama disease in mainland China. Amyotroph Lateral Scler. Epub ahead of print, 2009
5. Misra UK et al: A clinical, magnetic resonance imaging, and survival motor neuron gene deletion study of Hirayama disease. Arch Neurol. 62(1):120-3, 2005
6. Chen CJ et al: Hirayama flexion myelopathy: neutral-position MR imaging findings--importance of loss of attachment. Radiology. 231(1):39-44, 2004

TERMINOLOGY

- Osteitis deformans
- Chronic metabolic disorder of abnormal bone remodeling in adult skeleton

IMAGING

- Enlarged vertebra with trabecular coarsening and cortical thickening
  - Both vertebral body and neural arch involved
- Lumbar spine most common
- Picture frame vertebra
  - Central osteopenia
  - Coarse and sclerotic peripheral trabecular pattern
- Diffusely dense ivory vertebra
- Fibrovascular marrow in active phase
- Fatty marrow in mixed phase
- Blastic inactive phase
  - Marrow space low T1/T2 signal representing sclerosis-fibrosis

TOP DIFFERENTIAL DIAGNOSES

- Osteoblastic metastases
- Vertebral hemangioma

PATHOLOGY

- Sites of osseous involvement
  - Pelvis = spine > femur > skull > tibia > clavicle > humerus > ribs
  - Polyostotic, asymmetric > monostotic
- Possible viral etiology
  - Measles virus of Paramyxovirus family found in osteoclasts

CLINICAL ISSUES

- 20% asymptomatic
- Deep, dull bone pain
- Sarcomatous transformation: < 1%
- Myelopathy, cauda equina syndrome from canal narrowing

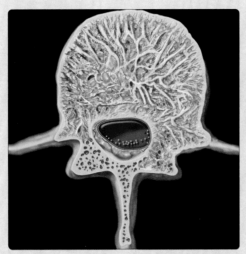
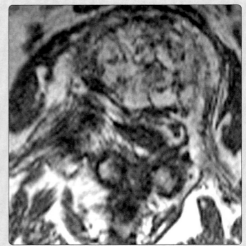

(Left) Axial graphic of pagetic vertebrae demonstrates an enlarged vertebral body, pedicles, and left facet with trabecular thickening and increased fatty marrow. Paget disease is a chronic metabolic disorder of abnormal bone remodeling and may virtually affect every bone in the skeleton. (Right) Axial T1WI MR through a lumbar vertebra shows coarse and irregular trabeculae with mild vertebral expansion. The pagetic bone marrow contains fatty areas with a heterogeneous distribution.

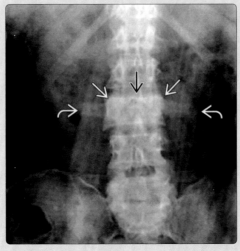
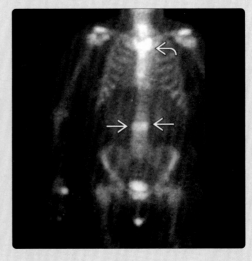

(Left) Anteroposterior radiograph depicts an enlarged L3 vertebral body ➡, pedicles ➡, and transverse processes ➡. Increased density gives the ivory vertebra appearance. The coarse and sclerotic peripheral trabecular pattern and central osteopenia gives the picture frame appearance. (Right) Anteroposterior bone scan reveals ↑ uptake in the L3 vertebra ➡. Increased uptake in the sternum ➡ is suspicious for Paget disease. Bone pain is common in the lumbar spine.

Bone Infarction

KEY FACTS

TERMINOLOGY

- Infarction of vertebral body cancellous bone and marrow secondary to systemic disease or aortic pathology
  - **Not** osteonecrosis (Kümmell disease)

IMAGING

- Well-defined, geographic signal abnormality, which tends to involve anterior 1/3 to 1/2 of vertebral body
- T2WI shows increased signal in multiple bodies with abrupt transition to normal marrow signal
- T1WI C+ shows markedly diminished enhancement of affected vertebral body areas
  - No associated epidural or paravertebral soft tissue
  - Rare to involve posterior elements

TOP DIFFERENTIAL DIAGNOSES

- Infarction secondary to underlying systemic disease
  - Sickle cell
  - Acute leukemia (ALL or AML)
    - SLE
    - Lymphoma
    - Transplantation with graft-vs.-host disease
- Infarction secondary to aortic disease
  - Dissection
  - Abdominal aortic surgery
- Metastatic disease marrow infiltration
- Leukemia or lymphoma marrow tumor infiltration
- Granulomatous or fungal infection

CLINICAL ISSUES

- Nonspecific back pain in setting of systemic illness

DIAGNOSTIC CHECKLIST

- Infarction as sign of systemic illness or malignancy, such as leukemia
- Associated with spinal cord infarction; useful as a confirmatory sign that nonspecific T2 hyperintensity in cord reflects infarction

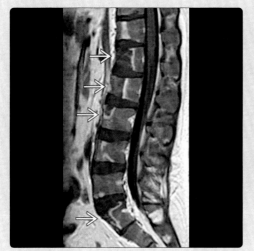

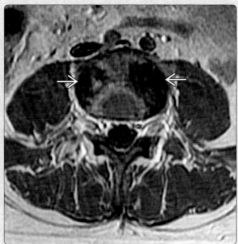

(Left) Sagittal T1WI C+ MR in a patient with a new diagnosis of lymphocytic leukemia shows multiple, well-defined, geographic foci of diminished enhancement ➡ in multiple vertebral bodies with a rim of increased enhancement. There is no associated soft tissue mass and no disc involvement. (Right) Axial T1WI C+ MR in a patient with multiple vertebral infarcts and a new diagnosis of acute leukemia (ALL) shows sharply marginated lesions in both right and left sides of the vertebral body ➡ with mild peripheral enhancement.

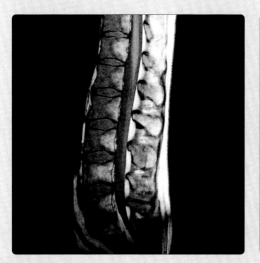

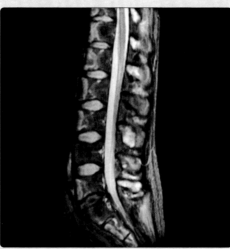

(Left) Sagittal T1WI MR shows multiple infarcts in a patient with ALL status post chemotherapy. Note well-defined low signal present in the anterior 1/2 of multiple vertebral bodies. (Courtesy M. Pathria, MD.) (Right) Sagittal T2WI FS MR in a patient with ALL status post chemotherapy shows focal, well-defined hyperintensity in the anterior 1/2 of multiple vertebral bodies, which also involves the sacrum. (Courtesy M. Pathria, MD.)

KEY FACTS

TERMINOLOGY

- Epidural ± paravertebral proliferation of hematopoietic tissue in response to profound chronic anemia
- Minimally enhancing isointense thoracic intra- or paraspinal masses with associated diffuse marrow hypointensity

IMAGING

- Midthoracic > cervical, lumbar
- CT
  - Soft tissue density, without bony erosion or calcification
- MR
  - T1: Isointense to cord
  - T2: Iso- to mildly hyperintense to cord

TOP DIFFERENTIAL DIAGNOSES

- Epidural/paraspinal metastasis
- Spinal epidural lymphoma
- Paravertebral phlegmon/abscess
- Peripheral nerve sheath tumor

- Epidural hematoma

PATHOLOGY

- Ectopic hematopoietic rests stimulated in response to chronic anemic states
  - Intermediate β-thalassemia: Most common
  - Sickle cell anemia
  - Polycythemia vera
  - Myelofibrosis with myeloid metaplasia

CLINICAL ISSUES

- Asymptomatic
- Back ± radicular pain
- Treatment includes
  - Radiation therapy
  - Intravenous steroids
  - Decompressive laminectomy with surgical resection
  - Transfusions
  - Hydroxyurea

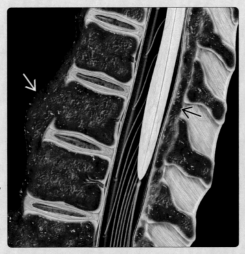

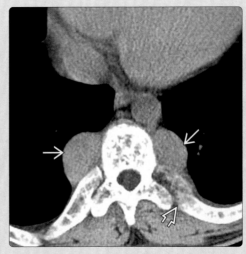

(Left) *Sagittal graphic of extramedullary hematopoiesis (EMH) depicts hematopoietic marrow extending into prevertebral ➡ and epidural space ➡. EMH is a common compensatory phenomenon to chronic hemolytic anemias.* (Right) *Axial NECT through the lower thoracic spine shows paraspinal soft tissue masses ➡ and medullary expansion of the vertebra and ribs ➡. With extramedullary hematopoiesis there is marrow expansion from severe anemia and paraspinal masses as extramedullary hematopoietic elements.*

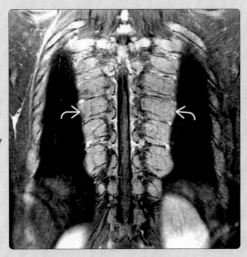

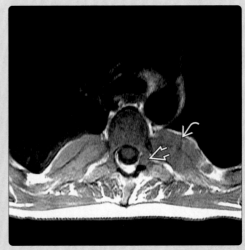

(Left) *Coronal T1WI C+ FS MR of the spine and paraspinal tissues demonstrates deposits of extramedullary hematopoiesis extending from the ribs ➡. Due to insufficient production of blood elements by the bone marrow, hematopoietic tissues at other sites proliferate to compensate for the circulatory demands for blood elements.* (Right) *Axial T1WI MR reveals foci of extramedullary hematopoiesis breaking through the vertebral bodies into the neural foramina ➡ from the ribs ➡.*

Tumoral Calcinosis

KEY FACTS

TERMINOLOGY

- Benign periarticular soft tissue hyperplasia, calcification

IMAGING

- Nonaggressive-appearing calcific mass centered about large synovial joints
- Predilection for large joints
  - Hip
  - Shoulder
  - Elbow
  - Spinal involvement uncommon
- Radiographs/CT
  - Calcific mass with clustered calcific aggregates surrounding joint
- T1/T2/STIR
  - Lobulated low-signal masses centered on facet joint
  - May extend into adjacent paraspinal soft tissue
  - Minimal enhancement

- May extend beyond midline to involve dorsal elements, ligamentum flavum

TOP DIFFERENTIAL DIAGNOSES

- Calcium pyrophosphate deposition disease
- Primary bone tumor
- Synovial chondromatosis
- Neuropathic joint
- Synovial cyst

PATHOLOGY

- Complication of chronic renal failure, on renal dialysis
- Familial tumoral calcinosis (FTC)
  - Normophosphatemic FTC
    - Likely related to mutations in gene encoding for SAMD9 protein
  - Hyperphosphatemic FTC
    - Increased renal absorption of phosphate due to loss-of-function mutations

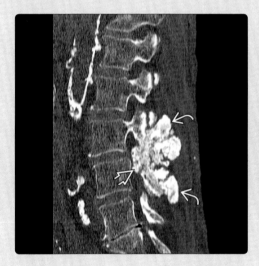

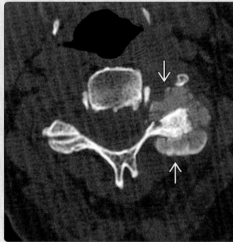

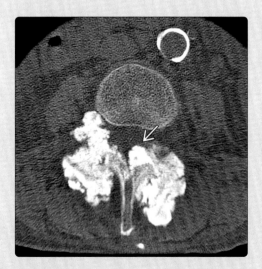

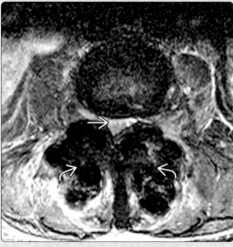

(Left) Sagittal lumbar CT shows mass-like calcifications involving posterior elements ➔. Calcified masses extend into the bony canal causing central canal encroachment ➔. Radiodense periarticular masses are usually calcium hydroxyapatite crystals surrounded by foreign body giant cell and histiocytic reaction. (Right) Axial NECT through the cervical spine shows lobulated density ➔ surrounding the facet joint with well-defined margins and no soft tissue component. (Courtesy N. Stence, MD.)

(Left) Axial bone CT reveals central canal encroachment ➔ due to copious posterior element calcifications. (Right) Axial T2WI MR exhibits hypointensity of these posterior element calcified masses ➔. There is moderate mass effect upon the nerve roots within the thecal sac ➔. Tumoral calcinosis is usually associated with hereditary disorders of calcium metabolism or renal dialysis. It also occurs in degenerated tissues in the absence of systemic disorders.

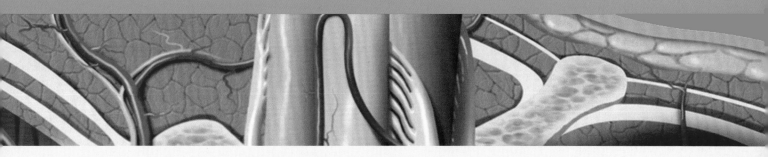

SECTION 9
Vascular Disorders

Terminology

Abbreviations: Anterior spinal artery (ASA), posterior spinal artery (PSA), artery of Adamkiewicz (AA)

Synonyms: Great anterior radicular artery, arteria radicularis magna = AA radicularis magna = AA

Imaging Anatomy

Vertebral Artery

The vertebra artery is divided into 4 segments. The **1st segment** (V1) of the vertebral artery extends from its origin to the point of entrance into the foramen of the cervical transverse process, which is usually the 6th body. The vertebral artery is usually the most proximal and largest branch off of the subclavian artery. Multiple variations in the anatomic course and origins of the vertebral arteries have been described. The most common variation in vertebral artery origin is in the origination from the proximal subclavian artery. The origin of the left vertebral artery from the aortic arch between the left common carotid artery and left subclavian artery has been described in 2.4-5.8% of cases. When there is an origin of the vertebral artery from the arch, the vertebral artery usually enters the foramen of the transverse process of the 5th cervical vertebrae. With a normal origin of the left vertebral artery from the subclavian artery, the vertebral artery enters the transverse foramen of the 6th cervical vertebrae in nearly 88% of cases. The site of entrance at the level of C4 is seen in 0.5%, C5 in 6.6%, and C7 in 5.4%. Rare examples of origins of the left vertebral artery from the left common carotid artery, or external carotid artery, have been described. Also rare are variations in the origin of the right vertebral artery (less than 1%) from the aorta, carotid arteries, or brachiocephalic arteries.

The **2nd segment** (V2) of the vertebral artery extends superiorly through the foramen of the transverse processes in a vertical course until it reaches the transverse process of C2. The **3rd segment** (V3) of the vertebral artery extends from the exit of C2 to its entrance into the spinal canal. After leaving the transverse foramen of C2, it courses laterally and posteriorly to pass through the transverse foramen of C1. The vertebral artery then extends posterior and medially in a horizontal groove on the upper surface of the posterior arch of C1. The vertebral artery turns abruptly as it nears the midline and pierces the posterior atlantooccipital membrane and enters into the vertebral canal. Anomalous connections in this region are uncommon but include the proatlantal intersegmental artery, which can communicate between the internal or external carotid artery and the vertebral artery at this level. Local duplication or fenestration of the V3 segment can occur. The occipital artery also can arise from the V3 segment. A persistent 1st intersegmental artery can occur where the vertebral artery courses below the C1 arch after exiting the transverse foramen of C2 and enters the spinal canal without passing through the C1 transverse foramen (3-4%). The origin of the posterior inferior cerebellar artery may also be anomalously low between C1 and C2.

The **4th segment** (V4) segment pierces the dura and extends through the foramen magnum where it lies anterior to the medulla and eventually joins the contralateral vertebral artery to form the basilar artery. Major branches arising off the vertebral artery include multiple muscular branches from the extracranial segments to supply the deep muscles of the neck and meningeal branches. The posterior meningeal branch arises from the vertebral artery above the level of C1 and below the foramen magnum and supplies the falx cerebelli and the medial portion of the dura of the occipital posterior fossa. Just before joining to form the basilar artery, each of the vertebral arteries gives off a branch that will become the ASA, which extends downward and medially to join in the midline with a corresponding branch from the other vertebral artery. The posterior spinal arteries can originate from the posterior inferior cerebellar arteries or from the intracranial portion of the vertebral arteries.

Spinal Arteries

The spinal cord circulation is derived from segmental branches off of the vertebral arteries as well as multiple radicular arteries arising from segmental vessels. These segmental vessels include the descending cervical, deep cervical, intercostal, lumbar, and sacral arteries. The ASA arises at the junction of the intradural segment of the vertebral arteries, caudal to the basilar artery. The ASA descends in the midline without interruption from the foramen magnum to the filum terminale. The ASA supply is reinforced by multiple segmental feeders. The segmental feeders give rise to sulcal, or central branches, which supply the anterior 2/3 of the cord. The anterior 2/3 includes the anterior horns, spinothalamic tracts, and corticospinal tracts. The ASA lies in the midline on a ventral aspect of the cord in the groove of the anterior median fissure. The posterior spinal arteries arise from the posterior rami of the vertebral artery or from the posterior inferior cerebellar artery.

The PSAs are a paired longitudinal system of vessels on the dorsal cord medial to the dorsal roots. These form a plexiform and variable network between the 2 dorsal arteries. The PSA supplies the posterior 1/3 of the cord, which includes supply to the posterior columns and a variable supply to the corticospinal tracts. Continuation of both the ASA and PSA supply is derived from segmental anastomoses. These segmental vessels arise as dorsal rami from vertebral, subclavian, thoracic intercostal, and lumbar intercostal arteries. The dorsal rami enter the canal through the neural foramen and then penetrate the dura and divide into 2 main branches: The dural artery, which supplies the nerve root sleeve and the dura, and the radiculomedullary branch. The radiculomedullary branch then divides into a radicular artery, which penetrates the subarachnoid space to supply the anterior and posterior roots. There is also a variable medullary artery branch, which joins the ASA and PSA. The radicular arteries arise from the division of the radiculomedullary arteries along the anterior and posterior nerve roots. The anterior radicular artery extends along the anterior surface of the spinal cord, while the posterior radicular artery likewise extends along the posterior cord surface.

The multiple fetal segmental vessels will regress with adulthood, leaving 2-14 (average 6) anterior radicular arteries persisting in the adult and 11-16 posterior radicular arteries in the adult. The major cervical radicular feeders to the spinal cord occur between the C5-C7 levels. There are 2-3 anterior cervical cord feeders that measure 400-600 microns in size. There are also 3-4 posterior cervical cord feeders, which are smaller in size, on the order of 150-400 microns. The V3 segment never gives rise to radiculomedullary branches. In the thoracic spine, there are 2-3 anterior thoracic cord feeding segmental vessels. These are usually left-sided and are on the order of 550-1200 microns in size. Small ventral feeding vessels may also be present on the order of 200 microns. There is an inverse relationship between the number and caliber of ventral radicular vessels. There "pauci-segmental" anatomy can occur with fewer vessels (< 5) with larger caliber or "plurisegmental" anatomy with more vessels with smaller caliber. The dominant thoracic anterior radicular artery is also called the **AA**. The AA tends to have a left-sided origin (73%) and arises from T9-T12 (62%), with less common origins in the lumbar region (26%) and from T6-T8 (12%). A major segmental feeder may also occur in the upper thoracic spine, often at the T5 level. This has been termed the artery of **von Haller**. The number of posterior thoracic cord feeding vessels varies from 9-12, with an average of 8. The posterior thoracic feeding vessels have no right-to-left lateralization. These vessels are on the order of 150-400 microns in size. The lumbosacral and pelvic regions have from 0-1 major feeding vessels to the spinal cord. The ASA ends at the conus with communicating branches (rami cruciantes) to the PSA. The posterior division of the iliac artery gives rise to the inferior and superior lateral sacral branches, which give rise to the spinal arteries via the anterior sacral foramen. The anterior division of the iliac artery gives rise to the inferior gluteal artery, which supplies the sciatic nerve. The posterior division of the internal iliac artery gives rise to the iliolumbar artery, which supplies the femoral nerve at the iliac wing level.

Spinal Veins

The veins of the spinal cord parallel the spinal arterial pattern. There is a very symmetrical pattern of venous drainage (compared with the highly asymmetrical arterial supply) with minimal anterior-to-posterior, right-to-left segmental variation. There are 2 sets of intrinsic radial draining veins, which drain into the anastomoses on the cord surface. The central group of veins provides for return of the anterior horns and surrounding white matter and drain into the central veins in the anterior median fissure. This forms the anterior median vein. Peripheral dorsal and lateral cord drainage is via the small, valveless radial vein plexus, which extends to the coronal venous plexus on the cord surface and then drains to the epidural venous plexus of Batson. The epidural plexus consists of anterior and posterior internal vertebral plexus components and connects with the superior and inferior vena cava, azygos and hemiazygos systems, and the intracranial dural sinuses. There are from 30-70 medullary radicular veins. The anterior median vein continues caudally along the filum terminale to the end of the dural sac. The coronal and median veins drain to the medullary veins, which leave the intradural space at the root sleeve and extend into the epidural plexus. Medullary veins have a functional valve-like mechanism at the dural margin, which prevents epidural reflux into the intradural space. There are no intradural valves present.

Embryology

The embryogenesis of the vertebral artery begins at approximately day 32 and is completed by day 40. The vertebral artery is formed from fusion of the longitudinal anastomosis that links cervical intersegmental arteries, which branch off of primitive paired dorsal aorta. The intersegmental arteries regress, except for the 7th vessel, which will come to form the proximal portion of the subclavian artery, including the origin of the vertebral artery. As the connections to the primitive dorsal aorta disappear, the vertebral artery takes shape and initially has a more beaded anastomotic appearance and a tortuous course. The basilar artery is formed by fusion of the 2 primitive vertebral arteries.

Spinal cord vessels originate from a capillary network on the ventral lateral surface of the cord connected with segmental aortic branches. Two primitive longitudinal systems are formed. By the end of the 2nd month, the ventrolateral systems transform into the longitudinal solitary anterior median ASA. The plexus-like pattern remains more prominent on the dorsal surface of the cord. The ASA formation is followed by a variable regression of segmental feeding vessels (initially 31) and is completed by the 4th month of gestation. The reduction is most pronounced in the thoracic and lumbar areas. Segmental arteries persist as intercostal and lumbar arteries. In the cervical spine, dorsal intersegmental anastomoses persist as components of the vertebral arteries. The ventral anastomoses persist as the thyrocervical trunk.

Selected References

1. Gailloud P: The artery of von Haller: a constant anterior radiculomedullary artery at the upper thoracic level. Neurosurgery. 73(6):1034-43, 2013
2. Eskander MS et al: Vertebral artery anatomy: a review of two hundred fifty magnetic resonance imaging scans. Spine (Phila Pa 1976). 35(23):2035-40, 2010
3. Becske T et al: The vascular anatomy of the vertebro-spinal axis. Neurosurg Clin N Am. 20(3):259-64, 2009
4. Bell R et al: Neurovascular anatomy: a practical guide. Neurosurg Clin N Am. 20(3):265-78, 2009
5. Debette S et al: Cervical-artery dissections: predisposing factors, diagnosis, and outcome. Lancet Neurol. 8(7):668-78, 2009
6. Goyal MS et al: The diagnosis and management of supraaortic arterial dissections. Curr Opin Neurol. 22(1):80-9, 2009
7. Johnson MH et al: Vascular anatomy: the head, neck, and skull base. Neurosurg Clin N Am. 20(3):239-58, 2009
8. Kim YK et al: Cervical artery dissection: pathology, epidemiology and management. Thromb Res. 123(6):810-21, 2009
9. Tubbs RS et al: Surgical anatomy and quantitation of the branches of the V2 and V3 segments of the vertebral artery. Laboratory investigation. J Neurosurg Spine. 11(1):84-7, 2009
10. Wang S et al: Anomalous vertebral artery in craniovertebral junction with occipitalization of the atlas. Spine (Phila Pa 1976). 34(26):2838-42, 2009
11. Bagheri SC et al: Penetrating neck injuries. Oral Maxillofac Surg Clin North Am. 20(3):393-414, 2008
12. Chen JW: Cervical spine injuries. Oral Maxillofac Surg Clin North Am. 20(3):381-91, 2008
13. Turan TN et al: Treatment of intracranial atherosclerotic stenosis. Rev Neurol Dis. 5(3):117-24, 2008
14. Schmidt WA: Takayasu and temporal arteritis. Front Neurol Neurosci. 21:96-104, 2006
15. Nelson PK et al: Vertebrospinal angiography in the evaluation of vertebral and spinal cord disease. Neuroimaging Clin N Am. 6(3):589-605, 1996

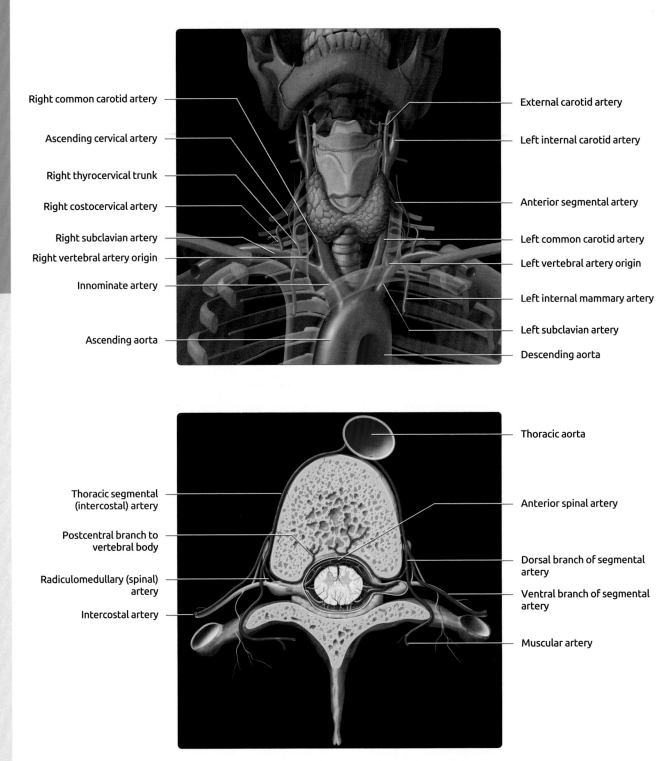

Right common carotid artery

Ascending cervical artery

Right thyrocervical trunk

Right costocervical artery

Right subclavian artery

Right vertebral artery origin

Innominate artery

Ascending aorta

External carotid artery

Left internal carotid artery

Anterior segmental artery

Left common carotid artery

Left vertebral artery origin

Left internal mammary artery

Left subclavian artery

Descending aorta

Thoracic aorta

Thoracic segmental (intercostal) artery

Postcentral branch to vertebral body

Radiculomedullary (spinal) artery

Intercostal artery

Anterior spinal artery

Dorsal branch of segmental artery

Ventral branch of segmental artery

Muscular artery

(Top) *AP graphic shows the aortic arch and arterial great vessels in red. The vertebral arteries give rise to the anterior and posterior spinal arteries. The ascending cervical arteries (branches of the thyrocervical trunks) give off anterior and posterior segmental medullary arteries that anastomose with the anterior spinal artery and posterior spinal artery on the cord surface. Complete spinal angiography includes evaluation of all these vessels.* **(Bottom)** *Axial graphic shows an overview of the arterial supply to the vertebral column and its contents, depicted here for the lower thoracic spine. A series of paired segmental arteries (cervical region arises from the vertebral and thyrocervical arteries, thoracic region are intercostal arteries, and lumbar region are lumbar arteries) divide into anterior and posterior branches. The posterior branch gives rise to a muscular branch, a branch to the vertebral body, and the radiculomedullary artery. The radiculomedullary artery enters the vertebral canal via the neural foramen.*

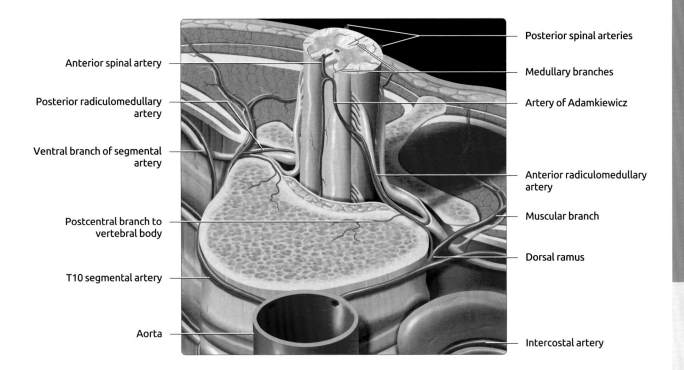

Posterior spinal arteries

Anterior spinal artery

Medullary branches

Posterior radiculomedullary artery

Artery of Adamkiewicz

Ventral branch of segmental artery

Anterior radiculomedullary artery

Postcentral branch to vertebral body

Muscular branch

T10 segmental artery

Dorsal ramus

Aorta

Intercostal artery

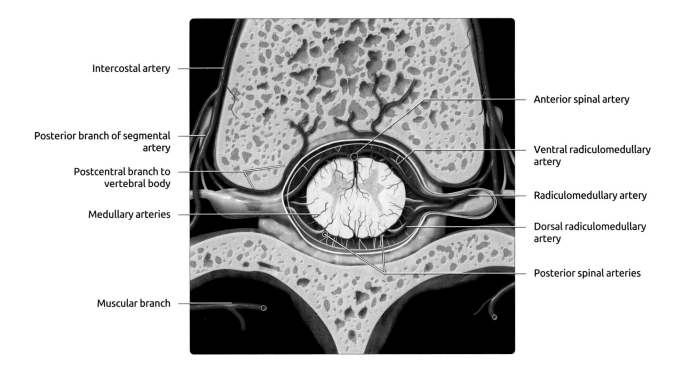

Intercostal artery

Anterior spinal artery

Posterior branch of segmental artery

Ventral radiculomedullary artery

Postcentral branch to vertebral body

Radiculomedullary artery

Medullary arteries

Dorsal radiculomedullary artery

Posterior spinal arteries

Muscular branch

(Top) *Oblique axial graphic rendering of T10 depicts segmental intercostal arteries arising from the lower thoracic aorta. The artery of Adamkiewicz is the dominant segmental feeding vessel to the thoracic cord, supplying the anterior aspect of the cord via the anterior spinal artery. Note its characteristic hairpin turn on the cord surface as it 1st courses superiorly, then turns inferiorly.* (Bottom) *Anterior and posterior radiculomedullary arteries anastomose with the anterior and posterior spinal arteries. Penetrating medullary arteries in the cord are largely end arteries with few collaterals. The cord watershed zone is at the central gray matter.*

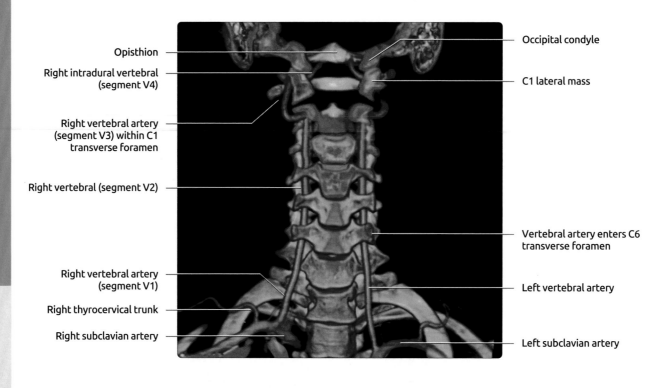

Opisthion — — Occipital condyle

Right intradural vertebral (segment V4) — — C1 lateral mass

Right vertebral artery (segment V3) within C1 transverse foramen —

Right vertebral (segment V2) —

— Vertebral artery enters C6 transverse foramen

Right vertebral artery (segment V1) — — Left vertebral artery

Right thyrocervical trunk —

Right subclavian artery — — Left subclavian artery

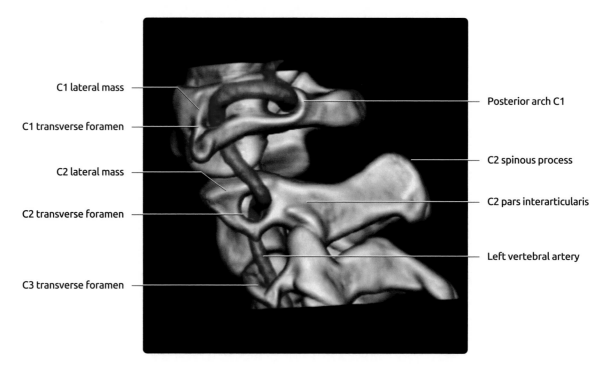

C1 lateral mass — — Posterior arch C1

C1 transverse foramen —

C2 lateral mass — — C2 spinous process

C2 transverse foramen — — C2 pars interarticularis

C3 transverse foramen — — Left vertebral artery

(Top) *AP volume-rendered image of a CTA shows the course of the vertebral arteries entering the transverse foramen and ascending to the foramen magnum. Both vertebral arteries in this patient enter the C6 level, but this can show wide normal variation. Left vertebral arteries arising from the arch enter more cephalad at C5.* **(Bottom)** *Lateral volume-rendered CTA shows the course of the distal left vertebral artery passing through C1 and horizontally oriented C2 transverse foramen.*

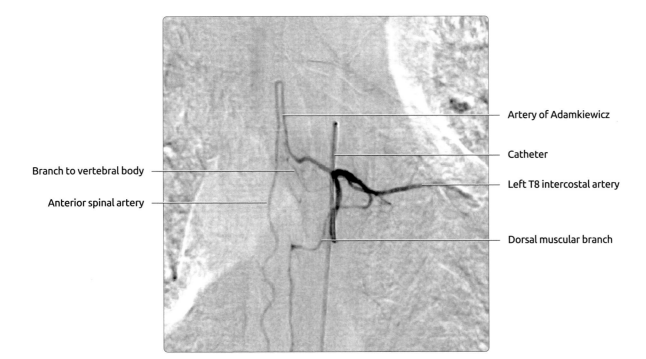

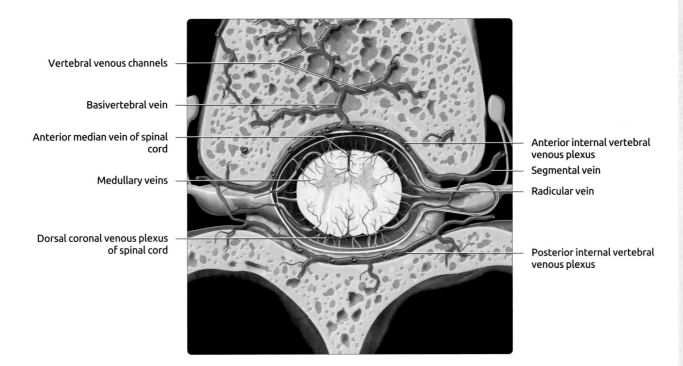

(Top) *AP view of a left T8 intercostal injection gives rise to the characteristic hairpin turn of the major segmental feeding vessel to the thoracic cord, the artery of Adamkiewicz. Extending inferiorly from the top of the hairpin turn is the anterior spinal artery, which supplies the anterior 2/3 of the cord.* **(Bottom)** *Magnified graphic of the internal vertebral venous plexus is shown. The radicular veins course along the dorsal and ventral rami, eventually draining into components of the anterior or posterior internal plexus and subsequently the segmental veins, which will drain into the superior or inferior vena cava.*

History

Development of the distal vertebral artery (VA) is classically defined by the works of Congdon (1922) and Padget (1948). Contributions of the lateral spinal artery (LSA) were initially defined by Kadyi (1889) but were more recently emphasized by Lasjuanias (1985) and Siclari (2007).

Imaging Anatomy

Three main longitudinal vascular axes supply blood to the spinal cord. Two of these axes are composed of the familiar single anterior spinal artery (ASA) and the 2 posterior spinal arteries (PSAs). The ASA is formed by the junction of small vessels arising from each of the intradural VAs and then extends as a continuous vessel along the ventral spinal cord in the ventral median sulcus. The PSAs arise from the extracranial VAs or from the posteroinferior cerebellar artery (PICA) proper and course along the posterolateral surface of the cord as more of an anastomotic chain or arterial plexus than as single dominant vessels (as is seen with the ASA).

In the upper cervical spine, the LSA is a 3rd longitudinal axis, complementing the ASA and PSA. The LSA lies on the lateral aspect of the spinal cord. This vessel is located ventral to the dorsal cervical roots and runs parallel to the spinal component of the spinal accessory nerve (CNXI). The cephalad extension of the LSA ends at the intradural VA (V4) at the C1 level, or at the PICA proper. The caudal limit of the LSA extends to C4 or C5 where the LSA turns posteriorly to the spinal roots and joins the PSA.

Embryology

The embryo develops 6 pairs of aortic arches. The arches undergo selective regression (apoptosis) with the residual arches forming the adult aortic arch and great vessels. Normally, the 1st and 2nd sets of arches regress, and the 3rd arches form the proximal internal carotid arteries (ICAs). The proximal 4th arch forms the right subclavian artery. The bulk of the left 4th arch regresses to end up forming a small portion of the adult arch between the left common carotid artery origin and left subclavian artery. The 5th arches regress. The 6th arch forms the right pulmonary artery and the ductus arteriosus.

Brain Vascular Development

Padget described 7 stages of development of the brain arteries. Briefly, stage 1 shows the forebrain and hindbrain vascular supply from the primitive carotid arteries via a series of transient carotid-vertebrobasilar connections (4- to 5-mm, 28-day embryo). The hindbrain is supplied by 3 presegmental arterial channels and 1 intersegmental channel. Two of the presegmental channels originate from the proximal ICA (trigeminal and otic) whereas the 3rd presegmental channel (hypoglossal) and the intersegmental channel (proatlantal) originate from the paired dorsal aorta. These 4 vascular channels supply paired longitudinal neural arteries (LNAs) that feed the hindbrain. These channels normally regress as the LNAs fuse in the midline to form the basilar artery (connecting cranially with the ICA and caudally with the longitudinal paravertebral anastomosis, which becomes the VAs). The carotid-vertebrobasilar connections are quite transient and exist for at most 8 days in the embryo before regressing (by stage 3).

Stage 2 (29 days) shows the posterior communicating arteries forming and the LNAs uniting to form the basilar artery. Stage 3 (32 days) shows a recognizable adult vascular configuration

with the basilar and vertebral arteries complete. The basilar artery has formed by fusion of the LNAs, and the VAs have formed from longitudinal paravertebral anastomosis between the C1 and C7 intersegmental arteries. Stage 4 (35 days) shows further development of the basilar and vertebral arteries with the appearance of rhombencephalic branches. Stage 5 (40 days) shows prominent choroidal arteries and development of the ventricular system (3rd, 4th, and lateral ventricles). Stages 6 (44 days) and 7 (52 days) show a mature vascular pattern with the new mesencephalic-PCA territory supplied by the vertebral and basilar arteries and not solely by the ICAs.

To summarize, the early posterior cranial circulation (4- to 5-mm embryo) is derived from bilateral LNAs, which are supplied by the trigeminal artery, otic artery, hypoglossal artery, proatlantal intersegmental artery, and cervical intersegmental arteries. The vertebral artery forms from a series of longitudinal anastomoses, which link the first 6 cervical intersegmental arteries. The proximal connections to the aorta of these intersegmental arteries regress with only the 6th intersegmental artery persisting as the adult subclavian artery.

Variations and Anomalies

Due to the complex embryology of the craniovertebral junction, a great number of variations occur in the course of the VAs. Overall, the most common variation is the direct origin from the aortic arch, which occurs in 2-6% of individuals. The level of entrance into the transverse foramen (V1 to V2 junction) occurs at the C6 level in 90-93% of individuals. Other sites of entrance into the transverse foramen can occur anywhere from the C3 level to the C7 level. C3 and C7 entrances are uncommon, each occurring in < 1% of individuals. C4-level entrance occurs in ~ 1% of individuals. The most common variation is the C5 entrance, occurring in 5% (on the left, this typically occurs in conjunction with the origin of the VA from the arch).

Loops of the VA within the neural foramen are common and may extend medially enough to become an inadvertent target during cervical spine surgery, particularly anterior cervical discectomies.

Carotid-Basilar Anastomoses

Persistent carotid-basilar anastomoses include the persistent trigeminal artery (common), hypoglossal artery (rare), persistent proatlantal intersegmental artery (rare), and persistent otic artery (extremely rare). Only the persistent hypoglossal and proatlantal (ProA) will be considered directly related to the craniovertebral junction.

The persistent hypoglossal artery is the 2nd most common persistent carotid-basilar anastomosis (the 1st being the persistent trigeminal artery). It normally is a very short-lived vessel, regressing before the 5th week. The vessel connects the distal ICA through the hypoglossal canal to give rise to the terminal segment of the VA. As is the case with most of the persistent vessels, the more proximal VAs are absent or hypoplastic.

The ProA is an embryonic vessel located between the most caudal presegmental artery (hypoglossal artery) and the 1st intersegmental artery (which accompanies the C2 root). It has its course between the C1 arch and the occipital bone, along with the C1 root. The ProA transiently supplies the basilar circulation before the development of the VAs. The branches of the ProA are incorporated into the adult basilar artery and ASA, and the distal segment of the adult VA (horizontal segment).

Fenestrations and Duplications

Fenestrations commonly occur along the course of the VAs, including the basilar artery. A duplicated VA is an uncommon anomaly. A fenestration has variable definitions in the literature but is generally considered to involve a single vessel whose main trunk divides into 2 parallel segments that may lie within or outside of the bony canal, depending upon the level of occurrence. Duplication should be applied when there are 2 distinct origins with fusion higher in the neck, outside of the bony canal.

Fenestrations occur related to abnormal fusion of the embryonic paired LNAs. The fusion of these vessels has been subdivided into 2 processes, called "longitudinal" and "axial" fusion. Longitudinal fusion is fusion in the midline of the 2 LNAs, whereas axial fusion is fusion of discrete cranial-caudal segments (trigeminal, carotid, and vertebral). Longitudinal nonfusion gives rise to basilar or distal vertebral fenestration. Fenestrations are typically most common in the caudal portion of the vessel. Axial nonfusion gives rise to discontinuous segments, such as a caudal vertebral segment that supplies only the PICA.

Duplications of the VAs at C1 can be related embryologically to persistence of either an intradural LSA segment or the PSA segment. These segments will split at the inferior C1-C2 level and have a superior course over the C1 arch and an inferior course caudal to the C1 arch.

C1-level duplications (or fenestrations) should be distinguished from a persistent 1st intersegmental artery. The 1st intersegmental artery is the continuation of the caudal normal-appearing VA below C2 within the transverse foramen. The persistent 1st intersegmental artery passes into the spinal canal at the C1-C2 level (below the C1 arch) and then extends superiorly to merge with the opposite VA to form the basilar artery. Persistent 1st intersegmental arteries are seen in 1-3% of individuals.

Posteroinferior Cerebellar Artery Origins

C1 origin of the PICA (low PICA) is a common variant that may occur related to anomalous development of the LSA or PSA. The PSA type of C1 origin has a typical hairpin course with a cranial loop before the vessel passes posteriorly and ascends to the cerebellum. The LSA variant of C1 origin ascends in a more ventral position (relative to the PSA variant) and does not have the loop.

C2 origins of the PICA may also relate to anomalous development of the LSA and PSA. Similar to the C1 PICA origin anatomy, the C2 origin related to the PSA has a hairpin cephalic loop and posterior position at the foramen magnum. This is an uncommon anomaly and is seen in < 1% of individuals.

Posteroinferior Cerebellar Artery Extradural Origins

PICA extradural origins are common and occur in 5-20% of cases. Extradural PICA origins tend to occur < 1 cm proximal to the site at which the VA penetrates the dura and tend not to have other extradural branches. In the extradural space, the PICAs course parallel to the VA and the C1 nerve, and the 3 structures together penetrate the dura. Intradurally, they remain lateral and posterior to the brainstem.

Selected References

1. Liu Y et al: Anomalous origin of bilateral vertebral arteries from the ICA: review of the literature and a case report. Ann Vasc Surg. 28(5):1319.e13-6, 2014

2. Uchino A et al: Fenestrations of the intracranial vertebrobasilar system diagnosed by MR angiography. Neuroradiology. 54(5):445-50, 2012

3. Uchino A et al: Vertebral artery variations at the C1-2 level diagnosed by magnetic resonance angiography. Neuroradiology. 54(1):19-23, 2012

4. Yamazaki M et al: Anomalous vertebral arteries in the extra- and intraosseous regions of the craniovertebral junction visualized by 3-dimensional computed tomographic angiography: analysis of 100 consecutive surgical cases and review of the literature. Spine (Phila Pa 1976). 37(22):E1389-97, 2012

5. Hong JT et al: Posterior C1 stabilization using superior lateral mass as an entry point in a case with vertebral artery anomaly: technical case report. Neurosurgery. 68(1 Suppl Operative):246-9; discussion 249, 2011

6. Pang D et al: Embryology and bony malformations of the craniovertebral junction. Childs Nerv Syst. 27(4):523-64, 2011

7. Tubbs RS et al: Persistent fetal intracranial arteries: a comprehensive review of anatomical and clinical significance. J Neurosurg. 114(4):1127-34, 2011

8. Lau SW et al: Study of the anatomical variations of vertebral artery in C2 vertebra with magnetic resonance imaging and its application in the C1-C2 transarticular screw fixation. Spine (Phila Pa 1976). 35(11):1136-43, 2010

9. Raybaud C: Normal and abnormal embryology and development of the intracranial vascular system. Neurosurg Clin N Am. 21(3):399-426, 2010

10. Ulm AJ et al: Normal anatomical variations of the V₃ segment of the vertebral artery: surgical implications. J Neurosurg Spine. 13(4):451-60, 2010

11. Wu A et al: Quantitative analysis of variants of the far-lateral approach: condylar fossa and transcondylar exposures. Neurosurgery. 66(6 Suppl Operative):191-8; discussion 198, 2010

12. Duan S et al: Imaging anatomy and variation of vertebral artery and bone structure at craniocervical junction. Eur Spine J. 18(8):1102-8, 2009

13. Johnson MH et al: Vascular anatomy: the head, neck, and skull base. Neurosurg Clin N Am. 20(3):239-58, 2009

14. Siclari F et al: Developmental anatomy of the distal vertebral artery in relationship to variants of the posterior and lateral spinal arterial systems. AJNR Am J Neuroradiol. 28(6):1185-90, 2007

15. Patel AB et al: Angiographic documentation of a persistent otic artery. AJNR Am J Neuroradiol. 24(1):124-6, 2003

16. Luh GY et al: The persistent fetal carotid-vertebrobasilar anastomoses. AJR Am J Roentgenol. 172(5):1427-32, 1999

17. Caldemeyer KS et al: The radiology and embryology of anomalous arteries of the head and neck. AJR Am J Roentgenol. 170(1):197-203, 1998

18. Lasjaunias P et al: The lateral spinal artery of the upper cervical spinal cord. Anatomy, normal variations, and angiographic aspects. J Neurosurg. 63(2):235-41, 1985

19. Padget DH: Designation of the embryonic intersegmental arteries in reference to the vertebral artery and subclavian stem. Anat Rec. 119(3):349-56, 1954

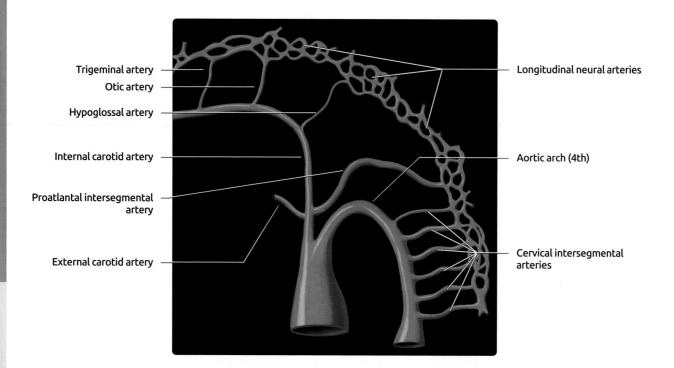

Trigeminal artery
Otic artery
Hypoglossal artery
Internal carotid artery
Proatlantal intersegmental artery
External carotid artery

Longitudinal neural arteries
Aortic arch (4th)
Cervical intersegmental arteries

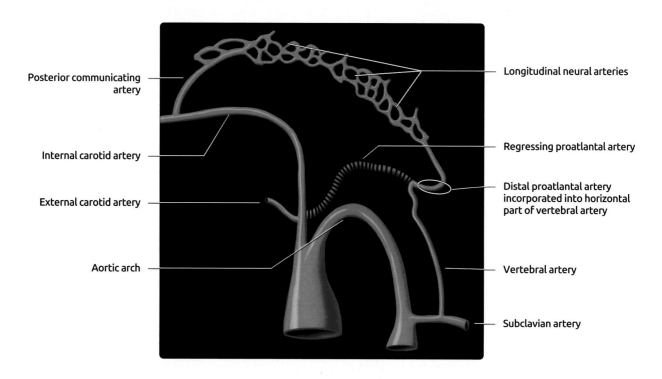

Posterior communicating artery
Internal carotid artery
External carotid artery
Aortic arch

Longitudinal neural arteries
Regressing proatlantal artery
Distal proatlantal artery incorporated into horizontal part of vertebral artery
Vertebral artery
Subclavian artery

(Top) *Schematic view of the embryonic circulation at the 4- to 5-mm stage shows 1 set of the paired longitudinal neural arteries, the aorta, and the cervical intersegmental arteries. The longitudinal neural arteries are supplied by the trigeminal artery, otic artery, hypoglossal artery, proatlantal intersegmental artery, and 6 cervical intersegmental arteries.* **(Bottom)** *Schematic view of embryonic circulation at the 7- to 12-mm stage shows 1 set of the paired longitudinal neural arteries, the aorta, and the cervical intersegmental arteries. The vertebral artery has now developed from the transverse anastomoses of the cervical intersegmental arteries, with the horizontal V3 segment being derived from the distal portion of the proatlantal artery. Failure of the proatlantal artery to regress (dashed vessel) gives rise to the persistent proatlantal artery. At this stage, the posterior communicating artery has formed, with regression of the trigeminal, otic, and hypoglossal arteries.*

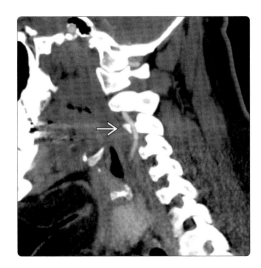

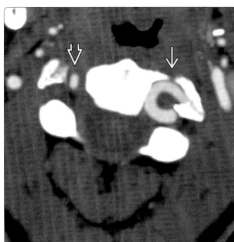

(Left) *Sagittal CTA demonstrates a variant entrance level for the vertebral artery at the C3 level* ➡. *The most common transverse foramen entrance site is C6 (> 90%) with the C3 level occurring in < 1%.* **(Right)** *Axial CTA shows an anatomic variant of a vascular loop involving the distal left vertebral artery at the C2 level* ➡. *The medial aspect of the loop extends into the left neural foramen. Contrast the left vertebral loop with the normal position of the right vertebral artery* ➡.

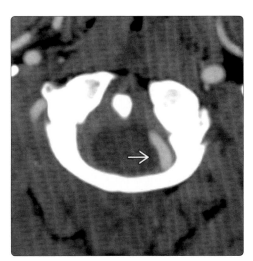

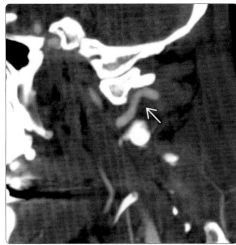

(Left) *Axial CTA shows the typical position within the spinal canal of a left persistent 1st intersegmental artery* ➡. *The artery supplies the typical distal vertebral distribution but enters the canal below the C1 arch level.* **(Right)** *Sagittal CTA demonstrates the typical position of a persistent 1st intersegmental artery at the C1-C2 level* ➡. *This variant may be problematic in an individual who requires C1-C2 fixation.*

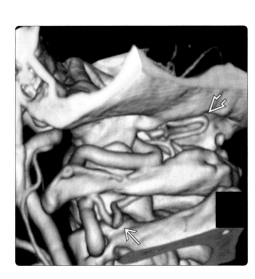

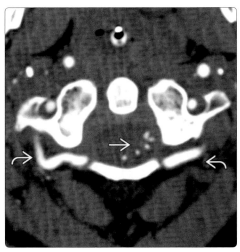

(Left) *Oblique 3D reformation shows a low C2 origin of the posteroinferior cerebellar artery (PICA)* ➡ *as a separate vessel off the vertebral artery. The distal PICA takes a course within the posterior aspect of the foramen magnum* ➡, *consistent with a "posterior spinal artery variety" of the low PICA.* **(Right)** *Axial CTA shows the intradural position of the more distal aspect of a low C2 PICA origin* ➡. *The vertebral arteries are in normal position bilaterally, coursing over the C1 arch* ➡.

Type 1 Vascular Malformation (Dural Arteriovenous Fistula)

TERMINOLOGY

- Synonyms: Type 1 spinal arteriovenous fistula (AVF), dural AVF, dural fistula
- Spinal arteriovenous (AV) fistula, present within dura, with intradural distended draining veins

IMAGING

- Cord enlarged, T2WI hyperintense, vessel flow voids on cord surface
- Multiple enhancing serpentine veins on cord surface
- Dynamic contrast-enhanced MRA capable of defining dilated intradural veins; very useful to guide catheter angiography
- Spinal catheter arteriography is gold standard for confirming diagnosis/treatment

TOP DIFFERENTIAL DIAGNOSES

- CSF pulsatile flow artifact
- Spinal cord tumor
- Spinal cord arteriovenous malformation
- Tortuous "redundant" roots from spinal stenosis
- Collateral venous flow

PATHOLOGY

- Venous hypertension from engorgement reduces intramedullary AV pressure gradient, causing reduced tissue perfusion and cord ischemia

CLINICAL ISSUES

- Most common presentation is progressive lower extremity weakness with both upper + lower motor neuron involvement
- Very rarely presents with subarachnoid hemorrhage
- Middle-aged male with progressive lower extremity weakness exacerbated by exercise
- Persistent edema and enhancement of cord can occur even with successful clinical treatment of fistula
- Treatment: Endovascular fistula occlusion with permanent embolic agents; surgical fistula obliteration

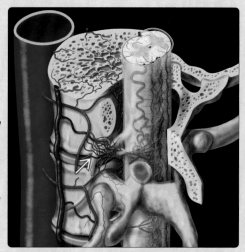
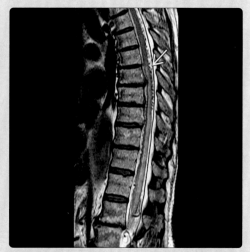

(Left) *Sagittal oblique graphic of the thoracic cord shows the site of a type 1 dural fistula at the dural root sleeve level* ➡️ *with secondary dilatation of intradural venous plexus due to an atrioventricular shunt.* (Right) *Sagittal T2WI MR shows central cord T2 hyperintensity (edema) related to venous hypertension from the peripheral fistula shunting, which typically spares the cord periphery. There are multiple serpentine intradural flow voids from the arterialized and distended venous plexus* ➡️.

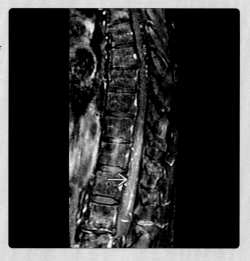
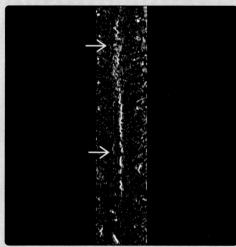

(Left) *Sagittal T1WI C+ FS MR shows ill-defined diffuse enhancement of the distal thoracic cord* ➡️ *in this case of type 1 dural fistula. Faint to moderate cord parenchymal enhancement is common with this lesion.* (Right) *Coronal reformat of double dose dynamic enhanced spinal MRA shows the dilated coronal venous plexus throughout the thoracic spine* ➡️.

Type 1 Vascular Malformation (Dural Arteriovenous Fistula)

TERMINOLOGY

Synonyms
- Type 1 spinal arteriovenous fistula (AVF), dural AVF (dAVF)
- Dural fistula; type 1 spinal vascular malformation; radiculomeningeal fistula

Definitions
- Spinal arteriovenous (AV) fistula, present within dura, with intradural distended draining veins

IMAGING

General Features
- Best diagnostic clue
  - Abnormally enlarged T2WI hyperintense distal cord covered with dilated pial vein flow voids
- Location
  - Intradural extramedullary flow voids (draining veins)

CT Findings
- CTA
  - Nidus in neural foramen shows focal enhancement with prominent intradural dilated veins

MR Findings
- T2WI
  - Cord enlarged, hyperintense
    - Multiple small abnormal vessel flow voids (dilated pial veins) on cord pial surface
    - Edema spares cord periphery
- T1WI C+
  - May show patchy, ill-defined enhancement within cord
- MRA
  - Dynamic contrast-enhanced MRA capable of defining dilated intradural veins; may guide catheter angiography

Angiographic Findings
- Spinal catheter arteriography is gold standard for confirming diagnosis
  - Permits identification of exact level of shunt
  - Provides precise localization of anterior spinal artery
  - Provides access for interventional therapy/embolization

DIFFERENTIAL DIAGNOSIS

CSF Flow Artifact
- Typically dorsal to cord on T2WI, ill-defined margins

Spinal Cord Tumor
- Distinguishable by imaging with intramedullary mass showing focal enhancement

Spinal Cord Arteriovenous Malformation
- Usually acute presentation (compared to insidious presentation of dAVF)

Tortuous "Redundant" Roots From Spinal Stenosis
- Distinguished by presence of severe central stenosis

Collateral Venous Flow
- Inferior vena cava occlusion may cause prominent intradural veins

PATHOLOGY

General Features
- Etiology
  - Fistula venous drainage gives increased pial vein pressure that is transmitted to intrinsic cord veins
  - Venous hypertension causes reduced tissue perfusion and cord ischemia

Staging, Grading, & Classification
- Anson-Spetzler classification: Type 1 spinal vascular malformation
- Spetzler 2002 classification: Intradural dorsal AVF

Gross Pathologic & Surgical Features
- Most commonly occurs at thoracolumbar level (T5-L3)
- Usually located either adjacent to intervertebral foramen or within dural root sleeve
- Arterial supply arises from dural branch of radicular artery

CLINICAL ISSUES

Presentation
- Most common signs/symptoms
  - Most common presentation is progressive lower extremity weakness with both upper + lower motor neuron involvement
  - Other signs/symptoms
    - Additional symptoms include back pain, bowel/bladder dysfunction, impotence
- Clinical profile
  - Middle-aged male with progressive lower extremity weakness exacerbated by exercise

Demographics
- Epidemiology
  - 80% of all spinal vascular malformations
  - 80% of patients are male

Natural History & Prognosis
- Slowly progressive clinical course over several years leading to paraplegia
- Cord ischemia reversible if treated early
- Bowel/bladder dysfunction and impotence rarely improve

Treatment
- Endovascular fistula occlusion with permanent embolic agents
- Surgical fistula obliteration
  - 40-60% improve following obliteration of fistula, 40-50% stabilize myelopathic symptoms
  - T2WI cord edema decreases over 1-4 months following successful embolization
  - Improved cord appearance on MR following treatment does not necessarily correlate with improved symptoms
  - Persistent edema and enhancement of cord can occur even with successful clinical treatment of fistula

SELECTED REFERENCES

1. Spetzler RF et al: Modified classification of spinal cord vascular lesions. J Neurosurg. 96(2 Suppl):145-56, 2002
2. Anson J et al: Classification of spinal arteriovenous malformations and implications for treatment. BNI Quarterly. 8: 2-8, 1992

(Left) *Sagittal T2WI MR shows the typical cord edema pattern of a spinal dural fistula with central cord T2 hyperintensity and multiple flow voids on the cord surface.* **(Right)** *Sagittal T1WI C+ FS MR shows the classic pattern of cord enhancement, which is ill-defined, diffuse, and without sharp margination* ➡.

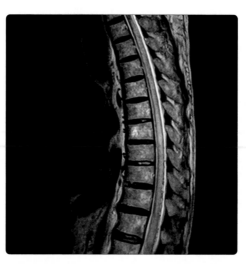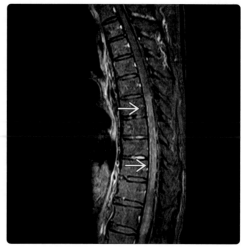

(Left) *Coronal reformat of dynamic enhanced MR angiography shows the abnormal cord surface vessels, and more precisely defines the site of the fistula on the left at T9* ➡ *as a more compact focus of vessels within the neural foramen.* **(Right)** *Catheter angiography with injection of the left T9 intercostal artery shows a type 1 fistula site at the neural foraminal level* ➡ *and flow into the dilated coronal venous plexus* ➡.

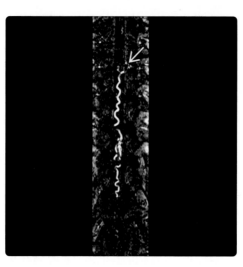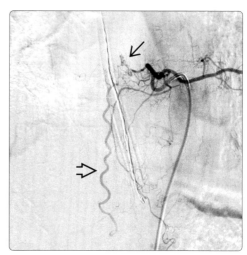

(Left) *Coronal reformat from a CTA shows a type 1 fistula in the right thoracic neural foramen* ➡ *with enlarged inferior draining veins* ➡. **(Right)** *Anteroposterior catheter angiography of the intercostal artery shows the peripheral fistula on the left* ➡ *draining centrally into the dilated venous plexus surrounding the cord.*

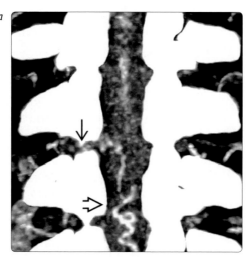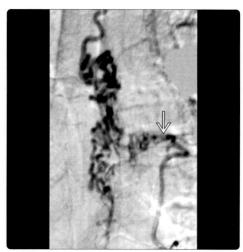

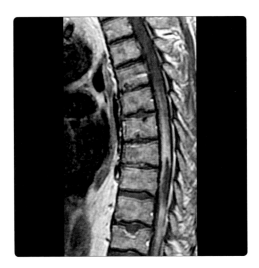

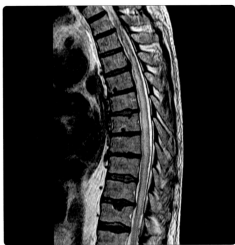

(Left) *Sagittal T1WI C+ MR in this case of type 1 fistula shows extensive confluent enhancement of the distal thoracic cord. The differential is extensive, including infectious and inflammatory etiologies, such as demyelinating disease.* (Right) *Sagittal T2WI MR in this case of type 1 fistula shows diffuse T2 hyperintensity throughout the thoracic cord with relative sparing of the cord periphery. There are no conspicuous flow voids on the dorsal cord periphery.*

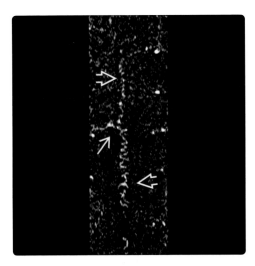

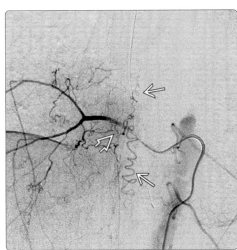

(Left) *Coronal reconstruction from a dynamic contrast-enhanced MRA data set shows the location of the fistula within the neural foramen ➡ and shunting to the dilated intradural spinal veins ⇛.* (Right) *Catheter angiogram shows shunting of contrast into the venous plexus surrounding the cord ➡ from the right-sided type 1 fistula ⇒.*

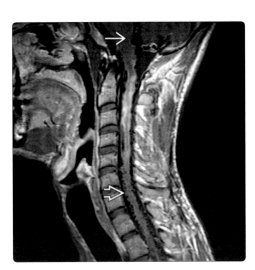

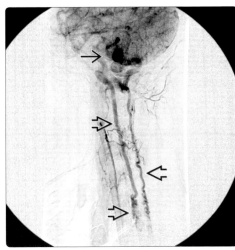

(Left) *Sagittal T1WI C+ MR demonstrates diffuse enhancement of the cord from the cervicomedullary junction to C5. This pattern mimics the look of spinal type 1 dural fistula, but myelopathy was caused by the posterior fossa fistula ➡ with caudal intraspinal venous drainage ⇛.* (Right) *Venous phase of the left vertebral injection shows a posterior fossa dural fistula ⇨ (Cognard type 5) supplied by meningeal branches with extensive intraspinal draining veins dorsal and ventral to the cord ⇨, a type 1 fistula mimic.*

Type 2 Arteriovenous Malformation

TERMINOLOGY

- Synonyms
  - Glomus-type arteriovenous malformation (AVM), plexiform AVM
- Direct arterial/venous communications forming compact nidus within cord

IMAGING

- Multiple, well-defined serpentine flow voids within substance of cord
- Large cord, heterogeneous signal (blood products), flow voids
- Dynamic-enhanced MRA capable of defining enlarged feeding arteries, nidus, and enlarged draining veins
- Supplied by anterior spinal artery &/or posterior spinal artery
  - Nidus drains to coronal venous plexus (on cord surface), which drains anterograde to extradural space

TOP DIFFERENTIAL DIAGNOSES

- Intramedullary neoplasm
- Cavernous hemangioma
- Type 4 perimedullary fistula
- Type 3 (juvenile) AVM
- Paraganglioma with large feeding vessels (rare)

PATHOLOGY

- Associated with cutaneous angiomas, Klippel-Trénaunay-Weber, Rendu-Osler-Weber syndromes
- Neurologic deterioration with subarachnoid hemorrhage, ischemia from vascular steal, cord compression, venous hypertension

CLINICAL ISSUES

- Subarachnoid hemorrhage most common symptom; pain, myelopathy
- Surgical resection + preop embolization (aneurysms, nidus)

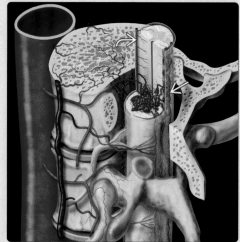

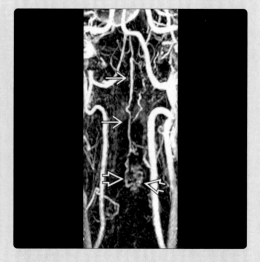

(Left) Sagittal oblique graphic of the thoracic cord shows a focal, compact intramedullary nidus of type 2 arteriovenous malformation (AVM) ➡ fed by branches from the anterior spinal artery ➡. (Right) Dynamic enhanced coronal MRA of the cervical spine allows high-resolution MRA within 30-60 seconds and illustrates the feeding anterior spinal artery ➡ extending inferiorly to the AVM nidus ➡.

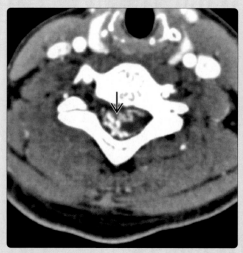

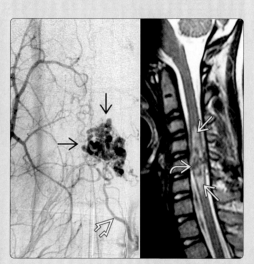

(Left) Axial CTA shows multiple serpentine enhancing vessels within substance of cervical cord, right side > left, representing the AVM nidus ➡. (Right) Anteroposterior DSA (left) demonstrates the compact AVM nidus ➡ involving the cervical cord. The draining vein is seen extending inferiorly to the cervical epidural plexus ➡. Sagittal T2WI MR (right) shows mild cord expansion with heterogeneous intramedullary T2 signal due to blood products ➡ and edema ➡.

Type 3 Arteriovenous Malformation

TERMINOLOGY

- Synonyms: Juvenile arteriovenous malformation (AVM); intramedullary extramedullary AVM
- Large, complex, intramedullary extramedullary AVM
  - Rarest of spinal AVMs (7%)

IMAGING

- Large complex nidus, multiple feeding vessels; may be intramedullary and extramedullary and even extraspinal

TOP DIFFERENTIAL DIAGNOSES

- Intramedullary neoplasm
  - Ependymoma: Heterogeneous (cysts, blood products)
  - Uncommon: Metastasis with hemorrhage (melanoma, renal cell)
- Cavernous angioma
- Type 4 perimedullary fistula
- Paraganglioma: Enhancing intradural extramedullary mass (rare)

PATHOLOGY

- Associated with **Cobb syndrome** (metameric vascular malformation with triad of spinal cord, skin, bone)
- Variety of vascular lesions may be present, including paravertebral and epidural hemangioma

CLINICAL ISSUES

- Progressive neurologic decline (weakness), subarachnoid hemorrhage
  - Pain in lower extremities or back; motor deficit
  - Poor prognosis for type 3 (juvenile) AVM

DIAGNOSTIC CHECKLIST

- Definition of intramedullary involvement is critical for classification, prognosis, treatment options
- CTA or dynamic MRA serves as localization tool prior to catheter angiography

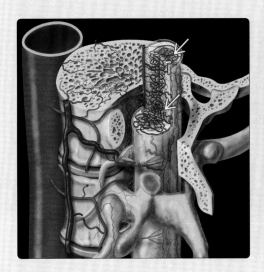

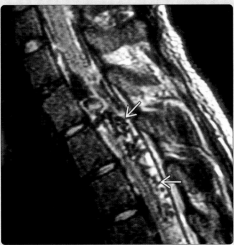

(Left) Sagittal oblique graphic of the thoracic cord shows a large, complex intramedullary nidus of a type 3 arteriovenous malformation (AVM) ➡ with multiple feeding vessels. (Right) Sagittal T2WI MR exhibits extensive flow voids ➡ involving a long segment of the cervical cord seen throughout the subarachnoid space. These lesions are fed by multiple arteries at multiple vertebral levels. An apoplectic presentation from subarachnoid hemorrhage or intramedullary hemorrhage is strongly associated with intramedullary AVMs.

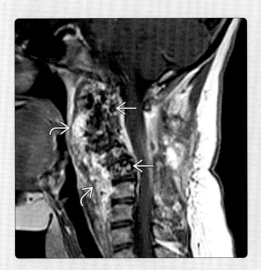

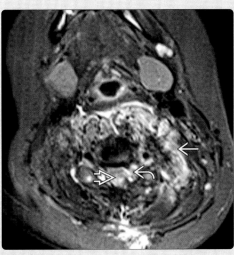

(Left) Sagittal T1WI C+ MR displays a vascular lesion composed of multiple flows in the cervical spine involving the vertebral bodies ➡ and prevertebral muscles ➡. (Right) Axial T1WI C+ FS MR in the same patient illustrates the intramedullary ➡, extramedullary ➡, and extradural ➡ components of this type 3 AVM. MR has the advantage of demonstrating the intraspinal vascular component as well as the extraspinal portion insinuating into the perivertebral space.

Type 4 Vascular Malformation (Arteriovenous Fistula)

TERMINOLOGY

- Synonyms: Perimedullary fistula; type 4 spinal vascular malformation, pial arteriovenous fistula (AVF)
- Direct intradural extramedullary arterial/venous communication from anterior or posterior spinal artery to draining vein without capillary bed

IMAGING

- Hyperintense cord + flow voids
- Intradural location for fistula, adjacent to cord
- Draining veins may be pronounced on dorsal or ventral surface of cord
- Feeding vessel from anterior or posterior spinal artery connects directly with spinal vein

TOP DIFFERENTIAL DIAGNOSES

- Normal CSF flow artifact
- Type 1 dural fistula
- Lumbar canal stenosis with tortuous intradural roots

- Intramedullary neoplasm

PATHOLOGY

- 4-A: Small AVF with slow flow, mild venous enlargement
- 4-B: Intermediate AVF, dilated feeding arteries; high flow rate
- 4-C: Large AVF, dilated feeding arteries; dilated, tortuous veins
- Associations
  - Hereditary hemorrhagic telangiectasia
  - Cobb syndrome
  - Klippel-Trénaunay-Weber syndrome

CLINICAL ISSUES

- > 90% of patients present with neurological deficits
  - Hemorrhage at presentation in 36%
- Embolization or surgical resection based upon anatomy and size: Surgical resection, surgical resection or embolization, embolization

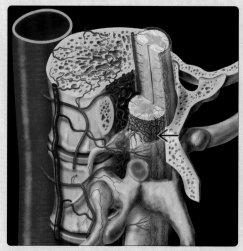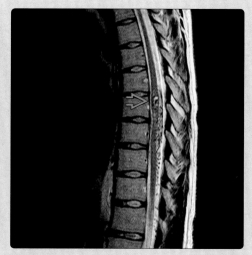

(Left) Coronal oblique graphic of the thoracic cord shows the intradural site of arteriovenous fistula (AVF, type 4) on the dorsal cord surface with diffuse venous engorgement ➡. A fistula is more typically along the ventral cord surface. (Right) Sagittal T2 MR shows multiple serpentine intradural extramedullary flow voids dorsal to the thoracic cord, plus focal cord abnormality ➡ due to a high-flow aneurysm.

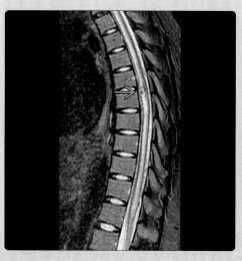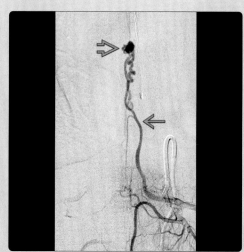

(Left) Sagittal STIR MR shows a long segment of cord hyperintensity with ill-defined flow voids along the ventral cord surface. There is a more focal area of low signal, which at angiography was a high-flow aneurysm ➡. (Right) AP view of a catheter angiogram (arterial phase) shows a prominent segmental feeder ➡ to the cord, which shunts into the coronal venous plexus, with no intervening nidus. There is high-flow aneurysm at the fistula site ➡.

Posterior Fossa Dural Fistula With Intraspinal Drainage

TERMINOLOGY

- Dural arteriovenous fistula (DAVF): Anomalous connection between dural arteries and venous sinuses &/or cortical veins without presence of normal intervening capillary bed
- Rare DAVF variant has preferential venous drainage inferiorly into spinal veins

IMAGING

- Increased T2 signal in upper cervical cord/medulla with abnormal perimedullary flow voids
- Fistula located in posterior fossa with symptoms related to site of venous drainage (myelopathy)
- Catheter angiography remains gold standard

TOP DIFFERENTIAL DIAGNOSES

- Spinal DAVF
  - Cord signal change and flow voids may look identical to posterior fossa DAVF with intraspinal drainage
- Demyelinating disease

- Cord enhancement and increased T2 signal but no abnormal perimedullary flow voids

CLINICAL ISSUES

- Myelopathy related to venous hypertension secondary to AV shunting and insufficient venous drainage of spinal cord
- Symptoms tend to be chronic and progressive
  - 25% have acute onset of neurological disorder
- Good prognosis for improvement of symptoms or complete recovery
- Occlusion/resection of fistula by endovascular means or open surgery

DIAGNOSTIC CHECKLIST

- Catheter angiography still required for exclusion of DAVF even if negative MRA
- DAVF clinical manifestations related to anatomical distribution of draining veins, not fistula site
- Cognard type V fistula presenting symptoms relate to dysfunction of spinal cord rather than brain

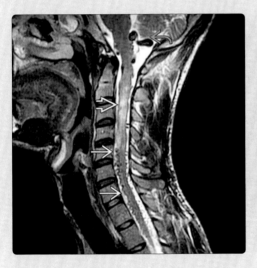

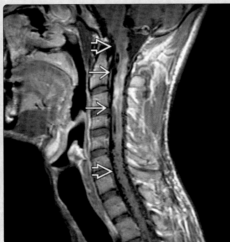

(Left) Sagittal T2WI MR shows extensive cord hyperintensity and mild fusiform cord expansion from C1 to C4 ➡. There are multiple abnormal pronounced perimedullary flow voids ➡. Dilated draining veins are present in the posterior fossa ➡. (Right) Following contrast administration, sagittal T1WI MR shows diffuse enhancement of the upper cervical cord from the cervicomedullary junction to C5 ➡. Multiple intradural extramedullary flow voids ➡ are present.

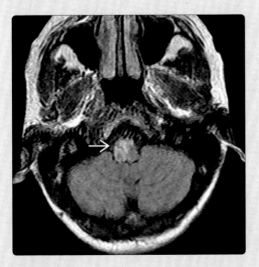

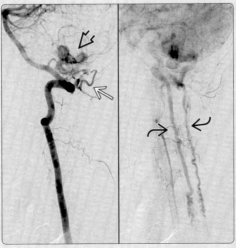

(Left) Axial FLAIR shows abnormal T2 hyperintensity within the right side of the medulla ➡. The diffusion study was normal (not shown). The abnormality within the medulla, coupled with the prominent veins, prompted the recommendation for a catheter angiogram to exclude a dural fistula. (Right) Arterial (left) and venous (right) phases of left vertebral injection show a dural fistula ➡ supplied by posterior meningeal branches ➡ with extensive intraspinal draining veins ➡ both dorsal and ventral to the cord.

TERMINOLOGY

- Vascular lesion with lobulated, thin, sinusoidal vascular channels and no interspersed neural tissue

IMAGING

- Locules of blood with fluid-fluid levels surrounded by very T2-hypointense rim
- Spinal cord uncommon site: 3-5% of all cavernous malformations (CMs)
- Round, heterogeneous signal abnormality, well-defined margins
- Brain MR to identify supratentorial lesions

TOP DIFFERENTIAL DIAGNOSES

- Intramedullary neoplasm
- Arteriovenous malformation
- Multiple sclerosis

PATHOLOGY

- Cervical (40%), thoracic (50%)

- Discrete, lobulated blue-reddish brown (mulberry-like) nodule
- Vascular spaces with single layer of endothelial cells
- No intervening neural tissue between vascular spaces
- Multiple (familial) CM syndrome (20%)
  - Familial CMs are at high risk for hemorrhage and formation of new lesions
  - Mutations in 3 genes (CCM1, CCM2, CCM3) implicated in familial forms

CLINICAL ISSUES

- Typically occurs in 3rd-6th decades
- M:F = 1:2
- Broad range of dynamic behavior (may progress, enlarge, or regress)
- Surgical resection is mainstay of symptomatic CM
- Variable outcomes in literature: 50-66% improve, 28% stabilize, and 6% deteriorate postoperatively

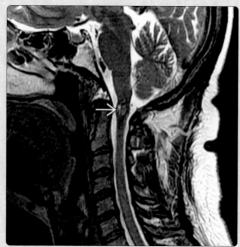

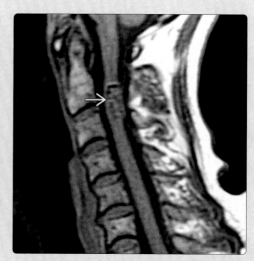

(Left) Sagittal T2WI MR shows a small heterogeneous intramedullary lesion ➡ at the C1 level. There is slight cord expansion but no adjacent edema. Mass effect & intrinsic cord edema generally occur with more acute hemorrhage. (Right) Sagittal T1WI MR shows the typical appearance of a cavernous malformation of the spinal cord. A heterogeneous, slightly expansile intramedullary lesion is seen at the C2-3 level ➡. A faint salt & pepper pattern is present from repeated hemorrhages & hemosiderin deposition.

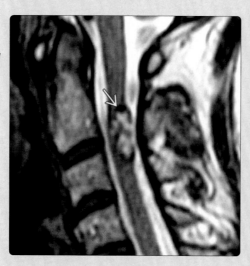

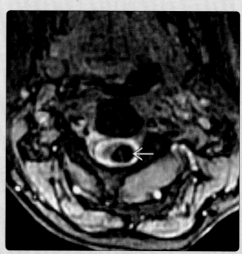

(Left) Sagittal T2WI MR depicts a classic, mixed hyperintense (popcorn or salt and pepper) lesion surrounded by a hypointense rim ➡ from hemosiderin. Cavernous malformation was found at surgery. (Right) Axial T2* GRE MR exhibits a cavernous malformation in the cervical cord as a large area of low signal from susceptibility artifact ➡ from the blood byproducts. There should be blooming of this type of lesion with longer echo times.

Spinal Artery Aneurysm

KEY FACTS

TERMINOLOGY

- Fusiform or saccular dilatation of artery supplying spinal cord, particularly anterior spinal artery but including radiculomedullary branches

IMAGING

- Catheter spinal angiography required for diagnosis

TOP DIFFERENTIAL DIAGNOSES

- Hemorrhage from intramedullary tumor
- Hemorrhage from spinal vascular malformation

PATHOLOGY

- Most commonly associated with spinal vascular malformations
- Coarctation of aorta
- Arteritis (including inflammatory etiologies, such as syphilis or mycotic)
- Fibromuscular dysplasia
- Pseudoxanthoma elasticum

- Klippel-Trenaunay-Weber syndrome
- Idiopathic
  - Tend to be fusiform in shape without defined neck (as seen commonly with intracranial aneurysms)
  - Often unrelated to arterial branching sites

CLINICAL ISSUES

- Presenting symptoms include back pain, headache, vomiting, weakness, paraparesis, and paralysis
- Treatment may include clipping if neck is present or trapping with occlusion of parent vessel or wrapping with muslin
- Isolated reports of coil embolization of spinal aneurysms
- Spontaneous regression reported in aneurysms with inflammatory etiology

DIAGNOSTIC CHECKLIST

- Unlike intracranial aneurysms, risk of surgical treatment of ruptured aneurysm may exceed expected benefit

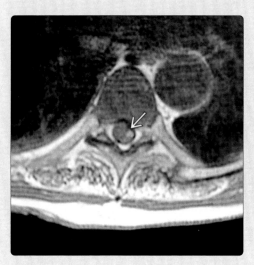

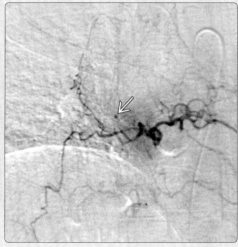

(Left) Axial T1WI MR shows high signal intensity blood throughout the subarachnoid space ➡ in this patient with spinal aneurysm. (Right) Anteroposterior catheter angiography with injection of the left-sided intercostal artery shows filling of a small anterior spinal aneurysm ➡.

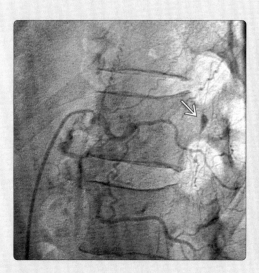

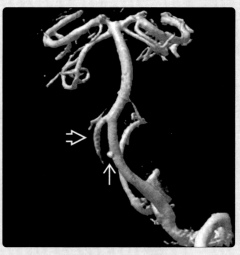

(Left) Lateral catheter angiography with injection of the thoracolumbar intercostal artery shows filling of a fusiform anterior spinal artery aneurysm ➡. (Right) Anteroposterior catheter angiography 3D spin study shows small outpouching of contrast off of the ventral medial aspect of the left vertebral artery due to an aneurysm at the origin of the anterior spinal artery ➡. There is a small amount of reflux extending down the right vertebral artery ➡.

TERMINOLOGY

- Spinal cord ischemia
- Cord infarction 2° to vessel occlusion (radicular artery)

IMAGING

- MR with contrast, + diffusion
- Hyperintensity on T2WI within cord; central owl's eye pattern
  - Slight cord expansion in acute phase
- Hyperintense central gray matter or entire cross-sectional area
- DWI: Hyperintense, as in brain infarcts

TOP DIFFERENTIAL DIAGNOSES

- Multiple sclerosis
- Transverse myelitis
- ADEM/viral myelitis
- Neuromyelitis optica
- Type I dural fistula

- Spinal cord neoplasm
- Radiation myelopathy

PATHOLOGY

- Up to 50% of cases have no known etiology
- Majority of known causes relate to aortic pathology
- Septicemia; systemic hypotension
- Blunt trauma with dissection
- Fibrocartilaginous embolism
- Iatrogenic; transforaminal steroid injection, selective root block

CLINICAL ISSUES

- Abrupt onset weakness, loss of sensation
- Rapid progression; maximum deficit within hours
- Poor prognosis, with permanent disabling sequelae
- Pain is frequent and disabling feature of cord infarct
- Treatment: Anticoagulation with heparin and aspirin; steroids; supportive care and rehabilitative physical therapy

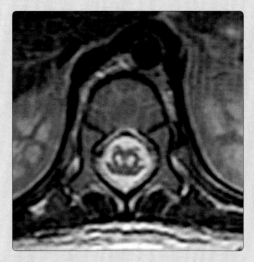
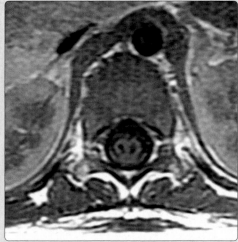

(Left) Axial T2WI MR in a case of hypoxic-ischemic encephalopathy (HIE) shows typical owl's eye abnormal hyperintensity within the central gray matter from chronic spinal cord infarction. (Right) Axial T1WI MR in case of severe HIE shows focal low signal within the central cord due to old infarction with myelomalacia.

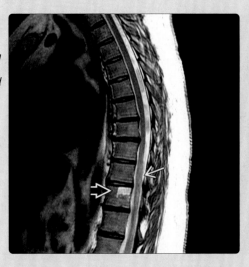
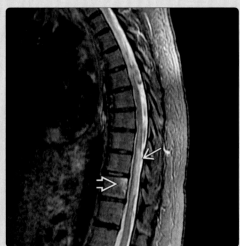

(Left) Sagittal T2 MR shows slight hyperintensity in the distal thoracic cord ⇒ in this patient with acute onset of leg weakness. There is a geographic region of increased signal ⇒ in the superior aspect of the thoracic vertebral body due to concomitant cord and vertebral body infarcts. (Right) Sagittal STIR MR shows the cord hyperintensity involving the mid and dorsal aspect of the thoracic cord ⇒ along with the vertebral body infarction ⇒. The classic anterior 2/3 of the cord involved is not always present.

TERMINOLOGY

- Hemorrhage into spinal subarachnoid space from variety of etiologies
  - Trauma (> 50%)
  - Aneurysmal subarachnoid hemorrhage (SAH) with spinal extension
  - Spinal arteriovenous malformations
    - Mainly types II, III, IVc, conus malformations
  - Tumor
  - Anticoagulant therapy
  - Infection (pneumococcal meningitis, herpes)
  - Systemic disease
  - Spinal artery aneurysm (rare)

IMAGING

- Fluid-fluid level within thecal sac
- Variable depending on stage of blood breakdown and byproducts
- Dynamic enhanced MRA useful as screen for spinal vascular malformation

TOP DIFFERENTIAL DIAGNOSES

- Epidural hemorrhage
- Subdural hemorrhage
- Intramedullary hemorrhage

PATHOLOGY

- Rare reports of cervical/thoracic arachnoiditis developing following spinal SAH

CLINICAL ISSUES

- Acute back or radicular pain ± signs of cord compression (numbness, weakness)
  - Spinal SAH characterized by sudden headache, acute sciatic pain, xanthochromic CSF, meningeal irritation, sensory deficit or paralysis
  - Massive spinal SAH may give acute cord compression, paraplegia, fecal and urinary incontinence

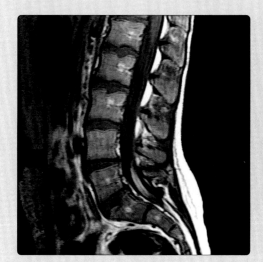
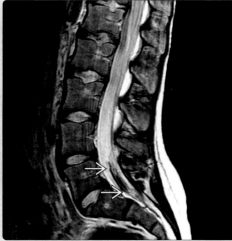

(Left) Sagittal T1WI MR of subarachnoid blood following an epidural blood patch, presumably related to an incorrect needle position, shows oblong focus of T1 hyperintensity within the distal thecal sac at the L5-S1 level due to methemoglobin. No epidural lesion is present. (Right) Sagittal T2WI MR of subarachnoid blood following an epidural blood patch, presumably related to an incorrect needle position, shows blood to be of low signal ➡. Epidural space is normal.

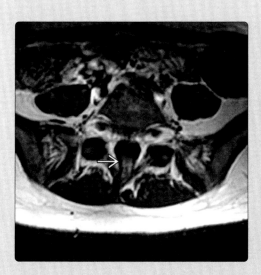
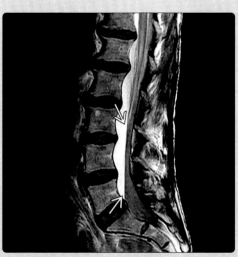

(Left) Axial T1WI MR of subarachnoid blood following an epidural blood patch shows focus of T1 hyperintensity within the distal thecal sac at the L5-S1 level ➡. (Right) Sagittal T2 MR shows the appearance of a large subarachnoid hemorrhage, which is layered within the thecal sac with a well-defined fluid-fluid level ➡.

KEY FACTS

TERMINOLOGY

- Hemorrhage build-up between dura and spine not caused by significant trauma or iatrogenic procedures

IMAGING

- Extradural multisegmental T1 hyperintense fluid collection
- Lentiform or biconvex
- T1WI acute: < 48 hours
  - Isointense > hypo-/hyperintense
- T1WI subacute and chronic
  - Hyperintense > isointense
- T2WI variably hyperintense

TOP DIFFERENTIAL DIAGNOSES

- Epidural metastasis
- Lymphoma
- Disc extrusion, migration
- Epidural abscess
- Subdural hematoma

PATHOLOGY

- Idiopathic: 40-50%
- Minor trauma
- Anticoagulation
- Coagulopathy
- Disc herniation
- Vascular anomaly

CLINICAL ISSUES

- Acute onset of neck, back pain, paraparesis, bowel or bladder dysfunction
- Severity and duration of neurologic deficit predictive of postoperative neurologic recovery
  - Return to neurologic baseline after surgery
    - 89-95% of patients with incomplete neurologic deficit vs. 38-45% of patients with complete impairment
  - Improved outcome when surgery performed ≤ 36 hours in patients with complete sensorimotor loss
    - ≤ 48 hours in patients with incomplete deficit

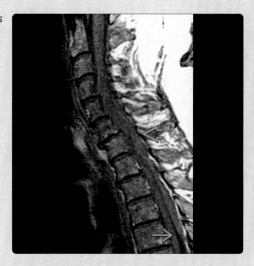
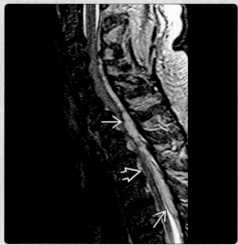

(Left) Sagittal T1WI MR shows an indistinct margin of the cervical cord due to an isointense mass within the dorsal epidural space ⮕. The location of the mass is best identified at the inferior margin as extradural ⮕. (Right) Sagittal T2WI MR shows a slightly heterogeneous, long segment hyperintense mass ⮕ within the posterior epidural space spanning the C2-T4 level. The cord is severely compressed and displaced anteriorly ⮕.

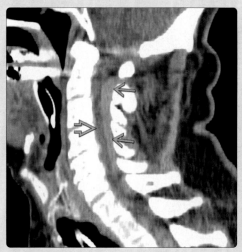
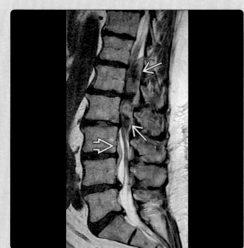

(Left) Sagittal NECT with a soft tissue window shows an extensive epidural hematoma ⮕ as slightly increased attenuation in the posterior canal with displacement of the cord anteriorly ⮕. (Right) Sagittal T2WI MR shows a larger cephalad extradural mass ⮕, which is mixed iso- and hypointense, displacing ventrally the cord and filum. A smaller caudal epidural hemorrhage shows mild effacement of the thecal sac at the L3-L4 level ⮕.

Subdural Hematoma

KEY FACTS

TERMINOLOGY

- Accumulation of blood between dura, arachnoid

IMAGING

- Intradural collection hyperintense on T1WI, predominantly hypointense on T2WI or gradient-echo imaging
- Thoracolumbar > lumbar or lumbosacral > cervical
- Clumped, loculated masses of hemorrhagic density/intensity

TOP DIFFERENTIAL DIAGNOSES

- Epidural hematoma
- Subdural abscess
- CSF leakage syndrome
- Spinal meningitis
- Idiopathic hypertrophic spinal pachymeningitis

PATHOLOGY

- Trauma

- Bleeding diathesis: 54% of reported cases
- Iatrogenic cause is factor in 2/3 of those with abnormal coagulation parameters
- Neoplasm
- Arteriovenous malformation
- Postoperative complication
- Spontaneous: 15%

CLINICAL ISSUES

- Acute onset of neck or back pain
- Radicular pain, bladder/bowel dysfunction
- Much less common than spinal epidural hematoma
- Treatment
  - May resolve spontaneously
  - Decompressive laminectomy with clot evacuation
    - Indicated by severe and progressive deterioration of neurologic symptoms

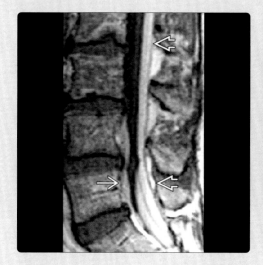

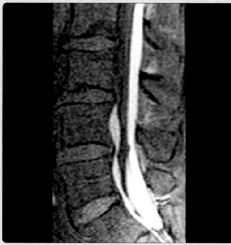

(Left) Sagittal T1WI MR without fat saturation shows prominent hyperintense linear collections both ventral ➡ and dorsal ➡ within the bony spinal canal with narrowing of the thecal CSF space. (Right) Sagittal T1WI MR with fat saturation shows hyperintense linear subdural blood collections both ventral and dorsal within the bony canal with marked narrowing of thecal CSF space. Iatrogenic cause is a factor in 2/3 of those with abnormal coagulation parameters.

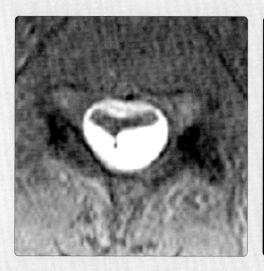

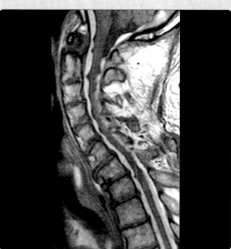

(Left) Axial T1WI FS MR shows the typical appearance of subdural hemorrhage with the well-defined outer margin bounded by the dura and an inner lobulated margin giving a Mercedes Benz sign. (Right) Sagittal T1WI MR in a patient with chronic neck pain demonstrates diffuse ventral and dorsal intraspinal hyperintense collections with intracranial extension.

Bow Hunter Syndrome

TERMINOLOGY

- Bow hunter stroke, positional occlusion of vertebral artery, rotational occlusion of vertebral artery
- Vertebrobasilar insufficiency secondary to mechanical occlusion or stenosis of vertebral artery during head rotation

IMAGING

- Occlusion or stenosis of vessel with head positional dependence based on ultrasound, MRA, CTA, or catheter angiography
- Along course of vertebral artery, typically at C1-C2 junction

PATHOLOGY

- Vertebral artery at C1-C2 particularly prone to mechanical compression
- May occur anywhere along vertebral course related to spondylosis, atlantoaxial instability, hypertrophy of atlantooccipital membranes, paravertebral muscle fascial bands

CLINICAL ISSUES

- Vertebrobasilar insufficiency
  - Motor or sensory deficits, ataxia, diplopia, dysarthria, dysmetria, vertigo, visual field deficit, cranial nerve dysfunction, syncope
- Treatment
  - Brace to restrict head motion, surgical fusion to prevent atlantoaxial rotation, vertebral artery decompression
  - Vertebral artery stenting

DIAGNOSTIC CHECKLIST

- Temporary positional occlusion of 1 vertebral artery during course of daily activities may be normal if asymptomatic
- Hypoplasia or stenosis of contralateral vertebral artery predisposes patients to vertebrobasilar ischemic attacks during head rotation

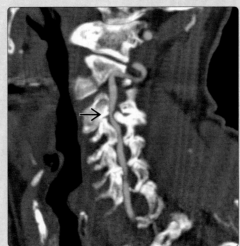
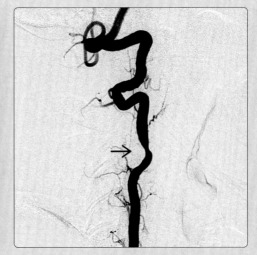

(Left) Coronal oblique CTA shows focal extrinsic narrowing of the left vertebral artery at the C3-C4 level due to facet degenerative hypertrophy and osteophyte formation ➡. (Right) Lateral catheter angiography in a neutral position shows moderate focal stenosis at the C3-C4 level due to osteophytic compression ➡.

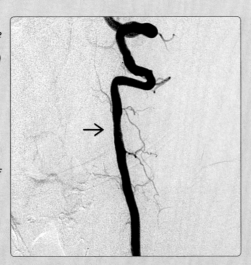
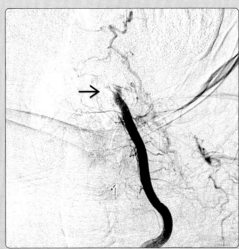

(Left) Anteroposterior catheter angiography with the head turned to the right (asymptomatic head turn side) shows a patent left vertebral with mild C3-C4 level narrowing ➡. (Right) Anteroposterior catheter angiography with the head turned to the left (symptomatic head turn side) shows occlusion of the vertebral artery at the level of the osteophytic compression ➡.

TERMINOLOGY

- Vertebral artery (VA) dissection
- Irregularity of VA contour from intimal tear or subadventitial hematoma

IMAGING

- **Stenoocclusive dissection**
  - Dissection to subintimal plane with vessel luminal narrowing or occlusion
- **Dissecting aneurysm**
  - Dissection into subadventitial plane with dilatation of outer wall
- Intramural hematoma is pathognomonic
  - Best seen as **bright crescent** on T1 fat-suppressed MR
- Conventional angiography is gold standard

TOP DIFFERENTIAL DIAGNOSES

- Extracranial atherosclerosis
- Fibromuscular dysplasia

- Miscellaneous vasculitis
- Congenital VA hypoplasia

PATHOLOGY

- **Traumatic** VA dissection
  - Direct or indirect arterial injury
- **Spontaneous** VA dissection
  - Many associations and predisposing factors

CLINICAL ISSUES

- Age: Adults < 45 years

DIAGNOSTIC CHECKLIST

- Check other vessels for 2nd dissection
- Look for suboccipital rind sign (hematoma without narrow lumen)
- Cerebellar infarction in young to middle-aged adults; need to exclude posterior inferior cerebellar artery infarction due to VA dissection

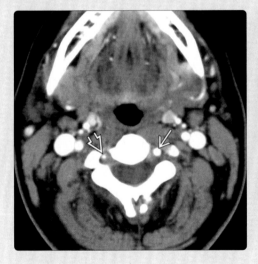

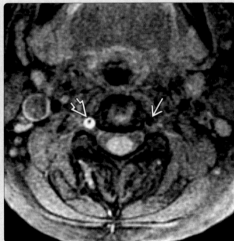

(Left) Axial CECT in a patient with idiopathic vertebral artery dissection demonstrates a normal caliber of the left vertebral artery ➡ and a narrowed, eccentric lumen of the right vertebral artery ➡. Note the normal and symmetric foramina transversarium. (Right) Axial T1 FS MR in the same patient reveals a hyperintense crescent of a mural hematoma ➡ with a small hypointense patent lumen. Contralateral vertebral artery shows no methemoglobin hyperintensity ➡. This is unilateral vertebral artery dissection.

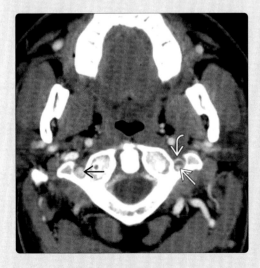

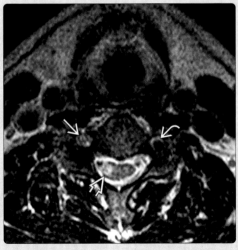

(Left) Axial CTA shows rim enhancement of the left vertebral artery ➡ with a low-density mural hematoma and contrast filling the narrowed lumen ➡. Subtle linear lucency in the right vertebral artery proved not to be a dissection flap ➡. (Right) Axial T2 MR in a patient with neck trauma and cervical fractures reveals traumatic vertebral artery dissection as loss of right vertebral flow void ➡, as compared to the normal left side ➡. Note right cervical hemicord hyperintensity from cord ischemia ➡.

TERMINOLOGY

- Internal carotid artery dissection (ICAD): Tear in internal carotid artery wall that allows blood to enter and delaminate wall layers

IMAGING

- CTA and MRA are typically 1st step in imaging evaluation
  - T1 MR with fat suppression is best sequence for **hyperintense mural hematomas**
- Pathognomonic findings of dissection: **Intimal flap** or **double lumen** (seen in < 10%)
- Aneurysmal dilatation (seen in 30%)
  - Commonly in distal subcranial segment of internal carotid artery (ICA)
  - Focal pseudoaneurysm is unusual
- ICAD most commonly originates in ICA 2-3 cm distal to carotid bulb and variably involves distal ICA
  - Stops before petrous ICA
- Angiography
  - Pathognomonic: Intimal flap + double lumen (true and false)
  - String sign: Long, tapered, usually eccentric and irregular stenosis distal to carotid bulb

TOP DIFFERENTIAL DIAGNOSES

- Fibromuscular dysplasia
- Carotid artery fenestration
- Traumatic ICA pseudoaneurysm
- Atheromatous plaque

CLINICAL ISSUES

- Ipsilateral pain in face, jaw, head or neck
- Oculosympathetic palsy (miosis and ptosis, partial Horner syndrome)
- Ischemic symptoms (cerebral or retinal TIA or stroke)
- Bruit (40%)
- Lower cranial nerve palsies (especially CNX)
- Pulsatile tinnitus

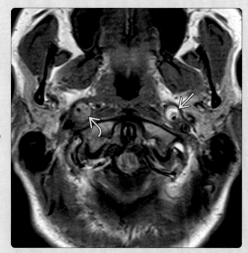
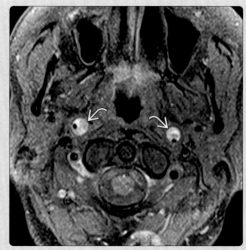

(Left) *Axial T1WI MR illustrates bilateral internal carotid artery dissections (ICADs) with isointense mural thrombus on the right ➡ and hyperintense mural thrombus on the left ➡. The residual lumens are markedly narrowed. Bilateral ICAD represents 4-16% of all dissections.* (Right) *Axial T1WI FS MR in the same patient demonstrates bilateral ICADs. The fat saturation increases the conspicuity of the methemoglobin in the mural thrombus ➡.*

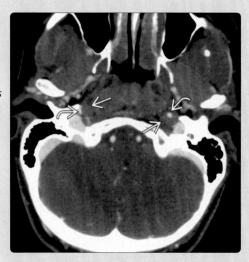
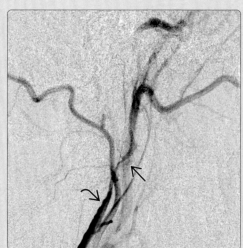

(Left) *Axial CTA displays soft tissue density ➡ narrowing the contrast-filled lumen of both internal carotid arteries (ICAs) ➡, compatible with mural thrombus. Intramural hematoma usually compresses the true lumen & causes enlargement of the external diameter.* (Right) *Lateral DSA exhibits a short segment of ICA narrowing ➡ due to dissection. Undulating irregularity of the proximal ICA ➡ may be due to vasospasm or standing wave artifact, which is induced by the angiography catheter & is related to injection speed.*

Fibromuscular Dysplasia

TERMINOLOGY

- Fibromuscular dysplasia (FMD)
- Arterial disease of unknown etiology affecting medium-sized and large arteries, most commonly in young to middle-aged women

IMAGING

- Multifocal ± bilateral cervical carotid or vertebral artery irregularity on CTA/MRA/DSA; string of beads appearance
- Location
  - Most commonly at C1-C2 levels
  - Carotid artery involved in 30% (bilateral in 65%)
  - Vertebral artery involved in 10%
- Morphological changes of FMD in carotid and vertebral artery circulations
  - Vessel beading/irregularities: String of beads appearance
  - Arterial stenosis without mural Ca++ as opposed to atherosclerotic vascular disease
  - FMD associations: Dissection, pseudoaneurysm, intracranial aneurysms
- Best imaging tool
  - CTA or MRA for noninvasive assessment
  - DSA for definitive diagnosis ± endovascular intervention

TOP DIFFERENTIAL DIAGNOSES

- Atherosclerosis
- Arterial dissection
- MRA motion artifact
- Standing waves

DIAGNOSTIC CHECKLIST

- String of beads is classic appearance on CTA/MRA/DSA of most common subtype (type 1)
- If FMD found in any artery, consider study of cervical and intracranial arteries for FMD ± associated saccular and pseudoaneurysms

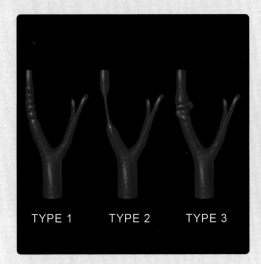

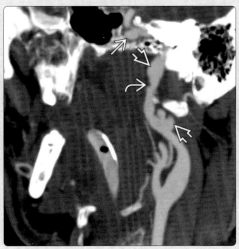

(Left) Graphic of carotid bifurcation shows the principal subtypes of fibromuscular dysplasia (FMD). Type 1 appears as alternating areas of constriction and dilatation, type 2 as tubular stenosis, and type 3 as focal corrugations ± diverticulum. (Right) Sagittal reformatted CTA reveals 2 pseudoaneurysms of the distal internal carotid artery (ICA) ➡. There is also a vascular outpouching of the petrous segment of the ICA ➡. Vascular irregularity with focal narrowing is also observed ➡.

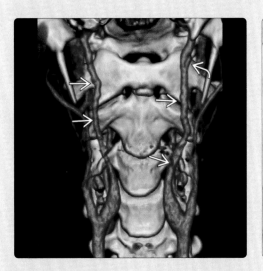

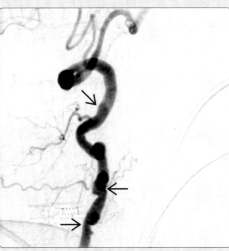

(Left) Coronal surface-rendered CTA demonstrates diffuse bilateral ICA irregularity ➡ with some areas showing the classic string of beads appearance. Note the small pseudoaneurysm ➡. (Right) Lateral angiographic image displays vertebral artery irregularity ➡. Histopathologically, FMD is heterogeneous with various degrees of collagen hyperplasia, internal elastic lamina rupture, and disorganization of the tunica media.

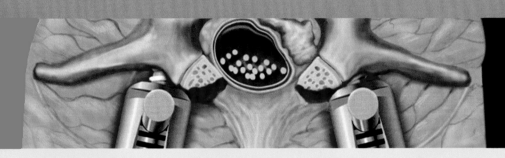

Terminology

Adverse event: Any unexpected or undesirable event occurring as a direct or indirect result of surgery.

Complication: Disorder related directly or indirectly to surgery; will change the expected outcome for the patient.

Medicolegal Issues

The literature evaluating malpractice litigation regarding spine surgery is limited, but important lessons can be learned from the available data. Rovit et al. evaluated claims against neurosurgeons in New York State from 1999 to 2003. Spine cases constituted 56% of malpractice allegations. It does not appear that malpractice exposure is limited by limiting the type of practice one has away from supposedly risky procedures, such as intracranial disease, complex spine cases, or emergency cases. Rather, the malpractice claims seem to be lumped into areas that are common and not complex, such as "routine" elective spine surgery. In that series, lumbar claims were more than 2x as common as cervical spine claims. The costs incurred are high, to say the least. Rovit found that $50 million was paid out for 280 cases closed against neurosurgeons during 5 years. Lawyers made $9 million. Epstein found that malpractice payouts for the cervical spine vary widely, with plaintiffs' verdicts receiving $4 million on average, settlements receiving $2.3 million, and defense verdicts receiving no compensation. This study also found 3 anticipated factors leading to cervical malpractice suits (negligent surgery, lack of informed consent, and failure to diagnose/treat). The unanticipated factor that was specific for cervical spine surgery was failure to brace.

The 1 area where relatively simple imaging can make a significant impact is wrong level surgery. Thoracic disc herniation localization is a prime example. This lesion is generally not apparent on plain films or intraoperative fluoroscopy, so direct localization is not possible, as may be with primary bone tumors and metastatic disease. Preoperative localization may be carried out by multiple techniques, extending from a skin scratch (indelible markers being not that indelible to surgical scrubbing) to placement of radiopaque markers within the soft tissues. This author's current favorite thoracic localization technique is placement of small gold beads at the thoracic pedicle/lamina junction at the appropriate level through an 18-gauge spinal needle using fluoroscopy. These types of beads were initially utilized for radiotherapy localization but work very well for general thoracic level localization. Correlation with CT &/or MR studies is mandatory. Counting is preferred from C2 down to the level of interest, given the frequency and confusing nature of lumbosacral transitional anatomy.

Blind Spots

Imaging of the postoperative spine is tough, both from the pathology standpoint and the sheer volume of data that needs to be evaluated, coupled with the bewildering array of hardware that seems to change daily. The problem is compounded for the imager by the lack of standards for approaches/hardware for even the most common of procedures. Lee et al. found that spine surgeons generally agree on when to operate in a particular clinical scenario but fail to agree on what type of procedures to perform. Specific choices are often related to surgeon familiarity and training and may not be easily generalized. Metal artifact seems ubiquitous and further confounds the quality of imaging for both CT and MR. Metal artifact suppression sequences are available for MR. While they do help, they are not a panacea, and degradation of image quality by metal is not going away.

There are no easy shortcuts to evaluate a postoperative CT or MR if useful information is to be gleaned. Every disc level needs to be evaluated with step-by-step inspection of the vertebral bodies, pedicles and posterior elements, and neural foramen and epidural space. Blind spots can develop, and having a specific search pattern can help to identify pathology. For instrumentation, each screw position must be evaluated and checked to see if it appropriately attaches to the fixation rod/plate and if the screw is appropriately positioned or if it has breeched the cortex. Are there screw breaks or rod fractures? Where are the graft positions? What is spinal alignment? Is the thecal sac decompressed, and what does the epidural space look like?

General knowledge of the previous surgical procedures that the patient has undergone is also essential for identifying complications. Knowing the surgery and its goals allows the imager to focus on the most common areas of complication given the operative approach to the pathology. If you do not know what a pedicle subtraction osteotomy (PSO) is, then you will not see the typical appearance of the vertebral body resection site. You cannot easily recognize what you do not know, and this extends to something as seemingly apparent as pedicles. Residents and fellows have stared at a lateral film of a PSO and not recognized that 1 level is lacking pedicles. Be particularly vigilant for double or staged procedures, which have an increased incidence of complications. One study of en bloc resections showed a 34% complication rate, the majority of them graded as "major," with a 2% mortality.

Selected References

1. Epstein NE: A review of medicolegal malpractice suits involving cervical spine: what can we learn or change? J Spinal Disord Tech. 24(1):15-9, 2011
2. Lee JY et al: Surgeons agree to disagree on surgical options for degenerative conditions of the cervical and lumbar spine. Spine (Phila Pa 1976). 36(3):E203-12, 2011
3. Epstein NE: A medico-legal review of cases involving quadriplegia following cervical spine surgery: is there an argument for a no-fault compensation system? Surg Neurol Int. 1:3, 2010
4. Lekovic GP et al: Litigation of missed cervical spine injuries in patients presenting with blunt traumatic injury. Neurosurgery. 60(3):516-22; discussion 522-3, 2007
5. Rovit RL et al: Neurosurgical experience with malpractice litigation: an analysis of closed claims against neurosurgeons in New York State, 1999 through 2003. J Neurosurg. 106(6):1108-14, 2007
6. Fager CA: Malpractice issues in neurological surgery. Surg Neurol. 65(4):416-21, 2006
7. Rampersaud YR et al: Intraoperative adverse events and related postoperative complications in spine surgery: implications for enhancing patient safety founded on evidence-based protocols. Spine (Phila Pa 1976). 31(13):1503-10, 2006
8. Goodkin R et al: Wrong disc space level surgery: medicolegal implications. Surg Neurol. 61(4):323-41; discussion 341-2, 2004
9. Malanga GA et al: Segmental anomaly leading to wrong level disc surgery in cauda equina syndrome. Pain Physician. 7(1):107-10, 2004
10. Dickman CA et al: Reoperation for herniated thoracic discs. J Neurosurg. 91(2 Suppl):157-62, 1999

Spine Surgery Malpractice Allegations

Lumbar Surgery	Cervical Surgery
Operation at wrong level	Operation at wrong level
Failure of fusion	Failure of fusion
Nerve root/cauda equina injury	Nerve root/cord injury
Durotomy/CSF leak	Infection/abscess
Infection	CSF leak
Hardware failure	Anterior displacement of graft
Failure to relieve pain	Injury to trachea/esophagus
Vascular/visceral injury	Recurrent laryngeal nerve palsy
Failure to remove disc completely	Failure to relieve pain
Inappropriate indication for operation	Inappropriate indication for operation
	Failure to remove disc
	Infected graft site

Adapted from Rovit RL et al: Neurosurgical experience with malpractice litigation: an analysis of closed claims against neurosurgeons in New York State, 1999 through 2003. J Neurosurg. 106(6):1108-14, 2007.

Cervical Spine Operations and Deficits Leading to Suits

Operations	Deficits
Most to Least	
Anterior cervical discectomy/fusion (1 level)	Quadriplegia
Posterior laminectomy/fusion	Paresis (other)
Anterior cervical discectomy/fusion (2 levels)	Pain
Posterior fusion alone	C5 root palsy
Anterior cervical fusion (3 or 4 levels)	Dysphagia
	Vocal cord paralysis
	Esophageal perforation

Adapted from Epstein NE: A medio-legal review of cases involving quadriplegia following cervical spine surgery: is there an argument for a no-fault compensation system? Surg Neurol Int. 1:3, 2010.

Overall Incidence of Adverse Events and Complications

Intraoperative Event	Adverse Event Incidence (%)	Complication Incidence (%)
Dural tear	8.3	1.6
Instrumentation	3.1	0.3
Massive blood loss	1.4	0.9
Anesthesia/medical	0.6	0.1
Anterior approach	2.1	0.0
Vertebral artery	1.4	0.0
Esophagus/pharynx	2.2	2.2
Sterile field contamination	0.3	0.1
Patient poisoning	0.3	0.0
Surgical instrument failure	0.1	0.0
Change of surgery plan	0.1	0.0

Adapted from Rampersaud YR et al: Intraoperative adverse events and related postoperative complications in spine surgery: implications for enhancing patient safety founded on evidence-based protocols. Spine (Phila Pa 1976). 31(13):1503-10, 2006.

Myelography Complications

TERMINOLOGY

- Minor complications
  - Post dural puncture headache (most common)
  - Incorrect needle position (subdural, epidural)
  - Transient neurologic sequela
  - Contrast reaction (minor)
- Major complications
  - CSF leak
  - Symptomatic spinal subdural or epidural hemorrhage
  - Contrast reaction (major)
  - Cord injury
  - Intracranial hemorrhage
  - Seizure
  - Paralysis
  - Death
- Delayed complications
  - Iatrogenic epidermoid

IMAGING

- Myelography technique
  - Monitor initial contrast injection fluoroscopically to confirm subarachnoid placement
  - Use smaller gauge, atraumatic needles
  - Replacing needle stylet before withdrawing helps to prevent headache
  - Fluoroscopic guidance for C1-C2 puncture, injection carefully monitored to avoid cord injection
  - Avoid hyperextension during cervical myelography: Rare cause of periprocedural cord injury
- Most common complications have no imaging findings

CLINICAL ISSUES

- Dural puncture headache usually begins by 3 days & lasts 3-5 days
- Nausea, vomiting, hearing loss, tinnitus, vertigo, dizziness, paresthesias

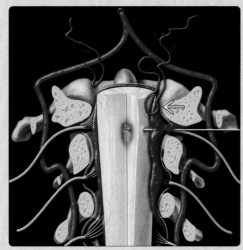
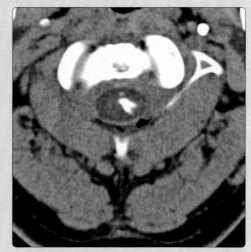

(Left) Coronal graphic shows complications of a C1-C2 puncture with cord injury from the needle as well as subarachnoid blood. Note the close proximity to the caudal loop of the posterior inferior cerebellar artery ➡. (Right) Axial CT following an attempted myelogram shows focal contrast within cord substance and a small amount of epidural gas.

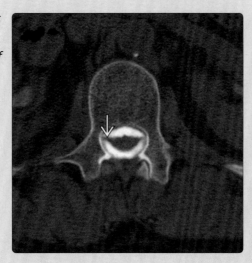
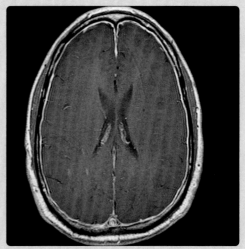

(Left) Axial post myelographic CT demonstrates contrast material that is subdural in location. Note the outlining of the dentate ligaments by contrast ➡. The well-defined outer margin (dura) allows differentiation from epidural injection. (Right) Axial contrast-enhanced T1WI MR of the brain shows diffuse, smooth pachymeningeal thickening and enhancement in this patient with intracranial hypotension following lumbar puncture.

Vertebroplasty Complications

IMAGING

- Extravasation of cement (into spinal canal, neural foramen, paravertebral spaces, epidural or paravertebral venous plexus) or pulmonary cement embolism
  - Improper needle placement
  - Inadequate intraprocedural monitoring of polymethylmethacrylate injection
  - Inadequate polymethylmethacrylate opacification
  - Low cement viscosity or too large of volume injected
  - Underlying neoplasm with deficient cortex
- New vertebral compression fracture adjacent to previously treated level
- Fat embolism
  - Branching or globular hyperdense material in lung parenchyma on fluoroscopy, radiography, or CT
- Vertebral osteomyelitis
  - Osseous destruction adjacent to polymethylmethacrylate

PATHOLOGY

- Adjacent compression fracture
  - 10-15% of treated patients
  - Controversial relationship to vertebroplasty
- Fat embolism
  - Embolism of fatty marrow displaced by polymethylmethacrylate injection

CLINICAL ISSUES

- Clinical presentation variable depending on complication type
- Symptomatic complications of vertebroplasty are rare
  - < 1% for osteoporotic compression fractures
  - 2-5% for treatment of osteolytic metastases

DIAGNOSTIC CHECKLIST

- Consider CT to investigate any unexpected peri- or postprocedural symptomatology

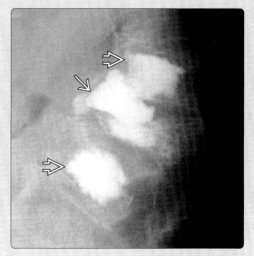

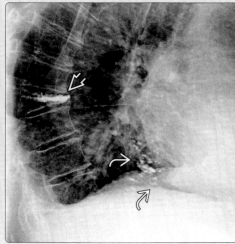

(Left) *Lateral radiograph shows a large volume of cement extending beyond the vertebral body into the disc interspace ➡ between 2 other vertebral bodies that were also treated, which contain cement within their confines ➡.* (Right) *Lateral radiograph shows a compression fracture of a midthoracic vertebral body treated with vertebroplasty ➡. Embolization of cement to the right lower lobe is seen as striated opacities projecting in the retrocardiac space ➡.*

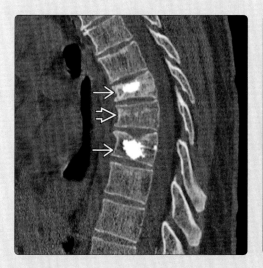

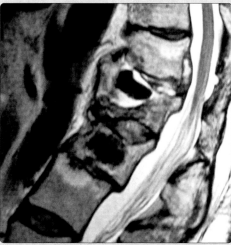

(Left) *Sagittal NECT shows bone cement from a prior 2-level vertebroplasty ➡. Imaging for acute back pain shows mild, acute compression fracture of T7 with horizontal sclerosis ➡ due to trabecular impaction.* (Right) *Sagittal T2WI MR shows high signal surrounding cement several weeks after vertebroplasty in a patient on chronic steroid therapy. Aspiration showed Staphylococcus aureus infection. (Courtesy S. Dunnagan, MD.)*

KEY FACTS

TERMINOLOGY

- Continued low back pain with or without radicular pain after lumbar surgery

IMAGING

- Stenosis: Trefoil appearance of lumbar canal on axial imaging
- Instability: Deformity increases with motion & time
- Recurrent herniation: Nonenhancing, well-defined mass arising out of intervertebral disc
- Fibrosis: Infiltration of epidural/perineural fat by enhancing soft tissue density (intensity)
- Arachnoiditis: Clumping, adhesion of cauda equina nerve roots
- Improper instrumentation placement

TOP DIFFERENTIAL DIAGNOSES

- Infection
  - Endplate destruction, disc T2 hyperintensity

- Tumor
  - Enhancing soft tissue mass
- Hemorrhage
  - Intermediate T1 signal acute-subacute age
- Pseudoarthrosis
  - Abnormal low T1 signal extending through disc, posterior elements, and ligaments

PATHOLOGY

- Multiple underlying etiologies for "late" failure
  - Foraminal/central stenosis (20-60%)
  - Pseudoarthrosis/instability (14%)
  - Recurrent herniation (7-12%)
  - Epidural fibrosis (5-25%)
  - Arachnoiditis

DIAGNOSTIC CHECKLIST

- Contrast-enhanced MR 96-100% accurate in detecting peridural fibrosis vs. recurrent herniation

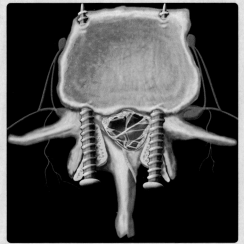

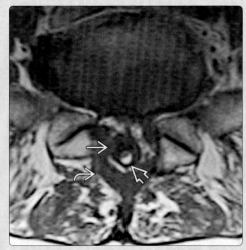

(Left) Axial graphic of the lumbar spine shows postoperative change with bilateral pedicle screws and left laminectomy defect. There is clumping of nerve roots, reflecting arachnoiditis. The screws are too anterior and have breached anterior vertebral body cortex. (Right) Axial T1WI MR shows a laminectomy at L5-S1. There is peripheral clumping of roots in the thecal sac due to arachnoiditis ➡. Note the droplet of T1 hyperintense Pantopaque ➡. Posterior epidural fibrosis is present ➡ at the laminectomy site.

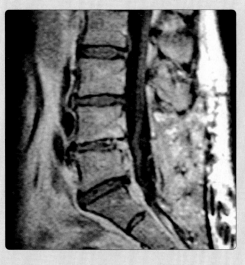

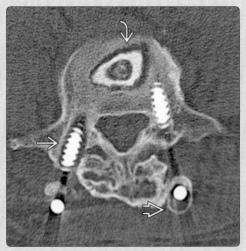

(Left) Sagittal T1WI C+ MR shows central clumping of intrathecal roots into a central rope-like mass, simulating low-lying cord. Note multilevel laminectomy defect and degenerative disc space enhancement, particularly at L4-5. (Right) Axial NECT shows bilateral loosened pedicle screws with prominent lucency surrounding the mid and distal aspects ➡. There are also lucency and bony remodeling surrounding the junction with the longitudinal rod ➡. Nonunion of the graft spanning L3-5 is shown with perigraft lucency ➡.

Epidural Abscess, Postop

TERMINOLOGY

- Spinal epidural abscess
- Extradural spinal infection with abscess formation

IMAGING

- MR
  - T1WI C+: Homogeneously or heterogeneously enhancing **phlegmon**
    - Peripherally enhancing necrotic **abscess**
- Fat saturation → STIR, T2WI FS, T1WI C+ FS
  - Increases lesion conspicuity by suppressing signal from epidural fat and vertebral marrow
- Signal alteration in spinal cord secondary to compression, ischemia, or direct infection
- Anterior epidural abscess arises from adjacent discitis & vertebral osteomyelitis
- Persistent epidural enhancement without mass effect after treatment

- Probable sterile granulation tissue or fibrosis, correlate with ESR, CRP for activity

TOP DIFFERENTIAL DIAGNOSES

- Extradural metastasis
- Epidural hematoma

PATHOLOGY

- *Staphylococcus aureus* most common in postoperative population, with *Enterococcus* next most frequent
- Predisposing factors
  - Intravenous drug abuse, immunocompromised state, diabetes mellitus, chronic renal failure, alcoholism, cancer, other chronic illnesses
  - Risk of epidural abscess in epidural anesthesia (5.5%)
    - Especially in presence of indwelling catheters

CLINICAL ISSUES

- 0.5% incidence of epidural abscess from epidural anesthesia for open aortic aneurysm repair

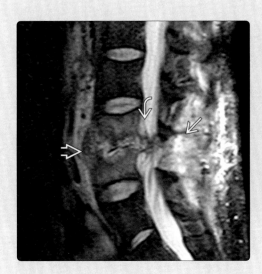

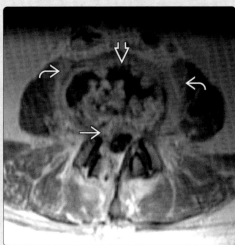

(Left) Sagittal T2WI MR shows dorsal soft tissue disruption from prior laminectomy ➡. There are classic changes of disc space infection at L4-5 with endplate destruction and T2 hyperintensity ➡ as well as ventral epidural abscess extension ➡. (Right) Axial T1WI C+ MR shows irregular enhancement and destruction of the endplates from disc space infection ➡. Paravertebral extension is seen into the psoas muscles ➡. Epidural phlegmon enhancement is present and compresses the thecal sac ➡.

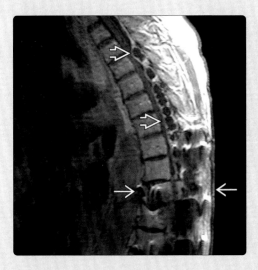

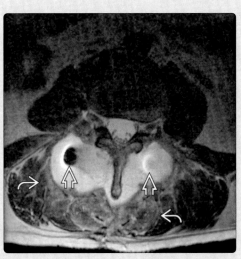

(Left) Sagittal T1WI C+ MR shows metal artifact from prior anterior and posterior fixation ➡. The large dorsal epidural loculated abscess ➡ shows peripheral enhancement with compression of the thecal sac and anterior cord displacement. (Right) Axial T2WI MR in patient status post posterior lumbar interbody fusion shows abscess collection surrounding the posterior spinal fusion hardware (metallic susceptibility ➡). Note edema in the paraspinal muscles ➡.

Disc Space Infection

TERMINOLOGY

- Bacterial suppurative infection of vertebrae and intervertebral disc

IMAGING

- Ill-defined hypointense T1 vertebral marrow with loss of endplate definition on both sides of disc
- Loss of disc height & abnormal disc signal
- Destruction of vertebral endplate cortex
- Vertebral collapse
- Paraspinal ± epidural infiltrative soft tissue ± loculated fluid collection
- Follow-up MR
  - Should focus on soft tissue findings
  - No single MR parameter is associated with clinical status

TOP DIFFERENTIAL DIAGNOSES

- Degenerative endplate changes
- Tuberculous vertebral osteomyelitis

- Spinal neuropathic arthropathy

PATHOLOGY

- Predisposing factors
  - Intravenous drug use
  - Immunocompromised state
  - Chronic medical illnesses (renal failure, cirrhosis, cancer, diabetes)
- *Staphylococcus aureus* is most common pathogen

CLINICAL ISSUES

- Acute or chronic back pain
- Focal spinal tenderness
- Fever
- ↑ ESR, ↑ CRP, ↑ WBC

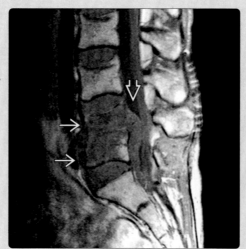
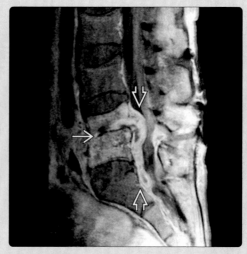

(Left) *Sagittal T1WI MR in a patient with a history of lumbar discectomy shows findings of disc space infection at L4-L5 with hypointense marrow ➡, vertebral collapse, endplate erosion, disc space loss, and epidural phlegmon ➡. (Right) Sagittal T1WI C+ MR demonstrates enhancing vertebral bodies and irregular enhancement of intervening disc ➡. There is an epidural abscess extending from L4-L5 to S1 ➡. Severe thecal sac compression is present at L4-L5.*

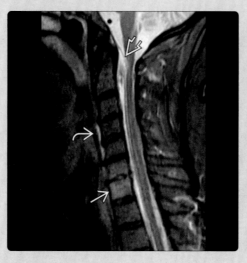
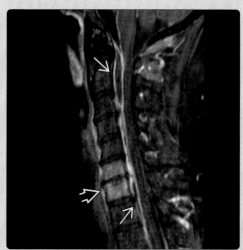

(Left) *Sagittal T2WI in cervical disc space infection with epidural abscess shows high signal in C6 and C7 bodies ➡ with prevertebral edema ➡. Abnormal signal is present ventral to the cord from the epidural abscess ➡. (Right) T1 C+ FS MR shows a ventral epidural abscess ➡ with mass effect upon the cord, which is displaced posteriorly. There is enhancement of the infected C6 and C7 bodies ➡.*

IMAGING

- MR
  - Diffuse, extensive subarachnoid enhancement
  - Smooth or irregular meningeal enhancement

TOP DIFFERENTIAL DIAGNOSES

- Carcinomatous meningitis
  - Focal or diffuse, sheet-like or nodular enhancement along cord or nerve roots
- Sarcoidosis
  - Leptomeningeal + nerve root enhancement mimics spinal meningitis
- Lumbar arachnoiditis
  - Empty sac sign with nerve roots adherent to periphery of thecal sac
- Guillain-Barré syndrome
  - Inflammatory demyelination typically following recent viral illness

PATHOLOGY

- Infection of CSF and meningeal coverings surrounding spinal cord
- Associated findings
  - Spondylodiscitis
  - Spinal epidural abscess
  - Blocked CSF flow → increased pressure within cord → syringomyelia

CLINICAL ISSUES

- Acute onset of fever, chills, headache, + altered level of consciousness

DIAGNOSTIC CHECKLIST

- Imaging often negative in early spinal meningitis
  - Positive in advanced bacterial meningitis or granulomatous infection
- Intravenous gadolinium increases sensitivity in detecting meningeal disease

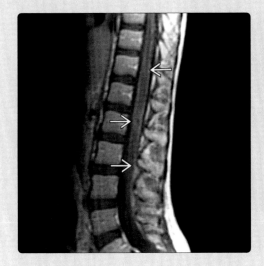

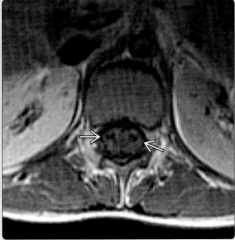

(Left) Sagittal T1WI C+ MR shows diffuse mildly irregular leptomeningeal enhancement ➡. No extradural or vertebral inflammatory changes are apparent. Abnormal contrast agent enhancement is noted on contrast-enhanced MR images in only 55-70% of patients with proven infectious meningitis; contrast-enhanced MR is particularly insensitive to viral meningitis. (Right) Axial T1WI C+ MR reveals diffuse nerve root enhancement ➡.

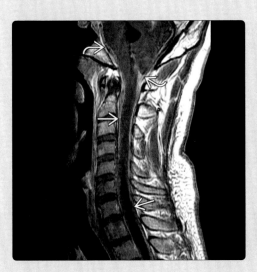

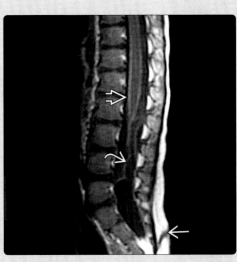

(Left) Sagittal T1WI C+ MR exhibits diffuse leptomeningeal enhancement ➡ extending into the posterior fossa ➡ in this patient with coccidioidomycosis. (Right) Diffuse pial and cauda equina enhancement is due to meningitis ➡. Minimal enhancement outlines an epidermoid ➡. There is a dorsal dermal sinus tract ➡ in the low sacral region.

CSF Leakage Syndrome

TERMINOLOGY

- Symptomatic leakage of CSF
- Postoperative, iatrogenic, or posttraumatic CSF leak, ± pseudomeningocele

IMAGING

- Intracranial findings
  - Smooth intracranial dural thickening
  - "Sagging" midbrain
  - Subdural hygromas
  - Subdural hematomas
  - Descent of cerebellar tonsils
- Spinal findings
  - Spinal hygromas
  - Dilatation of anterior epidural venous plexus, dural thickening/enhancement
  - Paraspinal fluid
  - Symmetric anterolateral epidural masses (dilated epidural veins)
  - Nerve root sleeve cysts/diverticula
- Radionuclide cisternography
  - Paucity or absence of radiotracer over cerebral convexities at 24-48 hours
  - Early washout
  - Early appearance in kidneys, bladder common
- Myelography/CT myelography
  - Demonstrate CSF leak site (arachnoid diverticula or ventral dural defect)

PATHOLOGY

- Low CSF volume secondary to leakage or overdrainage

CLINICAL ISSUES

- Autologous blood patch is mainstay
  - 15-30 mL, lumbar route
- Targeted blood patch or placement of fibrin glue if standard blood patch does not produce durable response
- Surgical dural closure or patching for identified leaks

(Left) Axial T1 C+ MR shows subdural effusions, small ventricles, and dural hyperemia in a patient with spontaneous intracranial hypotension. (Right) Axial CT myelography of the cervical spine shows leakage of contrast from the bilateral C5 nerve roots ➡ in this patient with spontaneous intracranial hypotension.

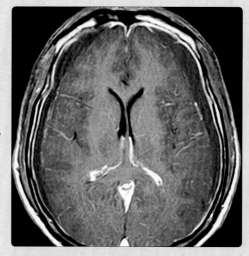
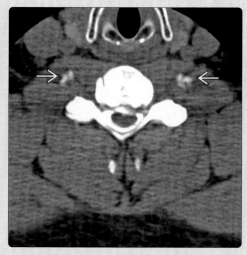

(Left) Axial CT myelogram shows extradural leakage into the ventral epidural space in the midthoracic spine ➡ in this patient with a fast thoracic CSF leak. (Right) Lateral thoracic view from a dynamic myelogram moving the contrast column toward the head shows the point of leakage ➡ from the ventral subarachnoid space through the dura and into the ventral epidural space.

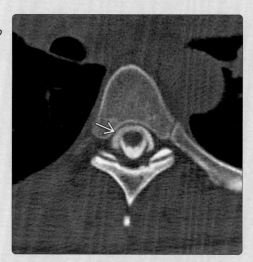
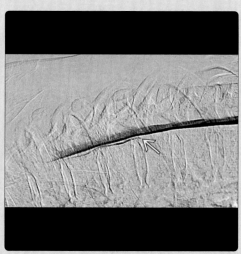

Pseudomeningocele

TERMINOLOGY

- Dural dehiscence, pseudocyst, CSF leak
- Spinal fluid collection contiguous with thecal sac, not lined with meninges

IMAGING

- CSF-filled spinal axis fluid collection with supportive postoperative or posttraumatic ancillary findings
- Most common location is dorsal to thecal sac at lumbar laminectomy site

TOP DIFFERENTIAL DIAGNOSES

- Paraspinous abscess
- Postoperative hematoma
  - Does not follow CSF signal on all pulse sequences
- Extradural spinal meningeal cyst
  - Nabors type 1
- True meningocele

- Disease or syndrome related, such as Marfan or neurofibromatosis type 1
- Plexiform neurofibroma

PATHOLOGY

- Posttraumatic
  - Most commonly following cervical root avulsion
  - May also see with posterior element fractures + dural laceration
- Postsurgical

CLINICAL ISSUES

- Commonly asymptomatic
- Nonspecific back pain
- Headache if associated with CSF hypotension

DIAGNOSTIC CHECKLIST

- Classic imaging appearance: CSF signal/density collection contiguous with thecal sac in correct clinical context

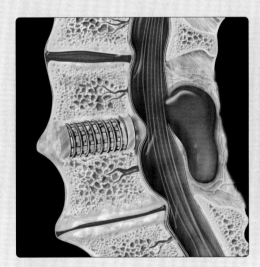

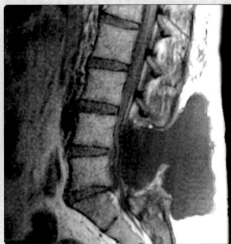

(Left) Sagittal graphic shows changes of L4-L5 interbody fusion with a cage. A large well-defined CSF collection extends into the dorsal soft tissue from the thecal sac from the site of operative dural tear. (Right) Sagittal T1WI MR shows a large CSF cyst at the surgical site extending dorsally from the dural sac into subcutaneous tissues. The CSF collection compresses the thecal sac at the L4 and L5 levels.

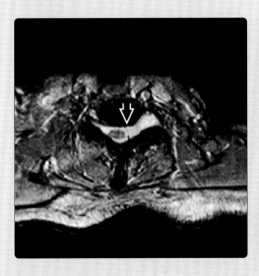

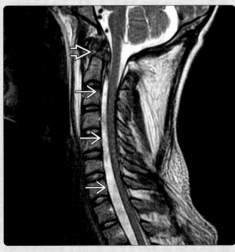

(Left) Axial T2* MR shows CSF signal pseudomeningocele extending out the neural foramina with septation separating the collections from the thecal sac ➡, reflecting old trauma and nerve root avulsion. (Right) Sagittal T2WI MR in a patient with C2 fracture ➡ and traumatic anterior cervical pseudomeningocele shows CSF signal collection anterior to the cord ➡ and with cord displacement. The surgery was pseudomeningocele decompression with discectomy at C5-C6, followed by C0-C2 fusion.

Direct Cord Trauma

TERMINOLOGY

- Iatrogenic surgical injury to spinal cord or root

IMAGING

- New T2 signal abnormality within cord following surgery
- Decreased T1W cord signal heralds poor prognosis

TOP DIFFERENTIAL DIAGNOSES

- Epidural hematoma
- Graft displacement
- Hardware malposition
- Bone impingement
- Cord infarction

PATHOLOGY

- Injury most likely during removal of posterior longitudinal ligament and posterior osteophytes during anterior cervical approach

CLINICAL ISSUES

- Variable incidence but < 1%
- Most common neurologic injuries
  - Radiculopathy (40%)
  - Permanent myelopathy (25%)
  - Recurrent laryngeal nerve palsy (17%)
- Root injury incidence is 4.6% after decompressive surgery for cervical myelopathy
- Root injury risk factors
  - Ossification of posterior longitudinal ligament
  - Older age
  - Increasing levels of decompression
- Treatment
  - Immediate imaging with MR or CT
  - Reexploration based on clinical and imaging findings
  - IV steroids (controversial, no clear evidence of efficacy)
  - Permissive hypertension

(Left) *Multilevel anterior cervical discectomy and fusion was attempted; during the procedure, somatosensory monitoring revealed cervical cord insult. The procedure was aborted and a posterior C2-C7 laminectomy was performed. Sagittal T2WI FS MR prior to surgery shows multilevel cervical spondylosis but no cord signal abnormality.* (Right) *Sagittal T2WI MR in the same patient immediately following surgery shows graft at C3-C4 ➡. Cord shows focal horizontal high signal from intraoperative trauma ➜.*

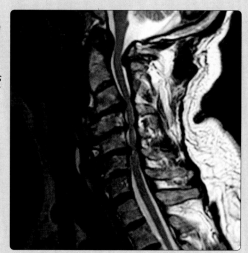
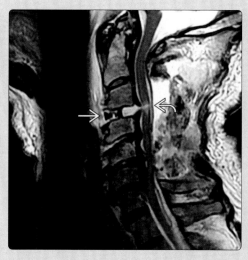

(Left) *Inadvertent intramedullary placement of a Baclofen catheter is seen on sagittal T2 MR study. The intramedullary location of the catheter ➡ is shown. High T2 signal cord edema surrounds the catheter ➜. (Right) Axial CECT study following myelogram shows posterior placement of the C5 screw ➡ related to ACDF, which is mildly effacing the ventral cord.*

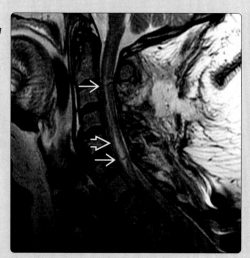
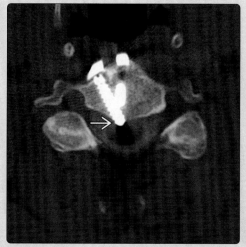

Vascular Injury

TERMINOLOGY

- Surgical traumatic injury to artery or vein
  - Vessel tear
  - Thrombosis
  - Dissection
  - Pseudoaneurysm

IMAGING

- Cervical surgery: Vertebral artery
  - Vertebral artery dissection or occlusion related to hardware malposition or direct injury
- Thoracic surgery
  - Aorta or intercostal arteries and esophagus for left-sided screws
- Lumbar anterior surgery
  - Iliac artery or vein

TOP DIFFERENTIAL DIAGNOSES

- Postoperative deep venous thrombosis

- Postoperative vasospasm
- Atherosclerotic stenosis
- Spontaneous dissection

PATHOLOGY

- **Vertebral injury**
  - Injury due to hardware malposition into course of vertebral artery (usually transverse foramen)
- **Common iliac vein**
  - Vein injury related to exposure at L4-5 and L5-S1
- **Iliac artery**
  - Usually results in thrombosis
- **Aortic abutment**
  - Seen in 2% of all malpositioned pedicle screws in 1 series
  - Screws in contact with major vessel (but not penetrating or deforming) may be observed
  - Screws placed for scoliosis surgery may move (plow) with direct vertebral rotation at time of surgery

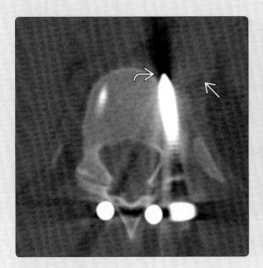

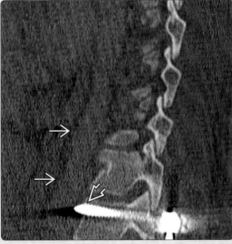

(Left) Axial NECT following surgery shows a left pedicle screw ➔ immediately adjacent to the aorta ➔, extending beyond the anterior vertebral body cortical margin. The patient was taken back to surgery and the screw backed out to appropriate depth. (Right) Sagittal NECT shows a left pedicle screw ➔ immediately adjacent to the aorta ➔, extending beyond the anterior vertebral body cortical margin.

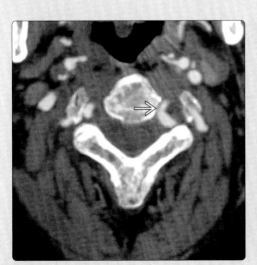

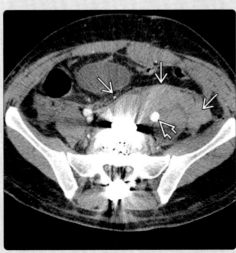

(Left) Axial CTA shows a anomalous course of a tortuous left vertebral artery entering into the left neural foramen ➔. (Right) CTA study in a patient with psoas and retroperitoneal hematoma following anterior interbody fusion at the L5-S1 level shows the large retroperitoneal hematoma ➔ extending circumferentially around the left iliac artery ➔.

Epidural Hematoma, Spine

TERMINOLOGY

- Hemorrhage build-up between dura & spine not caused by significant trauma/iatrogenic procedures

IMAGING

- Thoracic, lumbar > cervical
  - Lentiform or biconvex
- T1WI acute: < 48 hours
  - Isointense > hypo-/hyperintense
- T1WI subacute and chronic
  - Hyperintense > isointense
- T2WI heterogeneously hyperintense

TOP DIFFERENTIAL DIAGNOSES

- Epidural abscess
- Disc extrusion, migration
- Subdural hematoma
- Epidural fat lipomatosis
- Lymphoma

PATHOLOGY

- Idiopathic (40-50%)
- Minor trauma, anticoagulation, coagulopathy

CLINICAL ISSUES

- **Postoperative spinal epidural hematoma** < 1% incidence
  - Acute onset of neck, back pain
  - Progressive paraparesis
  - Bladder or bowel dysfunction
- Severity and duration of neurologic deficit predictive of postoperative neurologic recovery
  - Return to neurologic baseline after surgery
  - 89-95% of patients with incomplete neurologic deficit vs. 38-45% of patients with complete impairment
  - Improved outcome when surgery performed ≤ 36 hours in patients with complete sensorimotor loss
  - ≤ 48 hours in patients with incomplete deficit
- **Asymptomatic epidural hemorrhage common after surgery (33-100%)**

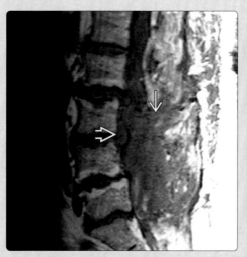
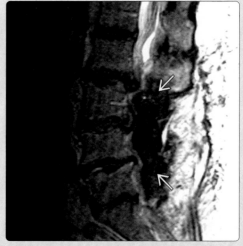

(Left) Sagittal T1WI MR shows a large lumbar laminectomy defect filled with intermediate signal ➡ and obscuring the normal CSF signal of the distal thecal sac. There is a large herniation at L3-L4 ⬌. (Right) Sagittal T2WI MR in the same patient shows marked diminished signal from the posterior epidural hemorrhage ➡, which severely compresses the thecal sac. Acute hemorrhage can have variable T2 signal and may also be hyperintense.

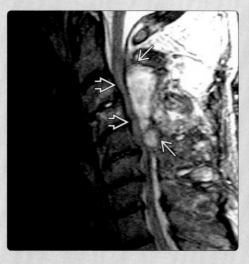
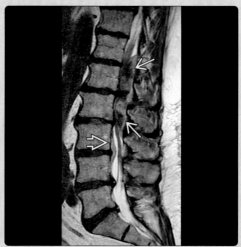

(Left) Sagittal T2WI MR shows a wide cervical laminectomy defect with intermediate signal filling the laminectomy defect ➡, which compresses the posterior thecal sac and cord ⬌. (Right) Sagittal T2WI MR shows a larger cephalad extradural mass ➡, which is mixed iso- and hypointense, ventrally displacing the cord and filum. Smaller caudal epidural hemorrhage shows mild effacement of the thecal sac at L3-L4 level ➡.

TERMINOLOGY

- Mechanical breakdown or malfunction of instrumentation

IMAGING

- **Fractured** or malpositioned metallic implant
- **Lucency** ± sclerosis along implant or at vertebral body-graft interface
- **Adjacent level** accelerated degenerative changes
- Soft tissue complications, marrow edema (suggesting segmental instability), or spinal cord injury
- Evaluation
  - Plain films excellent in evaluating vertebral alignment, instrumentation integrity, fusion status
  - Flexion-extension views if hardware failure present
  - CT evaluation if implant breakage suspected but not definitive on radiograph
    - Especially with complex constructs &/or in osteopenic patients
  - Enables accurate assessment of degree of osseous fusion; however, surgical exploration remains reference standard for evaluating fusion

PATHOLOGY

- Fibrous union may provide satisfactory stability in absence of radiographic osseous fusion

CLINICAL ISSUES

- Pain, tenderness, radiculopathy
- 2-45% reoperation rate for implant failure

DIAGNOSTIC CHECKLIST

- Compare with multiple prior studies to identify subtle progressive changes
- Failed fusion may indicate unsuspected ligamentous injury in trauma or tumor recurrence or progression

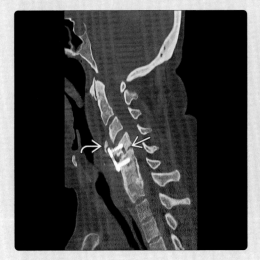

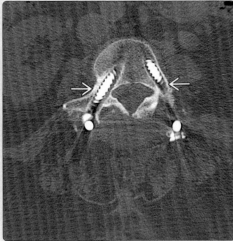

(Left) In this case, there is lack of fusion of the C4-C5 disc space ➡. Adjacent-level ossification within the first 12 postoperative months has a substantial likelihood of progression to advanced ossification by 24 months ➡. (Right) Axial NECT shows lucency and sclerosis along bilateral pedicle screw tracts ➡. Lucency suggests movement at the operated level and loosening of the screw. Such lucency is associated with delayed or failed fusion.

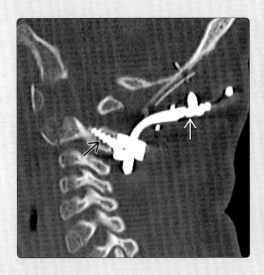

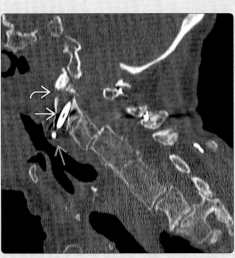

(Left) Sagittal NECT (bone window) in this child with Hurler syndrome shows that the fixation screws/plate ➡ have pulled away from the occipital bone. The proximal fixation screw in the C2 lateral mass ➡ is in the expected position. (Right) Sagittal NECT (bone window) shows a failed single screw fixation of a type II odontoid fracture ➡ with screw loosening ➡ as well as the screw backing out and extending into the retropharyngeal soft tissues ➡.

Complications

TERMINOLOGY

- Synonyms: Graft migration, graft displacement, graft extrusion
- Abnormal alignment, position, placement of graft or hardware ± associated neurologic deficit, instability, infection

IMAGING

- Plain films essential for rapid intraoperative/postoperative evaluation of graft position
- MDCT with reformats show graft position, endplate integrity, graft/vertebral body fractures
- Autogenous graft may show ↑ T1 signal with fatty marrow or ↓ signal due to edema
  - Allograft generally low signal
- T1WI C+ MR of little use in acute phase for graft malposition or epidural hemorrhage; mandatory if question of infection

TOP DIFFERENTIAL DIAGNOSES

- Abscess
- Hemorrhage
- Infarction
- Pseudoarthrosis

PATHOLOGY

- Graft migration rate ↑ with more levels of fusion
- ↑ graft migration with strut graft compared to interbody graft
- Graft migration occurs in 7% of cases after anterior cervical corpectomy

CLINICAL ISSUES

- May require reoperation for graft migration/extrusion/collapse
- New postoperative pain/focal deficit
- Rare respiratory distress

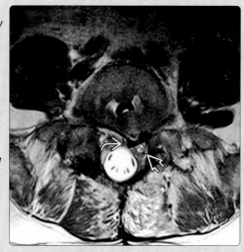

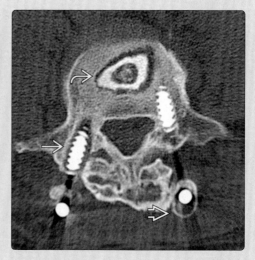

(Left) Axial T2WI MR in a patient following laminectomy and posterior lumbar interbody fusion shows posterior positioning of the lumbar interbody graft at the L4-L5 level ➡. The posterior margin of the graft contacts the dural margin and the exiting left L5 root ➡. (Right) Axial NECT in nonunion shows prominent lucency surrounding the bone graft ➡ and pedicle screws in the mid and distal aspects ➡. There is lucency and bony remodeling ➡ surrounding the junction with the longitudinal rod.

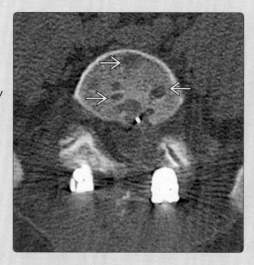

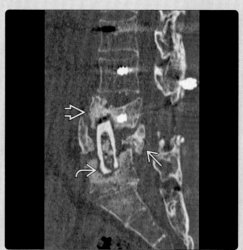

(Left) Axial NECT shows the effect of rhBMP-2 osseous remodeling with focal vertebral body bone resorption ➡. This appearance does not imply failure of fusion and generally will progress to solid fusion. (Right) Sagittal NECT shows the typical pattern of graft nonunion with lucency surrounding the graft placed at the L4 corpectomy site ➡. There is retropulsion of fracture fragment at L4 ➡ and collapse of the L3 body with sclerosis ➡.

TERMINOLOGY

- Recombinant human bone morphogenetic protein 2 (rhBMP-2)
  - Member of transforming growth factors-β super family of proteins
  - Used in surgery to decrease time of graft union and to reduce morbidity from nonunion
  - rhBMP-2 commercially supplied in USA as INFUSE bone graft (Medtronic; Minneapolis, MN)
  - rhBMP-7 commercially available as OP-1 putty (Olympus Biotech; Hopkinton, MA)

IMAGING

- Osteolysis seen as well-defined lucencies at vertebral endplates
- MR shows rounded low T1 signal, high T2 signal lesions along endplates
  - May mimic appearance of early postoperative infection
  - Usually involves adjacent vertebral bodies

TOP DIFFERENTIAL DIAGNOSES

- Heterotopic bone formation
  - Extradiscal, ectopic, and heterotopic bone production
  - Presumably occurs with BMP leakage from carrier into epidural space → canal or foraminal compression
- Resorption/osteolysis
  - Varying rates of occurrence of osteolysis (18-70%)
  - Lytic features resolve by 24 months, most by 9 months
- Subsidence/cage migration
  - Maximum osteolysis in first 12 weeks after surgery → cage at greatest risk for migration
- Hematomas/seromas
  - 5% of cases of posterolateral fusion in 1 series needed reoperation for exploration of painful seroma
- Soft tissue inflammation
  - rhBMP-2 not recommended for use in anterior cervical approach
  - > 20% of patients with neck swelling

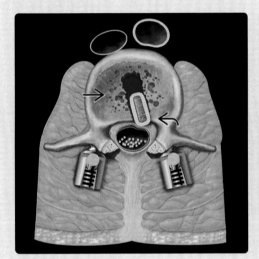

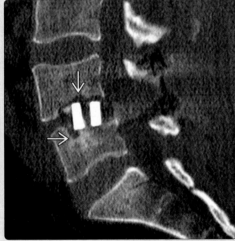

(Left) Axial graphic shows lysis of endplates ➡ associated with rhBMP-2 use in a posterior lumbar interbody fusion. There has been posterior migration of the interbody graft into the epidural space ➡. Maximum osteolysis occurs in the first 12 weeks after surgery. (Right) Sagittal CT shows lucency surrounding the graft ➡ in osteolysis related to bone rhBMP-2. This lucency might be concerning for infection or destruction but there is no sclerosis or soft tissue mass to suggest infection and the patient is asymptomatic.

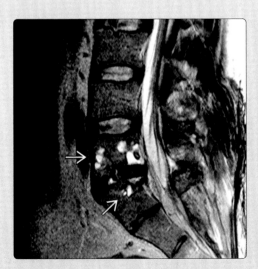

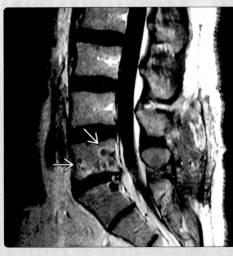

(Left) rhBMP-2 osteolysis is seen on this T2WI MR as multiple small, cystic-appearing lesions with T2 hyperintensity involving the L5 and S1 bodies ➡. Note the smooth margins with abrupt transition to more normal marrow signal and lack of adjacent marrow edema. (Right) Sagittal T1WI C+ MR in the same patient shows enhancement within several of the areas of lysis ➡, confirming their solid nature despite the T2 cystic appearance.

TERMINOLOGY

- Definition: Bone development in abnormal location
- Occurs in 3 main scenarios: rhBMP-2 related, TDR related, ACDF adjacent segment related

IMAGING

- Thin-section CT: High-attenuation bony osteophytes extending into canal or neural foramen with narrowing
- MR for definition of neural/thecal sac compression
- May be difficult to identify on T1WI if it contains fatty marrow mimicking adjacent fat signal

TOP DIFFERENTIAL DIAGNOSES

- Graft migration or extrusion
- Adjacent level degenerative change
- Myositis ossificans

PATHOLOGY

- **Osteobiologic related: Lumbar surgery**

- Extradiscal/ectopic/heterotopic bone formation presumably occurs when bone morphogenetic protein leaks from carrier into epidural space
- 75% incidence in 1 series of single-level posterior lumbar interbody fusion (PLIF)
- **Osteobiologic related: Cervical surgery**
- 11% of rhBMP-2 group vs. 6% in control group

CLINICAL ISSUES

- Majority of heterotopic ossification (HO) appears asymptomatic but symptomatic foraminal stenosis reported sporadically
- HO can be cause of new back pain and radiculopathy

DIAGNOSTIC CHECKLIST

- HO along PLIF or transforaminal lumbar interbody fusion path may be difficult to identify on axial images because it may be mistaken for normal pedicle
- Look closely at sagittal CT to identify bone projecting from disc level

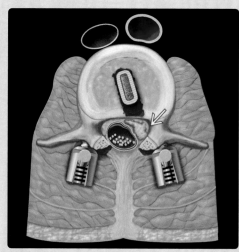
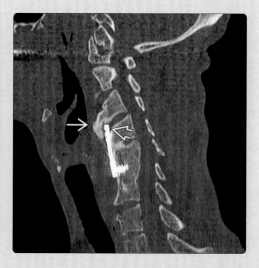

(Left) *Axial graphic shows heterotopic bone formation in a patient who has undergone a posterior lumbar interbody fusion. Bone formation is seen within the epidural space ➡ with mass effect upon the thecal sac. Heterotopic bone formation is highly correlated with the use of rhBMP-2.* (Right) *Sagittal NECT shows heterotopic ossification extending inferiorly from the C3 body ➡ to cover superior aspect of the C4 plate. This superior margin of the plate is malpositioned & extends to the disc level ➡.*

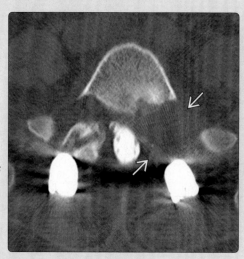
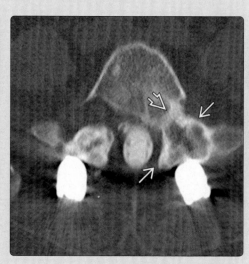

(Left) *Initial CT myelogram study shows a large facetectomy defect on the left at L5 ➡. Heterotopic bone formation mimics the appearance of facet joint in this patient status post facetectomy and posterior fusion.* (Right) *CT myelogram in the same patient performed 2 years later shows new heterotopic bone filling in the operative defect ➡, which has the outline of the prior facet joint margin. There is left foraminal stenosis ➡ from the heterotopic bone.*

Recurrent Disc Herniation

KEY FACTS

TERMINOLOGY

- Recurrent protrusion/extrusion
- Failed back surgery syndrome
- Focal extension of disc material beyond endplate margins at previously operated intervertebral disc level

IMAGING

- Nonenhancing, well-defined mass arising out of intervertebral disc
- Disc material shows no enhancement
- May enhance peripherally after intravenous contrast material due to granulation tissue or dilated epidural plexus
- Rare: Diffuse enhancement if associated with granulation tissue or if postcontrast imaging delayed
- Fat suppression of T1WI (pre-/postgadolinium) may increase sensitivity in detecting peridural fibrosis, differentiating fibrosis from disc

TOP DIFFERENTIAL DIAGNOSES

- Peridural fibrosis
  - Immediate homogeneous postcontrast enhancement
- Hemorrhage
- Abscess
- Osteophyte
- Synovial cyst/ganglion cyst
- Vertebral body/epidural tumor
  - Homogeneous enhancement

CLINICAL ISSUES

- Revision microdiscectomy with posterior lumbar interbody fusion/transforaminal lumbar interbody fusion vs. revision microdiscectomy
  - 30-35% success rate for repeat surgery (range: 12-100%)

DIAGNOSTIC CHECKLIST

- Best reoperative result in patients with herniation at new level away from operation site

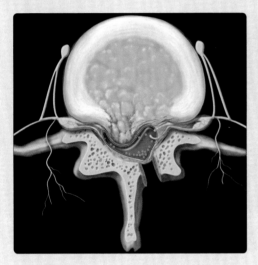

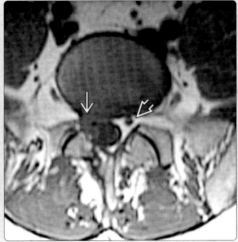

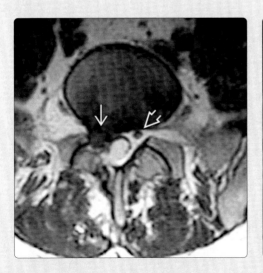

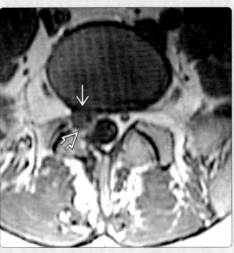

(Left) Axial graphic of the lumbar spine shows a left laminotomy defect. A large right paracentral herniation is present, compressing the thecal sac and roots adjacent to the site of the prior discectomy. (Right) Axial T1WI MR shows right-sided recurrent herniation as a focal epidural mass of intermediate signal with compression of the thecal sac ➡. The exiting right S1 root is obscured by the herniation. Note the normal position of the left S1 root ➡.

(Left) Axial T2WI MR shows right-sided recurrent extrusion ➡ as a focal low signal mass displacing the right S1 root and right lateral margin of the thecal sac. Note the normal left S1 root ➡. (Right) Axial T1WI C+ MR shows typical central lack of enhancement of herniation ➡ with peripheral enhancement of granulation tissue ➡.

TERMINOLOGY

- Scar formation within epidural space after lumbar surgery
- Part of failed back surgery syndrome (FBSS)

IMAGING

- Infiltration of epidural/perineural fat by enhancing soft tissue density (intensity)
- Variable signal intensity on T2WI
- Immediate homogeneous postcontrast enhancement

TOP DIFFERENTIAL DIAGNOSES

- Recurrent disc herniation
- Epidural abscess/phlegmon
- Pseudomeningocele
- Postoperative hemorrhage
- Arachnoiditis

PATHOLOGY

- Postoperative scarring is part of normal reparative mechanism
- May be asymptomatic; contribution to clinical symptoms controversial
- Up to 1/4 of all FBSS cases
- Most patients with some degree of fibrosis are asymptomatic

CLINICAL ISSUES

- Adult with gradual onset low back pain following initially successful disc surgery

DIAGNOSTIC CHECKLIST

- Identification of only epidural fibrosis in FBSS patient is contraindication to reoperation, yields poor reoperative result

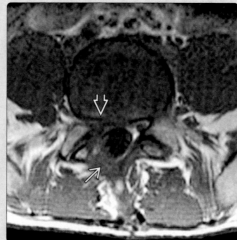
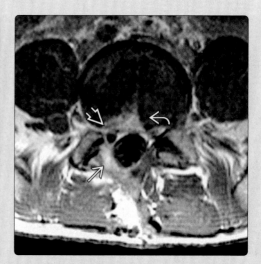

(Left) Axial T1WI MR shows a right laminectomy defect and extensive epidural fibrosis ➡ surrounding the right lateral and dorsal aspect of the thecal sac and the exiting root ➡. (Right) Axial T1WI C+ MR shows a right hemilaminectomy defect and diffuse enhancement of epidural fibrosis surrounding the right lateral aspect of the thecal sac ➡. The nerve root is seen as a nonenhancing structure within the fibrosis ➡. Enhancement continues into the operative defect in the disc ➡.

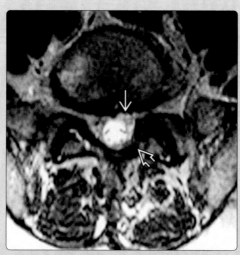
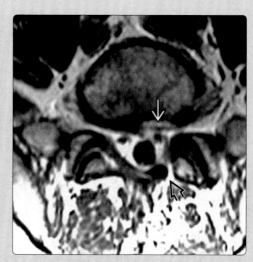

(Left) Axial T2WI MR a shows hemilaminectomy defect and absence of ligamentum flavum ➡. Epidural fibrosis surrounding the left S1 root shows slight increased signal relative to adjacent disc material ➡. (Right) Axial T1WI C+ MR shows a left hemilaminectomy defect ➡. A small amount of epidural fibrosis surrounds the exiting left S1 root, which diffusely enhances ➡, as does the operative defect in the posterior anulus.

TERMINOLOGY

- Postinflammatory changes usually involving cauda equina

IMAGING

- Thickening and clumping of nerve roots in cauda equina
- Adhesion of nerve roots to peripheral dura (empty sac sign)
- Soft tissue mass (pseudomass)
- Minimal to mild pial, dural enhancement
- Nerve root calcification (rare) or calcific mass (arachnoiditis ossificans)

TOP DIFFERENTIAL DIAGNOSES

- Spinal stenosis
- Cauda equina neoplasms
- Carcinomatous meningitis
- Intradural metastases

PATHOLOGY

- Inflammatory, collagenous mass

- Historically related to trauma or spinal meningitis, now more commonly associated with prior lumbar surgery

CLINICAL ISSUES

- Most common symptoms are chronic low back pain or leg pain (radicular or nonradicular)
  - Simulates spinal stenosis and polyneuropathy
- Less common are paraparesis, hypoesthesia, gait disorder, bowel/bladder dysfunction
- Treatment
  - Pain rehabilitation
  - Spinal cord stimulation

DIAGNOSTIC CHECKLIST

- Absent discrete nerve roots in thecal sac with clumping or empty sac sign highly suggestive of lumbar arachnoiditis
- Radiological findings may be present without clinical symptoms

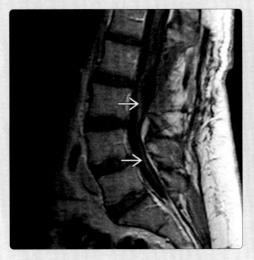

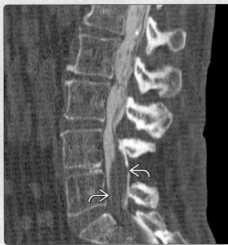

(Left) Sagittal T1 C+ MR shows clumping of the nerve roots of the cauda equina ➡. There is faint enhancement. A L2-L3 laminectomy defect is noted. (Right) Sagittal CECT myelography shows a large, mass-like filling defect in the caudal thecal sac (pseudomass) ➥ engulfing the cauda equina due to chronic changes of arachnoiditis.

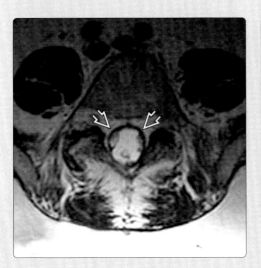

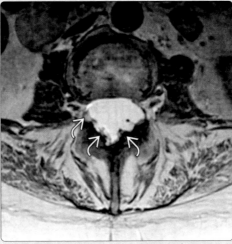

(Left) Axial T2WI MR shows diffuse thickening of the distal dural sac and clumping of the roots consistent with severe arachnoiditis. Note the thickening low signal dural margin suggestive of calcific arachnoiditis ➡. (Right) Axial T2WI MR in this patient with ankylosing spondylitis shows peripheral adhesion of the nerve roots to the margins of the thecal sac ➡, resulting in the empty sac sign of arachnoiditis. This pattern may cause cauda equina syndrome in patients with longstanding spondyloarthropathy.

Arachnoiditis Ossificans

TERMINOLOGY

- Intradural ossification associated with postinflammation adhesion and clumping of lumbar nerve roots

IMAGING

- Calcification morphology
  - Thin, linear
  - Mass-like, globular
- Calcific density on CT
  - Contrast may obscure calcifications on CT myelography
- T1WI: Areas of ossification are variable, mixed signal
  - Hypointense, isointense, or hyperintense
- T2WI: Linear or globular hypointensity if calcifications are present
  - Larger areas of ossification can occasionally be hyperintense on T2WI
- May exert mass effect on conus and cauda equina

PATHOLOGY

- Etiologies
  - Prior trauma
  - Spinal surgery
  - Subarachnoid hemorrhage
  - Pantopaque myelography
  - Spinal anesthesia
- Gross pathology: Calcified, inflammatory, collagenous mass

CLINICAL ISSUES

- No defining clinical symptomatology
  - Low back pain
  - Radicular or nonradicular leg pain
  - Paraparesis
  - Bladder and bowel dysfunction

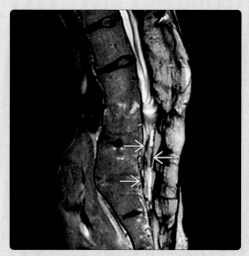
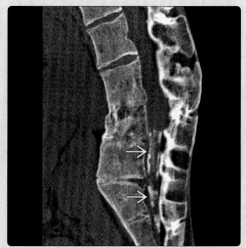

(Left) Sagittal T2WI MR through the lumbar spine shows a nodular hypointense signal along the margins of the caudal thecal sac ➡ due to calcific arachnoiditis. Note the prior multilevel anterior fusions. (Right) Sagittal NECT through the lumbar spine more clearly shows the coarse calcifications of the dura and thecal sac ➡. CT also shows intervertebral fusion at L3-L4, L4-L5, and L5-S1.

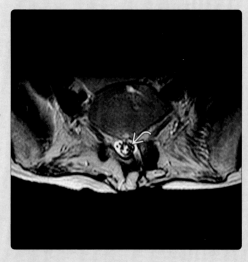
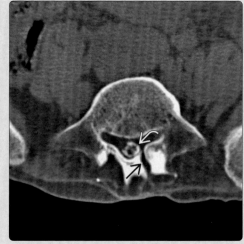

(Left) Axial T2WI MR again shows irregular hypointensity about the margins of the thecal sac ➡ due to dystrophic calcifications. (Right) Axial NECT shows coarse calcifications of the caudal thecal sac ➡. Also seen is a surgical defect of the left L5 lamina ➡.

Accelerated Degeneration

TERMINOLOGY

- Accelerated degeneration of disc space/facets at level(s) adjacent to surgical fusion
- Transitional degenerative syndrome, accelerated segmental degeneration, adjacent segment disease

IMAGING

- Degenerative disc/facet changes directly above or below fusion
  - Also occurs adjacent to congenital segmentation anomalies
- May show increased motion at degenerated level adjacent to fused segment
  - Flexion/extension views for definition of instability
- Plain films most economical way to demonstrate presence of adjacent segment degenerative changes and to serially follow for progression
- MR best identifies soft tissue abnormalities that are occult on plain film

TOP DIFFERENTIAL DIAGNOSES

- Disc space infection
- Pseudoarthrosis
- Spondylolysis
- Spondylolisthesis
- Normal postoperative changes

PATHOLOGY

- Produced by altered biophysical stresses from altered normal spinal motion
- Solid fusion alters biomechanics at adjacent mobile levels
- More common with multilevel fusion but also seen following single level fusion
- Presence of osteopenia at time of cervical surgery increases risk of adjacent segment degeneration

DIAGNOSTIC CHECKLIST

- Pseudoarthrosis if extensive signal abnormality involving anterior and posterior elements in horizontal fashion

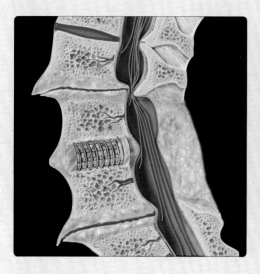

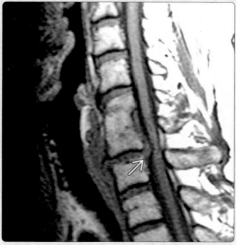

(Left) Sagittal graphic shows solid L4-L5 interbody fusion and laminectomy. Note severe disc degeneration at L3-L4 with spondylolisthesis, loss of disc height, osteophytes and central stenosis, and severe degeneration at L5-S1 due to altered biomechanics. (Right) Sagittal T1WI MR shows a solid fusion at C5-C6 with normal fatty marrow signal. There is disc degeneration at C6-C7 with decreased disc height and large disc extrusion compressing cord ➡.

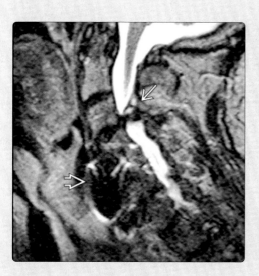

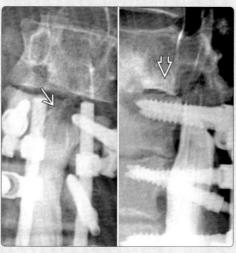

(Left) Sagittal T2WI MR shows a patient post C4-C7 fusion with anterior plating giving low signal artifact ➡. There is a large synovial cyst showing central hyperintensity at the C3-C4 level ➡. (Right) Anteroposterior myelography (left) shows block to contrast at L1-L2 ➡ at the upper margin of posterior fusion. Lateral view (right) shows contrast block and severe L1-L2 degeneration ➡.

TERMINOLOGY

- Deformity: Abnormality of alignment, angulation, or shape of vertebral column following surgery
  - May be associated with clinically significant findings such as instability

TOP DIFFERENTIAL DIAGNOSES

- Infection
- Tumor
- Degenerative instability
- Isthmic spondylolisthesis

PATHOLOGY

- Risk factors for deformity
  - Age (pediatric at increased risk), number of levels
  - Location of laminectomy
  - Intramedullary disease
  - Facet joint involvement
  - Bone density

- Preexisting degenerative disease risk factor for cervical deformity
  - 30% incidence of kyphosis in patients with straight spine
- Thoracolumbar junction
  - Particularly susceptible to deformity
- Spinal deformity reoperation complications as high as 33%
  - Implant failure
  - Adjacent segment degeneration (10%)
  - Pseudoarthrosis

CLINICAL ISSUES

- Surgery for progressive neurological decline, intractable pain, cosmetic appearance

DIAGNOSTIC CHECKLIST

- Thresholds for optimal correction of adult deformity include sagittal vertical axis < 50 mm, pelvic tilt < 25°, and pelvic incidence-lumbar lordosis < 10°

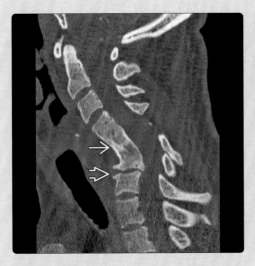
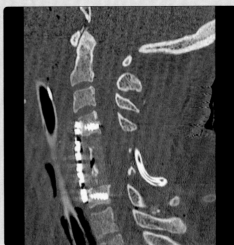

(Left) Sagittal NECT shows severe kyphotic deformity at site of anterior fusion ➡ at C5-C6 and adjacent segment degeneration ➡ at C6-C7. There had been prior laminectomy and posterior fusion. (Right) Sagittal NECT shows near normal alignment after 2 stages of surgery. The 1st stage was posterior osteotomies; the 2nd stage was anterior vertebrectomies with strut graft with plate/screws. The 3rd stage was posterior instrumented fusion (not shown).

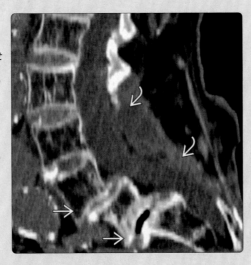
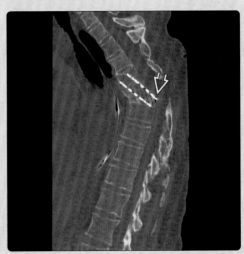

(Left) Sagittal NECT shows severe multilevel spondylolisthesis ➡ with multilevel laminectomy defect ➡. (Right) Sagittal CT shows increased kyphotic angulation in this patient following posterior laminectomy and corpectomy. Note the angulation of the cage with the displacement of the posterior superior margin into the canal ➡.

KEY FACTS

TERMINOLOGY

- Chronic progressive radiation myelitis
- Delayed radiation myelopathy

IMAGING

- Spindle-shaped cord swelling with irregular, focal rind of enhancement (early)
- Focal cord atrophy (late)
- Clinical signs may reflect longer segment of damage than demonstrated on MR

TOP DIFFERENTIAL DIAGNOSES

- Transverse myelitis
- Multiple sclerosis
- Spinal cord infarct
- Astrocytoma
- Syrinx

PATHOLOGY

- Demyelination, lipid-laden microphages, swollen astrocytes, endothelial damage, necrosis, local Ca^{++} deposition, hyalinosis of intramedullary vessel walls

CLINICAL ISSUES

- Onset of progressive numbness and weakness ± sphincter dysfunction 1 month → several years after fractionated radiotherapy
- Relentless progression without significant improvement in most cases

DIAGNOSTIC CHECKLIST

- Late focal atrophy at sites of previous enhancement
- Fatty marrow replacement in treatment field provides clue to etiology
- Pathologic cord changes not always visible on MR imaging

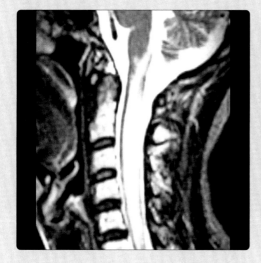
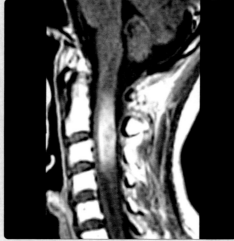

(Left) Sagittal T2WI MR in a patient following radiation therapy for head and neck squamous cell carcinoma demonstrates abnormal intramedullary T2 hyperintensity in conjunction with fatty marrow replacement, characteristic of postradiation vertebral and spinal cord changes. (Right) Sagittal T1WI C+ MR confirms abnormal spinal cord parenchymal enhancement in the area of greatest radiation myelopathic injury. Note also the marked T1 shortening in the vertebral marrow reflecting fatty replacement.

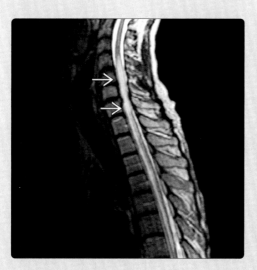
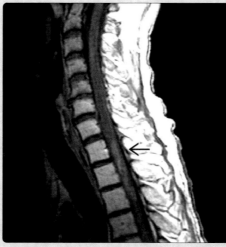

(Left) Sagittal T2WI MR following radiation treatment for melanoma shows extensive radiation myelopathy involving the cervical and thoracic cord with diffuse cord hyperintensity ➡. (Right) Sagittal T1 C+ MR in this patient with extensive radiation myelopathy involving cervical and thoracic cord following treatment for melanoma shows ill-defined mild enhancement of the upper thoracic cord from T1 to T3 ➡.

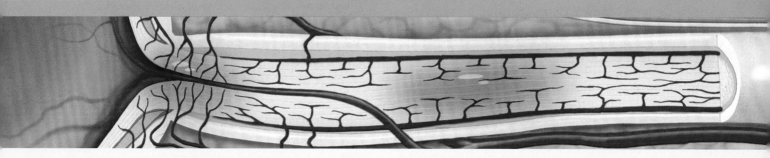

SECTION 11
Remote Complications

Terminology

Postoperative vision loss (POVL)

Ischemic optic neuropathy (ION)

General Medical Complications

Orthopedic surgery in total (including spine surgery) has a 1-5% incidence of cardiac death and nonfatal myocardial infarction. Studies have shown a 3.4% incidence of cardiac complications in spine surgery with a mortality as high as 70%. Highly functioning, cardiac asymptomatic patients who tolerate 4 metabolic equivalents (METS) do not seem to benefit from additional preoperative cardiac testing. For reference, 4 METS is equivalent to daily activities, including walking, eating, etc. Golf and climbing stairs requires more than 4 METS. Most postoperative myocardial infarctions occur in the first 48 hours after surgery. These are usually chest pain-free events with tachycardia.

Pulmonary Complications

Pulmonary complications such as atelectasis, pneumonia, respiratory failure, and bronchospasm are even more common than cardiac complications. Patient risk factors for pulmonary complications include COPD, stopping smoking < 8 weeks prior to surgery, continued smoking, surgery > 3 hours, albumin < 3 g/dL, and BUN > 30 mg/dL. Patients with COPD are 6x more likely to have complications. In 1 study of > 1,500 patients who underwent cervical corpectomy, pulmonary complications were the most common type (8.5%). Eighteen percent of patients in this study who underwent 3-level corpectomy had reoperation.

Surgical Complexity

More complex surgeries, not surprisingly, have more complications. One study of en bloc resections showed 34% had complications with > 2% mortality. Increased risk of complication in this group related to prior unsuccessful treatment or open biopsy, which contaminated the epidural space. Other factors that increased complication risk were multisegmental resections and double combined approaches. Devastating complications included 1 death due to vena cava injury and 2 late deaths from aortic dissections. General medical complications included myocardial infarction, pulmonary embolus, and renal failure. Ten percent of patients with a single posterior approach to tumor resection had a complication, whereas 48% of double-approach en bloc resections had a complication. Other risk factors include increasing age, American Society of Anesthesiologists class, history of disseminated cancer, and diabetes.

Remote Complication Categories

Remote complications can be viewed by the imager as either intuitive or nonintuitive.

Intuitive Remote Complications

Intuitive complications can be logically deduced from the nature of the surgery and the intraoperative adverse event. These tend to be easier to recognize because they flow from the procedure itself. For example, intracranial subdural hematoma might not be an obvious complication from physically remote spine surgery but not when placed into the framework of an intraoperative unintended durotomy with resultant CSF leak and intracranial hypotension. Cases of remote cerebellar hemorrhage may occur after uneventful spinal surgery when there is CSF loss. Again, intracranial hypotension with brain sagging is considered a possible mechanism for this complication. A distinct but seemingly related complication after uneventful spine surgery is described as pseudohypoxic brain swelling. This devastating (and potentially fatal) complication can occur in spinal surgery with minimal dural laceration and use of subfascial suction drains. Even in the most experienced surgical hands, unintended durotomy occurs at least in 1.6% of spine surgeries. An additional example of an intuitive type of complication is superior mesenteric artery (SMA) syndrome. SMA syndrome is a known complication of spine osteotomy. Although unusual, this makes sense given the marked change in alignment of the spine that occurs when closing the osteotomy with stretching of the ventral vessels.

Nonintuitive Remote Complications

Nonintuitive remote complications are ones that must be individually defined because one cannot logically deduce that they might occur. Examples of this type might be pancreatitis related to spine surgery and POVL. Why pancreatitis? No one really knows. Theories as to the cause of pancreatitis after spine surgery (particularly scoliosis surgery in children and adolescents) vary from nutritional status of the patient, intraoperative positioning, hypotension, and drug effect to derangement of the autonomic system affecting secretion of the gland.

Postoperative Vision Loss

Vision loss after surgery is a unique complication associated predominately with spine surgery. Factors affecting vision loss related to ION include increased duration of surgery, large degree of blood loss, and excessive use of replacement fluids. Patient positioning (head below heart level) seems also to be important. The incidence of POVL in all nonocular surgeries is estimated to be 1 in 60,000. However, the incidence in spine surgery is strikingly higher, on the order of 1 in 500. How can the imager be of help? The differential of POVL is 4-fold: External injuries such as corneal abrasion, central retinal artery occlusion, cortical blindness, and ION. Ophthalmologic examination allows the diagnosis of ION with classic fundal changes. Imaging is important to exclude cortical blindness with occipital infarction or more caudal causes of vessel injury such as vertebral dissection from cervical screw malposition.

Selected References

1. Malham GM et al: Anterior lumbar interbody fusion using recombinant human bone morphogenetic protein-2: a prospective study of complications. J Neurosurg Spine. 21(6):851-60, 2014
2. Willson MC et al: Postoperative spine complications. Neuroimaging Clin N Am. 24(2):305-26, 2014
3. Parpaley Y et al: Pseudohypoxic brain swelling (postoperative intracranial hypotension-associated venous congestion) after spinal surgery: report of 2 cases. Neurosurgery. 68(1):E277-83, 2011
4. Williams BJ et al: Incidence of unintended durotomy in spine surgery based on 108,478 cases. Neurosurgery. 68(1):117-23; discussion 123-4, 2011
5. Choi D et al: Outcome of 132 operations in 97 patients with chordomas of the craniocervical junction and upper cervical spine. Neurosurgery. 66(1):59-65; discussion 65, 2010
6. Dupanovic M et al: Management of the airway in multitrauma. Curr Opin Anaesthesiol. 23(2):276-82, 2010
7. Goepfert CE et al: Ischemic optic neuropathy: are we any further? Curr Opin Anaesthesiol. 23(5):582-7, 2010
8. Gonzalez-Garcia A et al: Ischemic optic neuropathy. Semin Ophthalmol. 25(4):130-5, 2010
9. He M et al: The use of diffusion MRI in ischemic optic neuropathy and optic neuritis. Semin Ophthalmol. 25(5-6):225-32, 2010
10. Lee LA et al: Postoperative ischemic optic neuropathy. Spine (Phila Pa 1976). 35(9 Suppl):S105-16, 2010
11. Miglis MG et al: Intracranial venous thrombosis after placement of a lumbar drain. Neurocrit Care. 12(1):83-7, 2010

12. Nasser R et al: Complications in spine surgery. J Neurosurg Spine. 13(2):144-57, 2010

13. Onishi E et al: Cerebral infarction due to an embolism after cervical pedicle screw fixation. Spine (Phila Pa 1976). 35(2):E63-6, 2010

14. Pierce V et al: Ischemic optic neuropathy after spine surgery. AANA J. 78(2):141-5, 2010

15. Radhakrishnan M et al: Perioperative stroke following anterior cervical discectomy. Br J Neurosurg. 24(5):592-4, 2010

16. Eskander MS et al: Injury of an aberrant vertebral artery during a routine corpectomy: a case report and literature review. Spinal Cord. 47(10):773-5, 2009

17. Kang BU et al: An analysis of general surgery-related complications in a series of 412 minilaparotomic anterior lumbosacral procedures. J Neurosurg Spine. 10(1):60-5, 2009

18. Morofuji Y et al: Remote cerebellar hemorrhage following thoracic spinal surgery. Neurol Med Chir (Tokyo). 49(3):117-9, 2009

19. Than KD et al: Postoperative management of incidental durotomy in minimally invasive lumbar spinal surgery. Minim Invasive Neurosurg. 51(5):263-6, 2008

20. Baig MN et al: Vision loss after spine surgery: review of the literature and recommendations. Neurosurg Focus. 23(5):E15, 2007

21. Cornips EM et al: Fatal cerebral and cerebellar hemorrhagic infarction after thoracoscopic microdiscectomy. Case report. J Neurosurg Spine. 6(3):276-9, 2007

22. Smith-Hammond CA et al: Prospective analysis of incidence and risk factors of dysphagia in spine surgery patients: comparison of anterior cervical, posterior cervical, and lumbar procedures. Spine (Phila Pa 1976). 29(13):1441-6, 2004

23. Ding R et al: Pneumonia in stroke patients: a retrospective study. Dysphagia. 15(2):51-7, 2000

24. Boriani S et al: Primary bone tumors of the spine. Terminology and surgical staging. Spine (Phila Pa 1976). 22(9):1036-44, 1997

25. Tomita K et al: Total en bloc spondylectomy. A new surgical technique for primary malignant vertebral tumors. Spine (Phila Pa 1976). 22(3):324-33, 1997

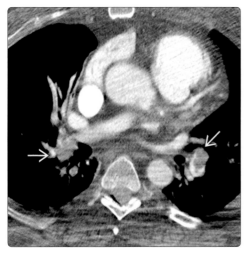

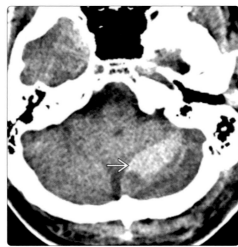

(Left) *This patient had resection of cervical schwannoma with preoperative left vertebral occlusion and tumor embolization. Postoperatively, the patient developed extensive pulmonary emboli* ➡, *as can be seen on this axial CECT.* (Right) *Postoperative cerebellar hemorrhage is shown on this axial noncontrast CT study as linear increased attenuation within the left cerebellum following spine surgery* ➡. *Remote cerebellar hemorrhage may be uni- or bilateral.*

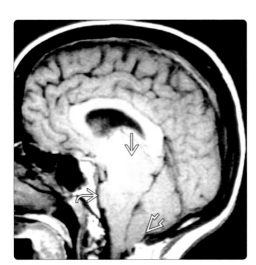

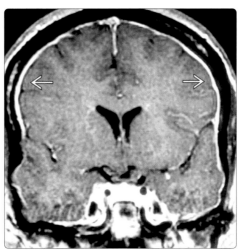

(Left) *Sagittal T1WI MR shows the typical appearance of severe intracranial hypotension and brain sag. Note the descent and distortion of the brainstem* ➡, *flattening of the pons against the clivus* ➡, *and low tonsils* ➡. (Right) *Coronal T1WI MR following contrast shows the typical diffuse dural enhancement* ➡ *of intracranial hypotension.*

Donor Site Complications

TERMINOLOGY

- **Graft characteristics**
  - Osteogenesis → create new bone
  - Osteoinduction → stimulate osteoblastic differentiation of progenitor cells
  - Osteoconduction → scaffold for bone deposition
- Graft needs porosity to enhance bony ingrowth (cancellous-type bone)
  - Also needs load-bearing capacity (cortical-type bone)
- **Autograft**
  - Gold standard, 77% mean arthrodesis rate
  - Biocompatible
  - No disease transmission
  - Nonimmunogenic
- **Graft morbidity**
  - 20-30% suffer persistent graft site pain
  - 15% numbness
  - 12% impaired ambulation

- Other complications
  - Infection (7%)
  - Hematoma
  - Pelvic fracture
  - Peritoneal perforation
  - Gait disturbance
  - Ureteral injury
  - Hernia
- **Allograft**
  - Avoids donor site morbidity
  - Has risk of disease transmission
  - 74% rate of arthrodesis
- **Synthetics**
  - Multiple types
    - Avoids donor site complications
    - Biocompatible
    - Limitless supply

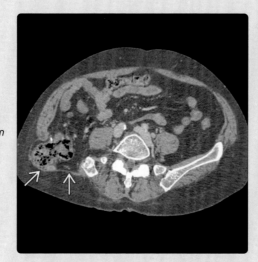
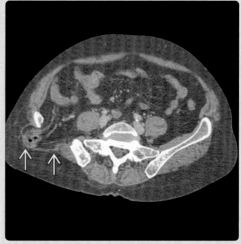

(Left) Axial bone CT of an unusual complication following large iliac bone graft harvest demonstrates protrusion of the colon and mesenteric fat through the large right iliac wing bone graft harvest site ➡. (Right) Axial CT in the same patient shows protrusion of the colon through the large right iliac wing bone graft harvest site ➡.

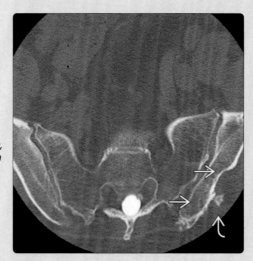
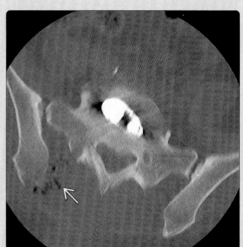

(Left) Axial NECT shows the typical appearance of an old iliac crest donor site with corticated margins ➡ and a small focus of heterotopic bone formation ➡. (Right) Axial NECT shows prior anterior lumbar interbody fusion with gas in the soft tissue adjacent to the right posterior iliac wing donor site, reflecting soft tissue infection ➡.

TERMINOLOGY

- Deep vein thrombosis: Condition where blood solidifies, producing blood clot (thrombus) within deep venous system, typically in lower limbs
- Can also be seen in upper limbs (especially related to central venous catheters)

IMAGING

- Filling defect in deep veins or pulmonary arteries
  - CT, MR, or contrast venogram, pulmonary CTA
- Noncompressible vein with intraluminal echoes on ultrasound examination
  - Duplex Doppler ultrasound 1st-line imaging tool; 90-100% sensitivity and specificity for acute deep vein thrombosis (DVT)
- CECT and CT/MR venography good noninvasive imaging tools
  - Assessment of pelvic veins and inferior vena cava; exclusion of pelvic and abdominal causes of DVT

- Conventional venography has 11% false-negative rate
  - Used in combination with catheter-directed or mechanical thrombolysis

TOP DIFFERENTIAL DIAGNOSES

- Interpretation errors
- Technical errors

CLINICAL ISSUES

- Acute DVT: Swollen, tender lower limb (swelling extent depends on DVT site), increased temperature
- Postthrombotic syndrome: Sequelae of DVT resulting from chronic venous obstruction &/or acquired incompetence of valves
  - Chronic leg swelling, ankle pigmentation, ulceration in lower calf and ankle (gaiter zone)
- Anticoagulation therapy for above knee DVT and PE; treatment for calf vein DVT controversial
- Heparin anticoagulation (unfractionated or low molecular weight) initial treatment for acute DVT

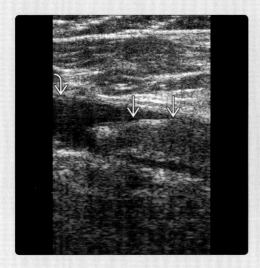
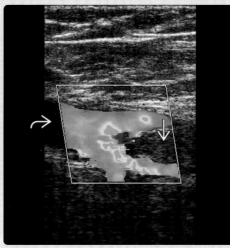

(Left) Grayscale ultrasound of the right upper thigh shows extensive echogenic thrombus ➡ in the lumen of the deep femoral vein ➡. This is a typical case of deep venous thrombosis. (Right) Color Doppler ultrasound of the right upper thigh shows extensive echogenic thrombus without flow ➡ in the lumen of the deep femoral vein, which shows color blood flow ➡. This is also a typical case of deep venous thrombosis.

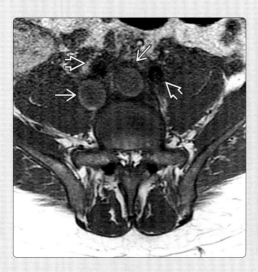
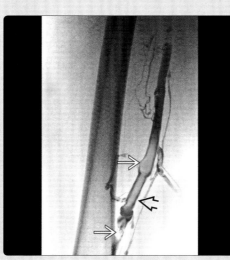

(Left) Axial T1WI MR at admission shows acute venous thrombosis with markedly distended iliac veins ➡ that lack the usual flow void. Note the normal arterial flow void of iliac arteries ➡. (Right) AP venogram shows extensive intraluminal filling defects ➡ in the superficial femoral vein of the thigh. A small amount of contrast ➡ outlines the thrombus with a resultant tram-track sign.

KEY FACTS

TERMINOLOGY

- Pulmonary arterial blockage with resultant segmental perfusion defect(s), most commonly caused by emboli arising from pelvic or lower extremity deep vein thrombosis

IMAGING

- Central low-density filling defect within pulmonary arteries on CTA or angiography
- CTA examination of choice
- CXR poor sensitivity and specificity
- V/Q scan highly sensitive but nonspecific

TOP DIFFERENTIAL DIAGNOSES

- Tumor thrombus
- Primary pulmonary artery sarcoma
- Pulmonary vasculitis
- Laminar flow artifact

CLINICAL ISSUES

- **Thromboembolism prophylaxis**
- Intermittent compression devices postoperatively
- Anticoagulation by either
  - Low-dose unfractionated heparin perioperatively
  - Low-molecular-weight heparin postoperatively
- **Risk factors for spine surgery**
  - Immobilization
  - Long operative times
  - Increased number of fused levels
  - Prone positioning with flexion of hips/knees
  - Spine distraction
  - Combined anterior/posterior surgery
- Anticoagulation is mainstay of treatment
  - Thrombolysis for severely symptomatic patients
  - Inferior vena cava filter if contraindications to drug therapy

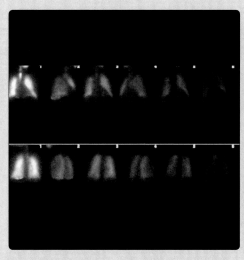
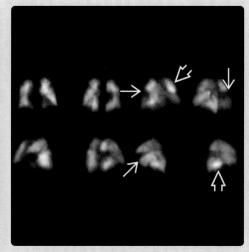

(Left) Ventilation study from a V/Q scan with findings of pulmonary embolism shows normal ventilation. Multiple segmental perfusion defects were also present. (Right) V/Q scan findings of pulmonary embolism in the same patient show high probability scan multiple segmental perfusion defects ➡ and areas of hyperperfusion ➡.

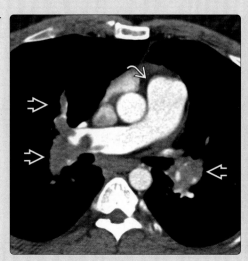
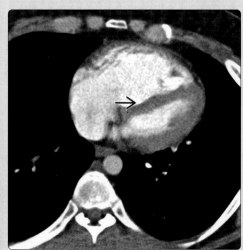

(Left) CECT reveals large lobar artery thrombi ➡ and enlargement of the main pulmonary artery relative to the ascending aorta ➡. (Right) Axial CECT shows marked increase in RV/LV ratio and flattening of the intraventricular septum ➡. The typical CT features of right heart strain and pulmonary arterial hypertension from pulmonary emboli are present.

Aspiration Pneumonia

TERMINOLOGY

- Aspiration pneumonia: Pulmonary infection caused by aspiration of colonized oropharyngeal secretions
- Aspiration pneumonitis: Acute lung injury caused by aspiration of materials inherently toxic to lungs (gastric acid, milk, mineral oil, and volatile hydrocarbons)
- Predisposing factors: Alcoholism, loss of consciousness, structural abnormalities of pharynx and esophagus, neuromuscular disorders, and deglutition abnormalities

IMAGING

- Gravity-dependent opacities
- Radiopaque material within airways (foreign body)
- Unilateral or bilateral airspace consolidation in dependent distribution
- Diffuse perihilar consolidation
- Consolidation with cavitation
- Airspace consolidation, solitary or multiple; gravitational distribution
- Atelectasis, segmental or lobar

TOP DIFFERENTIAL DIAGNOSES

- Diffuse bilateral opacities: Pulmonary edema, hemorrhage, diffuse alveolar damage
- Multifocal (patchy) airspace opacities: Organizing pneumonia, eosinophilic pneumonia, sarcoid, tuberculosis, vasculitis

PATHOLOGY

- Pulmonary edema, hyaline membrane formation, and alveolar hemorrhage (Mendelson syndrome)
  - Up to 50% death rate for patients who develop acute respiratory distress syndrome from Mendelson syndrome

CLINICAL ISSUES

- 300,000 to 600,000 cases per year in United States
- 5-15% of cases of community-acquired pneumonia

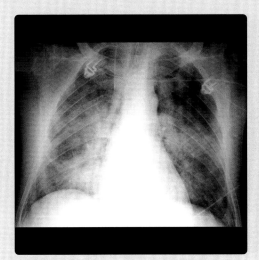

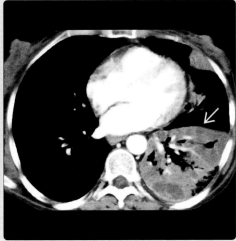

(Left) Anteroposterior radiograph shows extensive symmetrical bilateral consolidation after massive gastric aspiration. (Right) Axial CECT in the same patient shows left lower lobe homogeneous consolidation due to aspirated secretions and atelectasis ➔. The air bronchogram and opacified vessels give a CT angiogram sign.

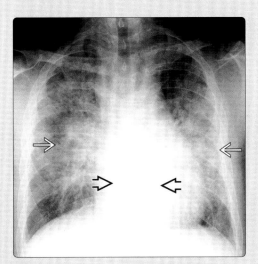

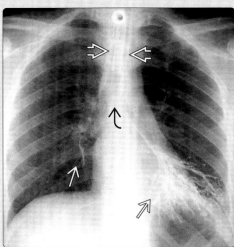

(Left) Frontal radiograph shows mediastinal widening ➔ from achalasia and diffuse central consolidation ➔ from massive aspiration. (Right) Inflated tracheostomy balloons do not necessarily prevent aspiration. This AP radiograph shows a tracheostomy tube in the normal position above the carina ➔ with the balloon inflated ➔. Swallowed barium passes the inflated balloon into both lower lobes ➔.

KEY FACTS

TERMINOLOGY

- Atherosclerotic plaque rupture followed by thrombosis and acute coronary occlusion leading to ischemic damage
  - Increased cardiac enzymes (troponin, CK, and CK-MB)
- Criteria for acute myocardial infarction
  - Detection of rise &/or fall of cardiac biomarker (cardiac troponin) with 1 value above 99th percentile limit with 1 of following (American Heart Association 3rd universal definition)
    - Symptoms of ischemia
    - New ST-segment T wave changes or new left bundle branch block
    - Development of pathological Q waves on ECG
    - Imaging evidence of new loss of viable myocardium or new wall motion abnormality
    - Intracoronary thrombus by angiography

IMAGING

- Coronary artery filling defect on coronary angiogram

- General findings
  - Diminished perfusion & function of affected area
  - Reduced regional contractility
  - Increased cell membrane permeability
  - Altered regional metabolism

TOP DIFFERENTIAL DIAGNOSES

- Old infarction
- Acute myocarditis
- Coronary vasospasm
- Unstable angina

CLINICAL ISSUES

- Chest pain: Substernal, pressing, occasionally radiating to left arm
- Associated with dyspnea, nausea, palpitations, radiation to jaw
- **Spine surgery-related < 1%**

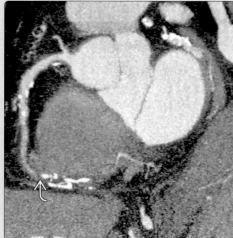
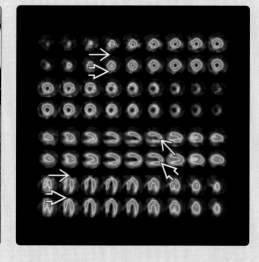

(Left) Oblique coronary CT angiogram shows occlusion of the distal right coronary artery ➡ with calcified and noncalcified plaque distal to occlusion. (Right) Stress and rest image of the left ventricular myocardium using Tc-99m tetrofosmin is shown. The stress images (top row) show perfusion defect located at the distal inferior wall and apex ➡ that normalizes at rest ➡. This reversible perfusion defect is consistent with stress-induced ischemia in this region.

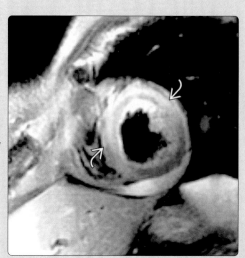
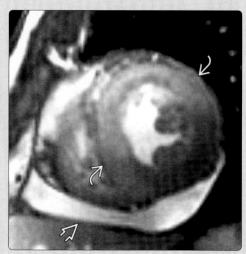

(Left) Short-axis T2WI FS MR shows an area of hyperintensity in the anterior and anterolateral walls ➡ (8 to 1 o'clock) representing myocardial edema in the setting of anterior acute myocardial infarction (AMI). (Right) Short-axis MR cine in systole shows area of hypokinesis in the anterior and anteroseptal walls associated with increased myocardial signal ➡ (edema) indicating AMI. Note the pericardial effusion ➡.

TERMINOLOGY

- Hypotensive cerebral infarction (HCI)
  - Infarction resulting from insufficient cerebral blood flow (CBF) to meet metabolic demands (low flow state)
  - Border zone or watershed infarction

IMAGING

- Best imaging tool
  - MR with DWI/ADC ± perfusion MR
- Cortical border zone (between major arterial territories)
  - Typically at gray-white matter junctions
  - Hypodensity between vascular territories
- White matter border zone (between perforating arteries)
  - Typically in deep white matter (centrum semiovale)
  - ≥ 3 lesions
  - Linear AP orientation → string of pearls appearance
  - If unilateral, look for stenosis of major vessel!
- Imaging recommendations
  - MR + GRE, DWI, MRA (both cervical, intracranial)
- ± perfusion MR (may show ↓ CBF to affected areas)
- NECT, perfusion CT, CTA if MR not available
- CTA/DSA > MRA for determining total vs. near-occlusion of internal carotid artery (ICA)

TOP DIFFERENTIAL DIAGNOSES

- Acute embolic cerebral infarction(s)
- Arteriosclerosis (small vessel disease)
- Posterior reversible encephalopathy (PRES)
- Vasculitis
- Pseudolaminar necrosis (other causes)

CLINICAL ISSUES

- Patient with high-grade ICA stenosis, transient hypotension leading to acute cerebral infarction
- Resuscitated patient with profound asphyxia or prolonged systemic hypotension
- Most common signs/symptoms
  - Altered mental status, coma

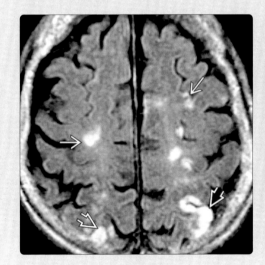
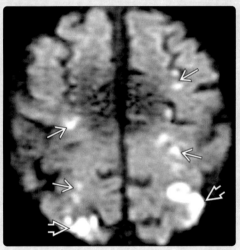

(Left) Axial FLAIR MR in a patient with transient global hypoperfusion secondary to a hypotensive episode shows multifocal hyperintensities along the cortical watershed zone ➡. Changes are most severe at the confluence of anterior cerebral artery, posterior cerebral artery, & middle cerebral artery cortical vascular territories ➡. (Right) DWI shows corresponding areas of restricted diffusion in watershed zones bilaterally ➡, most severe at trivascular confluence ➡. Diagnosis was hypotensive watershed cerebral infarctions.

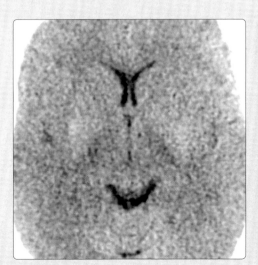
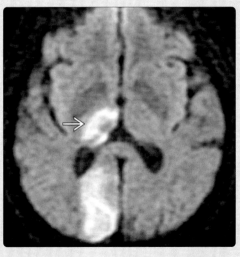

(Left) Axial NECT scan obtained a few hours after circulatory arrest and resuscitation shows diffuse cerebral edema with almost complete effacement of all gray-white matter interfaces in both the cortex and basal ganglia. The ventricles appear small and the sulci are inapparent. (Right) Axial DWI MR shows increased signal intensity from infarcts involving right thalamus ➡ and occipital lobe from basilar embolus. Lesions such as this should be excluded as a cause of postoperative vision loss.

Cerebellar Hemorrhage

TERMINOLOGY

- Remote cerebellar hemorrhage (RCH)
  - Following supratentorial craniotomy
  - Less often after spinal surgery
  - Remote to primary surgical site
  - No underlying pathologic lesion

IMAGING

- General features
  - Zebra sign (blood layered over cerebellar folia)
  - Location varies (in/over hemisphere, vermis)
  - Subarachnoid vs. superficial parenchymal bleed
  - Contralateral to side of surgery (29%)
  - Ipsilateral (22%)
  - Bilateral (33%)
  - Isolated vermian (9%)
- Imaging recommendations
  - NECT initial screen
  - MR ± contrast, MRA
  - Include T2* (GRE ± SWI)

TOP DIFFERENTIAL DIAGNOSES

- Hypertensive hemorrhage
- Coagulopathy-related spontaneous hemorrhage

PATHOLOGY

- CSF drainage → cerebellar "sagging" → vein stretching, bleeding
- RCH usually seen in immediate postoperative period
- Most occur within hours to 1 day postoperatively

CLINICAL ISSUES

- True incidence unknown (estimated at 0.3-4% of supratentorial craniotomies)
  - 0.08-0.29% after supratentorial craniotomy
- Occasionally asymptomatic, occult (not imaged)
- Death/disability in ~ 50% of cases
- Intervention for RCH rarely indicated

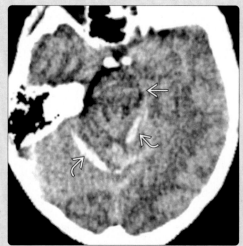

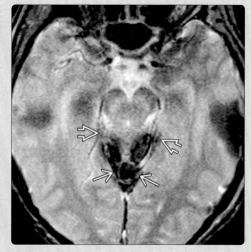

(Left) Axial NECT in a patient doing poorly immediately after surgery to resect a meningioma shows linear hemorrhages (zebra sign) bilaterally along the vermis ➡. This is a common pattern seen in remote cerebellar hemorrhage. Cisternal effacement is also present ➡. (Right) Axial T2* GRE MR in the same patient demonstrates bilateral blooming areas layering along the vermis ➡ and in the folia of the superior cerebellar hemispheres ➡ corresponding to the hemorrhage seen on prior CT.

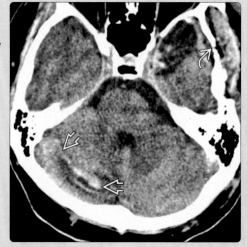

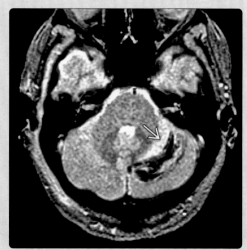

(Left) Axial NECT in a patient with an uneventful left temporal craniotomy ➡ for drainage of a left middle fossa arachnoid cyst with subdural hematoma shows a remote right cerebellar hemorrhage ➡. (Right) Axial T2* GRE MR shows hypointense signal in the cerebellar hematoma ➡ in this patient following frontal craniotomy. No other abnormalities were identified.

Intracranial Hypotension

KEY FACTS

TERMINOLOGY

- Headache caused by ↓ intracranial CSF pressure

IMAGING

- Classic imaging triad
  - Diffuse dural thickening/enhancement
  - Downward displacement of brain through incisura ("slumping" midbrain)
  - Subdural hygromas/hematomas
- Lack of 1 of 4 classic findings does not preclude diagnosis
- Dural enhancement is smooth, not nodular or "lumpy-bumpy"
- Veins, dural sinuses distended

TOP DIFFERENTIAL DIAGNOSES

- Meningitis
- Meningeal metastases
- Chronic subdural hematoma
- Dural sinus thrombosis
- Postsurgical dural thickening
- Idiopathic hypertrophic cranial pachymeningitis

CLINICAL ISSUES

- Severe headache (orthostatic, persistent, pulsatile, or even associated with nuchal rigidity)
- Uncommon: CN palsy (e.g., abducens), visual disturbances
- Rare: Severe encephalopathy with disturbances of consciousness
- Initial treatment: Lumbar or directed epidural blood patch
  - Spine surgery at leak site (imaging directed) if blood patch fails or acute clinical deterioration

DIAGNOSTIC CHECKLIST

- Frequently misdiagnosed; imaging is key to diagnosis
- Only rarely are **all** classic findings of intracranial hypotension present in same patient
- Look for enlarged spinal epidural venous plexi

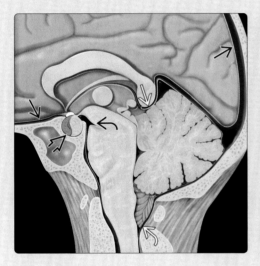

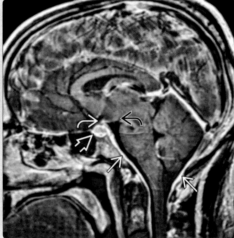

(Left) Intracranial hypotension (IH) with distended dural sinuses ➡, enlarged pituitary ➡, & herniated tonsils ➡ is shown. Central brain descent causes midbrain "slumping," inferiorly displaced pons, "closed" pons-midbrain angle ➡, & splenium depressing Vein of Galen junction ➡. (Right) Sagittal T1WI C+ FS MR shows dura-arachnoid venous engorgement ➡, enlarged pituitary ➡, & suprasellar cistern ➡ effacement by inferior hypothalamus displacement. The angle between midbrain & pons is decreased ➡.

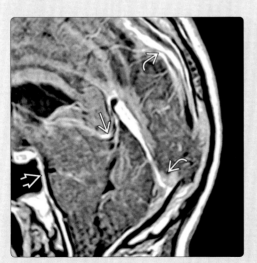

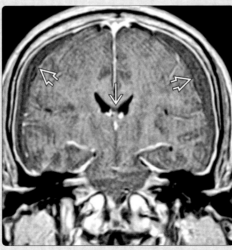

(Left) Sagittal T1WI C+ MR in a patient with life-threatening IH shows a "sagging" midbrain, dural thickening/enhancement ➡, distended torcular/superior sagittal/straight/transverse sinuses ➡, and downward herniation of the splenium ➡ causing an acute angle between ICV/V of G junction. (Right) Coronal T1WI C+ MR in same patient shows subdural fluid ➡, diffuse dural thickening/enhancement, and decreased angle between lateral ventricle roofs due to descent of central core brain structures ➡.

Remote Complications

IMAGING

- NECT as initial screen
  - Subdural hematoma (SDH)
    - Crescentic hyperdense extraaxial collection spread diffusely over convexity
    - Supratentorial convexity most common
    - May cross sutures, not dural attachments
  - Acute epidural hematoma
    - Biconvex extraaxial collection
    - May cross dural attachments, limited by sutures

TOP DIFFERENTIAL DIAGNOSES

- Hygroma
  - Clear CSF, no encapsulating membranes
- Effusion
  - Xanthochromic fluid secondary to extravasation of plasma from membrane; 1-3 days post trauma; near CSF density/intensity
- Empyema
  - Peripheral enhancement, hyperintensity on FLAIR and DWI; restricted diffusion

PATHOLOGY

- **Incidental durotomies occur in 1.7% of spine surgeries**
- Dural injury → intracranial hypotension → tearing of bridging veins → SDH
- Predisposing factors
  - Atrophy
  - Shunting (→ increased traction on superior cortical veins)
  - Coagulopathy (e.g., alcohol abuse) and anticoagulation

DIAGNOSTIC CHECKLIST

- Symptoms of persistent postural headache with nausea and vomiting after spinal intervention
  - Consider intracranial hypotension and SDH
- Wide window settings for CT increases conspicuity of subtle SDH
- FLAIR, T2* usually most sensitive sequences for SDH

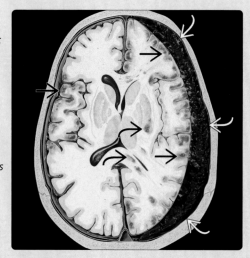

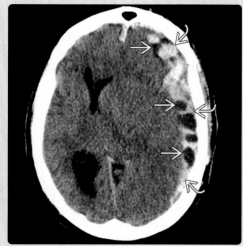

(Left) Axial graphic shows an acute subdural hematoma (SDH) ➔ compressing the left hemisphere and lateral ventricle resulting in midline shift. Note also the hemorrhagic contusions ➔ and diffuse axonal injuries ➔. Additional traumatic lesions are common in patients with SDHs. (Right) Axial NECT shows multiple low-attenuation foci ➔ within this hyperacute SDH ➔, findings consistent with active extravasation. Note the significant associated midline shift.

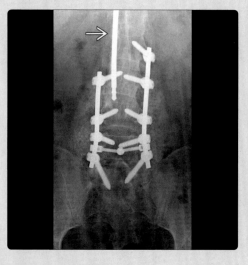

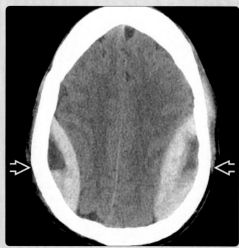

(Left) Postoperative film of intracranial epidural hematomas following lumbar surgery shows L2-S1 fusion with pedicle screws. Surgery was complicated by a large dural tear. Patient had history of remote scoliosis surgery ➔ with multilevel posterior fusion. (Right) Postoperative CT in the same patient shows large bilateral parietal epidural hematomas ➔. Epidural hematomas after lumbar surgery are very rare with only a few cases in the literature.

Retroperitoneal Hemorrhage

KEY FACTS

TERMINOLOGY

- Often misnomer: Most retroperitoneal hemorrhage is primarily in posterior abdominal wall musculature

IMAGING

- Major causes and CT findings
  - Coagulopathy or anticoagulation; high-density collection in retroperitoneum or body wall with cellular-fluid level (hematocrit sign)
  - Ruptured abdominal aortic aneurysm; large eccentric aneurysm with blood ± active extravasation contiguous with aorta
  - Renal tumors
  - Trauma
  - Vasculitis
- CT appearance of blood
  - Active bleeding
  - Linear or flame-like appearance **isodense** to enhanced vessels
  - Sentinel clot sign
    - Heterogeneous, high attenuation (60-80 HU)
    - Accumulates 1st near site of bleeding
    - Chronic, lower density (20-40 HU) more homogeneous lysed blood in adjacent spaces
- MR hyperacute phase (due to oxyhemoglobin)
  - T1WI: Slightly hypointense
  - T2WI: Hyperintense
- MR acute phase (due to deoxyhemoglobin)
  - T2WI: Markedly hypointense

TOP DIFFERENTIAL DIAGNOSES

- Retroperitoneal abscess
- Retroperitoneal sarcoma
- Asymmetrical muscles

CLINICAL ISSUES

- Often pain-free interval immediately after lumbar surgery with development of groin pain

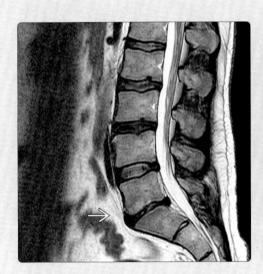

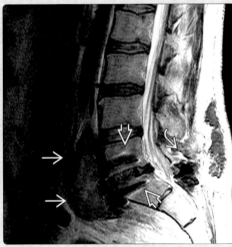

(Left) Sagittal MR prior to surgery shows disc degeneration at L5-S1 ➡. Psoas and retroperitoneal hematoma following anterior interbody fusion at the L5-S1 level can also be seen. (Right) Sagittal T2WI MR after surgery in the same patient shows a large, low-signal mass ventral to the operative site at L5-S1 ➡ from postoperative hemorrhage. Note low signal from the screw fixation ➡. The low signal within the posterior elements relates to an interspinous spacing device ➡.

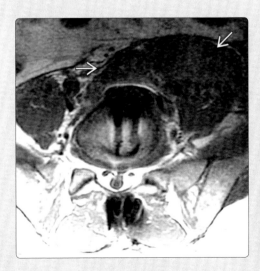

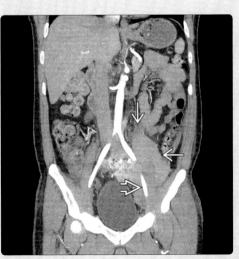

(Left) Axial MR in the same patient shows the large retroperitoneal hematoma ➡ extending eccentrically to the left. (Right) Coronal CTA study in the same patient shows the large retroperitoneal hematoma ➡ extending circumferentially around the left iliac artery ➡. The anterior approach to the lumbar spine shows a complication rate of 20%; 12% are major complications.

Retroperitoneal Lymphocele

TERMINOLOGY

- Definition: Pseudocyst formed when lymph leaks from disrupted lymphatics

IMAGING

- CT: Low-density pelvic or retroperitoneal fluid collection in postoperative patient
  - Along iliac vessels, paraaortic retroperitoneum, inguinal area
  - Unilocular or multilocular; round or oval
  - Calcification of wall is rare
  - Fat (chyle) within cyst
- MR: Homogeneous low intensity on T1WI, high on T2WI
- US: Anechoic or hypoechoic mass with acoustic enhancement
- May have dependent debris, septations

TOP DIFFERENTIAL DIAGNOSES

- Other pelvic cystic masses
  - Urinoma: Should fill with contrast on delayed contrast-enhanced CT or MR
- Bladder diverticulum: Fills with contrast on delayed imaging
- Lymphangioma (mesenteric cyst): Multiloculated
- Pseudomyxoma retroperitonei: Multicystic masses with thick walls

PATHOLOGY

- Occurs in up to 40% of patients undergoing hysterectomy, prostatectomy, or renal transplantation
- **Rare after anterior lumbar spine surgery ~ 0.3%**

CLINICAL ISSUES

- Most lymphoceles remain asymptomatic unless they become infected
- Percutaneous aspiration: Not definitive
- Long-term catheter drainage: Success in 50-87%
- Sclerotherapy: Success in 79-94%
- Surgical fenestration or marsupialization

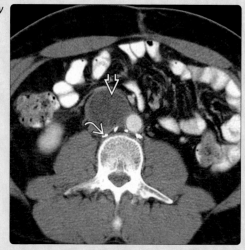

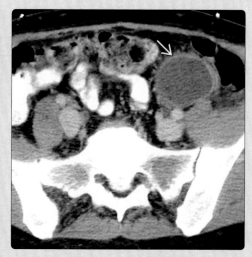

(Left) Well-defined low-density fluid collection ⇨ in the surgical bed following retroperitoneal lymph node dissection in a patient with testicular malignancy is shown. Note the surgical clips ➡. These usually develop within 2-4 weeks of surgery. (Right) This is the typical appearance of a retroperitoneal lymphocele caused by prior surgery. CECT shows a well-circumscribed, low-attenuation lesion in the left pelvis, which appeared postoperatively ➡.

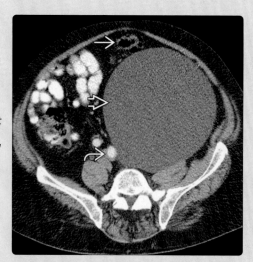

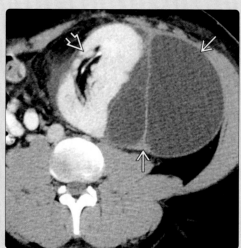

(Left) CECT shows a large retroperitoneal lymphocele ➡. The mass is cystic, well defined, and has an imperceptible wall. There is considerable mass effect on the descending colon ➡ and left common iliac artery ➡. (Right) Axial CECT in a patient with a lymphocele following renal transplantation shows a multiseptate mass ➡ compressing the renal allograft ➡.

KEY FACTS

TERMINOLOGY

- **Devastating vision loss related to operative event**
- Postoperative visual loss (POVL)
- Ischemic optic neuropathy (ION)
- Anterior ischemic optic neuropathy (AION)
- Posterior ischemic optic neuropathy (PION)
- Central retinal artery occlusion (CRAO)

TOP DIFFERENTIAL DIAGNOSES

- CRAO
  - Unilateral severe vision loss
- Cortical blindness
  - Procedures where there is high risk of emboli
  - Profound hypotension
- Pituitary apoplexy

CLINICAL ISSUES

- Highest incidence of ION after spine surgery 1:1,000
- **AION** → injury to optic nerve anterior to lamina cribrosa

- May have immediate POVL or period of normal vision with progressive loss
  - Blindness may be delayed from 48 hours to > 1 week after surgery
- **PION** → injury posterior to lamina cribrosa
  - PION most common cause of POVL where venous congestion occurs
  - Prone spine surgery
- Risk factors
  - Prolonged surgery in prone position (> 6 hours)
  - Venous congestion of head
  - Large intraoperative blood loss (> 1 liter)
  - Hypotension
- POVL → urgent ophthalmologic exam to exclude treatable causes
  - Direct globe injury, acute angle glaucoma, retinal detachment
  - Funduscopic exam also will diagnose untreatable vascular causes such as CRAO

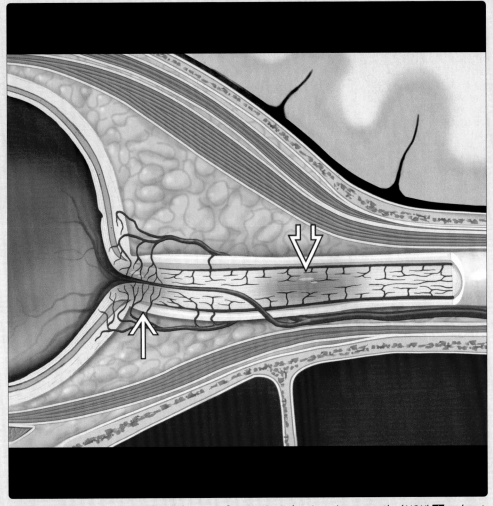

Sagittal graphic of the optic nerve shows the affected locations for anterior ischemic optic neuropathy (AION) ➡ and posterior ischemic optic neuropathy (PION) ➡. AION occurs at the nerve head, and the funduscopic examination shows swollen optic disc. PION is probably associated with intraoperative venous congestion and has a normal funduscopic examination.

IMAGING

- Diagnosis depends on high degree of suspicion and recognition of clinical features
  - Majority are due to esophageal instrumentation/anterior cervical spine surgery; confirmed by contrast esophagram or CT
- Cervical esophageal perforation (EP): Subcutaneous or interstitial emphysema; neck and mediastinum
- Thoracic EP
  - Chest film: Pneumomediastinum, pleural effusion
- EP of intraabdominal segment of distal esophagus
  - Abdominal plain film: Pneumoperitoneum
- EP near GE junction
  - Extravasated contrast from left lateral aspect of distal esophagus into mediastinum, pleural space, ± abdomen
- CT shows extraesophageal air in almost all cases, fluid and contrast medium in most
- Intramural EP: Extravasated gas and contrast remain within esophageal wall

- Much better prognosis
- Esophagography: Technique
  - Nonionic water-soluble contrast media initially, followed with barium if no leak or fistula seen
- Barium (or CT) may detect small leak not visible initially

TOP DIFFERENTIAL DIAGNOSES

- Postoperative state, esophagus
- Esophageal ulceration
- Tracheobronchial aspiration
- Esophageal diverticulum
- Boerhaave syndrome

CLINICAL ISSUES

- Surgical treatment
  - Cervical EP: Cervical mediastinotomy, open drainage
  - Thoracic EP: Immediate thoracotomy, primary closure of EP, mediastinal drainage

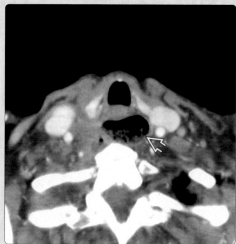
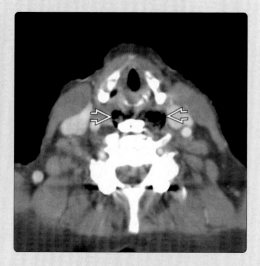

(Left) *Axial CECT of a hardware-induced fistula from the cervical esophagus into the retropharyngeal space shows air, fluid, and debris filling the retropharyngeal space ⟴ as a result of the fistula. At surgery, a rent in the back of the esophagus was caused by the surgical hardware.* (Right) *Axial CECT shows gas, fluid, and debris within the retropharyngeal space ⟴ as a result of a fistula connecting the esophagus to this space.*

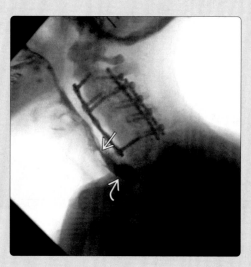
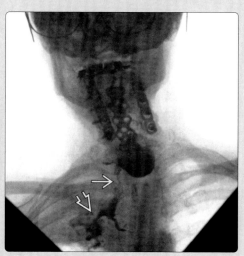

(Left) *Hardware-induced fistula from the cervical esophagus into the retropharyngeal space is shown. The fistula connection can be seen on the lateral esophagram image ⟴ with the retropharyngeal contrast visible below ⟴.* (Right) *AP esophagram of a hardware-induced fistula from the cervical esophagus with secondary fistulae to the neck and lung abscesses best delineates the inferolateral 2nd fistula ⟴ extending into the lung abscess cavity ⟴.*

Acute Pancreatitis

TERMINOLOGY

- Acute inflammatory process of pancreas with variable involvement of other regional tissues or remote organ systems

IMAGING

- Enlarged pancreas, fluid collections, and obliteration of fat planes
- ERCP: Communication of pseudocyst with main pancreatic duct (acutely)
- CT
  - Focal or diffuse pancreatic enlargement
  - Heterogeneous enhancement, nonenhancing necrotic areas

PATHOLOGY

- Etiology: Alcohol, gallstones, metabolic, infection, trauma, drugs

- Pathogenesis: Reflux of pancreatic enzymes, bile, duodenal contents, and increased ductal pressure
- Most important criteria: Presence and extent of necrotizing pancreatitis (nonenhancing parenchyma)

CLINICAL ISSUES

- **Pancreatitis is major cause of morbidity after spine fusion for scoliosis management**
  - Prevalence of > 30%
  - Higher risk patients: GERD with feeding difficulties and reactive airway disease
- Increased serum amylase and lipase
- Leukocytosis, hypocalcemia (poor prognostic sign)

DIAGNOSTIC CHECKLIST

- Bulky, irregularly enlarged pancreas with obliteration of peripancreatic fat planes, fluid collections, pseudocyst, or abscess formation
- Rule out other pathologies that can cause "peripancreatic infiltration"

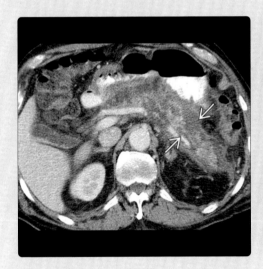

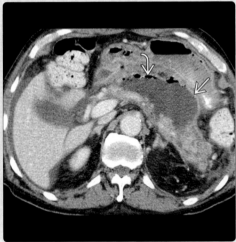

(Left) Axial CECT in an 82-year-old man with nausea, vomiting, and abdominal pain shows acute necrotizing pancreatitis. Note the heterogeneous and diminished enhancement of the pancreas ➡. (Right) Axial CECT 4 weeks later in the same patient reveals organized pancreatic necrosis ➡ or a pseudocyst within the body of the pancreas; the foci of gas ➡ likely represent a superimposed infection. Infected pancreatic necrosis is one of the most deadly complications of pancreatitis.

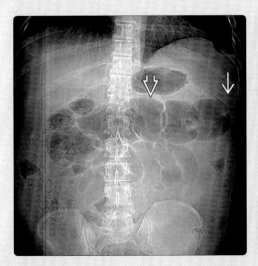

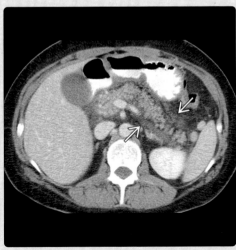

(Left) Supine radiograph shows dilation of the transverse colon ➡ with an abrupt "cutoff" at the splenic flexure ➡ due to spread of inflammation in this patient with pancreatitis. (Right) Axial enhanced CT shows the classic appearance for uncomplicated pancreatitis, demonstrating mild pancreatic enlargement and peripancreatic stranding and edema ➡.

Pseudomembranous Colitis (*Clostridium difficile*)

TERMINOLOGY

- Synonyms: Antibiotic colitis, *Clostridium difficile* colitis
- Acute inflammation of colon caused by toxins produced by *C. difficile* bacteria

IMAGING

- Best diagnostic clue: Marked submucosal edema over long segment of colon
- Location
  - Usually entire colon (pancolitis)
  - Rectum, sigmoid colon (80-90% of cases)
- Thumbprinting
  - Unusual, wide, transverse bands due to haustral fold thickening
- CECT
  - Accordion sign: Trapped enteric contrast between thickened colonic haustral folds
  - Target sign
  - Pericolonic stranding

- Best imaging tool: CECT with oral contrast
- Protocol advice: 150 mL IV contrast at 2.5 mL/sec with 5-mm collimation, 5-mm reconstruction interval

CLINICAL ISSUES

- Elderly at higher risk for developing pseudomembranous colitis and recurrent pseudomembranous colitis
- Clinical profile: Patient with history of watery diarrhea after antibiotic use or hospitalization
- Treatment in mild cases: Discontinue offending antibiotic therapy
- Severe cases
  - Metronidazole (drug of choice) or oral vancomycin
  - Fulminant and toxic megacolon: Colectomy

DIAGNOSTIC CHECKLIST

- Check history of antibiotic use or debilitating diseases
- Suspect in any hospitalized patient with acute colitis

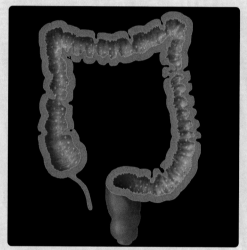
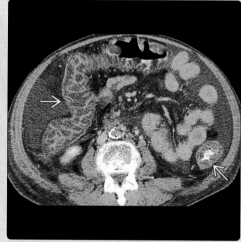

(Left) *Graphic demonstrates pancolitis with marked mural thickening and multiple, elevated, yellow-white plaques (or pseudomembranes).* (Right) *Axial CECT in a 62-year-old man who presented with diarrhea and dehydration demonstrates a classic case of pseudomembranous colitis. Note the severe bowel wall thickening throughout the entire colon →. Pseudomembranous colitis typically presents as a pancolitis, as in this example.*

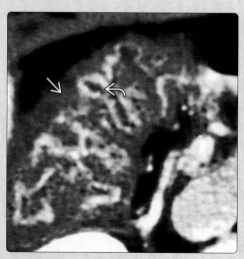
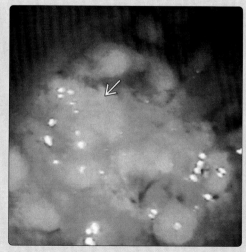

(Left) *Axial CECT in a 47-year-old man who had been taking antibiotics for 2 weeks for sinusitis now presents with a 2-day history of right lower quadrant pain, fever, and concern for appendicitis. Note the marked submucosal edema of the right colon → and the intense mucosal enhancement → (or accordion sign).* (Right) *Endoscopic photograph of the right colon in the same patient reveals the classic hyperemic mucosa and yellow plaques → characteristic of pseudomembranous colitis.*

Rhabdomyolysis

KEY FACTS

TERMINOLOGY

- Clinical and biochemical syndrome resulting from damage of integrity of skeletal muscle with release of toxic muscle cell components into circulation

IMAGING

- Increased T2 signal within affected skeletal muscle group
- May show patchy contrast enhancement
- Severe disease with myonecrosis shows peripheral enhancement with no central enhancement

PATHOLOGY

- **Major etiologies** include trauma (38%), including **prolonged immobilization for surgical procedures**, prolonged seizures, direct muscle injury
  - Ischemia (14%), including compression and vascular occlusion
  - Drug overdose (7%) and wide variety of drugs (including statins)

- **Risk factors for rhabdomyolysis** include surface area of muscle isolated and strained by retraction and surgical duration
  - Operative mean time in series of 5 affected patients was 420 minutes for minimally invasive spine surgery
- **Risk factors for acute renal failure** due to rhabdomyolysis
  - Presence of sepsis
  - Age > 70
  - Volume depletion
  - Degree of elevation of CPK, potassium, phosphorus

CLINICAL ISSUES

- Classic triad of muscle pain, weakness, and dark urine
- Treatment
  - Hydration with isotonic crystalloid
  - Treatment of acute renal failure (mannitol, diuretics)
- Life-threatening complications include acute renal failure, hyperkalemia, and cardiac arrest

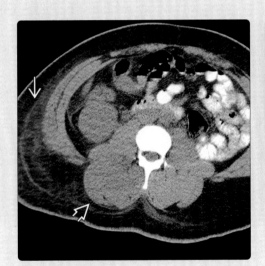
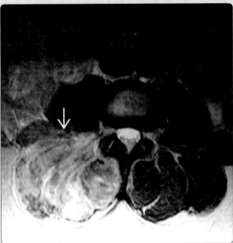

(Left) Axial NECT of rhabdomyolysis following the right lateral decubitus position shows enlargement of the right paraspinal muscles ➡ without abnormal attenuation. There is irregular reticulation of subcutaneous fat due to edema ➡. (Right) Axial T2WI MR shows diffuse hyperintensity of dorsal right paraspinal muscles ➡ with a sharp ventral margin. The patient was in a prolonged right decubitus position for surgery.

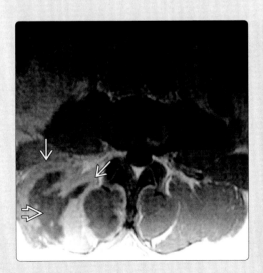
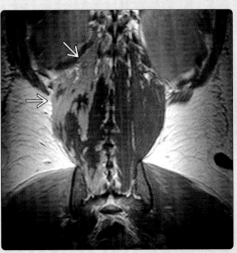

(Left) Axial T1 C+ MR shows diffuse and irregular muscle enhancement ➡ with a central nonenhancing component ➡. (Right) Coronal T1 C+ MR shows irregular abnormal enhancement of the right dorsal paraspinal muscles ➡ in contrast to normal left muscle signal intensity.

TERMINOLOGY

- Injury to bowel (duodenum, small bowel, colon)

IMAGING

- Best diagnostic clue: Bowel wall thickening, mesenteric infiltration ± extravasation of enteric or vascular contrast medium
- Best imaging tool: CECT
- CT findings
  - Sentinel clot sign: Localized > 60 HU mesenteric hematoma at site of bleeding
  - Bowel wall thickening > 3 mm (75% of transmural injuries)
  - Hemoperitoneum: Common in intraperitoneal bowel or mesenteric injury
  - Water-density peritoneal or interloop fluid

TOP DIFFERENTIAL DIAGNOSES

- Shock bowel

- Coagulopathy
- Vasculitis
- Ischemic enteritis

PATHOLOGY

- **Related to anterior lumbosacral surgery < 0.5%**
- Rare cases of perforation from migrated cage or graft

CLINICAL ISSUES

- Abdominal pain, distension, tenderness, and guarding
- Diagnostic peritoneal lavage: Severe injury if positive

DIAGNOSTIC CHECKLIST

- Check for motor vehicle accident history or other abdominal injury
- Image interpretation
  - CT evidence of extraluminal air/contrast, bowel wall thickening, free fluids, mesenteric stranding

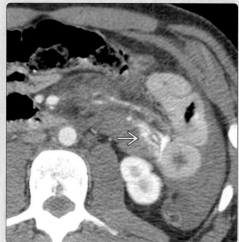
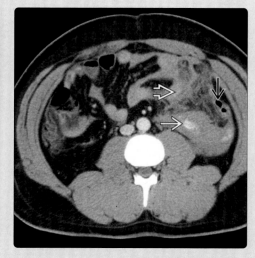

(Left) Axial CECT in a 24-year-old man presenting after a motorcycle collision demonstrates a hemoperitoneum in the left lower quadrant with active bleeding, as evidenced by the contrast extravasation ➡, which is a typical finding in intestinal trauma. (Right) Axial CECT shows mesenteric infiltration ➡ and active bleeding represented by extravasated contrast ➡; much of the bleeding is adjacent to descending colon ➡.

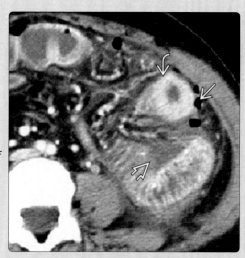
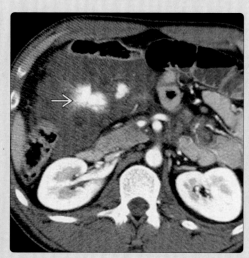

(Left) Axial CECT in a 19-year-old man presenting with abdominal pain after a motorcycle crash shows free air ➡, hyperdense bowel ➡, and a high-attenuation mesentery consistent with a hematoma ➡. Jejunal perforation was revealed at surgery. (Right) Axial CECT shows high-attenuation active bleeding into the mesentery of the right colon ➡, a characteristic finding in the setting of intestinal trauma.

Ureteral Trauma

TERMINOLOGY

- Injury of ureter from blunt, penetrating, or iatrogenic trauma

IMAGING

- Best imaging tools: CECT with CT urography for global view of abdomen and urinary tract
  - Antegrade or retrograde pyelography for detailed analysis of site and character of injury
- Sites of urine accumulation
  - Perirenal or subcapsular from blunt renal injury
  - Medial to ureteropelvic junction for proximal ureteral and ureteropelvic junction leaks
  - May enter peritoneal cavity (after penetrating trauma or laparotomy/laparoscopy)
- Ureteral strictures less accurately diagnosed by CT
  - Difficult to distinguish foci of ureteral spasm from peristalsis due to stricture

- Indirect signs of ureteral stricture: Delayed nephrogram, hydronephrosis
- Image-guided aspiration of fluid collection may identify fluid as urine and guide drainage

TOP DIFFERENTIAL DIAGNOSES

- Abdominal abscess
- Postoperative hematoma or seroma
- Postoperative edema

PATHOLOGY

- Iatrogenic trauma accounts for 80-90% of ureteral injuries
  - Open abdominal or gynecologic surgery (> 50%)
- **Spine surgeries such as total lumbar disc replacement and total disc replacement removal, revision lumbar arthrodesis**
  - Reported spine surgery complications include ureteral injury with nephrectomy

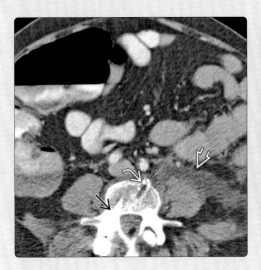

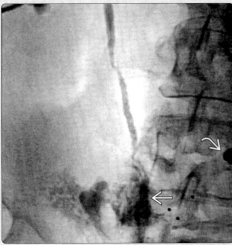

(Left) Axial CECT in a patient with ureteral perforation from spine surgery shows 1 of several metallic screws ➡ and the path of 1 that had been removed ➡. Note the water-density fluid collection ➡ in the retroperitoneum adjacent to the spine and psoas muscle. (Right) Antegrade pyelogram in the same patient shows transection of the distal left ureter ➡ as well as 1 of the metallic screws ➡. A nephrostomy catheter was subsequently placed.

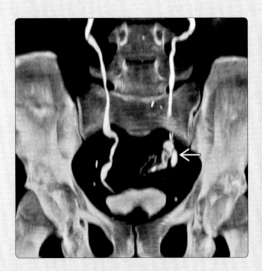

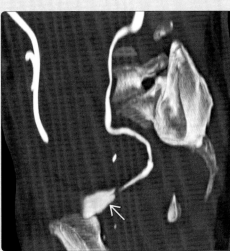

(Left) CT urography in the same patient shows extravasation of contrast-opacified urine ➡ from the transected ureter. Note that the more distal ureter is not opacified. The extravasated urine collected within the previously identified lentiform collection. (Right) Oblique CT urogram in the same patient clearly shows the extravasation of urine ➡ from the distal ureter.

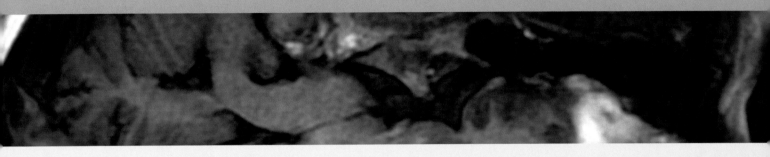

SECTION 12
Differential Diagnosis

DIFFERENTIAL DIAGNOSIS

Common

- Chiari 1 Malformation
- Chiari 2 Malformation
- Klippel-Feil Spectrum
- Atlantooccipital Assimilation

Less Common

- Basiocciput Hypoplasia
- Occipital Condylar Hypoplasia
- Atlas Hypoplasia
- Achondroplasia
- Down Syndrome

Rare but Important

- Syndromes With Vertebral Anomalies
  - 22q11.2 Deletion Syndrome (DiGeorge Syndrome)
  - Cleidocranial Dysplasia
  - Hajdu-Cheney Syndrome
  - Hemifacial Microsomia (Oculoauriculovertebral Dysplasia)
  - CHARGE Syndrome
  - Spondylocarpotarsal Synostosis Syndrome
  - Robinow Syndrome
  - Jarcho-Levin Syndrome

ESSENTIAL INFORMATION

Key Differential Diagnosis Issues

- **Basilar invagination** is term used for developmental anomalies of craniovertebral junction where odontoid has abnormal relationship to foramen magnum (prolapse)
  - Should be distinguished from **basilar impression**, which is characterized by acquired abnormal odontoid/foramen magnum relationship (rheumatoid arthritis, Paget, osteogenesis imperfecta)
- Basilar invagination variably associated with symptoms, brainstem compression
- Basilar invagination has been categorized by absence (type 1) or presence (type 2) of Chiari malformation
  - Has also been categorized by presence (type A) or absence (type B) of clinical/radiographic instability at craniovertebral junction

Helpful Clues for Common Diagnoses

- **Chiari 1 Malformation**
  - Key facts
    - Mismatch between posterior fossa size and cerebellar tissue
  - Imaging
    - Low-lying pointed cerebellar tonsils
    - Tonsils project ≥ 5 mm below foramen magnum
    - Often associated with syrinx, anomalies of 4th occipital sclerotome, and retroflexed odontoid
- **Chiari 2 Malformation**
  - Key facts
    - Nearly 100% with neural tube closure defect
  - Imaging
    - Small bony posterior fossa
    - "Notched" clivus
    - Large funnel-shaped foramen magnum

- Low-lying tentorium
- **Klippel-Feil Spectrum**
  - Key facts
    - Congenital spinal malformation characterized by segmentation failure of ≥ 2 cervical vertebrae ± thoracic, lumbar segmentation failure
    - Various syndromes (Turner and Noonan) associated but often clinically asymptomatic
  - Imaging
    - Single- or multiple-level congenital cervical segmentation and fusion anomalies
    - Associated abnormalities include odontoid dysplasia, basilar impression, C1 assimilation, and occipitocervical instability
- **Atlantooccipital Assimilation**
  - Key facts
    - Failure of C1 to correctly segment from occipital bone
  - Imaging
    - Atlas fusion to occipital bone
    - Wide variability ranging from partial to complete, uni- or bilateral

Helpful Clues for Less Common Diagnoses

- **Basiocciput Hypoplasia**
  - Key facts
    - Basiocciput derives from mesodermal cells of occipital somites and not from neural crest (as do facial bones)
    - Normal lower clivus formed from contributions of 4 occipital sclerotomes with upper portion formed from basisphenoid
  - Imaging
    - Truncated inferior margin with concave superior margin
- **Occipital Condyle Hypoplasia**
  - Key facts
    - Skull base is flattened with violation of Chamberlain line
  - Imaging
    - Wide variation in severity from minimal with no clinical impact to severe with basilar invagination
- **Atlas Hypoplasia**
  - Key facts
    - Hypoplasia usually involves posterior arch of C1, compressing cord and giving high cervical myelopathy
  - Imaging
    - Small C1 arch, which may be segmentally hypoplastic or aplastic, and posterior midline nonunion are common
    - Split atlas with midline anterior and posterior nonunion may be asymptomatic variant in adult
    - Fracture should be excluded
    - More aggressive work-up if identified in child with other associated vertebral anomalies
- **Achondroplasia**
  - Key facts
    - Foramen magnum stenosis is primary clinical concern with quadriparesis, feeding difficulty, and respiratory abnormalities
  - Imaging
    - Defects in enchondral bone formation with shortened basiocciput, short clivus

- **Down Syndrome**
  - Key facts
    - Atlantoaxial subluxation with transverse ligament laxity is key feature
    - Multiple other anomalies associated: Atlantooccipital instability, os odontoideum, odontoid hypoplasia, basiocciput hypoplasia, poster arch C1 hypoplasia
  - Imaging
    - Atlantodental instability in up to 40%, although 1% are symptomatic

Helpful Clues for Rare Diagnoses

- **22q11.2 Deletion Syndrome (DiGeorge Syndrome)**
  - Key facts: OMIM #188400
    - Rare congenital disease with symptoms including recurrent infections, heart defects, and characteristic facial features
  - Imaging
    - Platybasia and upper cervical spine anomalies are common (dysplastic atlas in 75%)
- **Cleidocranial Dysplasia**
  - Key facts: OMIM #119600
    - Autosomal dominant disorder with clavicular aplasia or hypoplasia, brachydactyly, dental anomalies, and vertebral anomalies
  - Imaging
    - Nonspecific vertebral and craniovertebral junction bony anomalies
- **Hajdu-Cheney Syndrome**
  - Key facts: OMIM #102500
    - Rare autosomal dominant disorder with dysmorphic facies, bowed long bones, and vertebral anomalies
  - Imaging
    - Progressive bone destruction with acroosteolysis and osteoporosis
- **Hemifacial Microsomia (Oculoauriculovertebral Dysplasia)**
  - Key facts: OMIM #164210
    - **Goldenhar** syndrome; oculoauriculovertebral dysplasia

---

    - Common birth defect involving 1st and 2nd branchial arch derivatives with highly variable phenotype
  - Imaging
    - Nonspecific vertebral and craniovertebral junction bony anomalies
- **CHARGE Syndrome**
  - Key facts: OMIM #214800
    - Coloboma, heart anomaly, choanal atresia, retarded growth and development, genital hypoplasia, and ear anomalies
  - Imaging
    - Basiocciput hypoplasia is common and may be severe
- **Spondylocarpotarsal Synostosis Syndrome**
  - Key facts: OMIM #272460
    - Congenital familial syndrome with extensive vertebral anomalies due to mutation in gene-encoding filamin B
  - Imaging: Platybasia and basilar invagination
- **Robinow Syndrome**
  - Key facts: OMIM #268310
    - Short-limbed dwarfism, dysmorphic facies, vertebral segmentation abnormalities, and hypoplastic genitalia due to mutation in *ROR2* gene
  - Imaging: Nonspecific segmentation anomalies
- **Jarcho-Levin Syndrome**
  - Key facts: OMIM #277300
    - Rib deformities and widespread vertebral segmentation anomalies related to mutation in *DLL3* gene
  - Imaging
    - Wide variability in phenotypes with Jarcho-Levin
    - Most severe form with "crab-chest," spondylocostal dysostosis

SELECTED REFERENCES

1. Wei G et al: Treatment of basilar invagination with Klippel-Feil syndrome: atlantoaxial joint distraction and fixation with transoral atlantoaxial reduction plate. Neurosurgery. 78(4):492-8, 2016
2. Dokai T et al: Posterior occipitocervical fixation under skull-femoral traction for the treatment of basilar impression in a child with Klippel-Feil syndrome. J Bone Joint Surg Br. 93(11):1571-4, 2011

Chiari 1 Malformation

Chiari 1 Malformation

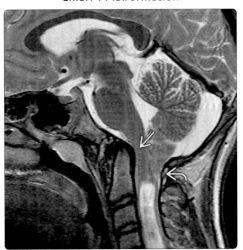
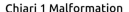

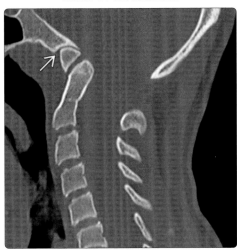

(Left) Sagittal T2WI MR shows a Chiari 1 malformation ➡ with the syrinx involving the upper cervical cord. There is basilar invagination with mild mass effect upon the medulla ➡. (Right) Sagittal midline bone CT in patient with Chiari 1 shows dens retroflexion. The anterior C1 ring is large and abnormally articulates with the remodeled clivus ➡. The odontoid tip is prolapsed cephalad to the foramen magnum.

Klippel-Feil Spectrum

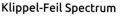

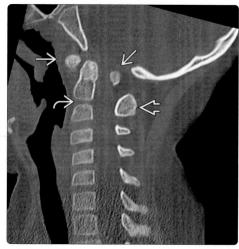

Klippel-Feil Spectrum

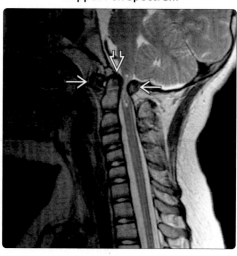

(Left) *Sagittal bone CT shows a thickened dysplastic appearance of the dens and C1 ring* ➡ *with the posterior C1 ring severely narrowing the central spinal canal. There is also narrowing of the C2-C3 disc space* ➡ *and fusion of the C2 and C3 spinous processes* ➡*. (Right) Sagittal T2WI MR shows dysplastic formation of the dens* ➡ *as well as an abnormal hypoplastic C1 ring* ➡ *resulting in severe spinal canal narrowing and cord compression with focal syrinx at the C1 level.*

Atlantooccipital Assimilation

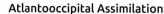

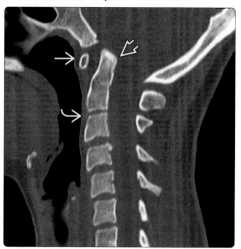

Atlantooccipital Assimilation

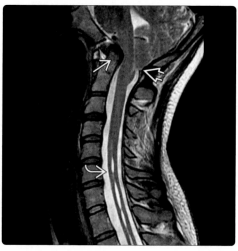

(Left) *Sagittal CT shows typical midline findings of assimilation of C1 into the occiput with a high riding C1 arch* ➡ *and upward translocation of the odontoid* ➡ *relative to the foramen magnum. Note the congenital fusion of C2-C3* ➡*. (Right) Sagittal T2 TSE MR shows upward displacement of the odontoid* ➡ *compressing the medulla with secondary Chiari 1 malformation* ➡ *due to the narrowed foramen magnum. Note the associated syrinx* ➡*.*

Atlantooccipital Assimilation

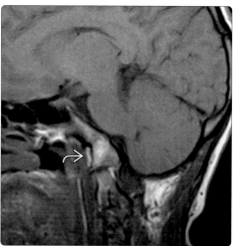

Atlantooccipital Assimilation

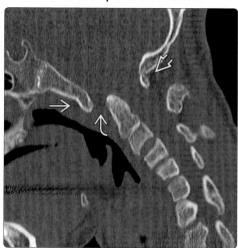

(Left) *Sagittal T1WI MR obtained off midline shows segmentation failure* ➡ *of the occipital condyles, which are fused to the C1 lateral masses. (Right) Sagittal CT study shows assimilation of the anterior C1 with the occiput* ➡ *and partial assimilation of the posterior arch* ➡*. There is a widened atlantodental interval* ➡ *and upward translocation of the odontoid with respect to the foramen magnum.*

Basiocciput Hypoplasia

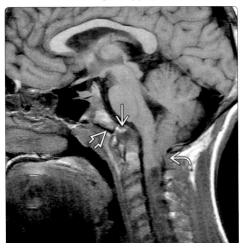

Basiocciput Hypoplasia

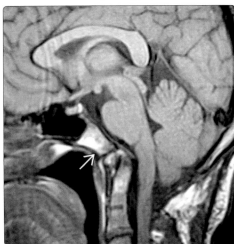

(Left) *Sagittal T1WI MR of atlantooccipital assimilation, basiocciput hypoplasia, and Chiari 1 malformation shows blunting of the clivus* ➡, *widening of the predental space* ➡, *and prolapse of the odontoid tip into the foramen magnum. The tonsils are low-lying* ➡, *and there is an upper cervical syrinx.* (Right) *Sagittal T1WI MR in atlantooccipital assimilation shows an abnormal truncated clivus* ➡ *and elongated odontoid process positioned cephalad to the foramen magnum (basilar invagination).*

Basiocciput Hypoplasia

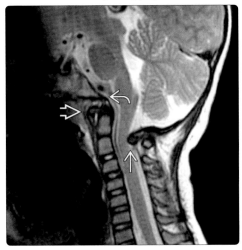

Atlas Hypoplasia

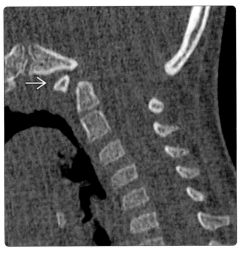

(Left) *Sagittal T2WI MR shows a shortened clivus* ➡ *and an abnormal C1 arch with the anterior arch too cephalad* ➡ *and the posterior arch too ventral* ➡. (Right) *Sagittal CT shows the typical appearance of a dysplastic (hypoplastic) C1 arch and the abnormal relationship of the anterior C1* ➡ *with the foramen magnum. The posterior C1 arch is not fused, so it is not visualized on this midline image.*

Atlas Hypoplasia

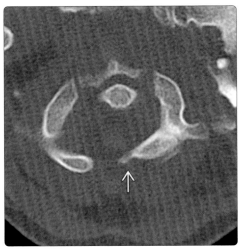

Syndromes With Vertebral Anomalies

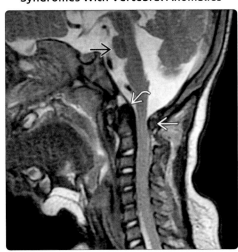

(Left) *Axial NECT shows an abnormal left posterior arch segment* ➡ *that narrows the spinal canal.* (Right) *Sagittal T2WI in a patient with a hypoplastic atlas and Marshall-Smith syndrome (accelerated skeletal maturation, failure to thrive, dysmorphic facial features) shows dorsal compression of the cervical spinal cord by the hypoplastic C1 posterior ring* ➡ *and invagination of the odontoid process* ➡. *The pons is hypoplastic* ➡.

DIFFERENTIAL DIAGNOSIS

Common
- Rheumatoid Arthritis
- Paget Disease
- Osteomalacia
  - Renal Osteodystrophy
  - Rickets
- Osteogenesis Imperfecta

Less Common
- Mucopolysaccharidoses
  - Hurler/Hunter
  - Morquio
- Ankylosing Spondylitis
- Osteomyelitis of Skull Base
- Neoplastic Destruction of Skull Base
- Hyperparathyroidism
- Fibrous Dysplasia

Rare but Important
- Syndromes With Metabolic Abnormalities
  - Metaphyseal Chondrodysplasia (Jansen Type)
  - Lowe Oculocerebrorenal Syndrome
- Chondrodysplasias
  - Schwartz-Jampel Syndrome
- SUNCT Syndrome

ESSENTIAL INFORMATION

Key Differential Diagnosis Issues
- **Basilar impression** is term used for **acquired** abnormalities of odontoid relationship with foramen magnum (bone softening at skull base)
- **Basilar invagination** is term used for **developmental** anomalies of craniovertebral junction where odontoid process has abnormal relationship to foramen magnum (prolapse)

Helpful Clues for Common Diagnoses
- **Rheumatoid Arthritis**
  - Key facts
    - Basilar impression is 1 of 3 directional instabilities that occur in rheumatoid arthritis (RA)
    - Other 2 are atlantoaxial subluxation and subaxial subluxation
  - Imaging
    - "Cranial settling" is term applied to basilar impression in RA
    - In cranial settling, skull and C1 ring move as unit with respect to C2 and rest of spine
    - Gives classic upward translocation of odontoid with low C1 ring due to transverse ligament incompetence
- **Paget Disease**
  - Key facts
    - Often asymptomatic involvement of skull base
    - M > F
    - Skull base is often only site of involvement
  - Imaging
    - May be multifocal disease with mixed sclerotic-lytic pattern
    - Expands bone; results in cotton wool appearance

- **Osteomalacia**
  - Key facts
    - Abnormal mineralization in trabecular and cortical bone
    - Most common cause: Renal osteodystrophy
    - Other causes: Malabsorption, liver disease, nutritional, abnormal vitamin D or phosphate metabolism, anticonvulsants, tumor induced
  - Imaging
    - Deformities due to bone softening: Basilar impression, vertebral endplate compressions, scoliosis
    - Long bones: Looser zones (e.g., Milkman fractures, pseudofractures)
- **Osteogenesis Imperfecta**
  - Key facts
    - Genetic disorder of type I collagen resulting in bone fragility
    - Associated anomalies include blue sclerae, early hearing loss, brittle teeth, thin fragile skin, and joint laxity
  - Imaging
    - Severe osteopenia, vertebral fractures, kyphoscoliosis

Helpful Clues for Less Common Diagnoses
- **Mucopolysaccharidoses**
  - Key facts
    - Heterogeneous group of inherited lysosomal storage disorders
  - Imaging
    - Craniovertebral junction stenosis, dens hypoplasia, ligamentous laxity, atlantoaxial instability, thickened dural ring at foramen magnum
- **Ankylosing Spondylitis**
  - Key facts
    - Early spine involvement
      - Squaring of vertebral bodies → corner erosions → "shiny corner" (corner sclerosis)
    - Late spine involvement
      - Widespread ankylosis ("bamboo spine")
    - Craniovertebral junction abnormalities may relate to accelerated degenerative change due to altered biomechanics of spine
  - Imaging
    - Severe degenerative change at C1-C2 junction due to abnormal stress from caudal bony fusion
    - C0-C1 joint with collapse of C1 lateral mass and upward translocation of odontoid
- **Osteomyelitis of Skull Base**
  - Key facts
    - *Staphylococcus aureus* most common in USA
    - *Mycobacterium tuberculosis* most common worldwide for C1-C2 joint infection
  - Imaging
    - Soft tissue mass and bone destruction at C1-C2 level
- **Neoplastic Destruction of Skull Base**
  - Key facts
    - Patient with known malignant neoplasm
  - Imaging
    - Lytic destructive lesion of skull base
    - Look for associated soft tissue mass
    - Check for multiple lesions

- **Hyperparathyroidism**
  - ○ Key facts
    - Primary: Due to parathyroid adenoma, hyperplasia, or carcinoma
    - Secondary: Due to renal failure or, rarely, intestinal malabsorption
  - ○ Imaging
    - Osteopenia
    - Resorption of secondary trabeculae (interlinking, nonweight-bearing trabeculae)
    - Rare: Brown tumor (osteoclastoma)
- **Fibrous Dysplasia**
  - ○ Key facts
    - Relatively common lesion of occiput and sphenoid
  - ○ Imaging
    - Ground-glass matrix is classic appearance
    - Often hypointense on T2WI MR; shows intense enhancement on T1WI

Helpful Clues for Rare Diagnoses

- **Metaphyseal Chondrodysplasia (Jansen Type)**
  - ○ Key facts: OMIM #156400
    - Hypercalcemia and hypophosphatemia occur without parathyroid abnormalities
  - ○ Imaging
    - Short stature, short bowed limbs, clinodactyly, small mandible
- **Lowe Oculocerebrorenal Syndrome**
  - ○ Key facts: OMIM #309000
    - Mutation in *OCRL1* gene (phosphatidylinositol 4,5-biphosphate 5-phosphatase deficiency)
  - ○ Imaging
    - Cataracts, mental retardation, vitamin D-resistant rickets, amino aciduria
- **Schwartz-Jampel Syndrome**
  - ○ Key facts
    - Very rare; also called Stüve-Wiedemann syndrome
    - Joint contractures, bone dysplasia, small stature
  - ○ Imaging
    - Multiple skeletal abnormalities

- **SUNCT Syndrome**
  - ○ Key facts
    - **S**hort-lasting **u**nilateral **n**euralgiform headache with **c**onjunctival injection and **t**earing
    - Short attacks of severe pain with autonomic symptoms (e.g., tearing, rhinorrhea, conjunctival injection)
    - May be caused by variety of intracerebral tumors and posterior fossa deformities
  - ○ Imaging
    - Necessary to exclude posterior fossa pathology

SELECTED REFERENCES

1. Botelho RV et al: Angular craniometry in craniocervical junction malformation. Neurosurg Rev. 36(4):603-10; discussion 610, 2013
2. Brockmeyer DL: The complex Chiari: issues and management strategies. Neurol Sci. 32 Suppl 3:S345-7, 2011
3. Krauss WE et al: Rheumatoid arthritis of the craniovertebral junction. Neurosurgery. 66(3 Suppl):83-95, 2010
4. Smoker WR et al: Imaging the craniocervical junction. Childs Nerv Syst. 24(10):1123-45, 2008
5. Riew KD et al: Diagnosing basilar invagination in the rheumatoid patient. The reliability of radiographic criteria. J Bone Joint Surg Am. 83-A(2):194-200, 2001
6. Nanduri VR et al: Basilar invagination as a sequela of multisystem Langerhans' cell histiocytosis. J Pediatr. 136(1):114-8, 2000
7. Smoker WR: MR imaging of the craniovertebral junction. Magn Reson Imaging Clin N Am. 8(3):635-50, 2000
8. Crockard HA: Transoral surgery: some lessons learned. Br J Neurosurg. 9(3):283-93, 1995
9. Zeidman SM et al: Rheumatoid arthritis. Neuroanatomy, compression, and grading of deficits. Spine (Phila Pa 1976). 19(20):2259-66, 1994
10. Rajshekhar V et al: Haemangioma of the skull base producing basilar impression. Br J Neurosurg. 3(2):229-33, 1989
11. Sherk HH: Atlantoaxial instability and acquired basilar invagination in rheumatoid arthritis. Orthop Clin North Am. 9(4):1053-63, 1978

Rheumatoid Arthritis

Rheumatoid Arthritis

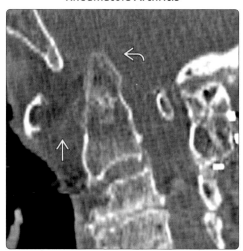

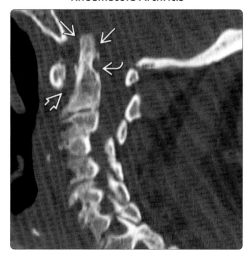

(Left) Sagittal bone CT shows an odontoid tip projecting through the foramen magnum ⇗ (cranial settling). The anterior C1-odontoid distance ⇒ is increased (normal distance < 2 mm at inferior aspect of C1 arch). (Right) Sagittal NECT shows cranial settling with upward translocation of the odontoid process relative to the foramen magnum ⇒. There are also dense erosions ⇗ and increased atlantodental interval ⇒.

Differential Diagnosis

(Left) *Sagittal T1WI C+ MR shows the typical appearance of a severe basilar impression with flattening of the anterior skull base (platybasia) ➡ and upward displacement of the odontoid process ➡ and posterior skull base ➡. **(Right)** Coronal T1 C+ MR shows a basilar impression due to bony softening of the skull base with upward displacement of the skull base and mild effacement of the temporal lobes ➡.*

Paget Disease

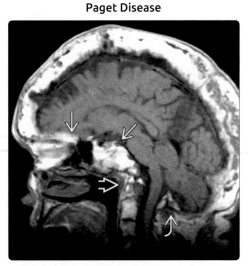

Paget Disease

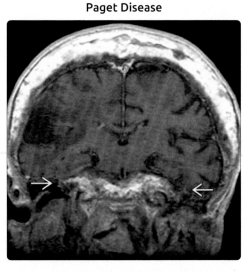

(Left) *Sagittal T1WI MR shows heterogeneous increased signal from an expanded clivus ➡ due to Paget disease. There is upward displacement of the odontoid process ➡ relative to the Chamberlain line ➡ as well as Chiari 1 malformation and cervical syrinx. **(Right)** Sagittal NECT reconstruction shows a horizontal orientation of the clivus (platybasia) ➡ and protrusion of the dens into the foramen magnum (basilar impression) ➡.*

Paget Disease

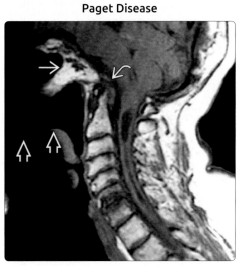

Osteogenesis Imperfecta

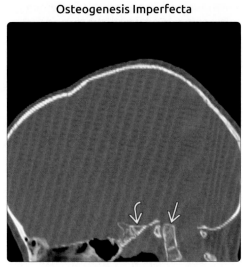

(Left) *Sagittal T1WI MR shows horizontal clivus orientation ➡ and upward protrusion of the dens into the foramen magnum ➡. Note the associated angular deformity of the brainstem ➡. A large, heterogeneous extraaxial subdural hematoma is present ➡. **(Right)** Axial T1WI MR shows a soft tissue component of the infection involving the basion ➡ and anterior arch of C1 with a phlegmon adjacent to the cervicomedullary junction ➡.*

Osteogenesis Imperfecta

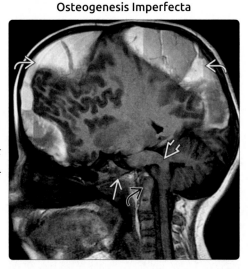

Osteomyelitis of Skull Base

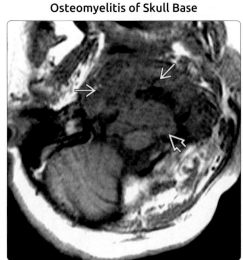

Osteomyelitis of Skull Base

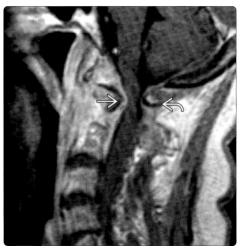

Osteomyelitis of Skull Base

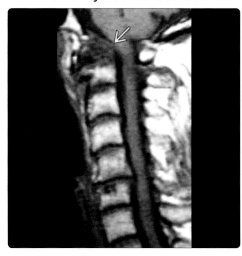

(Left) *Sagittal T1WI C+ MR shows diffuse enhancement of the phlegmon and destruction of the C2 body with soft tissue extension. The subluxation causes anterior cord compression from the C2 body ➡ and posterior cord compression due to posterior arch C1 compression ➡.* (Right) *Sagittal T1WI MR in partially treated C1-C2 Staphylococcus aureus osteomyelitis shows abnormal low signal involving a partially collapsed odontoid process that has migrated superiorly to compress the ventral medulla ➡.*

Osteomyelitis of Skull Base

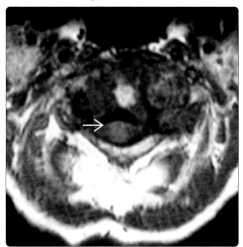

Neoplastic Destruction of Skull Base

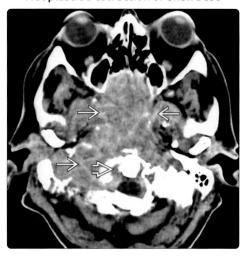

(Left) *Axial T1WI MR in this case of partially treated C1-C2 joint osteomyelitis shows the abnormal odontoid process with adjacent phlegmon and a compression on the cervicomedullary junction ➡.* (Right) *Axial NECT shows a destructive mass ➡ involving the skull base, C1, and adjacent nasopharynx in a patient with multiple myeloma and plasmacytoma. There is upward translocation of the odontoid process ➡ with basilar impression.*

Neoplastic Destruction of Skull Base

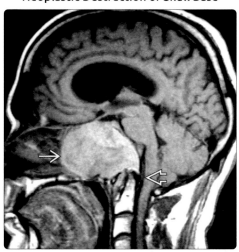

Fibrous Dysplasia

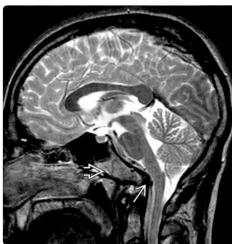

(Left) *Sagittal T1W MR shows a very large mass ➡ expanding the clivus in a patient with plasmacytoma. The plasmacytoma is nearly isointense to the brain on T1 images. There is basilar impression ➡ due to the generalized softening of the skull base.* (Right) *Sagittal FS T2WI MR shows an abnormally sloped and expanded clivus with mild platybasia due to fibrous dysplasia ➡. Also note the anomalous spur of dense cortical bone that projects dorsally, indenting the dura at the cervicomedullary junction ➡.*

DIFFERENTIAL DIAGNOSIS

Common

- Cranial Settling
- Basilar Invagination
- Basilar Impression
- Platybasia

ESSENTIAL INFORMATION

Key Differential Diagnosis Issues

- **Cranial Settling**
  - Defined as **subtype of basilar impression** occurring in rheumatoid arthritis (RA)
    - Cranial settling diagnosed when 2 conditions are met: (1) Superior aspect of dens is even with or above McRae line (foramen magnum), unless there is marked dental erosion, and (2) anterior arch of C1 assumes an abnormally low position in relation to C2 (cranial settling is also known as vertical atlantoaxial subluxation)
    - Skull and C1 ring move as unit with respect to C2 and rest of spine
    - Shows classic upward translocation of odontoid with low C1 ring due to transverse ligament incompetence
  - Erosive changes of atlantal lateral masses result in downward telescoping of atlas onto axis body
    - Anterior displacement of atlantal posterior arch
    - Ventral and dorsal cervicomedullary compression
  - Clark station is determined by dividing odontoid process into 3 equal parts in sagittal plane
    - If anterior ring of atlas is level with middle 3rd (station II) or caudal 3rd (station III) of odontoid process, basilar impression is present
  - McGregor line is line drawn on midline image from hard palate to base of occiput
    - Cranial settling of occiput is defined as migration of odontoid more than 4.5 mm above McGregor line

- Redlund-Johnell measurement is distance between midpoint of caudal end plate of C2 to McGregor line (value of < 34 mm in men and 29 mm in women is considered abnormal)
- **Basilar Invagination**
  - **Developmental** anomaly of craniovertebral junction where odontoid process has abnormal relationship to foramen magnum (prolapse)
  - Has been categorized by absence (type 1) or presence (type 2) of Chiari malformation
- **Basilar Impression**
  - **Acquired** abnormality of odontoid position with respect to foramen magnum resulting from bone softening or ligamentous laxity at skull base
  - 1 of 3 directional instabilities that occur in RA
    - Other 2 instabilities: Atlantoaxial subluxation and subaxial subluxation
- **Platybasia**
  - Abnormal flattening of skull base
  - Determined through lines from nasion to dorsum sellae and from dorsum sella to basion
  - Generally associated with abnormalities such as Chiari malformations but not clinically significant

SELECTED REFERENCES

1. Krauss WE et al: Rheumatoid arthritis of the craniovertebral junction. Neurosurgery. 66(3 Suppl):83-95, 2010
2. Mouchaty H et al: Craniovertebral junction lesions: our experience with the transoral surgical approach. Eur Spine J. 18 Suppl 1:13-9, 2009
3. Smoker WR et al: Imaging the craniocervical junction. Childs Nerv Syst. 24(10):1123-45, 2008
4. Caird J et al: Preoperative cervical traction in cases of cranial settling with halo ring and Mayfield skull clamp. Br J Neurosurg. 19(6):488-9, 2005
5. Goel A et al: Atlantoaxial joint distraction for treatment of basilar invagination secondary to rheumatoid arthritis. Neurol India. 53(2):238-40, 2005
6. Nannapaneni R et al: Surgical outcome in rheumatoid Ranawat Class IIIb myelopathy. Neurosurgery. 56(4):706-15; discussion 706-15, 2005
7. Goel A et al: Craniovertebral realignment for basilar invagination and atlantoaxial dislocation secondary to rheumatoid arthritis. Neurol India. 52(3):338-41, 2004
8. Nguyen HV et al: Rheumatoid arthritis of the cervical spine. Spine J. 4(3):329-34, 2004

(Left) Sagittal NECT shows cranial settling with upward translocation of the odontoid process ➡. There are also dens erosions ➡ and increased atlantodental interval ➡. Note the low position of C1 ring relative to the C2 body. (Right) Sagittal T2WI MR study shows compression of the cord at the C1 level due to cranial settling and atlantodental instability with ventral and dorsal compression ➡.

Cranial Settling

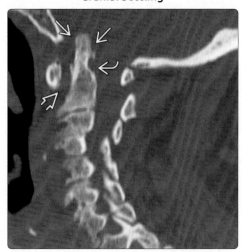

Cranial Settling

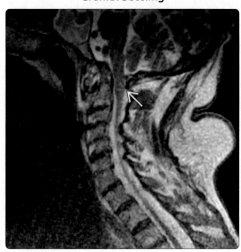

Cranial Settling

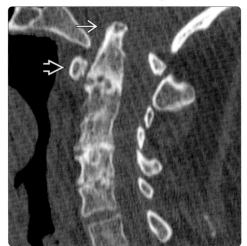

Cranial Settling

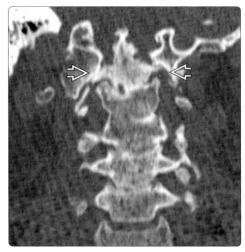

(Left) *Sagittal NECT shows rheumatoid cranial settling with upward translocation of the odontoid process* ➡ *into the foramen magnum and abnormal relationship between the skull base and C1. There are typical erosive changes in the odontoid process and subaxial erosions. Note the caudal position of C1 relative to C2 body* ➡. (Right) *Coronal NECT shows rheumatoid cranial settling with upward prolapse of the odontoid into the foramen magnum and collapse of the lateral masses of C1* ➡.

Basilar Invagination

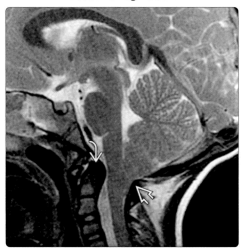

Basilar Invagination

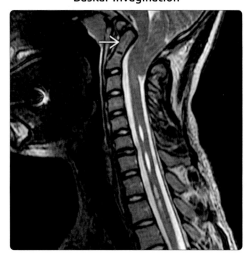

(Left) *Sagittal T2WI MR shows Chiari 1 malformation with inferior descent of the abnormally pointed ectopic cerebellar tonsils* ➡ *through the foramen magnum. The odontoid process* ➡ *is also retroflexed, and the clivus is mildly hypoplastic.* (Right) *Sagittal T2WI MR shows severe Chiari 1 malformation with contributory craniovertebral segmentation anomalies and syringomyelia. There is striking odontoid process retroflexion* ➡ *and upward positioning.*

Basilar Impression

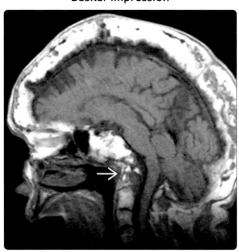

Platybasia

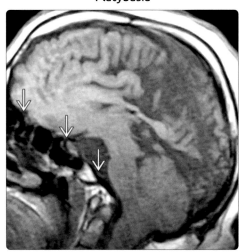

(Left) *Sagittal T1WI shows the typical pattern of basilar impression with Paget disease due to bone softening of the skull base, causing relative upward prolapse of the odontoid process* ➡. (Right) *Sagittal T1WI shows basilar invagination in a patient with Chiari 2 malformation who also has platybasia* ➡.

Differential Diagnosis

DIFFERENTIAL DIAGNOSIS

Common

- Chiari 1 Malformation
- Chiari 2 Malformation
- Klippel-Feil Spectrum
- Paget Disease
- Osteomalacia
- Osteogenesis Imperfecta

Less Common

- 22q11.2 Deletion Syndrome

ESSENTIAL INFORMATION

Key Differential Diagnosis Issues

- **Platybasia** is defined as abnormal flattening of skull base
  - Occurs in various congenital disorders but usually as secondary or associated finding; typically has no clinical impact
    - Often associated with basilar invagination
  - Associated with rise in odontoid and craniocervical junction above palatine line, which may favor transnasal approach to skull base
- Variable methods of measurement
  - Angle at junction of lines from nasion to central aspect of pituitary fossa and from pituitary fossa to basion on plain films
    - Normal: 130°-140° (Welcher basal angle)
    - Abnormal: > 140° (flattening)
  - Angle at junction of lines from nasion to dorsum sella and from dorsum sella to basion (along posterior margin of clivus) on MR images
    - Adults: 129° ± 6°; children: 127° ± 5°

Helpful Clues for Common Diagnoses

- **Chiari 1 Malformation**
  - Key facts: Mismatch between posterior fossa size and cerebellar tissue volume
  - Imaging: Tonsils project ≥ 5 mm below foramen magnum

- **Chiari 2 Malformation**
  - Key facts: Nearly 100% have neural tube closure defect
  - Imaging: Small posterior fossa, "notched" clivus, low-lying tentorium
- **Klippel-Feil Spectrum**
  - Key facts: Congenital spinal malformation characterized by segmentation failure of ≥ 2 cervical vertebrae ± thoracic or lumbar segmentation failure
  - Imaging: Single- or multilevel congenital cervical segmentation and fusion anomalies
    - Associated abnormalities include odontoid dysplasia, basilar impression, C1 assimilation, occipitocervical instability
- **Paget Disease**
  - Key facts: Often asymptomatic involvement of skull base (often only site of involvement); M > F
  - Imaging: May be multifocal disease with mixed sclerotic-lytic pattern
    - Expands bone; results in cotton wool appearance
- **Osteomalacia**
  - Key facts: Abnormal mineralization in trabecular and cortical bone
  - Imaging: Deformities due to bone softening: Basilar impression, vertebral endplate compressions, scoliosis
- **Osteogenesis Imperfecta**
  - Key facts: Genetic disorder of type I collagen resulting in bone fragility
  - Imaging: Severe osteopenia, vertebral fractures, kyphoscoliosis

Helpful Clues for Less Common Diagnoses

- **22q11.2 Deletion Syndrome**
  - Key facts: OMIM #188400 (DiGeorge syndrome)
  - Imaging: Platybasia and upper cervical spine anomalies common (dysplastic atlas in 75%)

SELECTED REFERENCES

1. Dasenbrock HH et al: Endoscopic image-guided transcervical odontoidectomy: outcomes of 15 patients with basilar invagination. Neurosurgery. 70(2):351-9; discussion 359-60, 2012

Chiari 1 Malformation

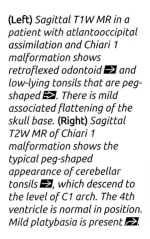

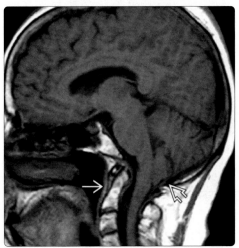

Chiari 1 Malformation

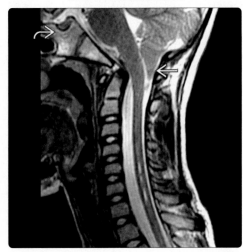

(Left) Sagittal T1W MR in a patient with atlantooccipital assimilation and Chiari 1 malformation shows retroflexed odontoid ➡ and low-lying tonsils that are peg-shaped ➡. There is mild associated flattening of the skull base. (Right) Sagittal T2W MR of Chiari 1 malformation shows the typical peg-shaped appearance of cerebellar tonsils ➡, which descend to the level of C1 arch. The 4th ventricle is normal in position. Mild platybasia is present ➡.

Chiari 2 Malformation

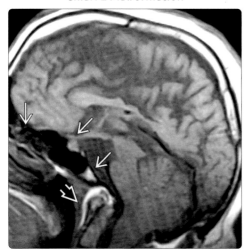

Klippel-Feil Spectrum

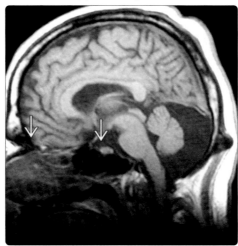

(Left) Sagittal T1WI in a patient with Chiari 2 malformation shows flattening of the Welcher basal angle ➡ and basilar invagination ⇉ with upward prolapse of the odontoid process into the foramen magnum. (Right) Sagittal T2WI MR in a child with Klippel-Feil spectrum and basilar invagination shows flattening of the skull base ➡ and upward migration of the odontoid process ⇉ into the foramen magnum with cord compression.

Klippel-Feil Spectrum

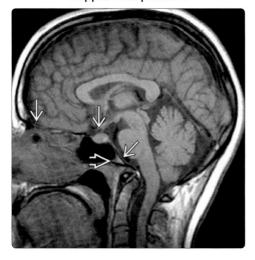

Klippel-Feil Spectrum

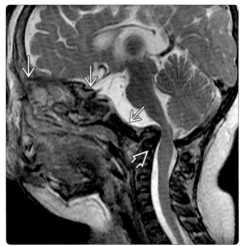

(Left) Sagittal T1WI MR in a patient with C0-C1 assimilation, retroflexed odontoid, and C2-C3 fusion shows associated flattening of the skull base angle ➡ and short, truncated clivus ⇉. (Right) Sagittal T1WI MR shows severe flattening of the Welcher basal angle ➡ in a patient with multiple vertebral segmentation anomalies.

Osteogenesis Imperfecta

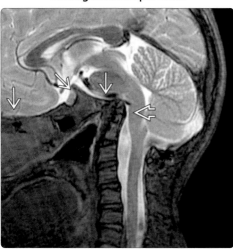

Osteogenesis Imperfecta

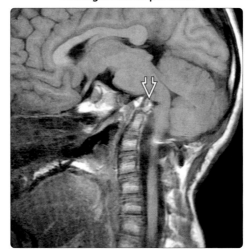

(Left) Sagittal T2WI MR shows basilar impression in osteogenesis imperfecta with platybasia ➡ and upward displacement of the odontoid process ⇉ into the foramen magnum, producing ventral cervicomedullary compression. (Right) Sagittal T1WI MR shows severe basilar impression related to osteogenesis imperfecta with the odontoid process ⇉ projecting into the foramen magnum, producing ventral cervicomedullary compression.

DIFFERENTIAL DIAGNOSIS

Common

- Metastasis, Skull Base
- Fibrous Dysplasia, Skull Base
- Paget Disease, Skull Base
- Chordoma, Clivus
- Multiple Myeloma, Skull Base
- Plasmacytoma, Skull Base
- Chondrosarcoma, Skull Base
- Pneumatization Arrest, Sphenoid

Less Common

- Langerhans Histiocytosis, Skull Base
- Arachnoid Granulations, Dural Sinuses
- Osteomyelitis, Skull Base
- Meningioma, Skull Base

Rare but Important

- Giant Cell Tumor, Skull Base
- Cephalocele, Skull Base
- Ecchordosis Physaliphora
- Pseudotumor, Skull Base

ESSENTIAL INFORMATION

Key Differential Diagnosis Issues

- Lesion may be focal, diffuse, localized, or part of systemic disease
- Variable presentation of skull base lesion
  - Headache, cranial neuropathy
  - May be incidental imaging finding
- Imaging strategy
  - CT and MR often complementary
    - CT best demonstrates aggressive or benign bone features
    - MR may have characteristic signal intensity or enhancement

Helpful Clues for Common Diagnoses

- **Metastasis, Skull Base**
  - Key facts
    - Central skull base is most frequent site
    - Most often prostate, breast, and lung carcinoma
  - Imaging
    - CT: Lytic, destructive, or sclerotic
    - MR: Variable signal, usually enhances
- **Fibrous Dysplasia, Skull Base**
  - Key facts
    - Benign expansile bone anomaly
    - Prone to enlarge during childhood
  - Imaging
    - CT: Characteristic ground-glass appearance; may narrow foramina and fissures
    - MR: Heterogeneous, mass-like lesion
    - T2: Ground-glass hypointense, lucent hyperintense, variable enhancement
- **Paget Disease, Skull Base**
  - Key facts
    - Chronic bone disorder with abnormal bone breakdown and formation
  - Imaging
    - CT: Sclerotic expansion of bone with cotton wool texture ± lytic areas
    - MR: T2 mainly low, lytic areas bright
- **Chordoma, Clivus**
  - Key facts
    - Benign but locally aggressive primary tumor of notochord remnants
    - From sphenooccipital synchondrosis
  - Imaging
    - CT: Lytic destructive midline sphenoid mass ± irregular bone spicules
    - MR: Characteristic high T2 signal, heterogeneous enhancement
- **Multiple Myeloma, Skull Base**
  - Key facts
    - Focal mass of malignant plasma cells
    - More frequently seen in calvarium
  - Imaging
    - CT
      - Multiple well-defined lytic lesions
- **Plasmacytoma, Skull Base**
  - Key facts
    - Isolated tumor of malignant plasma cells
  - Imaging
    - CT: Solitary lesion, bony lysis
    - MR: T2 intermediate signal; moderate enhancement
- **Chondrosarcoma, Skull Base**
  - Key facts
    - Malignant cartilaginous neoplasm
    - Arises from petroclival synchondrosis
  - Imaging
    - CT: Destructive mass at junction of sphenoid and temporal bones
    - Arcs and whorls of calcification
    - MR: T2 bright, intense enhancement
- **Pneumatization Arrest, Sphenoid**
  - Key facts
    - Incidental lesion of basisphenoid
  - Imaging
    - CT: Nonexpansile with sclerotic margin
    - Contains fat and curvilinear calcification
    - MR: Heterogeneous, often focal T1 fat

Helpful Clues for Less Common Diagnoses

- **Langerhans Histiocytosis, Skull Base**
  - Key facts
    - Proliferation of bone marrow-derived Langerhans cells and eosinophils
    - Skull base involvement more often with multifocal or acute disseminated forms
  - Imaging
    - Nonspecific destructive soft tissue mass
- **Arachnoid Granulations, Dural Sinuses**
  - Key facts
    - Usually incidental imaging finding
  - Imaging
    - More numerous around dural sinuses
    - CT: Small, well-defined "pits" in skull base
    - MR: Often subtle, focal T2 hyperintensity

- **Osteomyelitis, Skull Base**
  - Key facts
    - Primary bone infection, acute or chronic
  - Imaging
    - CT: Permeative lytic when acute; chronic may be lytic or lytic-sclerotic
    - MR: Marrow replacement, enhancement; often extensive involvement of dura
- **Meningioma, Skull Base**
  - Key facts
    - Dural-based, benign extraaxial tumor
    - May occur as intraosseous lesion
  - Imaging
    - CT: Bony changes may be hyperostosis, erosion, or permeative destruction
    - MR: Bone and thick dura enhance

Helpful Clues for Rare Diagnoses

- **Giant Cell Tumor, Skull Base**
  - Key facts
    - Benign long bone tumor
    - Skull base
      - □ Sphenoid and temporal bones
    - Can be locally aggressive &/or recur
  - Imaging
    - CT: Destructive mass with focally interrupted, thinned cortical shell
    - MR: Scant matrix, larger lesions more heterogeneous, marked enhancement
- **Cephalocele, Skull Base**
  - Key facts
    - Skull base defect with protrusion of meninges ± neural tissue
  - Imaging
    - CT: Focal bone defect
    - MR: Dura, CSF, ± neural elements
- **Ecchordosis Physaliphora**
  - Key facts
    - Notochordal remnant exophytic from dorsal aspect of clivus

- Imaging
  - CT: Soft tissue density lesion
  - MR: T1 low, T2 high, no enhancement
- **Pseudotumor, Skull Base**
  - Key facts
    - Idiopathic inflammatory lesion
    - Inflammatory cells and variable fibrosis
  - Imaging
    - CT: Soft tissue mass, permeative bone
    - MR: Enhancing infiltrative process, T2 hypointense, T1 iso- to hypointense

SELECTED REFERENCES

1. Mathur A et al: Imaging of skull base pathologies: Role of advanced magnetic resonance imaging techniques. Neuroradiol J. 28(4):426-37, 2015
2. Walcott BP et al: Chordoma: current concepts, management, and future directions. Lancet Oncol. 13(2):e69-76, 2012
3. Adamek D et al: Ecchordosis physaliphora: a case report and a review of notochord-derived lesions. Neurol Neurochir Pol. 45(2):169-73, 2011
4. Alonso-Basanta M et al: Proton beam therapy in skull base pathology. Otolaryngol Clin North Am. 44(5):1173-83, 2011
5. Chamoun RB et al: Management of skull base metastases. Neurosurg Clin N Am. 22(1):61-6, vi-ii, 2011
6. Koutourousiou M et al: Skull base chordomas. Otolaryngol Clin North Am. 44(5):1155-71, 2011
7. Lui YW et al: Sphenoid masses in children: radiologic differential diagnosis with pathologic correlation. AJNR Am J Neuroradiol. 32(4):617-26, 2011
8. Nuñez S et al: Midline congenital malformations of the brain and skull. Neuroimaging Clin N Am. 21(3):429-82, vii, 2011
9. Scholz M et al: Skull base approaches in neurosurgery. Head Neck Oncol. 2:16, 2010
10. Kastrup O et al: Neuroimaging of infections of the central nervous system. Semin Neurol. 28(4):511-22, 2008
11. Welker KM et al: Arrested pneumatization of the skull base: imaging characteristics. AJR Am J Roentgenol. 190(6):1691-6, 2008
12. Dubrulle F et al: Extension patterns of nasopharyngeal carcinoma. Eur Radiol. 17(10):2622-30, 2007
13. Noël G et al: Chondrosarcomas of the base of the skull in Ollier's disease or Maffucci's syndrome–three case reports and review of the literature. Acta Oncol. 43(8):705-10, 2004
14. St Martin M et al: Chordomas of the skull base: manifestations and management. Curr Opin Otolaryngol Head Neck Surg. 11(5):324-7, 2003
15. Wallace RC et al: Posttreatment imaging of the skull base. Semin Ultrasound CT MR. 24(3):164-81, 2003

Metastasis, Skull Base

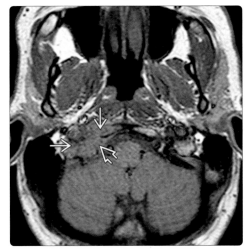

Fibrous Dysplasia, Skull Base

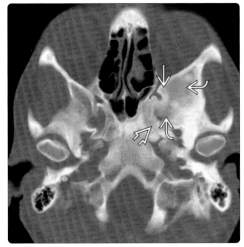

(Left) Axial T1WI MR in a patient with a history of lung cancer and a new right CNXII palsy shows focal loss of bright marrow signal at the right skull base ➡ with abnormal tissue around the hypoglossal canal ➡. (Right) Axial bone CT demonstrates that the greater wing ➡ has the characteristic ground-glass appearance with areas of dense sclerosis and other areas of greater lucency ➡. Note the narrowed vidian canal ➡.

(Left) *Axial bone CT shows a diffuse cotton wool appearance of the entire skull base with expansion of the squamous temporal bone ➡, petrous apex ➡, and occipital bone ➡. Note also the stapes prosthesis on the right ➡, which was placed for conductive hearing loss.* (Right) *Axial T2WI MR shows an expansile, hyperintense mass ➡ arising in the clivus and eroding the posterior clival cortex ➡. The mass otherwise has more benign, well-defined contours as it extends anteriorly to involve the longus capitis muscles.*

Paget Disease, Skull Base

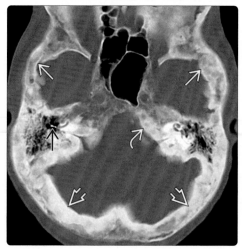

Chordoma, Clivus

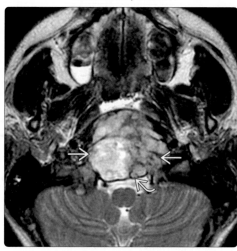

(Left) *Axial bone CT shows multiple tiny lytic lesions ➡ in the skull base with sharply demarcated borders. Note the additional lesion in the occipital bone ➡. Lesions of this size are easily overlooked, especially without a bone algorithm CT.* (Right) *Axial T2WI FS MR reveals a large central skull base mass ➡, which expands bone and appears to extend laterally to the cavernous sinuses. The mass is homogeneous and has intermediate signal intensity.*

Multiple Myeloma, Skull Base

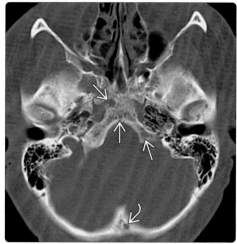

Plasmacytoma, Skull Base

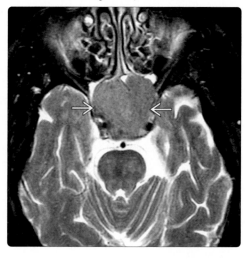

(Left) *Axial T2WI MR through the skull base demonstrates a markedly high signal intensity tumor ➡ involving the right petrous apex and extending into the cerebellopontine angle cistern. The location suggests chondrosarcoma arising from petroclival synchondrosis.* (Right) *Axial bone CT in a younger patient shows a large paramedian lytic lesion of the right basiocciput and a petrous bone with chondroid calcifications ➡.*

Chondrosarcoma, Skull Base

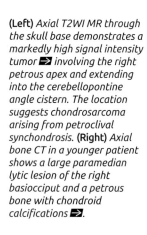
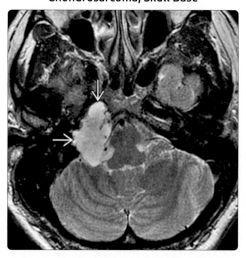

Chondrosarcoma, Skull Base

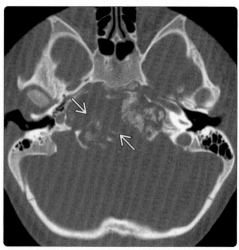

Pneumatization Arrest, Sphenoid

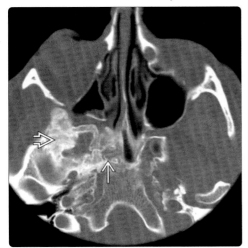

Langerhans Histiocytosis, Skull Base

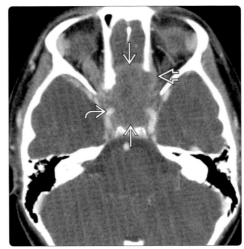

(Left) Axial bone CT reveals a benign hyperdense appearance of the sphenoid body ➡ and greater wing ➡, mimicking fibrous dysplasia but without the significant expansion seen with fibrous dysplasia. (Right) Axial CECT shows a nonspecific but destructive lesion ➡ of the central and anterior skull base with invasion to the orbits ➡ bilaterally. The tumor surrounds carotid arteries ➡, indicating involvement of cavernous sinuses bilaterally also. The key to the diagnosis is that this is a pediatric patient.

Osteomyelitis, Skull Base

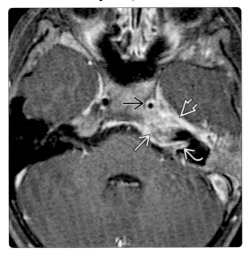

Meningioma, Skull Base

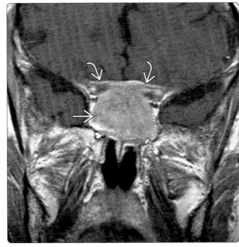

(Left) Axial T1 C+ FS MR in a patient with Gradenigo syndrome shows extensive enhancement of the petrous apex ➡ but also adjacent dural reflections. There is involvement of middle fossa dura ➡ and dura of internal auditory canal ➡, as well as spasm of the adjacent internal carotid artery ➡. (Right) Coronal T1 C+ MR demonstrates a homogeneously enhancing mass centered in the sphenoid bone ➡. The key to the diagnosis is the presence of overlying dural thickening and enhancement ➡.

Giant Cell Tumor, Skull Base

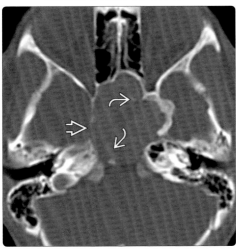

Ecchordosis Physaliphora

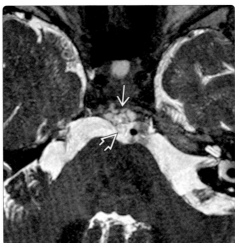

(Left) Axial bone CT reveals a thin, irregularly sclerotic "eggshell" of the cortex. Expansile margins suggest a benign process. Focal areas of bone dehiscence ➡ and matrix calcifications are evident ➡. (Right) Axial T2WI MR demonstrates a subtle, well-defined bilobed lesion ➡ arising from the dorsal clivus and extending into the prepontine cistern ➡, although not causing any deformity of the pons.

DIFFERENTIAL DIAGNOSIS

Common

- Acquired Tonsillar Herniation
- Chiari 1 Malformation
- Chiari 2 Malformation
- Meningioma, Clivus
- Rheumatoid Arthritis, Adult
- Schwannoma, Jugular Foramen

Less Common

- Chordoma, Clivus
- Ependymoma
- Chondrosarcoma, Skull Base
- Retroodontoid Pseudopannus
- Hemangioblastoma
- Calcium Pyrophosphate Dihydrate Deposition Disease (CPPD)
- Metastasis, Skull Base

Rare but Important

- Fusiform Aneurysm, ASVD
- Fusiform Aneurysm, Non-ASVD
- Brainstem Glioma, Pediatric
- Epidermoid Cyst
- Neurenteric Cyst

ESSENTIAL INFORMATION

Key Differential Diagnosis Issues

- Foramen magnum (FM): Posterior skull base aperture in occipital bone
  - Transmits medulla oblongata, vertebral arteries, and CNXI
- Lesions of FM can be intraaxial, extraaxial, and bony skull base in origin
- Cisternal magna: Skull base cistern between medulla anteriorly and occiput posteriorly

Helpful Clues for Common Diagnoses

- **Acquired Tonsillar Herniation**
  - Key facts: Secondary to posterior fossa mass effect or severe hydrocephalus
    - May also be secondary to CSF leak with intracranial hypotension ("sagging brain")
  - Imaging: Cerebellar tonsils → into FM
    - Cisterna magna obliterated
    - 4th ventricle obstruction → hydrocephalus
- **Chiari 1 Malformation**
  - Key facts
    - May be incidental
  - Imaging: Small posterior fossa
    - Low-lying "pegged" tonsils
    - Tonsils > 5 mm below FM
- **Chiari 2 Malformation**
  - Key facts: Complex hindbrain malformation + lumbar myelomeningocele
    - "Beaked" tectum, "towering" cerebellum, dysgenic corpus callosum
  - Imaging: Tonsillar ectopia
    - Straw-like 4th ventricle; hydrocephalus

- **Meningioma, Clivus**
  - Key facts: Older, female patients
    - Tends to encase and narrow vessels
  - Imaging: Enhancing dural-based mass with tails; extends through FM when clival
    - CT: High-density lesion ± Ca^{++}
    - MR: Low signal on T2 MR
- **Rheumatoid Arthritis, Adult**
  - Key facts
    - Inflammatory pannus in retroodontoid soft tissues
  - Imaging: Odontoid erosions common
    - CT: Cranial settling in severe cases
    - MR: Markedly hypointense on T2; T1 variable; enhances
- **Schwannoma, Jugular Foramen**
  - Key facts: Arises from CNIX-CNXI
    - Cisternal component may involve FM
    - May arise primarily within FM
  - Imaging: Fusiform jugular foramen mass
    - CT: Smooth enlargement of jugular foramen
    - MR: Enhances; high T2 signal; intramural cysts

Helpful Clues for Less Common Diagnoses

- **Chordoma, Clivus**
  - Key facts: Midline mass; exophytic
    - Extension into prepontine cistern "thumbs" pons
  - Imaging: Lower clival location extending to FM
    - CT: Irregular destructive mass lesion within clivus
    - MR: Characteristic high T2 signal; intensely enhancing
- **Ependymoma**
  - Key facts: Soft tumor, "squeezes out" 4th ventricle foramina
    - 2/3 infratentorial, 4th ventricle
  - Imaging: Heterogeneously enhancing 4th ventricle mass
    - Inferiorly extending tumor in FM
- **Chondrosarcoma, Skull Base**
  - Key facts: Chondroid malignancy; petrooccipital fissure most common
  - Imaging: 50% chondroid Ca^{++} (CT)
    - MR: Destructive, enhancing, T2 hyperintense tumor
    - When large, affects FM
- **Retroodontoid Pseudopannus**
  - Key facts: Calcific debris arising posterosuperior to C1-C2
    - Associated with degenerative arthritis, gout, CPPD
  - Imaging: Look for medullary or cervical cord compression
    - CT: Calcifications of ligaments and within joint capsule
    - MR: Low signal intensity mass behind odontoid
- **Hemangioblastoma**
  - Key facts: Associated with von Hippel Lindau
    - 80% cerebellar hemispheres, 15% vermis, 5% medulla, 4th ventricle
  - Imaging: Cystic cerebellar mass + enhancing mural nodule (60%)
    - 40% solid mass
- **Calcium Pyrophosphate Dihydrate Deposition Disease (CPPD)**
  - Key facts: Calcium pyrophosphate dihydrate deposition disease
  - Imaging: Retroodontoid mass may cause instability ± cervical cord compression

- **Metastasis, Skull Base**
  - Key facts: Involvement of occiput by bony metastatic lesion
  - Imaging: Irregular bone destruction ± soft tissue mass
    - When large, compresses brainstem

Helpful Clues for Rare Diagnoses

- **Fusiform Aneurysm, ASVD**
  - Key facts
    - Aneurysm of distal vertebral artery or proximal basilar artery
  - Imaging
    - CT: Lamellated layers of calcific and noncalcific thrombus; residual lumen
    - MR: Flow-related changes of lumen with varying age thrombus in wall, prominent phase artifact from aneurysm pulsation
    - MRA: Shows residual lumen
    - High T1 signal thrombus may be mistaken for lumen blood flow on TOF studies
- **Fusiform Aneurysm, Non-ASVD**
  - Key facts: Associated with collagen vascular diseases, other vasculopathies
  - Imaging
    - CT: Shows fusiform enlargement of vessel involved
    - MR: Layered thrombus or enlarged vessel
- **Brainstem Glioma, Pediatric**
  - Key facts: Infiltrative glioma, typically low grade, involving medulla and pons
  - Imaging: Enlarged brainstem
    - Usually no enhancement
    - High T2 and FLAIR signal
    - Lobulated ventral margin (exophytic)
- **Epidermoid Cyst**
  - Key facts: Ectodermal rest in cistern
    - Cerebellopontine angle 40-50%, 4th ventricle 15-20%
  - Imaging: CSF-like, lobular, extraaxial
    - DWI shows hyperintensity
    - Insinuates into cisterns
    - Encases nerves/vessels

- **Neurenteric Cyst**
  - Key facts: Developmental lesion resulting in intradural midline cystic mass
  - Imaging: Smooth extraaxial mass at skull base
    - Ventral to brainstem
    - Iso- to hyperintense to CSF on T1
    - High T2 signal; conspicuous on FLAIR

SELECTED REFERENCES

1. Lucas JW et al: Endoscopic endonasal and keyhole surgery for the management of skull base meningiomas. Neurosurg Clin N Am. 27(2):207-14, 2016
2. Jansen MH et al: Diffuse intrinsic pontine gliomas: a systematic update on clinical trials and biology. Cancer Treat Rev. 38(1):27-35, 2012
3. Poretti A et al: Neuroimaging of pediatric posterior fossa tumors including review of the literature. J Magn Reson Imaging. 35(1):32-47, 2012
4. Starke RM et al: Gamma knife surgery for skull base meningiomas. J Neurosurg. 116(3):588-97, 2012
5. Walcott BP et al: Chordoma: current concepts, management, and future directions. Lancet Oncol. 13(2):e69-76, 2012
6. Gutierrez J et al: Dolichoectasia-an evolving arterial disease. Nat Rev Neurol. 7(1):41-50, 2011
7. Ishiyama G et al: Vertebrobasilar infarcts and ischemia. Otolaryngol Clin North Am. 44(2):415-35, ix-x, 2011
8. Khatua S et al: Diffuse intrinsic pontine glioma-current status and future strategies. Childs Nerv Syst. 27(9):1391-7, 2011
9. Koutourousiou M et al: Skull base chordomas. Otolaryngol Clin North Am. 44(5):1155-71, 2011
10. Lee CJ et al: Treatment of vertebral disease: appropriate use of open and endovascular techniques. Semin Vasc Surg. 24(1):24-30, 2011
11. Mattle HP et al: Basilar artery occlusion. Lancet Neurol. 10(11):1002-14, 2011
12. Oakes WJ: Chiari malformation Type I. J Neurosurg. 115(3):645; discussion 645-6, 2011
13. Fraser JF et al: Endoscopic endonasal transclival resection of chordomas: operative technique, clinical outcome, and review of the literature. J Neurosurg. 112(5):1061-9, 2010
14. Fangusaro J: Pediatric high-grade gliomas and diffuse intrinsic pontine gliomas. J Child Neurol. 24(11):1409-17, 2009
15. Sievert AJ et al: Pediatric low-grade gliomas. J Child Neurol. 24(11):1397-408, 2009
16. Johnson MD et al: New prospects for management and treatment of inoperable and recurrent skull base meningiomas. J Neurooncol. 86(1):109-22, 2008
17. Sekhar LN et al: Meningiomas involving the clivus: a six-year experience with 41 patients. Neurosurgery. 27(5):764-81; discussion 781, 1990

Acquired Tonsillar Herniation

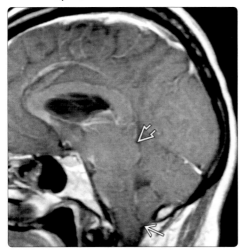

Chiari 1 Malformation

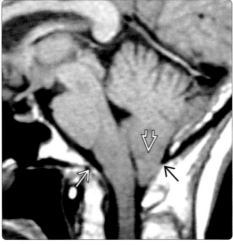

(Left) *Sagittal T1WI MR reveals acquired tonsillar herniation ➡ as a result of intracranial hypotension with the "slumping" midbrain ➡ squeezing the pons inferiorly.* (Right) *Sagittal T1WI MR shows a Chiari 1 malformation demonstrating tonsillar herniation. The tonsils ➡ protrude through the foramen magnum, below an imaginary line drawn between the basion ➡ and opisthion ➡.*

Chiari 2 Malformation

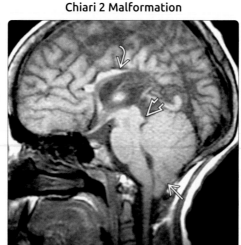

Meningioma, Clivus

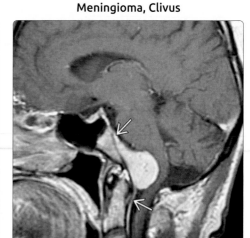

(Left) *Sagittal T1WI MR shows caudal descent of the cerebellar tissue and 4th ventricle* ➡ *associated with callosal dysgenesis* ➡. *Abnormal tectum, or beaking* ➡, *is an important associated finding.* **(Right)** *Sagittal T1WI C+ MR demonstrates a homogeneously enhancing meningioma with conspicuous dural "tails"* ➡ *along the anterior margin of the foramen magnum.*

Rheumatoid Arthritis, Adult

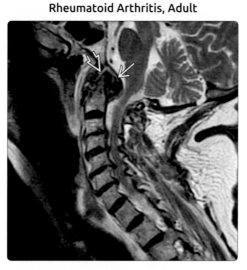

Schwannoma, Jugular Foramen

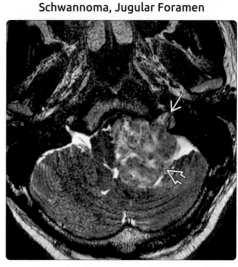

(Left) *Sagittal T2WI MR reveals a large amount of rheumatoid pannus* ➡ *with effacement of the spinal canal and posterior displacement of the lower medulla. The odontoid process is abnormally "pointed" and eroded* ➡. **(Right)** *Axial T2WI MR shows a jugular foramen schwannoma with a very large cisternal component* ➡ *displacing the medulla and filling the basal cistern. Note that the left jugular foramen is filled by a schwannoma* ➡.

Chordoma, Clivus

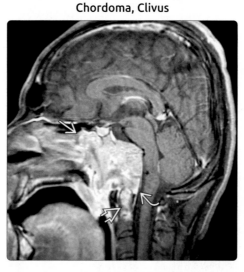

Chordoma, Clivus

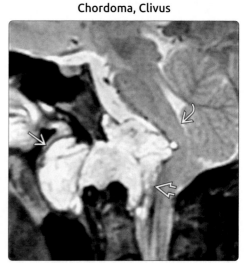

(Left) *Sagittal T1WI C+ MR shows a very large enhancing chordoma of the clivus with involvement of the sphenoid sinus* ➡ *and C2 vertebra* ➡ *with extension into the posterior fossa and foramen magnum* ➡. **(Right)** *Sagittal T1WI FS MR reveals a hyperintense midline chordoma arising from the inferior clivus, projecting anteriorly into the nasopharynx* ➡ *and posteriorly into the foramen magnum* ➡. *Note the medullary compression* ➡.

Ependymoma

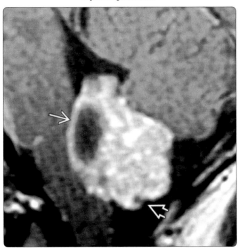

Calcium Pyrophosphate Dihydrate Deposition Disease (CPPD)

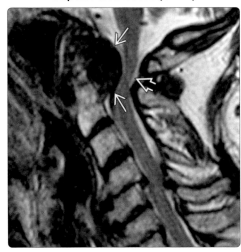

(Left) *Sagittal T1WI C+ MR shows an enhancing ependymoma ➡ projecting from the inferior 4th ventricle into the superior foramen magnum ➡. **(Right)** Sagittal T2WI MR shows CPPD involvement of the upper cervical spine with an associated low-signal mass ➡ compressing the lower medulla ➡. Pseudopannus is nonspecific with differential diagnoses that include degenerative arthritis, calcium pyrophosphate dihydrate deposition disease, and gout.*

Fusiform Aneurysm, ASVD

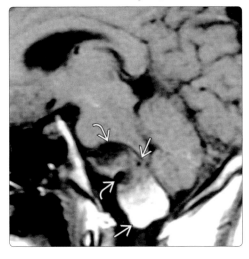

Fusiform Aneurysm, Non-ASVD

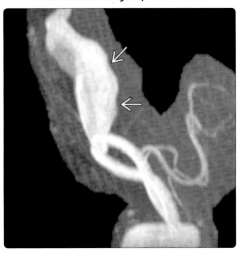

(Left) *Sagittal T1WI MR shows a mixed signal intensity extraaxial mass ➡. An extraaxial lesion with evidence of flow and thrombosis is strongly suggestive of aneurysm. Only small residual flow voids are seen on this sagittal image ➡. **(Right)** Sagittal MRA depicts a fusiform nonatherosclerotic aneurysm of the basilar artery in an adolescent male. The vessel wall is somewhat irregular ➡ but without stenosis.*

Brainstem Glioma, Pediatric

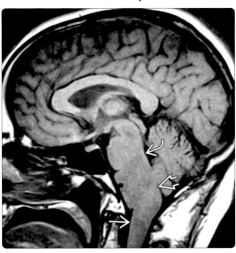

Neurenteric Cyst

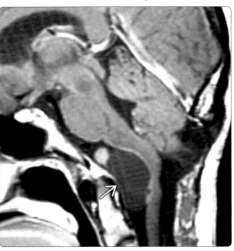

(Left) *Sagittal T1WI MR shows a markedly expanded upper cervical cord ➡, medulla ➡, and inferior pons ➡ resulting from an infiltrative mass isointense to the brainstem. Brainstem gliomas often smoothly enlarge the brainstem. **(Right)** Sagittal T1WI C+ MR shows an extraaxial mass ➡ in the anterior foramen magnum elevating and displacing the medulla. This neurenteric cyst is slightly hyperintense compared to cerebrospinal fluid and was conspicuous on FLAIR (not shown).*

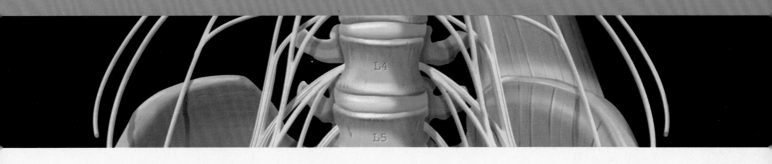

SECTION 13
Peripheral Nerve and Plexus

Terminology

Nerve rootlets: Individual neural filaments of dorsal and ventral roots directly exiting from spinal cord

Nerve roots: Composed of multiple individual dorsal or ventral nerve rootlets
- Dorsal sensory roots exit from dorsolateral cord and have cell bodies within dorsal root ganglion (DRG)
- Ventral motor roots arise from anterior cord gray matter and have cell bodies within cord

DRG: Dorsal nerve root sensory ganglion, resides in neural foramen

Spinal nerve (proper): Union of dorsal and ventral nerve roots
- 31 nerve pairs (8 cervical, 12 thoracic, 5 lumbar, 5 sacral, and 1 coccygeal)
- Proper spinal nerve is short in length, bifurcates into ventral and dorsal rami

Ramus: 1st spinal nerve branch
- Larger ventral primary ramus supplies ventral musculature and facets
- Smaller dorsal primary ramus supplies paraspinal muscles and part of facet

Peripheral nerve: Combination of 1 or more rami into single neural conduit

Plexus: Neural network of anastomosing nerves

Imaging Anatomy

Cervical Plexus
The cervical plexus forms from the ventral rami of C1-C4 and, variably, a C5 minor branch. It has ascending superficial, descending superficial, and deep branches that supply nuchal muscles, the diaphragm, and cutaneous head/neck tissues.

Brachial Plexus
The brachial plexus (BP) forms from the ventral rami of C5-T1 and variably from minor branches of C4 or T2. The BP contributes to several nerves originating above the BP proper, including the dorsal scapular nerve, long thoracic nerve, nerves to scalene/longus colli muscles, and a branch to the phrenic nerve. The remaining minor and all major terminal nerve branches arise from the BP proper. Depending on the cranial or caudal variation of the nerves supplying the BP, it can be defined as prefixed or postfixed. A prefixed BP has a large contribution from C4 with or without a small contribution from T1. A postfixed BP has a large contribution from T2 and little to no communication with C5.

Anatomically, the BP is classically divided sequentially (proximal to distal) into 5 segments: Roots/rami, trunks, divisions, cords, and terminal branches. The roots/rami originate directly from the spinal cord levels C5 to T1. The 3 trunks include the superior or upper (C5-C6), middle (C7), and inferior or lower (C8, T1) trunks. Important minor nerves arising directly from the trunks include the suprascapular nerve and nerve to subclavius muscle. Two divisions are described: Anterior division innervates anterior (flexor) muscles and posterior division innervates posterior (extensor) muscles. No named minor nerves arise directly from the anterior or posterior divisions. The 3 cords include the lateral cord (anterior divisions of superior, middle trunks) that innervates anterior (flexor) muscles, the medial cord (anterior division of inferior trunk) that innervates anterior (flexor) muscles, and the posterior cord (posterior divisions of all 3 trunks) that innervates posterior (extensor) muscles. The cords branch to form several important named terminal peripheral nerve branches.

Clinically, the BP is divided into 3 discrete segments based on anatomic relationship to the clavicle. These include the supraclavicular (roots, trunks), retroclavicular (divisions), and infraclavicular (cords, terminal branches) plexus.

Lumbar Plexus
The lumbar plexus derives from the L1-L4 ventral rami and a minor branch from T12. Important named minor nerve branches include the iliohypogastric, ilioinguinal, genitofemoral, lateral femoral cutaneous (L2-L3), and superior (L4-S1) and inferior (L5-S2) gluteal nerves. Important major nerve branches include the femoral (posterior division L2-L4) and obturator (anterior division L2-L4) nerves (Table 2).

Lumbosacral Trunk
The lumbosacral trunk (LST) is derived from the ventral rami of L4 (minor branch) and L5, and it is easily followed on axial imaging as it transits along the ventral surface of the sacral ala to join the sacral plexus in the pelvis.

Sacral Plexus
The sacral plexus is composed of the LST, S1-S3 ventral rami, and a minor branch from S4. The sacral rami and LST converge into the upper sacral neural band (LST and S1-S3) that forms the sciatic nerve and the lower sacral neural band (S3-S4) that forms the pudendal nerve.

Coccygeal Plexus
The coccygeal plexus converges from the S5 ventral ramus, Cx1, and a minor branch of S4. The major named branch is the anococcygeal nerve.

Anatomy-Based Imaging Issues

Normal Nerve Findings
Surrounding perineural fat provides excellent visualization of nerves and allows them to be easily distinguished from adjacent soft tissues. The normal peripheral nerve is a round/ovoid shape with well-defined internal fascicular architecture. Normal nerve fascicles are uniform in size and shape, and this characteristic fascicular pattern helps distinguish peripheral nerves from other lesions, such as schwannoma or a ganglion cyst, which also demonstrate high intrinsic T2 signal intensity.

Intrafascicular signal intensity is determined predominately by endoneurial fluid and axoplasmic water, whereas the interfascicular signal is dominated by fibrofatty connective tissue that is amenable to fat suppression. Therefore, normal nerve fascicles are isointense to adjacent muscle tissue on T1WI and mildly hyperintense relative to muscle interspersed within hypointense fibrofatty connective tissue on fat-saturated T2WI or STIR MR. No abrupt change in nerve caliber or course should be observed in an anatomically normal nerve.

Abnormal Nerve Findings
The acutely abnormal nerve demonstrates 1 or more of the following findings: Segmental nerve enlargement, disruption of nerve anatomic continuity, T2 signal intensity approaching that of regional blood vessels on fat-saturated T2WI or STIR sequences, or disruption or distortion of normal fascicular architecture. Entrapped or scarred nerves may show abrupt change in caliber or course.

The abnormal nerve, therefore, remains isointense on T1WI but becomes increasingly hyperintense to muscle on T2WI. In the setting of injury, it is postulated that increased endoneurial free water content alters the normal signal characteristics of peripheral nerves. The cause of abnormal high signal on T2WI and STIR sequences is not definitively known, but it has been speculated that edema from increased endoneurial fluid due to disordered endoneurial fluid flow or local venous obstruction may explain abnormal T2 hyperintensity. Alterations in axoplasmic flow may also produce increased signal. Axoplasmic flow is impeded by nerve compression, and increased axoplasm proximal and distal to the injury site may produce T2 hyperintensity.

Imaging Pitfalls

It can sometimes be difficult to distinguish peripheral nerve from adjacent vascular structures, particularly if the abnormal nerve displays high T2 signal intensity. Vessels demonstrate internal flow voids, branch at large angles, and show intense contrast enhancement. On the other hand, nerves do not show flow voids, branch at relatively acute angles, enhance minimally, and display a discrete distinctive fascicular architecture on transverse imaging.

Clinical Implications

High-resolution MR technique readily identifies the large major nerves and major plexi and permits visualization of their internal neural anatomy. Conversely, smaller major and essentially all minor peripheral nerves are too small to directly visualize.

Successful peripheral nerve imaging requires a strong working knowledge of normal plexus and nerve anatomy. Additionally, peripheral nerve imaging is time consuming and necessitates constraining the imaging volume to clinically relevant regions rather than general "screening" surveys. It is critical to have all pertinent clinical and electrodiagnostic data available to appropriately constrain imaging volume and help detect subtle abnormalities.

Differential Diagnosis

Normal Nerve/Plexus

The normal nerve/plexus shows normal course, caliber, contour, and internal fascicular architecture. Consider myopathic or other nonneural etiology in symptomatic patients.

Nerve/Plexus Mass

Neural neoplasms are most commonly of neural sheath origin. Consider solitary or plexiform neurofibroma, schwannoma, or malignant peripheral nerve sheath tumor. Less common considerations include neurolymphomatosis and peripheral nerve metastasis.

Trauma

Etiologies include traction (stretch or avulsion), laceration (projectile, fracture fragment, sharp object), or direct compression (hematoma, fracture).

MR is sensitive for the detection, and in some cases, discrimination of all 3 described peripheral nerve injury levels. **Neurapraxia**, the least severe type of injury, is characterized by focal damage to the myelin sheath without axonal disruption and manifests as identifiable but swollen and hyperintense nerve fascicles. **Axonotmesis** is an intermediate level of crush or traction injury that produces axonal disruption and subsequent wallerian degeneration but leaves the Schwann cells and endoneurium intact. Axonotmesis will display a homogeneously increased signal intensity nerve with

loss of fascicular architecture at the injury site. **Neurotmesis**, the most severe form of nerve injury, cannot always be distinguished from axonotmesis in the cases of functional rather than anatomical transaction but may display axonal disruption with discontinuity of some or all of the surrounding connective tissues and subsequent wallerian degeneration in definitive cases.

Entrapment Syndrome

Neural compression occurs at characteristic locations. These injuries are often, but not always, related to poor ergonomics or overuse injuries.

Hereditary Motor and Sensory Neuropathy

Inherited peripheral nerve disorders are characterized by abnormally enlarged peripheral nerves (usually palpable if not deep) and variable clinical neuropathy presentations. Some demonstrate the characteristic onion bulb appearance on micropathology following nerve biopsy, reflecting recurrent episodes of demyelination and remyelination. The most common hereditary motor and sensory neuropathy disorder is Charcot-Marie-Tooth, which has characteristic clinical manifestations and may involve the cauda equina, peripheral nerves, or both.

Infection/Inflammation

Myriad pathological etiologies and clinical manifestations characterize this diverse group of disorders. Important causes include syphilis (tabes dorsalis), leprosy, infectious neuritis (usually viral), and sarcoidosis. Immune-mediated noninfectious disorders include postviral or vaccination (Guillain-Barré syndrome), chronic immune demyelinating polyneuropathy, and idiopathic brachial plexitis (Parsonage-Turner syndrome).

Drug/Toxic Injury

Neural injuries have been linked to vinca alkaloids, therapeutic gold, amiodarone, dapsone, thalidomide, and lead or mercury intoxication.

Vascular Insult

Injury may result from either nerve ischemia related to peripheral vascular disease or vascular trauma or sequelae of vasculitis. The most common vasculitis etiologies are diabetes, Churg-Strauss, polyarteritis nodosa, and Wegener granulomatosis.

Selected References

1. Chhabra A et al: Peripheral nerve injury grading simplified on MR neurography: as referenced to Seddon and Sunderland classifications. Indian J Radiol Imaging. 24(3):217-24, 2014
2. Crush AB et al: Malignant involvement of the peripheral nervous system in patients with cancer: multimodality imaging and pathologic correlation. Radiographics. 34(7):1987-2007, 2014
3. Demehri S et al: Conventional and functional MR imaging of peripheral nerve sheath tumors: initial experience. AJNR Am J Neuroradiol. 35(8):1615-20, 2014
4. Pham M et al: Peripheral nerves and plexus: imaging by MR-neurography and high-resolution ultrasound. Curr Opin Neurol. 27(4):370-9, 2014
5. Sureka J et al: MRI of brachial plexopathies. Clin Radiol. 64(2):208-18, 2009
6. Bowen BC et al: Plexopathy. AJNR Am J Neuroradiol. 29(2):400-2, 2008
7. Hof JJ et al: What's new in MRI of peripheral nerve entrapment? Neurosurg Clin N Am. 19(4):583-95, vi, 2008
8. Kim S et al: Role of magnetic resonance imaging in entrapment and compressive neuropathy—what, where, and how to see the peripheral nerves on the musculoskeletal magnetic resonance image: part 2. Upper extremity. Eur Radiol. 17(2):509-22, 2007
9. Castillo M: Imaging the anatomy of the brachial plexus: review and self-assessment module. AJR Am J Roentgenol. 185(6 Suppl):S196-204, 2005

Brachial Plexus Major Nerves

Nerve	Definition	Motor/Sensory Innervation	Important Branches
Radial nerve	Terminal branch of posterior brachial plexus cord	Innervates extensor muscles of arm and forearm (triceps, brachioradialis, extensor forearm muscles)	Most important branch is posterior interosseous nerve
Median nerve	Terminal branch arises from both lateral and medial brachial plexus cords	Innervates flexor muscles of forearm and thumb as well as 1st and 2nd lumbricals	Most important branch is anterior interosseous nerve
Ulnar nerve	Terminal branch of medial brachial plexus cord	Innervates flexor carpi ulnaris, 3rd and 4th lumbricals, and majority of intrinsic hand muscles	
Musculocutaneous nerve	Terminal branch of lateral brachial plexus cord	Innervates flexor muscles of arm (coracobrachialis, biceps, and brachialis)	
Axillary nerve	Terminal branch of posterior brachial plexus cord	Innervates deltoid and teres minor muscles	

Lumbosacral Plexus Major Nerves

Nerve	Definition	Motor/Sensory Innervation
Obturator nerve	Terminal branch of lumbar plexus (anterior division)	Innervates thigh adductor muscles
Femoral nerve	Terminal branch of lumbar plexus (posterior division)	Innervates iliacus, psoas, and quadriceps muscles
Sciatic nerve	Largest peripheral nerve branch of sacral plexus	Innervates posterior thigh (biceps femoris, semitendinosus, semimembranosus, adductor magnus) and all leg muscles (via tibial and common peroneal nerve)
Common peroneal nerve	Major anterior terminal branch of sciatic nerve	Innervates anterior leg muscles; superficial peroneal nerve innervates peroneus muscles, extensor digitorum brevis; deep peroneal nerve innervates tibialis anterior, extensor digitorum longus, extensor hallucis longus muscles
Tibial nerve	Major posterior branch of sciatic nerve	Innervates posterior leg muscles (gastrocnemius, soleus, tibialis posterior, flexor digitorum longus, flexor hallucis longus)

High-Resolution MR Protocols

MR Pulse Sequence	Technical Parameters	Technical Comments
Coronal T1WI MR	3- to 4-mm slice thickness, 20- to 24-cm FOV, no interslice gap	Direct coronal plane, not oblique
Coronal fat-saturated T2WI or STIR MR	3- to 4-mm slice thickness, 20- to 24-cm FOV, no interslice gap	Direct coronal plane, not oblique
Direct axial or sagittal oblique T1WI MR	5- to 7-mm slice thickness, 16- to 20-cm FOV, no interslice gap	Sagittal oblique plane oriented perpendicular to plexus
Direct axial or sagittal oblique fat-saturated T2WI or STIR MR	5- to 7-mm slice thickness, 16- to 20-cm FOV, no interslice gap	Sagittal oblique plane oriented perpendicular to plexus
Coronal and axial fat-saturated T1WI C+ MR (optional)	Same planes as unenhanced imaging sequences	Use if suspected or confirmed mass or infection

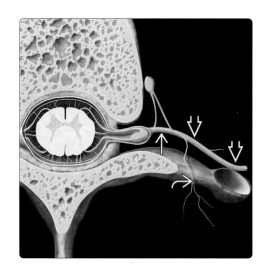

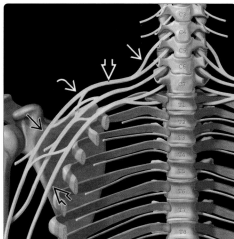

(Left) *Axial graphic of the thoracic spine shows formation of a typical spinal nerve from dorsal and ventral rootlets to form the spinal nerve proper ➡. The short spinal nerve bifurcates into large ventral ➡ and small dorsal primary rami ➡.* (Right) *Coronal graphic shows the classic anatomic classification of the 5 brachial plexus sections from proximal to distal: Roots ➡ (technically ventral primary rami) of C5-T1, trunks ➡, divisions ➡, cords ➡, and terminal major branches ➡ are shown.*

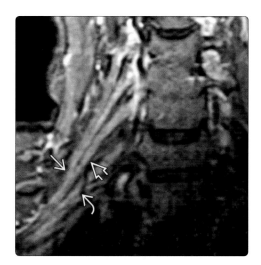

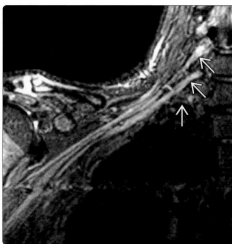

(Left) *Coronal STIR MR of the upper right brachial plexus depicts normal mildly hyperintense brachial plexus roots/rami of C5 to T1. C5 and C6 form the superior (upper) trunk ➡, C7 the middle trunk ➡, and C8 and T1 the inferior (lower) trunk ➡.* (Right) *Coronal STIR MR of the lower right brachial plexus demonstrates normal C7, C8, and T1 roots/rami ➡ sequentially forming trunks, divisions, and cords. The normal brachial plexus courses retroclavicular into the axilla.*

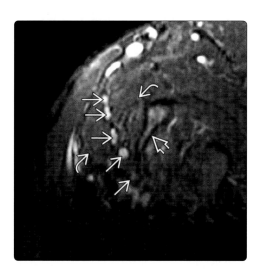

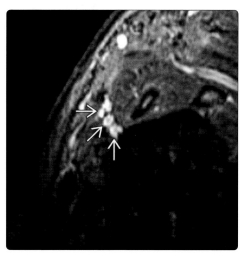

(Left) *Sagittal oblique STIR MR demonstrates the ventral primary rami ➡ of C5 through T1 proximal to the trunks. C8 exits above the 1st rib ➡, whereas T1 exits below. The brachial plexus is "sandwiched" between the anterior and middle scalene muscles ➡.* (Right) *Sagittal oblique STIR MR distal to the root level shows formation of the upper, middle, and lower trunks ➡ arranged in a vertical line between the scalene muscles.*

Peripheral Nerve and Plexus

TERMINOLOGY

- Synonym: Pancoast tumor
- Benign or malignant neoplasm extending to superior thoracic inlet with (1) severe shoulder/arm pain along C8, T1, T2 nerve trunks, (2) Horner syndrome, and (3) weakness + atrophy of intrinsic hand muscles (Pancoast syndrome)

IMAGING

- Soft tissue apical lung mass with variable extension into chest wall, adjacent bone destruction, brachial plexus invasion

TOP DIFFERENTIAL DIAGNOSES

- Metastatic disease
- Other thoracic tumors (besides non-small cell lung carcinoma)
- Brachial plexus neural tumors
- Hematologic neoplasms
- Radiation fibrosis

- Vascular (venolymphatic) malformation
- Infection

PATHOLOGY

- Bronchogenic carcinomas may arise from either upper lobe
- Invades parietal pleura, endothoracic fascia, subclavian vessels, brachial plexus, vertebral bodies, and upper ribs
- Non-small cell lung carcinoma most frequent etiology

CLINICAL ISSUES

- Clinical findings determined by tumor location relative to scalene muscles
- Severe shoulder and arm pain
- Pulmonary symptoms uncommon early in disease course

DIAGNOSTIC CHECKLIST

- Apical lung mass with bone destruction = bronchogenic carcinoma until proven otherwise
- Rare benign tumors or infection may mimic lung carcinoma

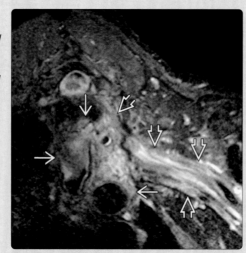
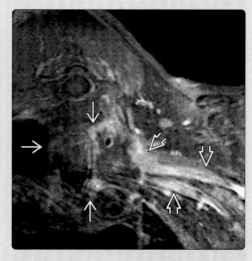

(Left) Coronal STIR MR of a patient with non-small cell lung carcinoma, arm pain, and weakness shows extensive architectural distortion of the lung apex by a peripheral lung mass ➡ with extension along the brachial plexus elements ➡. (Right) Coronal T1 C+ FS MR of the same patient demonstrates a heterogeneously enhancing apical lung neoplasm ➡ with tumor extension ➡ along the lower brachial plexus elements.

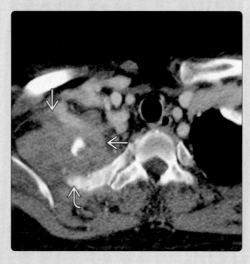
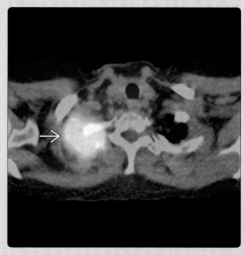

(Left) Axial CECT demonstrates a soft tissue mass ➡ involving the right upper lobe with extension beyond the chest wall, producing destruction of the right T1, T2 ribs ➡. (Right) Axial PET (FDG) CT fusion image reveals marked hypermetabolic radiotracer uptake within the right upper lobe bronchogenic carcinoma ➡.

Thoracic Outlet Syndrome

TERMINOLOGY

- Neural, venous, &/or arterial compressive syndrome at thoracic outlet
- Diagnosis made by 1 of 3 methods (by event, affected structure, or compression cause)

IMAGING

- ± cervical rib, elongated C7 transverse process
- ± brachial plexus compression/distortion, scalene muscle inflammation, abnormal vascular flow voids at thoracic outlet
- Positional occlusion or narrowing of subclavian artery with arm hyperabduction, external rotation

TOP DIFFERENTIAL DIAGNOSES

- Primary and secondary plexus tumors
- Radiation plexopathy
- Trauma

PATHOLOGY

- Cervical ribs, abnormal transverse processes, fibrous bands, scalene compression of thoracic outlet contents

CLINICAL ISSUES

- "True" neurological thoracic outlet syndrome: Intermittent arm pain, numbness, and weakness with hyperabduction, external rotation
  - Pain in shoulder, proximal upper extremity → neck
  - Paresthesias, numbness in forearm/hand
- Vascular thoracic outlet syndrome: Paresthesias 2° to arterial or venous ischemia
  - Obliteration of brachial, radial pulses with arm hyperabduction and elevation

DIAGNOSTIC CHECKLIST

- Subclavian artery aneurysm, subclavian vein thrombosis, or brachial plexus compression at thoracic outlet strongly suggest thoracic outlet syndrome

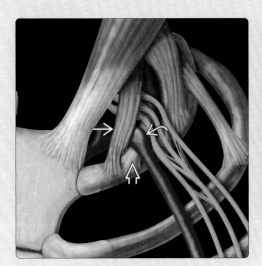
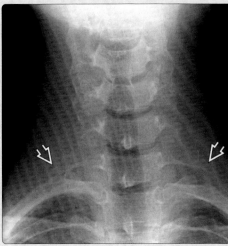
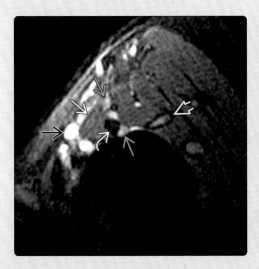
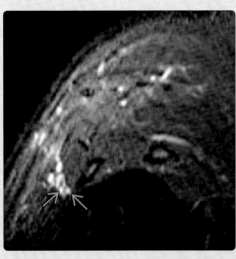

(Left) Coronal graphic of the thoracic outlet demonstrates brachial plexus compression + a subclavian artery aneurysm ➡ arising secondary to the C7 cervical rib ➡ and anterior scalene muscle ➡ compression. (Right) Anteroposterior radiograph demonstrates bilateral rudimentary C7 cervical ribs ➡. The right cervical rib articulates with the 1st thoracic rib.

(Left) Sagittal oblique STIR MR shows normal anatomy of the interscalene triangle: Brachial plexus trunks ➡, anterior ➡ and middle scalene muscles, subclavian artery ➡, subclavian vein ➡, and 1st thoracic rib ➡. (The anterior is to the left per radiologic convention.) (Right) Sagittal oblique STIR MR (in a professional drummer) through the thoracic outlet shows mild T2 hyperintensity of some fascicles within the lower trunk ➡, correlating with the clinical presentation with lower brachial plexopathy.

TERMINOLOGY

- Secondary muscle injury resulting from denervation following nerve injury

IMAGING

- **Acute denervation**
  - Muscle appears normal on T1WI
  - Diffusely increased signal intensity on T2WI, STIR
  - Mild, homogeneous enhancement with gadolinium
- **Chronic denervation**
  - Fatty atrophy evident on T1WI
  - Muscle volume decreased
  - Denervation edema often persists for prolonged period

TOP DIFFERENTIAL DIAGNOSES

- Disuse atrophy
- Muscle trauma
- Muscle inflammation or infection
- Radiation myopathy

PATHOLOGY

- Nerve tumor, infection, autoimmune neuritis, peripheral neuropathy or injury

CLINICAL ISSUES

- Weakness, muscle volume loss in distribution of injured nerve
  - May be painful
- Acute denervation may partially or totally recover depending on nerve injury severity
- Chronic denervation changes permanent

DIAGNOSTIC CHECKLIST

- Distribution of muscle signal abnormalities indicates location of nerve lesion
- Obtain fluid-sensitive sequence that shows muscle of concern in cross section

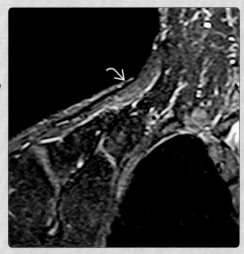

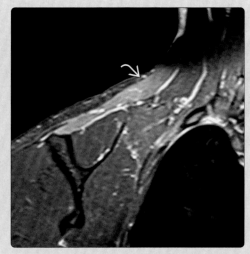

(Left) Coronal STIR MR shows denervation edema ➡ of the trapezius, which is innervated by the spinal accessory nerve. This nerve can be traumatized by carrying heavy loads on the shoulder. (Right) Coronal T1WI C+ FS MR in the same patient shows uniform enhancement ➡ of the affected muscle. Muscle tears, in contrast, have a heterogeneous appearance.

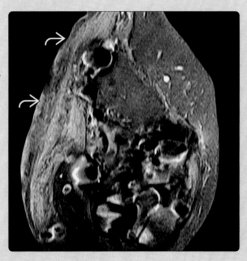

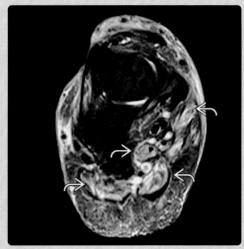

(Left) Axial T2WI FS MR shows a free muscle flap ➡ to the leg. The muscle shows severe, diffuse edema with a few streaks of fat interspersed. This is an expected finding and should not be confused with infection. (Right) Coronal T2WI FS MR shows denervation edema ➡ throughout the intrinsic muscles of the foot. Denervation edema due to diabetes primarily involves the feet. It tends to be streakier and less homogeneous than denervation from other causes.

Brachial Plexus Traction Injury

TERMINOLOGY

- Synonyms: Brachial plexus stretch injury, brachial plexus avulsion, avulsion pseudomeningocele
- Stretch injury or avulsion of ≥ 1 cervical roots, brachial plexus

IMAGING

- Stretch injury: Enlargement, abnormal edema of neural elements
- Avulsion: Abnormal CSF signal intensity within empty thecal diverticulum
- Obstetric brachial plexus palsy: C5-C6 roots (Erb-Duchenne palsy, 80%) > C8-T1 nerve roots (Klumpke palsy, 20%)

TOP DIFFERENTIAL DIAGNOSES

- Nerve sheath tumor
- Lateral meningocele
- Nerve root sleeve cyst

PATHOLOGY

- Adults: Majority posttraumatic injuries 2° to high-energy force
- Infants: 2° to excessive traction on plexus during difficult delivery (breech or forceps)

CLINICAL ISSUES

- Pain, paralysis of ipsilateral limb ± phrenic nerve palsy
- Complete brachial plexus avulsion produces useless "flail arm"
- Clinical incomplete paralysis possible with complete root avulsion(s) because of redundant muscle innervation from multiple roots

DIAGNOSTIC CHECKLIST

- Familiarity with normal brachial plexus anatomy essential for MR interpretation
- Muscle denervation pattern predicts abnormal nerves

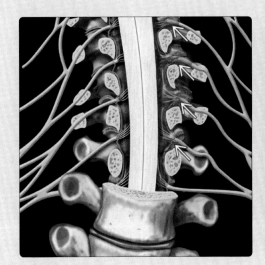

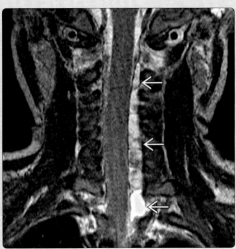

(Left) Coronal graphic demonstrates posttraumatic avulsion of left C5-C8 nerve roots ➡ producing local hemorrhage at the site of root injury and associated pseudomeningoceles. (Right) Coronal T2WI MR in a patient with posttraumatic paralyzed "flail arm" demonstrates an extensive extradural CSF signal intensity collection admixed with blood products ➡, representing CSF leakage following avulsion of multiple nerve roots, displacing the spinal cord to the right.

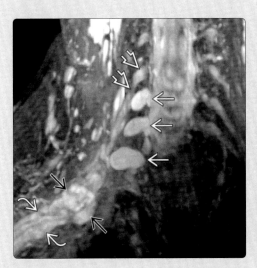

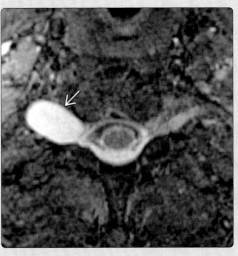

(Left) Coronal STIR MR in a patient with severe brachial plexus traction injury shows avulsion pseudomeningoceles of right C6, C7, and C8 roots ➡. The C5 root is attenuated with abnormally ↑ signal (incomplete stretch injury) ➡. The avulsed nerve roots have formed a "retraction ball" ➡, with abnormal enlargement and T2 hyperintensity of the distal (denervated) plexus ➡. (Right) Axial STIR MR confirms the CSF signal and lack of demonstrable neural elements within the right C7 pseudomeningocele ➡.

Idiopathic Brachial Plexus Neuritis

TERMINOLOGY

- Parsonage-Turner syndrome

IMAGING

- Can affect any muscle innervated by brachial plexus
  - Most common: Rotator cuff, deltoid, biceps, triceps
- Denervation edema is earliest finding
  - Diffuse, homogeneous high signal on T2WI, STIR throughout affected muscle
- Fatty atrophy occurs in chronic denervation
  - Uncommonly seen
- Often muscles innervated by 2 or more different peripheral nerves are affected

TOP DIFFERENTIAL DIAGNOSES

- Cervical radiculopathy
- Suprascapular nerve entrapment
- Brachial plexus neoplasm
- Brachial plexus or cervical nerve root avulsion
- Radiation neuritis/myositis
- Quadrilateral space syndrome
- Pancoast tumor
- Muscle injury

PATHOLOGY

- Often associated with viral or bacterial infection
- Can also be posttraumatic or postsurgery occurrence

CLINICAL ISSUES

- Sudden onset of pain, followed by weakness, paresthesias
- M > F
- Most cases resolve in 3 months to 2 years
- Physical therapy to preserve range of motion

DIAGNOSTIC CHECKLIST

- Often unexpected finding on shoulder MR performed to evaluate weakness, pain
- Abnormal muscle signal often involves > 1 peripheral nerve distribution

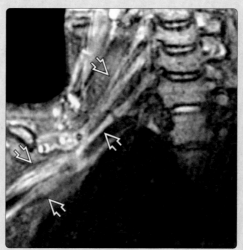
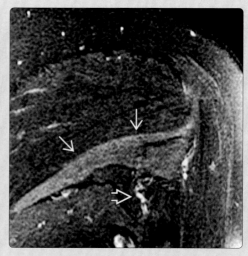

(Left) Coronal STIR MR shows diffusely increased signal intensity in brachial plexus ➡ due to idiopathic brachial neuritis. (Right) Coronal oblique T2WI MR shows denervation edema of the teres minor ➡ due to brachial neuritis. Edema is homogeneous and uniform, and there is no disruption of muscle fibers. Quadrilateral space ➡ shows no evidence of the mass involving axillary nerve. Whenever denervation edema is seen, a search should be made for nerve mass or extrinsic compression.

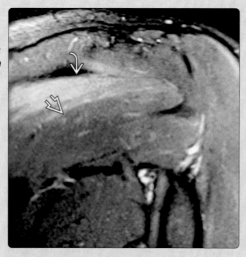
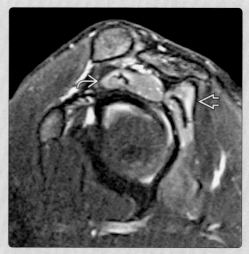

(Left) Coronal oblique T2WI MR shows diffuse increase in signal intensity throughout superior fibers of infraspinatus muscle ➡. The inferior portion of the muscle ➡ is spared. Unusual distributions of denervation edema are common in brachial neuritis. (Right) Sagittal T2WI MR shows diffusely abnormal signal intensity in the infraspinatus ➡ and supraspinatus muscles ➡. Differential diagnosis in this case includes suprascapular nerve entrapment.

Traumatic Neuroma

TERMINOLOGY

- Amputation neuroma (stump neuroma)
  - Subtype of traumatic neuroma following traumatic or surgical amputation
- Morton neuroma: Traumatic neuroma between metatarsal heads

IMAGING

- Bulbous enlargement of nerve
- Enlargement of nerve fascicles
- Normal signal intensity on T1WI
- Intermediate to high signal intensity on T2WI, STIR
- Avid enhancement after gadolinium enhancement
- Any site of nerve injury or surgery

TOP DIFFERENTIAL DIAGNOSES

- Benign or malignant peripheral nerve tumor
- Perineural cyst
  - Eccentric to nerve, no enhancement

- Ganglion cyst
  - Associated with tendon, no enhancement
- Soft tissue metastasis or recurrent malignancy
- Neuritis

PATHOLOGY

- Secondary to nerve injury: Amputation, crush injury, deep burns, minor trauma, nerve compression
- All elements of nerve present in neuroma in addition to scar tissue

CLINICAL ISSUES

- Severe pain or paresthesias
- Arises 1-12 months after nerve injury
- As many as 1/4 of amputees develop stump neuroma

DIAGNOSTIC CHECKLIST

- May be mistaken for recurrent sarcoma

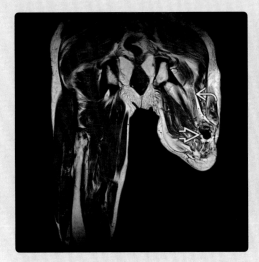

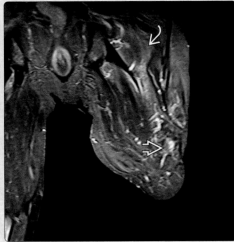

(Left) Coronal T1WI MR in a patient status post above-knee amputation for trauma shows the sciatic nerve ➡ terminating in a large stump neuroma ⇉. (Right) Coronal STIR MR in the same patient nicely demonstrates the stump neuroma ⇉. The normal sciatic nerve ➡ is much less visible than on T1WI, as it blends with fat. T1W images are best for locating normal nerves, since the nerves' low signal intensity is conspicuous against the adjacent high signal intensity fat.

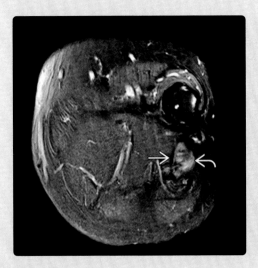

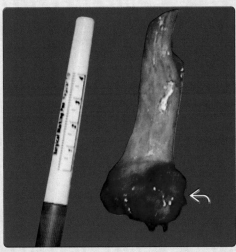

(Left) Axial T1WI C+ FS MR in the same patient shows marked enlargement of the abnormal sciatic nerve at the neuroma site. The separate tibial ➡ and peroneal ➡ nerves are distinctly seen. (Right) Surgical photograph of a resected stump neuroma illustrates bulbous enlargement of a nerve stump tip ➡ gradually tapering proximally into normal nerve.

KEY FACTS

TERMINOLOGY

- Synonyms: Radiation-induced plexitis, radiation-induced fibrosis

IMAGING

- Smooth, diffuse T2 hyperintensity ± enhancement of multiple plexus elements
- Upper brachial plexus (BP) (C5-C7) > lower BP (C8, T1) following radiation therapy (XRT) for breast and lung cancer, lymphoma
- Lumbosacral plexus following XRT for prostate, colorectal, and gynecologic tumors and lymphoma

TOP DIFFERENTIAL DIAGNOSES

- Malignant brachial plexus infiltration
- Plexiform neurofibroma
- Plexus traction injury

PATHOLOGY

- Direct cell damage 2° to ionizing radiation and radiation-induced vascular damage to vaso nervosum
- Modified LENT-SOMA scale (brachial plexopathy)
  - Grade 1: Mild sensory deficits, no pain
  - Grade 2: Moderate sensory deficits, tolerable pain, mild arm weakness
  - Grade 3: Continuous paresthesia with incomplete paresis
  - Grade 4: Complete paresis, severe pain, muscle atrophy

CLINICAL ISSUES

- Pain, paresthesia, motor deficits of ipsilateral extremity
- Prognosis variable; related to dose delivered to plexus, severity of nerve injury

DIAGNOSTIC CHECKLIST

- Correctly diagnosis to avoid inappropriate additional radiation therapy

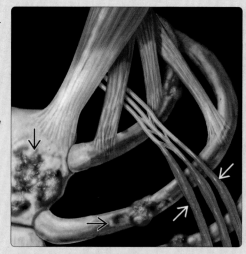
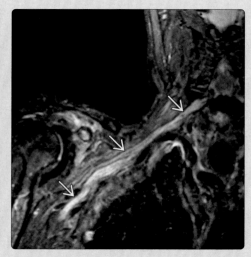

(Left) Coronal graphic of the left brachial plexus in a breast cancer patient with skeletal metastases ⇨ following radiation therapy demonstrates diffuse swelling of irradiated brachial plexus elements ➜. Segmental involvement of all neural elements in the radiation field is characteristic of radiation plexopathy. (Right) Coronal STIR MR (3 years post radiation for breast cancer with vague arm symptoms) shows diffuse, smooth, abnormal brachial plexus T2 hyperintensity ➜. No nodal mass was evident.

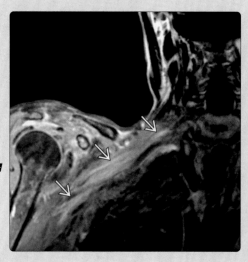
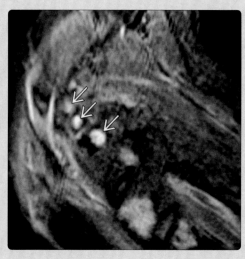

(Left) Coronal T1WI C+ FS MR (3 years post radiation for breast cancer with vague arm symptoms) reveals only mild patchy plexus enhancement ➜. No nodular mass lesion or enhancement was present, a finding that would imply neoplastic infiltration. (Right) Sagittal oblique STIR MR shows that abnormal T2 hyperintensity in the upper plexus ventral primary rami ➜ preserves fascicular architecture. Plexus nodal tumor invasion more commonly involves the lower plexus because of axillary nodal location.

TERMINOLOGY

- Grouping of benign and malignant primary tumors of peripheral nerves

IMAGING

- Mass associated with peripheral nerve
  - Schwannoma: Round mass, eccentric to nerve
  - Neurofibroma: Fusiform, cord-like, or lobulated mass centered on nerve
  - Plexiform neurofibroma: Arborizing tangle of lobular masses
  - Malignant peripheral nerve sheath tumor: Round, ovoid, fusiform, or lobulated
- Low signal intensity on T1WI, PDWI
- Intermediate to high signal intensity on T2WI, STIR
- Avid enhancement with gadolinium
- Muscles innervated by nerve often show denervation changes

TOP DIFFERENTIAL DIAGNOSES

- Traumatic neuroma
- Hemangioma
- Neuritis
- Other soft tissue sarcomas
- Metastases, soft tissue
- Lymphoma

PATHOLOGY

- Malignant degeneration seen in neurofibroma but rare in schwannoma

CLINICAL ISSUES

- Palpable mass, often painful
- May cause weakness in distribution of affected nerve

DIAGNOSTIC CHECKLIST

- Imaging cannot reliably distinguish between benign and malignant nerve sheath tumors

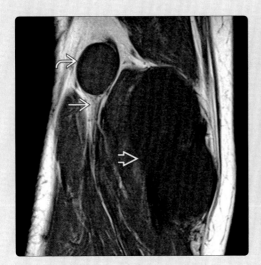
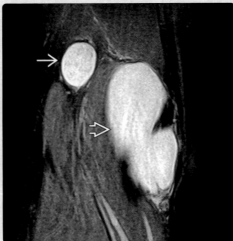

(Left) Coronal T1WI MR demonstrates a large mass ➡ arising from the peroneal nerve ➡. The mass has the same signal intensity as the adjacent popliteal cyst ➡. (Right) Coronal PD FSE FS MR in the same patient confirms that both the tumor ➡ and fluid ➡ have a similar degree of minimal signal heterogeneity. It can be challenging to discern these tumors from cysts even with MR.

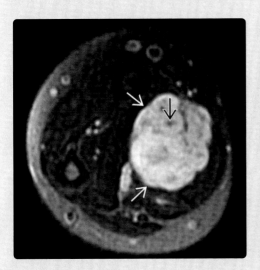
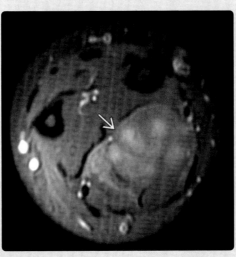

(Left) Axial T2 FS MR reveals marked T2 hyperintensity characteristic of neural sheath tumor in a large median nerve mass ➡. Note the characteristic target appearance ➡ of plexiform neurofibroma. (Right) Axial T1 C+ FS MR confirms the typical heterogeneous, relatively understated enhancement (compared to schwannoma) within the large median nerve plexiform neurofibroma ➡.

Peripheral Neurolymphomatosis

TERMINOLOGY

- Synonyms: Peripheral neurolymphomatosis (NL), perineural lymphomatosis
- Perineural plexus or peripheral nerve lymphomatous infiltration

IMAGING

- Diffusely infiltrating plexus or peripheral nerve lesion in patient with lymphoma
  - Abnormal nerve T2 hyperintensity
  - Disruption/distortion of normal neural fascicular morphology
  - Variable enhancement

TOP DIFFERENTIAL DIAGNOSES

- Peripheral nerve metastasis
- Chronic inflammatory demyelinating polyneuropathy
- Hypertrophic neuropathy
- Nerve/plexus stretch injury

PATHOLOGY

- Perineural lymphomatous nerve infiltration produces thickened neural elements

CLINICAL ISSUES

- Pain ± motor weakness, sensory deficit
- Progressive sensorimotor neuropathy ± plexopathy
- Relentlessly progressive; variable response to chemotherapy, radiotherapy

DIAGNOSTIC CHECKLIST

- Careful evaluation of NL patients often reveals evidence for subclinical systemic lymphoma
- Imaging findings are often subtle
  - Carefully scrutinize clinically abnormal nerves and plexi for thickening, abnormal T2 signal
  - High index of suspicion important for recognition

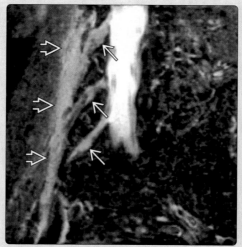

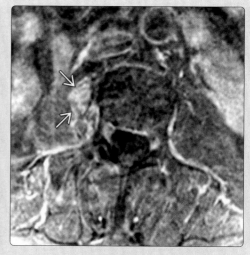

(Left) Coronal STIR MR in a patient with stage IV thoracic lymphoma, progressive leg atrophy, and pain demonstrates abnormal L2-L4 nerve root and dorsal root ganglia ➡ hyperintensity and enlargement. Also present is concomitant abnormal thickening and T2 hyperintensity of the right lumbar plexus ➡. (Right) Axial T1WI C+ MR in the same patient reveals abnormal thickening and avid enhancement of the infiltrated right lumbar plexus ➡.

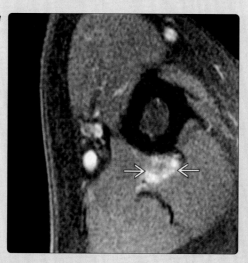

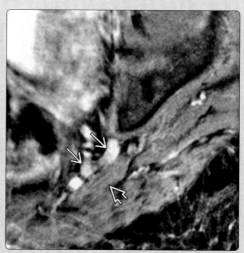

(Left) Axial T1WI C+ FS MR in a patient with non-Hodgkin lymphoma, systemic metastases with progressive arm pain, and weakness demonstrates an ill-defined, enhancing infiltrative mass ➡ centered within the left radial nerve neurovascular bundle near the humeral spiral groove. (Right) Sagittal oblique T1WI C+ FS MR in a patient with known lymphoma and progressive left sciatic neuropathy demonstrates abnormal left sciatic nerve enlargement and avid enhancement ➡ at the piriformis muscle ➡ level.

Hypertrophic Neuropathy

KEY FACTS

TERMINOLOGY

- Clinically and genetically heterogeneous group of inherited disorders with focal or diffuse peripheral nerve enlargement
- Hereditary motor-sensory neuropathy (HMSN)
  - HMSN I (Charcot-Marie-Tooth syndrome type I, CMT1)
  - HMSN II (neuronal-type peroneal muscular atrophy, CMT2)
  - HMSN III (Dejerine-Sottas disease, hypertrophic neuropathy of infancy, congenital hypomyelinating neuropathy)

IMAGING

- Focal or diffuse fusiform peripheral nerve enlargement
  - Peripheral nerves ± intradural nerve roots
- Acute &/or chronic muscle denervation changes
- Best imaging tool: High-resolution MR neurography

TOP DIFFERENTIAL DIAGNOSES

- Guillain-Barré syndrome
- Chronic inflammatory demyelinating polyneuropathy
- Nerve sheath tumor

PATHOLOGY

- Hypertrophic nerve roots, peripheral nerves
- Histologic shows demyelination, remyelination + "onion bulb" formations (HMSN I)

CLINICAL ISSUES

- Distal extremity muscle weakness/atrophy (motor > sensory), foot deformities
- Back/lower extremity radicular pain ± myelopathy
- Sensory loss, focal tenderness, dysesthesias

DIAGNOSTIC CHECKLIST

- Consider HMSN when abnormally enlarged peripheral nerves identified on MR

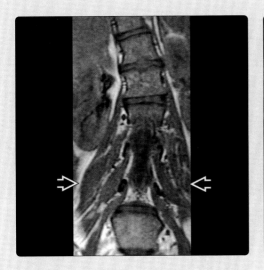
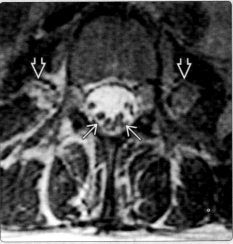

(Left) Coronal T1WI MR in a patient with Charcot-Marie-Tooth and painful scoliosis demonstrates convex left scoliosis and bilateral abnormal fusiform enlargement of the extradural spinal nerve roots and lumbar plexus ➡. (Right) Axial T2WI MR in the same patient confirms abnormal enlargement and T2 hyperintensity of the bilateral extradural lumbar nerve roots ➡ as well as aberrant enlargement of the intradural cauda equina nerve roots ➡.

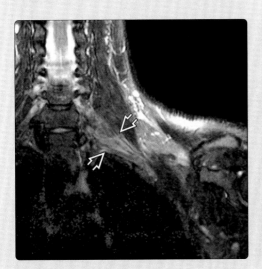
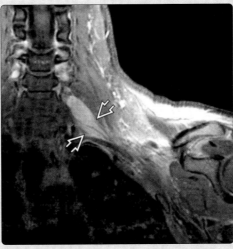

(Left) Coronal STIR MR (unknown type, hypertrophic neuropathy, left arm pain and weakness) demonstrates abnormal fusiform enlargement of the left proximal brachial plexus C7 and C8 roots/rami ➡. (Right) Coronal T1WI C+ FS MR in the same patient of the left brachial plexus confirms fusiform enlargement and diffuse homogeneous nerve enhancement within the left proximal brachial plexus C7 and C8 roots/rami ➡.

TERMINOLOGY

- Synonyms: Femoral neuropathy, femoral mononeuropathy, femoral nerve (FN) palsy
- FN entrapment or injury 2° to direct trauma, compression, stretch injury, or ischemia

IMAGING

- Nerve enlargement ± loss of internal fascicular architecture, ↑ T2 hyperintensity
- Injury most common in psoas muscle body, iliopsoas groove, or femoral canal

TOP DIFFERENTIAL DIAGNOSES

- Neoplastic FN infiltration
- Nerve sheath tumor
- Lumbosacral disc syndromes
- Lumbar plexopathy

PATHOLOGY

- Reported causes include self-retaining retractor, thigh tourniquet, traumatic injury, heparin anticoagulation (retroperitoneal hematoma), arterial catheterization complication, obstetrical complication, diabetic neuropathy

CLINICAL ISSUES

- Acute symptom onset, pain/weakness in FN distribution, diminished/absent knee jerk reflex, thigh muscle atrophy
- Severe back/groin pain (retroperitoneal hematoma)
- Recovery is rule over days → months

DIAGNOSTIC CHECKLIST

- Femoral neuropathy is uncommon
- Look carefully for lesion or hematoma in iliopsoas groove or femoral canal

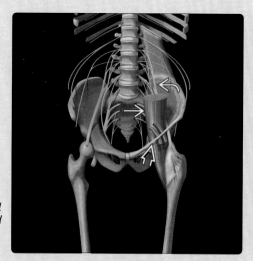
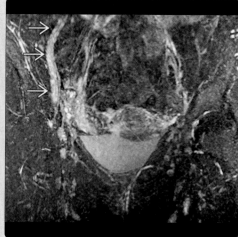

(Left) Coronal graphic shows the normal course of the femoral nerve ➡ relative to the psoas muscle ➡ and inguinal ligament ➡. The femoral nerve produces multiple peripheral branches to the anterior thigh muscles. (Right) Coronal STIR MR (femoral neuropathy postsurgical herniorrhaphy) depicts marked enlargement and T2 hyperintensity of the right femoral nerve ➡, with abrupt transition at the right groin. In this case, the femoral nerve was accidentally ligated during herniorrhaphy.

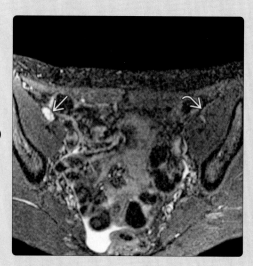
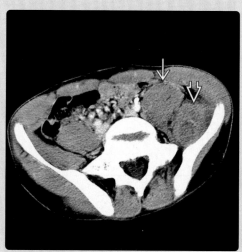

(Left) Axial STIR MR (femoral neuropathy postsurgical herniorrhaphy) through the pelvis confirms that the right femoral nerve ➡ in the iliopsoas groove is markedly enlarged with discrete T2 hyperintense fascicles (compared with the normal left femoral nerve ➡). (Right) Axial CECT (severe hemophilia) depicts large left iliacus ➡ and psoas ➡ hematomas. Femoral neuropathy occurs from compression of the adjacent femoral nerve, which runs along the psoas muscle and iliopsoas groove.

Ulnar Neuropathy

TERMINOLOGY

- Synonyms: Ulnar nerve (UN) entrapment, cubital tunnel syndrome
- Partial fixation, compression, or distortion of UN

IMAGING

- UN enlargement ± abnormal T2 hyperintensity, architectural distortion
- Most commonly occurs within cubital tunnel (elbow); uncommon at Guyon tunnel (wrist) or brachial plexus

TOP DIFFERENTIAL DIAGNOSES

- Acute direct nerve trauma
- Idiopathic brachial plexitis (Parsonage-Turner syndrome)
- Nerve sheath tumor
- Enlarged perineural vein
- Medial epicondylitis

PATHOLOGY

- Edematous/indurated UN ± thickened retinaculum, fibrous infiltration, fascicular atrophy/loss
- ± anconeus epitrochlearis, enlarged medial triceps head

CLINICAL ISSUES

- Symptoms range from mild transient paresthesias of 4th and 5th digits → claw hand/digits, intrinsic muscle atrophy
- ± severe elbow/wrist pain radiating proximally or distally

DIAGNOSTIC CHECKLIST

- Focal nerve enlargement, abnormal T2 hyperintensity distal to medial epicondyle
- Search for anatomic abnormalities (enlarged triceps medial head or anconeus muscle, osteophyte, thickened retinaculum)
- Electromyography: Helps localize most likely level of nerve injury

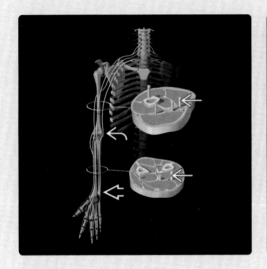

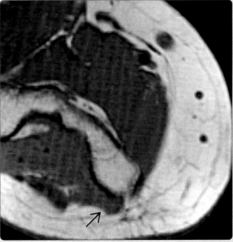

(Left) Coronal graphic of the right upper extremity demonstrates the normal course of the ulnar nerve ➡ (yellow). Vulnerable locations to injury include the cubital tunnel ➡ at the medial elbow and Guyon canal ➡ at the medial wrist. (Right) Axial T1WI MR of the right elbow demonstrates mild abnormal enlargement and rounded configuration of the right ulnar nerve ➡ within the cubital tunnel.

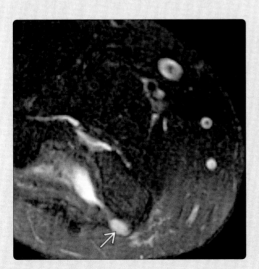

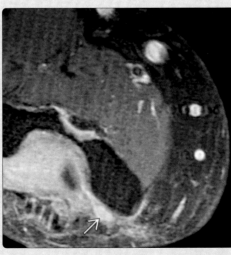

(Left) Axial T2WI FS MR of the right elbow demonstrates mild enlargement and abnormal T2 hyperintensity of the right ulnar nerve ➡ with complete loss of internal fascicular architecture, indicating an axonotmetic or neurotmetic injury rather than the less severe neuropraxic injury. (Right) Axial T1WI C+ FS MR of the right elbow confirms diffuse abnormal enhancement of the mildly enlarged right ulnar nerve ➡. Note also mild edema and inflammation in the adjacent soft tissues.

KEY FACTS

TERMINOLOGY

- Suprascapular nerve impingement with muscle denervation

IMAGING

- Suprascapular nerve impingement may occur at either spinoglenoid or suprascapular notch
- Spinoglenoid notch: Between neck and blade of scapula, roofed by spinoglenoid ligament
  - Entrapment affects infraspinatus muscle only
- Suprascapular notch: At superior border of scapula, roofed by superior transverse ligament
  - Entrapment affects both supraspinatus and infraspinatus muscles
- Denervation edema is 1st sign on MR
  - Uniformly increased signal intensity of muscle
- Fatty atrophy occurs later

TOP DIFFERENTIAL DIAGNOSES

- Cervical radiculopathy

- Parsonage-Turner syndrome (brachial neuritis)
- Rotator cuff tear
- Traction neuropathy
- Neural tumor

PATHOLOGY

- Paralabral cyst due to tear of posterosuperior glenoid labrum
- Mass or venous varicosities compressing nerve
- Posttraumatic scar or heterotopic ossification

CLINICAL ISSUES

- Young or middle-aged patients, M > F
- Overhead throwing athletes

DIAGNOSTIC CHECKLIST

- Denervation edema best seen on sagittal fluid-sensitive sequences

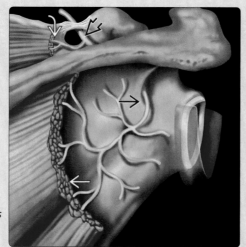
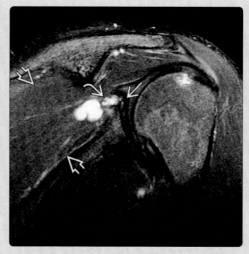

(Left) Coronal graphic shows a suprascapular nerve coursing through the suprascapular notch ➡, after which it gives rise to motor branch to supraspinatus muscle ➡. The nerve then passes through the spinoglenoid notch ➡ and innervates the infraspinatus muscle ➡. (Right) Coronal T2WI FS MR shows an elongated, multilocular cyst ➡ extending from a posterosuperior glenoid labral tear ➡ through the spinoglenoid notch. The infraspinatus muscle ➡ shows a mild, homogeneous increase in signal intensity.

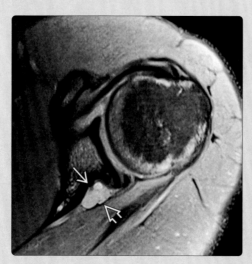
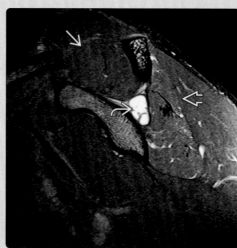

(Left) Axial PD FSE FS MR in the same patient shows the cyst ➡ at the level of the spinoglenoid notch ➡. Denervation edema is less visible on this sequence than on T2 FS or STIR. (Right) Sagittal T2WI FS MR in the same patient shows the cyst ➡ at the spinoglenoid notch. The sagittal image most readily shows the abnormal signal intensity of the infraspinatus ➡ relative to the supraspinatus ➡ muscle.

Median Neuropathy

TERMINOLOGY

- Pronator syndrome: Nerve entrapment at pronator teres
- Carpal tunnel syndrome: Nerve entrapment at carpal tunnel

IMAGING

- Nerve enlargement distal to region of entrapment
  - Fascicles indistinct
- Perineural enhancement
- ± mass compressing nerve
- Denervation changes in muscles distal to entrapment

TOP DIFFERENTIAL DIAGNOSES

- Cervical radiculopathy
- Tenosynovitis
- Peripheral nerve sheath tumor
- Thoracic outlet syndrome

PATHOLOGY

- Overuse
- Arthritis
- Tumors
- Fractures
- Anatomic variants

CLINICAL ISSUES

- Tinel sign: Tingling along course of nerve when nerve tapped at point of entrapment
- Electrodiagnosis standard for diagnosis

DIAGNOSTIC CHECKLIST

- Imaging diagnosis challenging
  - Nerve normally high signal intensity (in carpal tunnel) on FSE T2WI
  - Nerve normally flattened at level of hook of hamate
- Diagnosis usually made on EMG, not MR

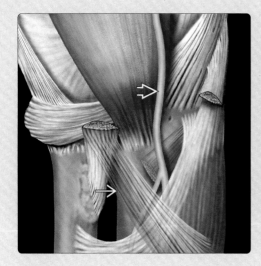

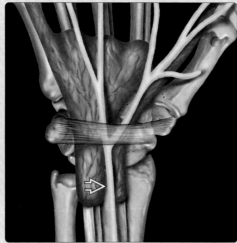

(Left) Graphic of the anterior elbow shows the median nerve ⇨ passing anterior to the brachialis muscle. It extends between the heads of the pronator teres and beneath the biceps aponeurosis ⇨. Entrapment of the nerve in this region is rare compared to carpal tunnel syndrome. It usually presents with numbness with repeated pronation/supination of the forearm. (Right) Coronal graphic of carpal tunnel shows the median nerve ⇨ at the ventral margin of the carpal tunnel, superficial to the flexor tendons.

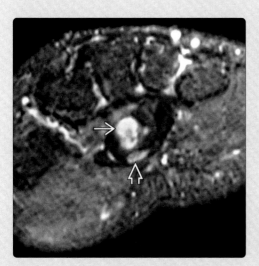

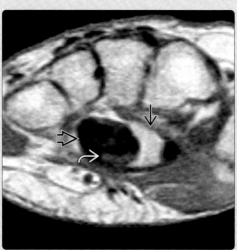

(Left) Axial T2 FS MR performed at the wrist demonstrates a ganglion cyst ⇨ in the carpal tunnel, exerting mass effect on the median nerve ⇨. (Right) Axial T1WI MR reveals a lipoma ⇨ within the carpal tunnel. The flexor tendons ⇨ are displaced ulnarly, and the median nerve ⇨ is compressed.

TERMINOLOGY

- Synonyms: Common peroneal nerve (CPN) palsy, CPN entrapment
- Common peroneal nerve entrapment at fibular head

IMAGING

- CPN swelling, abnormal T2 hyperintensity
  - Fascicular architecture preserved in milder cases (neuropraxic injury)
  - Loss of internal fascicular architecture in more severe cases (axonotmetic, neurotmetic)
- EMG: Anterior compartment (tibial anterior, peroneus longus muscles) muscle denervation
- Nerve conduction velocity: Conduction block at fibular head

TOP DIFFERENTIAL DIAGNOSES

- Ganglion cyst
- Viral neuritis
- Nerve sheath tumor

- Direct acute CPN trauma

PATHOLOGY

- Usual etiology is entrapment or sequelae of continued pressure on CPN at fibular head level
- Edematous/indurated CPN ± thickened "fibular tunnel" at surgery

CLINICAL ISSUES

- Foot drop, sensory abnormality along anterolateral leg
- Prognosis variable; frequently good recovery following conservative management
- Surgical decompression reserved for recalcitrant cases

DIAGNOSTIC CHECKLIST

- Focal CPN enlargement, abnormal T2 hyperintensity at fibular head suggests CPN neuropathy
- MR more sensitive for detecting acute than chronic nerve injuries

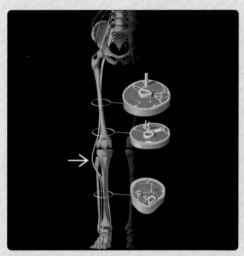
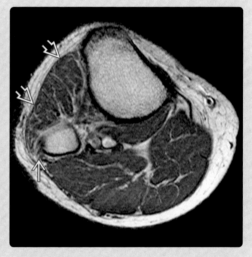

(Left) Coronal graphic depicts the normal course of the common peroneal nerve (CPN) originating from the sciatic nerve, around the fibular head, into the leg. Note the vulnerable position of the CPN as it courses around the fibular head ⟹. (Right) Axial T1WI MR demonstrates atrophy and fatty infiltration of the right anterolateral compartment muscles ⟹ innervated by the CPN. Mild fascicular enlargement within the right CPN ⟹ is not as conspicuous on T1WI as it is on T2WI FS MR or STIR MR.

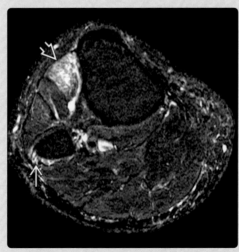
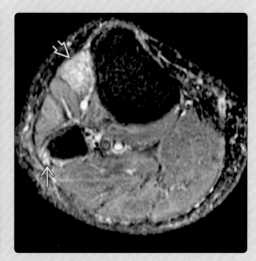

(Left) Axial T2WI FS MR reveals abnormal T2 hyperintensity in some of the anterolateral compartment muscles ⟹, confirming ongoing denervation superimposed on chronic denervation. The right CPN ⟹ is mildly enlarged, with swollen, hyperintense fascicles. (Right) Axial STIR MR confirms abnormal T2 hyperintensity in some anterolateral compartment muscles ⟹. The CPN ⟹ shows mild enlargement and abnormal T2 signal intensity with preservation of intrinsic fascicular architecture.

Tibial Neuropathy

KEY FACTS

TERMINOLOGY

- Tarsal tunnel syndrome

IMAGING

- Denervation of affected plantar intrinsic muscles
  - Uniform high signal intensity on fluid-sensitive sequences
- Mass in tarsal tunnel
  - Ganglion cyst: Follows fluid signal intensity, homogeneous, ± thin rim of enhancement with gadolinium
  - Nerve sheath tumor: Round or ovoid shape, often shows tail where it arises from nerve, diffuse enhancement
  - Venous varicosities: Serpentine, enlarged vessels in tarsal tunnel, can be followed beyond tunnel
- Scar: Amorphous material around tibial nerve
- Osseous impingement: Fracture malunion, subtalar coalition

TOP DIFFERENTIAL DIAGNOSES

- Radiculopathy
- Diabetic neuropathy
- Calcaneal stress fracture
- Isolated fatty atrophy of plantar muscles

PATHOLOGY

- Up to 50% of cases are idiopathic

CLINICAL ISSUES

- Burning, tingling pain, numbness at plantar aspect of foot

DIAGNOSTIC CHECKLIST

- Fatty atrophy of plantar intrinsic muscles can be incidental finding, increasing with age
- Intramuscular edema is most reliable sign of muscle denervation

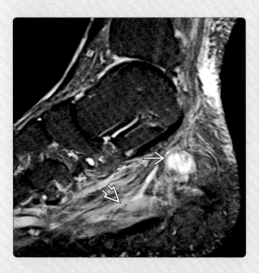

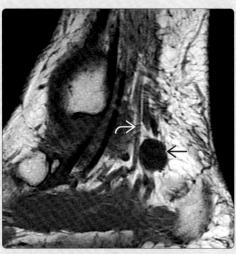

(Left) Graphic shows that the inferior flexor retinaculum ➔ forms a superficial border of the tarsal tunnel and the floor is composed of the talus & calcaneus. The tibial nerve is vulnerable to compression from behind the medial malleolus to the midfoot. The lateral calcaneal nerve ➔ arises in the proximal tarsal tunnel. The tibial nerve divides into the medial ➔ and lateral ➔ plantar nerves. (Right) Sagittal T1WI MR shows a mass ➔ in the tarsal tunnel. The mass has a small tail ➔, characteristic of nerve sheath tumors.

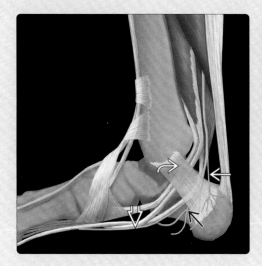

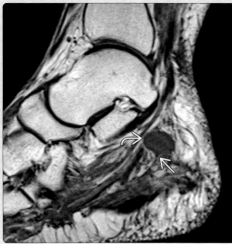

(Left) Sagittal STIR MR in the same patient shows that the mass ➔ is heterogeneously high in signal intensity. The degree of heterogeneity is greater than expected for a synovial cyst. There is denervation edema in the abductor hallucis muscle ➔. (Right) Sagittal T1WI MR shows a lobular ganglion cyst ➔ in the tarsal tunnel adjacent to the posterior tibial vein ➔. (This patient presented with tibial neuropathy.)

SECTION 14
Image-Guided Procedures

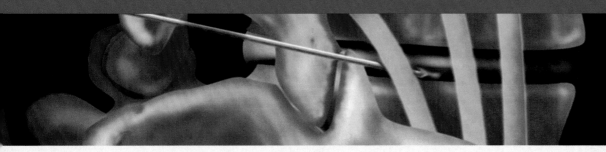

Medial Branch Block, Cervical Spine

KEY FACTS

TERMINOLOGY

- Selective anesthesia of cervical nerve medial branch in diagnosis of cervical facet joint pain

PREPROCEDURE

- Facet joint pain
  - Useful in selecting patients for medial branch radiofrequency ablation procedure
  - Need to block level above and below facet joint for effective anesthesia

PROCEDURE

- Preferred patient position: Supine
- Preferred imaging plane: True lateral view
- C2/3: 3rd occipital nerve block
  - Target: Immediately above and below C2/3 facet joint
- C3/4-C6/7 MBB
  - Target: Midportion of articular pillar above and below facet joint

- C8 MBB
  - Target: Junction of superior articular process and T1 transverse process

POST PROCEDURE

- Document pain before, during, and after injection
  - < 100% pain relief decreases likelihood of successful rhizotomy
- If corticosteroid injected, maximal benefit will be in 48-72 hours

OUTCOMES

- Possible problem: Failure of pain relief
- Complications
  - Stroke
  - Dural puncture: Spinal cord injury, CSF leak
  - Ataxia (upper cervical injections, particularly C2/3)
  - Phrenic nerve blockade (C3/4, C4/5, C5/6)

Radiographic Target

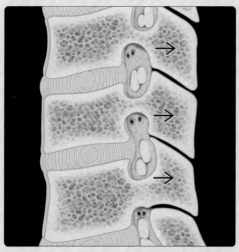

Needle Position

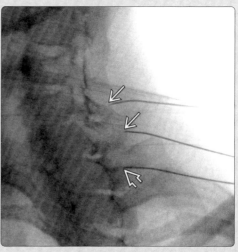

(Left) *Parasagittal graphic shows the radiographic target for a C3-C7 medial branch block at the midportion of the articular pillar* ⟹ *above and below the facet joint. A direct lateral approach or posterolateral approach can be utilized.* (Right) *Oblique fluoroscopic image shows the needle tip against the cortex at the midpoint of the articular pillar* ⟹ *for C6 and C7 medial branch block (MBB) vs. at the junction of the T1 superior articular process and transverse process* ⟹ *for C8 MBB.*

Needle Placement: PA View

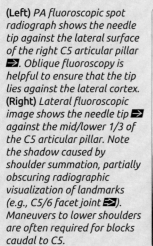

Shoulder Summation Artifact

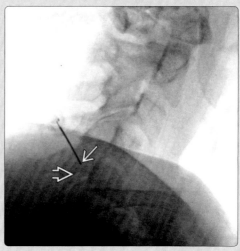

(Left) *PA fluoroscopic spot radiograph shows the needle tip against the lateral surface of the right C5 articular pillar* ⟹. *Oblique fluoroscopy is helpful to ensure that the tip lies against the lateral cortex.* (Right) *Lateral fluoroscopic image shows the needle tip* ⟹ *against the mid/lower 1/3 of the C5 articular pillar. Note the shadow caused by shoulder summation, partially obscuring radiographic visualization of landmarks (e.g., C5/6 facet joint* ⟹). *Maneuvers to lower shoulders are often required for blocks caudal to C5.*

TERMINOLOGY

Abbreviations

- Medial branch block (MBB)

Definitions

- Selective anesthesia of cervical nerve medial branch(es) in diagnosis of cervical facet joint pain

PREPROCEDURE

Indications

- Chronic cervical pain
  - Referable to facet joints
  - Not referable to cervical nerve root dermatome
  - Useful in selecting patients for medial branch radiofrequency ablation procedure

Contraindications

- Severe allergy to injectate component(s)
- Coagulopathy
  - Patients undergoing anticoagulation or antiplatelet therapy

Getting Started

- Things to check
  - Correct level(s)
    - Effective block requires injection of levels above and below facet joint
      - E.g., C3/4 facet joint requires block of both C3 and C4 medial branches
  - Laboratory data
    - Assess coagulation parameters as indicated
- Medications
  - ± corticosteroid
    - Used for therapeutic block
  - Long-acting anesthetic
    - Combined with corticosteroid for therapeutic block
  - Short-acting anesthetic
    - Local anesthesia
  - Myelography-safe contrast

PROCEDURE

Patient Position/Location

- Best procedure approach
  - Supine
    - True lateral fluoroscopic view
    - For lower cervical levels, shoulders may obscure view
  - Some prefer lateral decubitus view
    - Side to be injected is up

Procedure Steps

- Perform preprocedure "time-out"
  - Verify correct patient
  - Correct side to be injected
  - Correct procedure
  - All necessary equipment is available
- Conscious sedation as indicated
- Carefully determine correct level(s) and mark skin
  - C2/3: 3rd occipital nerve block

- Radiographic target immediately above and below C2/3 facet joint
  - 1 needle tip will contact C2 inferior articular process cortex just above facet joint
  - Another needle tip will contact C3 superior articular process immediately posterior to midportion of facet joint on true lateral view
- C3/4-C6/7 MBB
  - Radiographic target is midportion of articular pillar above and below facet joint
- C8 MBB
  - Radiographic target is junction of superior articular process and transverse process of T1
- Provide local anesthetic
- Advance spinal needle under intermittent fluoroscopy
- Remove stylette and observe needle hub for blood
- Attach contrast tubing/syringe and gently aspirate to confirm extravascular placement
- Inject small amount of contrast during fluoroscopy
- Attach injectate syringe and inject slowly

Findings and Reporting

- Level(s) injected
- Pain scale before, during, and after injection(s)

POST PROCEDURE

Expected Outcome

- Significant reduction in pain corresponding to facet joint(s) injected
  - May be short duration of pain relief with anesthetic only
  - If corticosteroid injected, maximal benefit will be in 48-72 hours
- Verification of pain-generating level suggested by clinical examination
- < 100% pain relief decreases likelihood of successful rhizotomy

Things to Avoid

- Intravascular injection
- Suboptimal needle positioning (false-negative/false-positive block)

OUTCOMES

Problems

- Failure of pain relief
  - Technical failure
    - Incorrect level injected
    - Injection not correctly localized to medial branch
  - Clinical failure
    - Facet joint not source of pain
- Vasovagal reaction

Complications

- Most feared complication(s)
  - Stroke
    - Vertebral artery injection
    - Air embolism if introduced during contrast injection
  - Dural puncture
    - Spinal cord injury
    - Cerebrospinal fluid leak

Facet Joint Injection, Cervical Spine

TERMINOLOGY

- Anesthetic ± corticosteroid injection into cervical facet joint
  - Diagnostic study for pain referable to cervical facet joint

PREPROCEDURE

- Indications
  - Chronic or acute on chronic cervical facet osteoarthritis
  - Posttraumatic osteoarthritis
- Preprocedure imaging
  - Correlate imaging abnormality with patient symptoms
  - Assess degree of bone overgrowth and best place to access joint

PROCEDURE

- Supine, decubitus, or prone depending on level to be injected/anatomic relationships
- Craniocervical junction
  - Occiput/C1: Lateral approach with patient supine or decubitus

- C1/C2: Posterior approach with patient prone
- CT imaging is preferred by some interventionalists in upper cervical region
- Subaxial cervical spine (C3-C7): Generally lateral approach with patient supine or decubitus

POST PROCEDURE

- Reproduction of pain with injection
  - Concordant or discordant pain
  - Pain intensity before, during, and after injection

(Left) *Sagittal graphic shows the oblique orientation of the subaxial cervical facet joints ➡. Note the relationship of the vascular structures ➡ to the exiting nerve roots ➡ within the cervical neural foramina.* (Right) *Anteroposterior fluoroscopic spot radiograph obtained after needle placement ➡ within the left C1/2 facet joint with confirmatory contrast injection shows a linear, smooth contrast collection ➡ characteristic of an intraarticular injection.*

Normal Anatomy

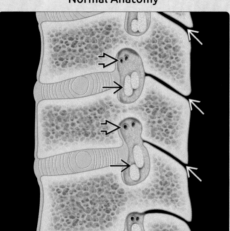

Intraarticular Injection: AP View

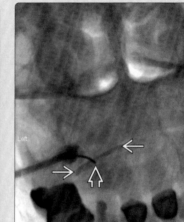

(Left) *AP view during right C6/7 facet injection shows the needle hub ➡ superimposed on the needle shaft in a "down the barrel" view of the needle. Note the contrast ➡ spreading away from the needle tip and along the anomalous course of the facet joint ➡.* (Right) *Lateral fluoroscopic radiograph in a postoperative patient shows the needle tip within the facet joint ➡ entering from a lateral approach. Note contrast spreading throughout the joint space in a linear fashion with some pooling in the inferior recess ➡.*

Intraarticular Injection: AP View

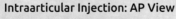
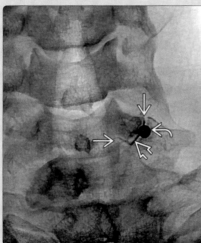

Needle Placement: C3/4 Facet Injection

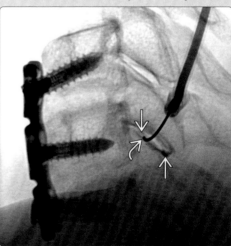

TERMINOLOGY

Definitions

- Anesthetic ± corticosteroid injection into cervical facet joint

PREPROCEDURE

Indications

- Chronic cervical facet osteoarthritis

Contraindications

- Local or systemic infection
- Allergy to injectate

Getting Started

- Things to check
  - Coagulation parameters
    - In anticoagulated patients
      □ Prothrombin time, activated partial thromboplastin time, international normalized ratio, platelet count
      □ Complete blood count (CBC) (platelets, hemoglobin, hematocrit)
  - Informed consent

PROCEDURE

Patient Position/Location

- Best procedure approach
  - Supine or prone depending on level to be injected/anatomic relationships
    - Craniocervical junction
      □ Occiput/C1: Lateral approach
      □ C1/2: Most amenable to posterior approach with patient prone
    - Subaxial cervical spine (C3-C7): Lateral approach
      □ Patient may be positioned supine or decubitus with affected side up
    - In mid to lower cervical spine, shoulders are often problematic
    - In severely degenerated subaxial cervical facet joints
      □ Prone or lateral positioning with targeting of inferior joint recess
      □ May require CT guidance to achieve intraarticular needle positioning
      □ Rotational flat-panel imaging/angiographic CT can also be performed (if equipment available)

Procedure Steps

- Procedural "time out"
  - Correct patient, level, and side(s) for injection
- Some advocate use of conscious sedation
  - Patient reaction to procedure must be reliably determined throughout procedure
  - Nonsedated patients can provide more reliable assessment of pain before, during, and after injection
- Perform sterile prep, drape, local anesthetic
- Slowly advance needle under intermittent fluoroscopy to facet joint
  - Must avoid puncture of spinal canal
- If bone is encountered prior to entering joint space, stop and assess tip placement
  - Often lower 1/3 of joint space is easier to access

- "Walk" needle gently to joint space
- Feel "pop" into joint space
- Remove stylette
  - Observe hub of needle to ensure no return of blood
- Attach preloaded, air-free contrast syringe and extension tubing
  - Aspirate gently to confirm extravascular needle tip position
- Inject only enough contrast to confirm intraarticular needle tip position
- Remove contrast tubing, and attach injectate syringe
  - Quickly remix injectate prior to injection
- Inject slowly, as patient will likely experience significant reproduction of pain
  - Note patient pain before, during, and immediately following injection

Alternative Procedures/Therapies

- Radiologic
  - Median branch block
  - Epidural steroid injection
  - Selective nerve root block

POST PROCEDURE

Expected Outcome

- Reproduction of pain with injection
- Improvement in pain following injection

OUTCOMES

Problems

- Failure to improve/alleviate clinical symptoms
  - Technical failure
    - Incorrect level injected
      □ Multiple level injection may be necessary
    - Extraarticular injection
  - Clinical failure
    - Incorrect level determined by clinical exam
    - Facet joint not source of patient pain
- Vasovagal reaction

Complications

- Most feared complication(s)
  - Vascular injury/stroke
  - Spinal cord injury
    - Direct puncture
    - Compression from hematoma
  - Meningitis

SELECTED REFERENCES

1. Manchikanti L et al: Comprehensive review of neurophysiologic basis and diagnostic interventions in managing chronic spinal pain. Pain Physician. 12(4):E71-120, 2009
2. Boswell MV et al: A systematic review of therapeutic facet joint interventions in chronic spinal pain. Pain Physician. 10(1):229-53, 2007
3. Boswell MV et al: Accuracy of precision diagnostic blocks in the diagnosis of chronic spinal pain of facet or zygapophysial joint origin. Pain Physician. 6(4):449-56, 2003

Selective Nerve Root Block, Cervical Spine

TERMINOLOGY

- Selective anesthesia of cervical nerve root at level of neural foramen

PREPROCEDURE

- Radiculopathy corresponding to cervical dermatome

PROCEDURE

- Target
  - Superior articular process of same number vertebra as nerve being injected (nerve comes out 1 level above)
  - At level of superior articular facet, deflect needle anteriorly into neural foramen
  - Verify needle tip placement within neural foramen in frontal and lateral projections
- Slowly inject iodinated contrast to confirm correct needle placement if no contraindication
  - Should see contrast track along nerve root

- May see contrast track beneath pedicle and into epidural space (transforaminal epidural steroid injection)
- Should **not** see vascular enhancement, contrast pooling, or feathering within skeletal muscle
- Use nonparticulate steroid preparation to minimize vascular complications
- Alternative procedure: Interlaminar epidural steroid injection

POST PROCEDURE

- Pain assessment
  - Note pain before, during, and after injection and whether characteristic pain was reproduced

OUTCOMES

- Vasovagal reaction
- Most feared complications
  - Stroke, spinal cord puncture, hematoma

Anatomy: Coronal Graphic

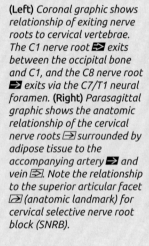

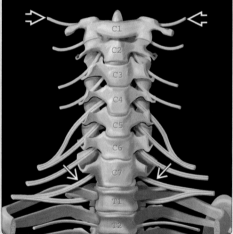

(Left) Coronal graphic shows relationship of exiting nerve roots to cervical vertebrae. The C1 nerve root ➡ exits between the occipital bone and C1, and the C8 nerve root ➡ exits via the C7/T1 neural foramen. (Right) Parasagittal graphic shows the anatomic relationship of the cervical nerve roots ➡ surrounded by adipose tissue to the accompanying artery ➡ and vein ➡. Note the relationship to the superior articular facet ➡ (anatomic landmark) for cervical selective nerve root block (SNRB).

Anatomy: Sagittal Graphic

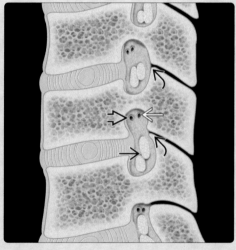

C6 Selective Root Block

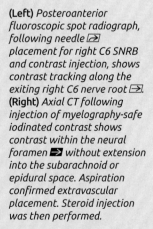

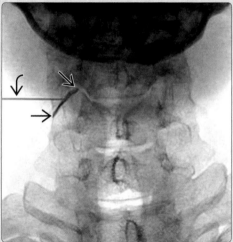

(Left) Posteroanterior fluoroscopic spot radiograph, following needle ➡ placement for right C6 SNRB and contrast injection, shows contrast tracking along the exiting right C6 nerve root ➡. (Right) Axial CT following injection of myelography-safe iodinated contrast shows contrast within the neural foramen ➡ without extension into the subarachnoid or epidural space. Aspiration confirmed extravascular placement. Steroid injection was then performed.

Contrast Injection

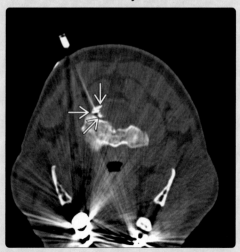

TERMINOLOGY

Synonyms

- Cervical selective nerve root block (CSNRB)

Definitions

- Selective anesthesia of cervical nerve root at level of neural foramen

PREPROCEDURE

Indications

- Radiculopathy, chronic neck pain
- Acute exacerbation of chronic neck pain

Contraindications

- Local or systemic infection
- Coagulopathy
- Allergy to injectate
- Relative: Iodinated contrast allergy, pregnancy, active hepatitis

Getting Started

- Things to check
  - Prior imaging: Causative lesion; multilevel vs. single-level disease
  - Coagulation parameters as indicated
  - Informed consent
- Medications
  - Corticosteroid
  - Short- and long-acting anesthetic
  - Iodinated contrast (myelography-safe)

PROCEDURE

Patient Position/Location

- Best procedure approach
  - Supine position
    - Visualizing mid to lower cervical spine on lateral fluoroscopy may be difficult due to shoulder position
      - Have patient hold each end of rolled sheet pulled taught against feet with knees flexed at ~ 45°
      - Holding sheet, extend knees to use legs to hold shoulders stretched downward
  - Lateral approach
    - Must have true lateral fluoroscopic view of cervical vertebrae
    - Align vertebral and facet joint margins
  - Target
    - Superior articular process of same number vertebra as nerve being injected (nerve comes out 1 level above)
    - At level of superior articular facet, deflect needle anteriorly into neural foramen
- "Time out"
  - Verify correct patient, procedure, and side to be injected
  - Verify all necessary equipment is readily available

Procedure Steps

- Verify needle trajectory to target in PA and lateral projections
- Intermittently advance needle, and verify under fluoroscopy until anterior margin of superior articular process is reached
- Deflect needle tip anteriorly, and advance slowly into neural foramen
  - Be prepared for patient to jump &/or vocalize if nerve root is hit
- Verify needle tip placement within neural foramen in frontal and lateral projections
- Remove stylette, and observe hub for blood
- Slowly inject iodinated contrast to confirm correct needle placement if no contraindication
  - Should see contrast track along nerve root
  - May see contrast track beneath pedicle and into epidural space (transforaminal epidural steroid injection)
  - Should **not** see vascular enhancement, contrast pooling, or feathering within skeletal muscle
- Attach 3-mL syringe containing injectate
- Inject slowly: Use nonparticulate steroid preparation
  - If not possible to inject due to resistance from contrast, attach 1-mL syringe containing portion of injectate, and inject to clear contrast from needle
- Remove needle, and obtain hemostasis

Findings and Reporting

- Change in patient's pain following injection
- Whether epidural injection was also noted during contrast injection
- Any complications

Alternative Procedures/Therapies

- Radiologic
  - Interlaminar epidural steroid injection
    - Bilateral, multifactorial stenosis affecting multiple nerve roots

POST PROCEDURE

Expected Outcome

- Improvement in pain

Things to Do

- Remind patient of potential late complications
- Remind patient to log pain/relief of pain between clinical visits (pain diary)
- Establish follow-up

OUTCOMES

Problems

- Vasovagal reaction

Complications

- Most feared complication(s)
  - Intravascular injection/stroke
  - Spinal cord injury/intraspinal hematoma
- Other complications
  - Bleeding, infection, nerve root injury

KEY FACTS

TERMINOLOGY

- Percutaneous injection of glucocorticoid into cervical epidural space
  - Interlaminar: Approach epidural space between lamina
  - Transforaminal: Approach epidural space via neural foramen

PREPROCEDURE

- Indication
  - Cervical pain &/or cervical radiculopathy
- Coagulopathy
- Preprocedure imaging
  - Assess adequate epidural space to accommodate needle placement/injection

PROCEDURE

- Loss of resistance/free injection of saline reveals tip in epidural space (or intrathecal)
  - Inject contrast to verify needle tip placement

POST PROCEDURE

- Expectation
  - Improvement in, or eradication of, pain at level of injection
  - Steroid may take 48-72 hours to reach maximum therapeutic effect

OUTCOMES

- Most feared complications
  - Direct spinal cord injury or intraspinal hematoma
  - Intrathecal injection of anesthetic/respiratory paralysis

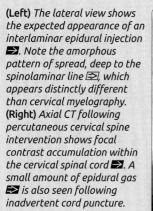

(Left) Sagittal graphic of the cervical spine and cervical spinal cord shows a thin layer of epidural fat ➡ representing the epidural space just deep to the spinous processes/spinolaminar line ➡. (Right) Anteroposterior fluoroscopic spot radiograph shows the needle tip near the midline in the cervical epidural space, entering from an interlaminar approach. Contrast typically shows Christmas tree appearance and outlines the epidural space ➡. Note the lamina ➡ and spinous process ➡ at the level of puncture.

Normal Anatomy

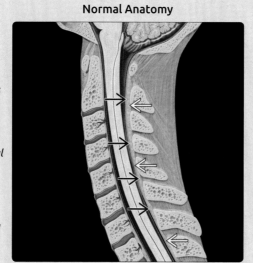

Needle Placement: Epidural Injection

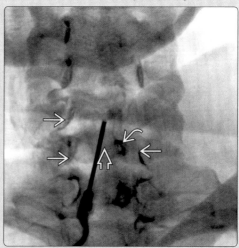

(Left) The lateral view shows the expected appearance of an interlaminar epidural injection ➡. Note the amorphous pattern of spread, deep to the spinolaminar line ➡, which appears distinctly different than cervical myelography. (Right) Axial CT following percutaneous cervical spine intervention shows focal contrast accumulation within the cervical spinal cord ➡. A small amount of epidural gas ➡ is also seen following inadvertent cord puncture.

Cervical Epidurogram: Lateral View

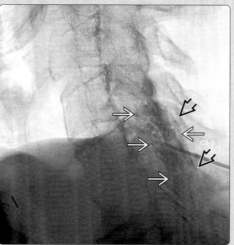

Complication: Cord Puncture

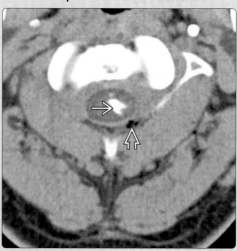

TERMINOLOGY

Abbreviations

- Epidural steroid injection

Definitions

- Injection of corticosteroid percutaneously into epidural space
  - Interlaminar: Approach epidural space between lamina (C7-T1 level preferred)
  - Transforaminal: Approach epidural space via neural foramen

PREPROCEDURE

Indications

- Cervical pain &/or cervical radiculopathy

Contraindications

- Coagulopathy
- Systemic or localized infection at site of planned injection
- Allergy to injectate

Getting Started

- Medications
  - Corticosteroid
    - Long-acting anesthetic not injected, as respiratory paralysis may result
  - Short-acting local anesthetic

PROCEDURE

Patient Position/Location

- Best procedure approach
  - Prone
    - Slight angulation of AP fluoroscopy tube for delineation of lamina/interlaminar space
    - True lateral fluoroscopy helpful for needle depth

Procedure Steps

- Preprocedure "time out": Correct patient, side of injection, and procedure
- Position patient as comfortably as possible with supporting pillows
  - Conscious sedation is generally not provided, as it is believed to be safer for patient to be alert and fully able to notify interventionalist immediately of new or unusual pain during procedure
- Angle fluoroscopy tube to maximize visualization of interlaminar space
- Mark correct level at cephalad margin of lamina near junction with spinous process
- Create skin wheal, and carefully anesthetize deeper subcutaneous tissues
- Place epidural needle into subcutaneous tissue with curved tip projecting cephalad
- Slowly advance needle to lamina under intermittent imaging
- Once lamina is reached, carefully direct needle tip cephalad and "walk" off cephalad edge of lamina
- Attach glass syringe containing preservative-free saline
- Slowly advance epidural needle, testing with gentle plunging of glass syringe while slowly advancing
  - Loss of resistance/free injection of saline reveals tip in epidural space (or intrathecal)
- Attach contrast syringe/tubing to needle
- Warn patient, then inject contrast to verify needle tip placement within epidural space
- Once confirmed, document with radiographic images
- Mix, then attach injectate syringe
- Warn patient, then slowly inject, noting intensity and character of pain produced

Findings and Reporting

- Character and severity of patient pain before, during, and after procedure

Alternative Procedures/Therapies

- Radiologic
  - Selective nerve root block
    - Generally for 1- or 2-level unilateral or 1-level bilateral radicular symptoms
- Surgical
  - Decompression
- Other
  - Neurolysis
  - Percutaneous disc ablation/discectomy

POST PROCEDURE

Expected Outcome

- Improvement in or eradication of pain at level of injection
  - Patients often describe numbness/heaviness in side injected
- Pain may increase as local and long-acting anesthetic wear off
  - Steroid may take 48-72 hours to reach maximum therapeutic effect

Things to Do

- Assess patient after injection, and assist from table when ready
  - Patients can often be discharged within 30 minutes after procedure if feeling well

OUTCOMES

Problems

- Failure of injection to provide symptomatic relief
  - Relief may not be experienced for 48-72 hours following injection

Complications

- Most feared complication(s)
  - Spinal cord puncture/cord hematoma
  - Compressive epidural hematoma
  - Intrathecal injection of anesthetic/respiratory paralysis

SELECTED REFERENCES

1. Huston CW: Cervical epidural steroid injections in the management of cervical radiculitis: interlaminar versus transforaminal. A review. Curr Rev Musculoskelet Med. 2(1):30-42, 2009
2. Kim KS et al: Fluoroscopically guided cervical interlaminar epidural injections using the midline approach: an analysis of epidurography contrast patterns. Anesth Analg. 108(5):1658-61, 2009
3. Malhotra G et al: Complications of transforaminal cervical epidural steroid injections. Spine (Phila Pa 1976). 34(7):731-9, 2009

Image-Guided Procedures

TERMINOLOGY

- Selective anesthesia of thoracic spinal nerve medial branch in assessment of thoracic facet joint pain

PREPROCEDURE

- Thoracic facet joint pain
  - Confirm clinical suspicion (diagnostic)
  - Evaluate likelihood of successful facet neurolysis
- Preprocedure imaging

PROCEDURE

- Target
  - Immediately above transverse process/superior articular process junction
    - Be sure to avoid lung
  - Carefully approach medial branch as close as possible to lateral aspect of superior articular process
- Record pain score
  - Before, during, and after injection for each level

POST PROCEDURE

- Expected outcome: Significant reduction in pain associated with target facet joint
  - < 100% pain reduction reduces likelihood of successful neurolysis

OUTCOMES

- Problem: Failure of pain reduction
  - Facet joints not sole pain generator
  - Inaccurate needle placement
- Complications
  - Vasovagal reaction
  - Pneumothorax
  - Spinal/nerve cord injury
- Alternative procedures
  - Physical therapy
  - Neurolysis
  - Thoracic facet joint injection(s)

Anatomy

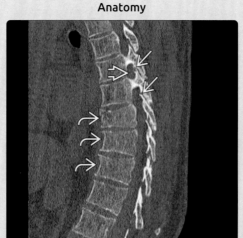

Needle Placement: Oblique View

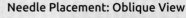
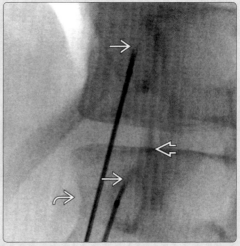

(Left) Sagittal CT shows hypertrophic changes of thoracic facet joints with bony overgrowth ➡ encroaching on the dorsal aspect of the neural foramina ➡. Note the anterior compression fractures ➡. (Right) Oblique view shows the needle tip ➡ directed toward the junction of the superior articular process ➡ and transverse process ➡. Oblique view should provide excellent visualization of the "Scotty dog." At higher levels, careful attention to lung margins is essential.

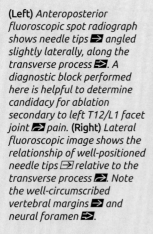

Needle Placement: Frontal View

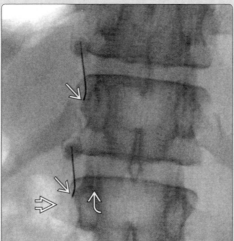

Needle Placement: Lateral View

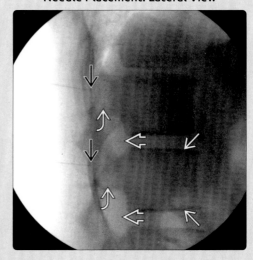

(Left) Anteroposterior fluoroscopic spot radiograph shows needle tips ➡ angled slightly laterally, along the transverse process ➡. A diagnostic block performed here is helpful to determine candidacy for ablation secondary to left T12/L1 facet joint ➡ pain. (Right) Lateral fluoroscopic image shows the relationship of well-positioned needle tips ➡ relative to the transverse process ➡. Note the well-circumscribed vertebral margins ➡ and neural foramen ➡.

TERMINOLOGY

Abbreviations

- Superior articular process (SAP)

Definitions

- Selective anesthesia of thoracic spinal nerve medial branch in assessment of thoracic facet joint pain

PREPROCEDURE

Indications

- Thoracic facet joint pain
  - Confirm clinical suspicion (diagnostic)
    - Clinical exam often unreliable in assessment of facet joint pain
  - Determine likelihood of successful facet neurolysis
- Acute or chronic thoracic back pain
- Facet joint osteoarthritis

Contraindications

- Coagulopathy
- Local or systemic infection

Getting Started

- Things to check
  - Laboratory data
    - Signs of infection or impaired coagulation
  - Informed consent
- Medications
  - Short-acting anesthetic
  - Long-acting anesthetic
  - ± corticosteroid
  - Iodinated contrast (myelography-safe)

PROCEDURE

Patient Position/Location

- Best procedure approach
  - Prone
    - Target is junction of superior articular process and transverse process
      - Carefully approach medial branch as close as possible to lateral aspect of superior articular process

Procedure Steps

- Create skin wheal with local anesthetic and anesthetize subcutaneous tissues
- Anchor 22-gauge spinal needle in subcutaneous tissue and check trajectory under fluoroscopy or CT
- Carefully advance needle under intermittent imaging guidance
  - Be sure to avoid lung
- Target
  - Immediately above transverse process/SAP junction
- Remove stylette and observe hub for blood
  - If blood present, reposition needle slightly
  - If no blood, proceed
- Attach injectate syringe
- Record patient's pain
  - Before, during, and after injection

- Repeat steps for each additional level as indicated

Findings and Reporting

- Level(s) injected
- Pain score
  - Before, during, and after injection for each level
- Component(s) of injectate
- Complications

Alternative Procedures/Therapies

- Radiologic
  - Thoracic facet joint injection(s)
- Surgical
  - Fusion
- Other
  - Neurolysis
  - Conservative management
  - Physical therapy

POST PROCEDURE

Expected Outcome

- Significant reduction in pain associated with target facet joint
  - < 100% pain reduction reduces likelihood of successful neurolysis

Things to Do

- Ensure that clinical follow-up is established
- Remind patient to keep a pain diary until next clinic visit

Things to Avoid

- Bathing for 48-72 hours

OUTCOMES

Problems

- Vasovagal reaction
- Failure of pain reduction
  - Facet joints not sole pain generator
  - Inaccurate needle placement

Complications

- Most feared complication(s)
  - Pneumothorax
  - Dural puncture
    - Spinal cord injury
    - Epidural/subdural hematoma
  - Meningitis
- Other complications
  - Bleeding
  - Local infection
  - Nerve root injury

SELECTED REFERENCES

1. Atluri S et al: Systematic review of diagnostic utility and therapeutic effectiveness of thoracic facet joint interventions. Pain Physician. 11(5):611-29, 2008
2. Manchikanti L et al: Effectiveness of thoracic medial branch blocks in managing chronic pain: a preliminary report of a randomized, double-blind controlled trial. Pain Physician. 11(4):491-504, 2008
3. Verrills P et al: The incidence of intravascular penetration in medial branch blocks: cervical, thoracic, and lumbar spines. Spine (Phila Pa 1976). 33(6):E174-7, 2008

KEY FACTS

TERMINOLOGY

- Injection of long-acting anesthetic ± corticosteroid into thoracic facet joint

PREPROCEDURE

- Preprocedure imaging
  - Correlate level with prior imaging
    - Evaluate for 12 ribs &/or transitional vertebral anatomy
- Indications for procedure and future treatment plan
  - Is facet joint injection or medial branch block more appropriate?

PROCEDURE

- Fluoroscopy
  - Align margins of facet joint to maximize visualization of joint space
  - Contrast is useful to evaluate intraarticular injection during fluoroscopy-guided facet injection

- CT
  - Gantry angulation may be necessary to "open" facet joints
  - Sagittal reformats helpful for determining correct level and angulation of needle

POST PROCEDURE

- Improvement/relief of pain referable to facet joint(s) injected
  - < 100% pain relief decreases likelihood of successful outcome following facet neurolysis/radiofrequency ablation

OUTCOMES

- Most feared complications
  - Spinal cord/nerve root injury
  - Pneumothorax
  - Epidural hematoma

Degenerated Facets

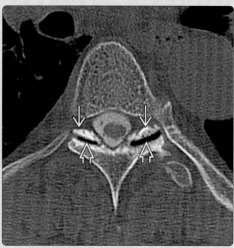

Needle Placement

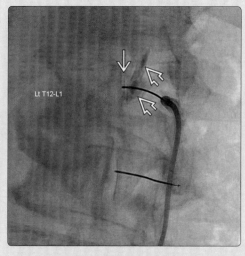

(Left) *Image from an axial CT myelogram shows characteristic findings of facet joint osteoarthritis, including sclerosis with irregularity of the facets* ➡ *and vacuum phenomenon within the joint space(s)* ➡. (Right) *Oblique view obtained during left-sided injection shows extraarticular contrast* ➡ *from earlier injection with intraarticular opacification* ➡ *after the needle was advanced into the joint space.*

Intraarticular Needle Placement

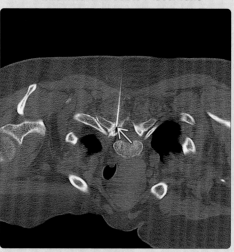

Intraarticular Needle Placement

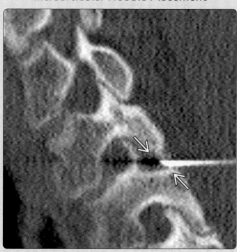

(Left) *Axial NECT shows the position after "walking" the needle slightly lateral and cephalad, at which time the needle was felt to "pop" into the joint space. This image now confirms that the needle tip lies within the facet joint* ➡. (Right) *Sagittal reformatted NECT confirms intraarticular needle tip placement* ➡ *as seen in the previous axial image. Two planes of imaging are very helpful for confident determination of needle tip positioning, particularly if contrast injection is not being performed.*

TERMINOLOGY

Abbreviations

- Facet joint injection (FJI)

Definitions

- Injection of long-acting anesthetic ± corticosteroid into thoracic facet joint

PREPROCEDURE

Indications

- Thoracic facet joint osteoarthritis
  - Chronic or acute exacerbation of thoracic facet joint pain

Contraindications

- Coagulopathy
- Local or systemic infection
- Severe allergy to components of injectate

Getting Started

- Things to check
  - Preprocedure imaging
    - Look for facet joint degenerative changes, correlate correct level
  - Indications for procedure/plan for definitive treatment
    - Median branch block vs. FJI
  - Coagulopathy
  - Informed consent

PROCEDURE

Patient Position/Location

- Best procedure approach
  - Prone

Equipment Preparation

- Fluoroscopy
  - Align margins of facet joint to maximize visualization of joint space
- CT
  - Gantry angulation may be necessary to "open" facet joints

Procedure Steps

- Procedure "time out"
- Carefully determine correct level for injection
- Mark skin, and perform sterile prep and drape
- Apply local anesthetic, and assess trajectory to facet joint with fluoroscopy or CT
- Place spinal or Chiba needle into dorsal subcutaneous tissue, and reassess trajectory to facet joint
- Under intermittent fluoroscopy or CT imaging, advance needle until "pop" into joint or firm bone is felt
- Assess needle placement on oblique and lateral fluoroscopy or CT
- If necessary, "walk" needle into facet joint, and reassess with imaging
- Attach contrast syringe/tubing
  - Useful to evaluate extravascular, intraarticular injection during fluoroscopy-guided facet injection
  - ± for CT-guided injection
- Aspirate gently to confirm extravascular, then slowly inject contrast to confirm intraarticular needle tip placement
  - Inject minimal amount of contrast to confirm needle position
- Mix injectate, attach, then slowly inject facet joint
  - 0.5-1.5-mL injection volume is generally sufficient
- Note symptoms during and after injection

Alternative Procedures/Therapies

- Radiologic
  - Medial branch block
- Surgical
  - Fusion

POST PROCEDURE

Expected Outcome

- Improvement/relief of pain referable to facet joint(s) injected
  - < 100% pain relief decreases likelihood of successful outcome following radiofrequency ablation

OUTCOMES

Problems

- Failure of pain relief
  - Facet joint not pain generator
  - Wrong level(s) injected
  - Extraarticular injection
- Vasovagal reaction

Complications

- Most feared complication(s)
  - Spinal cord/nerve root injury
  - Pneumothorax
  - Epidural hematoma
- Other complications
  - Bleeding
  - Infection

SELECTED REFERENCES

1. Peterson C et al: Evidence-based radiology (part 1): is there sufficient research to support the use of therapeutic injections for the spine and sacroiliac joints? Skeletal Radiol. 39(1):5-9, 2010
2. Sehgal N et al: Systematic review of diagnostic utility of facet (zygapophysial) joint injections in chronic spinal pain: an update. Pain Physician. 10(1):213-28, 2007
3. Boswell MV et al: Accuracy of precision diagnostic blocks in the diagnosis of chronic spinal pain of facet or zygapophysial joint origin. Pain Physician. 6(4):449-56, 2003

Selective Nerve Root Block, Thoracic Spine

TERMINOLOGY

- Selective corticosteroid and long-acting anesthetic injection of thoracic nerve root at level of neural foramen

PREPROCEDURE

- Indications
  - Thoracic radiculopathy
  - Persistent pain after vertebroplasty/kyphoplasty
  - Neoplastic compression of thoracic nerve root

PROCEDURE

- Use nonparticulate steroid to minimize vascular risk
- C-arm angulation must permit visualization of medial pleural surface of lung during procedure
- CT offers improved soft tissue and lung visualization
  - Sagittal/coronal reformatted CT may facilitate difficult needle placement

POST PROCEDURE

- Report pain intensity before, during, and after injection

OUTCOMES

- Expected: Significant improvement in pain
- Potential problem: Failure of pain relief
  - Technical failure: Injection not properly localized or wrong level injected
  - Clinical failure: Thoracic nerve root not sole pain generator
- Most feared complications
  - Vascular injury
    - Spinal cord ischemia from compromise of artery of Adamkiewicz
  - Pneumothorax, dural puncture
  - Spinal cord puncture or compression secondary to hematoma

---

Cervical Root Numbering

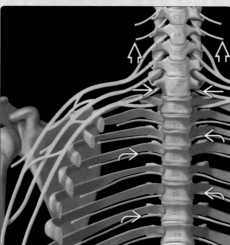

Vertebral Body Numbering

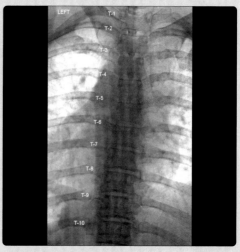

(Left) Coronal graphic depicts the cervical nerve roots ➡ exiting above their corresponding pedicle, while thoracic (and lumbar) nerve roots ➡ exit below. Note the C8 nerve roots ➡. (Right) Anteroposterior fluoroscopic spot radiograph was obtained prior to thoracic spine intervention. Careful numbering of the ribs or vertebrae after assessing the entire spine for transitional anatomy is critical.

Foraminal Injection: Transforaminal Epidural Steroid Injection

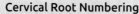
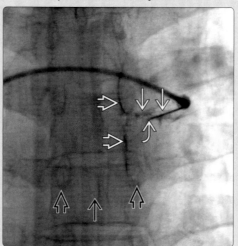

Needle Placement: CT

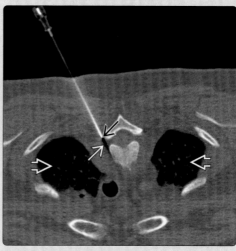

(Left) Fluoroscopic spot radiograph after needle placement ➡ shows contrast within right thoracic neural foramen ➡. Note linear extension along exiting nerve root and medial extension into epidural space ➡. Note also the pedicles ➡ and spinous process ➡. (Right) Axial NECT shows the needle tip ➡ placed at the posterior margin of the neural foramen ➡. Note dramatically improved visualization of lungs ➡ and other soft tissue structures with CT-guided thoracic procedures.

TERMINOLOGY

Abbreviations
- Selective nerve root block (SNRB)

Definitions
- Selective corticosteroid and long-acting anesthetic injection of thoracic nerve root at level of neural foramen

PREPROCEDURE

Indications
- Thoracic radiculopathy
  - Thoracic spine degenerative disease
  - Posttraumatic osteoarthritis
  - Persistent pain after vertebroplasty/kyphoplasty
  - Neoplastic compression of thoracic nerve root

Contraindications
- Coagulopathy
- Evidence of local or systemic infection
- Severe allergy to components of injectate

Preprocedure Imaging
- Evaluate causes of pain
  - e.g., nerve root displacement/compression by degenerative or neoplastic disease
- Gain familiarity with patient-specific anatomic relationships
  - Vertebral or facet joint fusion anomalies
    - Severe hypertrophic facet changes may make access to neural foramen challenging
  - Transitional lumbosacral anatomy
    - Must carefully assess anatomy to ensure injection is at correct level
  - Cervical ribs
    - Must carefully assess anatomy to ensure injection is at correct level
  - Scoliosis
    - May require change in patient positioning

Getting Started
- Things to check
  - Laboratory data
    - Evidence of coagulopathy
    - Evidence of infection/inflammation
      - White blood cell count (WBC), recent febrile illness, cultures if available
  - Informed consent
- Medications
  - Short- and long-acting anesthetic
  - Corticosteroid
  - Radiographic contrast (myelography-safe)

PROCEDURE

Patient Position/Location
- Best procedure approach
  - Prone

Procedure Steps
- Procedure "time out"
  - Correct patient
  - Correct side
  - Correct procedure
  - All necessary equipment present
- Carefully determine correct level
  - Nerve root exits beneath pedicle of same numbered thoracic vertebra
- Mark skin, allowing for needle trajectory that is medial to pleural margin
- Perform sterile prep and drape
- Create skin wheal, and anesthetize deep subcutaneous tissues
- Anchor 22-gauge needle in subcutaneous tissue
- Carefully advance needle under intermittent imaging guidance
  - Alternating oblique, AP, and lateral fluoroscopy to ensure knowledge of needle depth and relationship of needle to pleural surface
- If bone is reached, reassess with imaging, and "walk" needle into foramen
  - Most frequent barrier is needle placement against facet (posterior or superficial to neural foramen)
- When needle slips into foramen, reassess with imaging
  - Tip should be beneath lateral pedicle cortex on frontal radiograph and in foramen on lateral view
  - Always assess for evidence of pneumothorax
- Inject contrast slowly
  - Look for vascular enhancement/flow
  - Contrast should outline nerve
  - Look for signs of transforaminal epidural steroid injection
    - Contrast spreading beneath/medial to pedicle into epidural space
- Remove contrast syringe/tubing, and attach injectate syringe
  - Mix injectate immediately prior to attaching
- Slowly inject injectate
  - Determine pain intensity (1-10) during and after injection

POST PROCEDURE

Expected Outcome
- Significant improvement in pain corresponding to nerve root(s) injected
  - May take 48-72 hours for corticosteroid to take full effect

OUTCOMES

Complications
- Most feared complication(s)
  - Pneumothorax
  - Dural puncture
  - Vascular injury
    - Spinal cord ischemia

SELECTED REFERENCES
1. Boezaart AP et al: Paravertebral block: cervical, thoracic, lumbar, and sacral. Curr Opin Anaesthesiol. 22(5):637-43, 2009
2. Eckel TS et al: Epidural steroid injections and selective nerve root blocks. Tech Vasc Interv Radiol. 12(1):11-21, 2009
3. Boswell MV et al: Interventional techniques: evidence-based practice guidelines in the management of chronic spinal pain. Pain Physician. 10(1):7-111, 2007

Image-Guided Procedures

TERMINOLOGY

- Injection of glucocorticoid/long-acting anesthetic into thoracic epidural space via interlaminar or transforaminal approach

PROCEDURE

- Interlaminar epidural steroid injection (ESI)
  - Define margins of lamina and interlaminar space
- Transforaminal ESI
  - Ensure good visualization of neural foramen on true lateral view
- Benefit of CT
  - Improved visualization of osseous structures in severely osteopenic patients
  - Improved visualization of pleura/medial chest cavity

POST PROCEDURE

- Expectation

- Improvement in pain, or cessation of pain, following injection
- Things to do
  - Establish clinical follow-up, and have patient maintain pain diary
  - Remind patient to expect full benefit of injection over next 24-48 hours

OUTCOMES

- Most feared complications
  - Intraarterial injection: Spinal cord ischemia
  - Spinal cord puncture/hematoma
  - Compressive epidural hematoma
  - Pneumothorax

Normal Anatomy

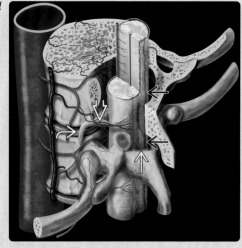

Normal Anatomy

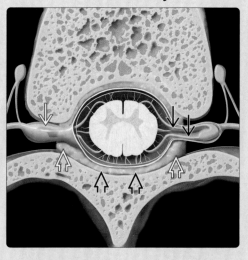

(Left) Graphic shows the spinal cord ➡ and the relationship of vascular structures ➡ to exiting nerve roots ➡. Interlaminar epidural steroid injection (ESI) approach is at the junction of the lamina and spinous process ➡. (Right) Axial graphic demonstrates relationship of nerve roots ➡ and nerve root sleeve ➡ to neural foramen. Optimal needle tip placement for transforaminal ➡ or interlaminar ➡ ESI is shown.

Frontal Oblique Epidurogram

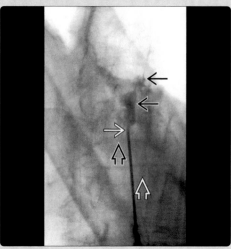

Lateral Epidurogram

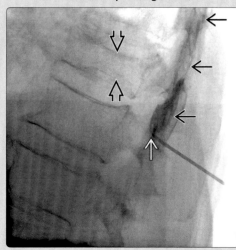

(Left) Oblique fluoroscopic spot radiograph shows the needle tip in the interlaminar space ➡ with contrast tracking cephalad in the thoracic epidural space ➡. Note the superior margin of the lamina ➡ and spinous process ➡. (Right) A lateral fluoroscopic spot radiograph shows the needle tip positioned within the thoracic epidural space ➡. Contrast ➡ is seen tracking cephalad within the epidural space with an amorphous appearance characteristic of epidural injections. Note the vertebral compression fracture ➡.

TERMINOLOGY

Abbreviations

- Thoracic epidural steroid injection

Definitions

- Injection of corticosteroid/long-acting anesthetic into thoracic epidural space via interlaminar or transforaminal approach

PREPROCEDURE

Indications

- Thoracic radiculopathy at > 1 level
- Persistent pain following vertebroplasty/kyphoplasty

Contraindications

- Coagulopathy
- Local or systemic infection
- Allergy to injectate

Getting Started

- Things to check
  - Clinical indication
    - Correlation between pain and level chosen for injection
  - Diagnostic imaging
    - Adequate epidural fat/space for needle placement
  - Laboratory
    - Coagulopathy
    - Infection
  - Informed consent
- Medications
  - Glucocorticoid
  - Long- and short-acting anesthetic
  - Myelography-safe iodinated contrast for fluoroscopy-guided injection

PROCEDURE

Patient Position/Location

- Best procedure approach
  - Prone
    - Pillow placement beneath patient (kyphosis) may improve visualization of interlaminar space
    - Interlaminar: Define margins of lamina and interlaminar space
    - Transforaminal: Ensure good visualization of neural foramen on true lateral view; triangulate trajectory between frontal and lateral views keeping medial to avoid lung
  - Benefit of CT
    - Improved visualization of osseous structures in severely osteopenic patients
    - Improved visualization of pleura/medial chest cavity

Procedure Steps

- Procedure "time out": Verify correct patient, procedure, and side
- Perform sterile prep and drape, local anesthetic
- **Interlaminar**
  - Carefully assess trajectory intermittently while advancing needle tip to level of superior lamina
  - Very slowly advance needle under intermittent imaging until loss of resistance is noted on plunging glass syringe
  - Once loss of resistance occurs, attach contrast tubing and inject contrast to confirm needle tip placement in epidural space
  - Attach injectate syringe, and inject slowly
- **Transforaminal**
  - Carefully assess trajectory needed on biplane fluoroscopy or CT to reach superomedial neural foramen
  - Slowly advance 22-gauge spinal needle under intermittent imaging guidance
    - Placing gentle curve 20-30° in distal needle often facilitates placement within neural foramen
  - When approaching foramen, warn patient of possible sudden pain in case needle contacts exiting nerve
  - When needle lies within medial neural foramen, remove stylette, and attach air-free contrast extension tubing
  - Slowly inject contrast to confirm tracking into epidural space
  - Obtain image to document needle tip placement
  - Attach injectate syringe, and slowly inject

Alternative Procedures/Therapies

- Radiologic
  - Selective nerve root block
- Surgical
  - Decompression

POST PROCEDURE

Expected Outcome

- Improvement in or cessation of pain following injection

Things to Do

- Help patient to sitting posture
- Establish clinical follow-up, and have patient maintain pain diary
- Remind patient to expect full benefit of injection over next 24-48 hours

OUTCOMES

Problems

- Failure of pain relief

Complications

- Most feared complication(s)
  - Intraarterial injection: Spinal cord ischemia
  - Spinal cord puncture/hematoma
  - Pneumothorax
- Other complications
  - Bleeding, infection, nerve injury

SELECTED REFERENCES

1. Georgy BA: Interventional techniques in managing persistent pain after vertebral augmentation procedures: a retrospective evaluation. Pain Physician. 10(5):673-6, 2007
2. Botwin KP et al: Adverse effects of fluoroscopically guided interlaminar thoracic epidural steroid injections. Am J Phys Med Rehabil. 85(1):14-23, 2006

KEY FACTS

TERMINOLOGY

- Selective anesthesia of lumbar nerve medial branch in diagnostic evaluation of lumbar facet joint pain

PREPROCEDURE

- Facet joint pain
  - Useful in selecting patients for medial branch radiofrequency ablation procedure

PROCEDURE

- Target: Junction of superior articular process and transverse process
  - Medial branch is numbered along with exiting lumbar nerve root
  - L5 medial branch innervates inferior L4/5 and superior L5/S1 facet joint
- Patient positioning
  - Prone: Angulate C-arm such that "eye" of "Scotty dog" is well visualized

POST PROCEDURE

- Expectation
  - Significant reduction in facet joint pain
  - < 100% pain relief decreases likelihood of successful rhizotomy
    - Injection of superior and inferior rami essential to effectively block nervous supply to facet joint

OUTCOMES

- Failure of pain relief
  - Incorrect level or poor needle placement
  - Facet joint may not be source of pain
- Complications
  - Intravascular injection: Spinal cord ischemia
  - Dural puncture: Cauda equina injury, meningitis

Dorsal Ramus Medial Branch

Needle Placement: Lateral View

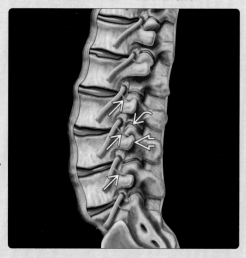
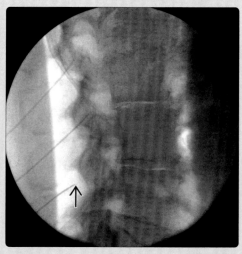

(Left) Sagittal graphic shows the dorsal ramus medial branch ➡ in the osseous groove at the junction of the superior articular process ➡ and transverse process ➡, immediately above the pedicle. (Right) Lateral fluoroscopy shows an L3 needle ➡ that is superficially located. Lateral fluoroscopy is useful during needle placement to ensure that bone is reached at an appropriate depth. Single-plane imaging is deceptive, and care must be taken to ensure safe needle depth.

Needle Placement: AP View

Needle Position: AP View

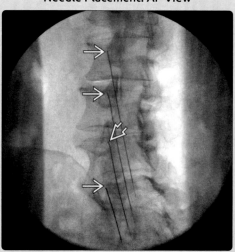
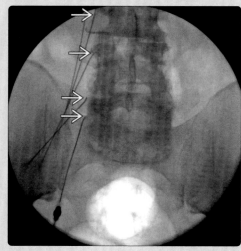

(Left) Oblique fluoroscopic spot radiograph shows successful needle placement for L2, 3, and 5 medial branch blocks ➡. Medial L4 needle tip is not optimal ➡. (Right) Anteroposterior fluoroscopic spot radiograph shows the needle tips ➡ at the expected location of the right L2, L3, L4, and L5 medial branches. Note that the target point of L5 dorsal ramus is at the lateral junction of the S1 superior articular process and sacral ala. Compare with previous oblique view.

TERMINOLOGY

Definitions

- Selective anesthesia of lumbar nerve medial branch in diagnostic evaluation of lumbar facet joint pain

PREPROCEDURE

Indications

- Chronic lower back pain
- Facet joint pain
  - Useful in selecting patients for medial branch radiofrequency ablation (RFA) procedure

Contraindications

- Allergy to injectate
- Coagulopathy
- Local or systemic infection
- Relative contraindication
  - Pregnancy

Getting Started

- Medications
  - ± corticosteroid
  - Long-acting anesthetic
  - Short-acting anesthetic
  - Iodinated contrast (myelography-safe) is optional

PROCEDURE

Patient Position/Location

- Best procedure approach
  - Prone
    - Pillow or bumper beneath patient may be useful for stable positioning/patient comfort
    - Angulate C-arm such that "eye" of "Scotty dog" is well visualized
  - Target
    - Junction of superior articular process (SAP) and transverse process
    - Medial branch is numbered along with exiting lumbar nerve root
      □ L5 medial branch innervates inferior L4/5 and superior L5/S1 facet joint

Procedure Steps

- Procedure "time out"
  - Correct patient, procedure, side, and levels of intervention
- Optimize C-arm angulation, 10-15° toward side of injection
- Perform sterile prep and drape
- Provide local anesthetic
- Insert 22-gauge spinal needle into subcutaneous tissue
- Advance needle under intermittent fluoroscopy
  - T12/L1-L4/L5
    - Target junction of SAP and transverse process (small osseous groove)
  - L5 dorsal ramus
    - Target junction of S1 SAP and sacral ala
- When bone is reached, turn bevel down (away from neural foramen)
  - Gently aspirate to confirm extravascular

- Inject small amount of contrast
  - If desired to confirm needle tip placement/extravascular injection
- Place needles at additional levels as indicated
- Attach injectate syringe, and inject slowly
  - Assess pain with each injection

Findings and Reporting

- Level(s) injected
- Pain scale and character before and after injection(s)

Alternative Procedures/Therapies

- Radiologic
  - Lumbar facet joint block
  - Lumbar epidural steroid injection
- Other
  - Neurolysis
    - RFA
    - Cryoablation

POST PROCEDURE

Expected Outcome

- Significant reduction in pain corresponding to facet joint injected
  - < 100% pain relief decreases likelihood of successful rhizotomy
    - Injection of superior and inferior rami essential to effectively block nervous supply to facet joint

OUTCOMES

Problems

- Failure of pain relief
  - Incorrect level or poor needle placement
  - Facet joint may not be source of pain

Complications

- Most feared complication(s)
  - Intravascular injection
    - Spinal cord ischemia
  - Dural puncture
    - Spinal cord or cauda equina injury
    - Meningitis
- Other complications
  - Bleeding
  - Infection
  - Nerve root injury

SELECTED REFERENCES

1. Chou R et al: Nonsurgical interventional therapies for low back pain: a review of the evidence for an American Pain Society clinical practice guideline. Spine (Phila Pa 1976). 34(10):1078-93, 2009
2. Lee CJ et al: Intravascular injection in lumbar medial branch block: a prospective evaluation of 1433 injections. Anesth Analg. 106(4):1274-8, table of contents, 2008
3. Manchikanti L et al: Lumbar facet joint nerve blocks in managing chronic facet joint pain: one-year follow-up of a randomized, double-blind controlled trial: Clinical Trial NCT00355914. Pain Physician. 11(2):121-32, 2008
4. Verrills P et al: The incidence of intravascular penetration in medial branch blocks: cervical, thoracic, and lumbar spines. Spine (Phila Pa 1976). 33(6):E174-7, 2008

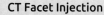

KEY FACTS

TERMINOLOGY

- Injection of corticosteroid and anesthetic into lumbar facet joint

PREPROCEDURE

- Facet joint osteoarthritis
- Synovial cyst causing neurologic symptoms

PROCEDURE

- Prone
- Angle C-arm or PA fluoroscopy tube slightly toward side of joint to be injected
  - Generally, lower 1/3 of joint is most amenable to needle entry/injection in arthritic joint
- Ensure proper level
- Slowly inject only enough contrast to confirm that needle tip is in joint space
- Note pain scale and pain characteristics
  - Before, during, and after injection

- Synovial cyst therapeutic rupture
  - May require significant injection pressure
  - See sudden spread of contrast into epidural space

OUTCOMES

- Failure to alleviate pain
  - Wrong level injected
  - Injection extraarticular
  - Facet joint not source of pain
  - May require multilevel injections
- Most feared complications
  - Thecal sac puncture, cord injury, meningitis
- Other complications
  - Nerve root injury, bleeding, infection

CT Facet Injection

Needle Positioning: Frontal Oblique View

(Left) *Axial NECT shows the needle tip ➡ at the superolateral margin of the right L4/5 facet joint. Note that the needle is nearly within the plane of the image and that the needle tip casts a dark artifact ➡. (Right) Oblique fluoroscopic radiograph shows a 22-gauge spinal needle passing between adjacent articular facets ➡ into the right L4/5 facet joint ➡. Correlation with lateral imaging is helpful in determining depth. A "pop" is felt upon penetration of the joint capsule.*

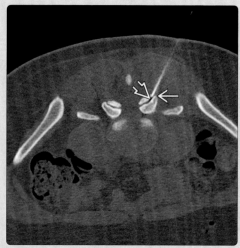

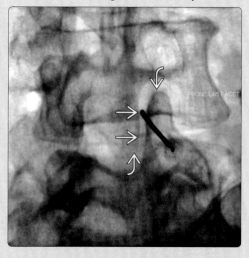

Mixed Intra-/Extraarticular Injection: AP Oblique View

Contrast Injection: Facet Joint and Synovial Cyst

(Left) *Fluoroscopic spot radiograph obtained during lumbar facet joint injection shows contrast ➡ about the joint; particularly note linear craniocaudal extension of contrast ➡, which is characteristic of an intraarticular injection. (Right) AP fluoroscopic spot radiograph shows contrast opacification within the facet joint extending caudally into a focal collection consistent with a synovial cyst ➡.*

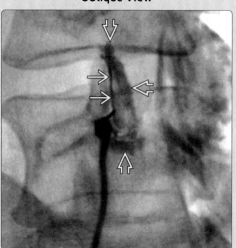

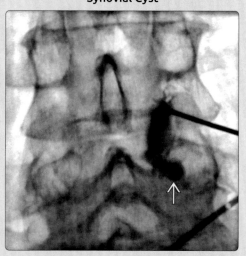

TERMINOLOGY

Abbreviations

- Facet joint injection (FJI)

Definitions

- Injection of corticosteroid ± anesthetic into lumbar facet joint

PREPROCEDURE

Indications

- Facet joint osteoarthritis
- Synovial cyst causing neurologic symptoms

Contraindications

- Local or systemic infection
- Coagulopathy
- Allergy to injectate

Getting Started

- Things to check
  o Imaging of facet joint for pathology and anatomic relationships
  o Informed consent
  o Laboratory: Coagulation parameters

PROCEDURE

Patient Position/Location

- Best procedure approach
  o Prone
    – Angle C-arm or PA fluoroscopy tube slightly toward side of joint to be injected
    – May need slight cranial angulation as well to optimize joint visualization
    – Generally, lower 1/3 of joint is most amenable to needle entry/injection in arthritic joint
      □ Inferior recess may be only accessible site for injection in severely arthritic joint

Procedure Steps

- Ensure correct spine level for injection
- Target lower 1/3 of joint space
  o Often, arthritic joints will have redundancy inferiorly, creating more accessible joint space
- Perform sterile prep and drape
- Apply local anesthetic
- Place spinal needle into subcutaneous tissue, and confirm trajectory with imaging
- Advance until bone is reached or feel needle advance into joint space
- If reach bone, "walk" needle into joint
- Attach preloaded contrast tubing and syringe
- Slowly inject only enough contrast to confirm needle tip in joint space
- Remix and attach injectate syringe
- Slowly inject
- Note patient's symptoms during and immediately following injection
- **Synovial cyst therapeutic rupture**
  o Same steps as FJI

- o Alternate approach is interlaminar puncture of cyst
  – CT guidance suggested for translaminar approach
- o Patient will often feel "pop" with cyst rupture
  – May require significant injection pressure
  – Can be quite painful for patient
- o Interventionalist will see sudden spread of contrast into epidural space with cyst rupture

Alternative Procedures/Therapies

- Radiologic
  o Medial branch block
  o Epidural steroid injection
  o Percutaneous facet joint fusion

POST PROCEDURE

Expected Outcome

- Improved pain symptoms

Things to Do

- Help patient from procedure table
- Establish follow-up
- Remind patient to keep pain diary until next clinic appointment

Things to Avoid

- Strenuous activity for remainder of day
- Bathing for 48 hours

OUTCOMES

Problems

- Failure to alleviate pain
  o Technical failure
    – Wrong level injected
    – Injection extraarticular
  o Clinical failure
    – Facet joint not source of pain
      □ May require multilevel injections
    – Multifactorial pain

Complications

- Most feared complication(s)
  o Thecal sac puncture
    – Cord injury
    – Meningitis
    – Cerebrospinal fluid leak
- Other complications
  o Bleeding
  o Infection
  o Nerve injury

SELECTED REFERENCES

1. Datta S et al: Systematic assessment of diagnostic accuracy and therapeutic utility of lumbar facet joint interventions. Pain Physician. 12(2):437-60, 2009
2. Martha JF et al: Outcome of percutaneous rupture of lumbar synovial cysts: a case series of 101 patients. Spine J. 9(11):899-904, 2009

Selective Nerve Root Block, Lumbar Spine

TERMINOLOGY

- Selective corticosteroid and long-acting anesthetic injection of lumbar nerve root at level of neural foramen

PREPROCEDURE

- Imaging
  - Single or multilevel involvement

PROCEDURE

- Carefully determine correct level(s) for injection
  - Nerve root exits below pedicle of same numbered vertebral body
- 2 approaches for lumbar selective nerve root block
  - Angle C-arm toward side to be injected and target beneath pedicle/"eye" of "Scotty dog"
  - Using AP projection, mark skin 6-8 cm lateral to neural foramen and determine trajectory to foramen
- Assess pain score/reproduction of pain before, during, and after injection

- Findings and reporting
  - Pain before, during, and after injection
  - Was pain reproduced by procedure?
  - Level(s) injected including injectate volume and medications injected

POST PROCEDURE

- Expectation
  - Significant reduction in pain following injection (may take 48-72 hours)

OUTCOMES

- Most feared complications
  - Dural puncture (spinal cord injury, meningitis, CSF leak)
  - Vascular injury/intravascular injection (spinal cord ischemia)
- Problems
  - Failure of pain relief
  - Vasovagal reaction

Anatomy

Intraforaminal and Epidural Injection

(Left) Sagittal T1-weighted MR shows hyperintense fat ➡ in the neural foramina surrounding the lumbar nerve roots. The nerve root is located superiorly ➡, like thoracic nerves. Cervical nerves are located inferiorly. (Right) AP spot radiograph shows the needle tip ➡ deep within the neural foramen beneath the central aspect of the pedicle ➡ with contrast within the left L5 neural foramen ➡ as well as a large volume of contrast extending into the right dorsolateral epidural space from the L4-S1 levels ➡.

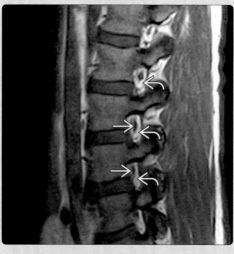

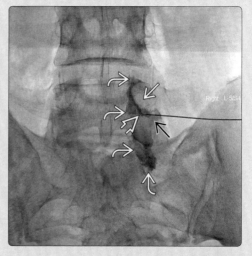

Needle Placement: Oblique View

Intraforaminal and Epidural Injection

(Left) Oblique "Scotty dog" view of the lumbar spine allows targeting of the neural foramen beneath the pedicle/"eye" ➡, and then advance the needle parallel to the imaging beam ➡. Intermittent lateral imaging is essential to determine needle depth. (Right) AP image from another patient shows the expected linear appearance of contrast tracking along the exiting lumbar nerve root ➡. In addition, there is contrast extending slightly above the neural foramen, medial to the pedicle, into the epidural space ➡.

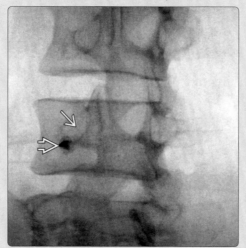

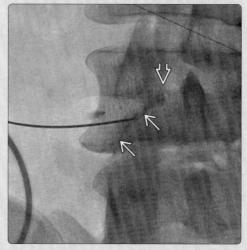

TERMINOLOGY

Abbreviations

- Selective nerve root block (SNRB), epidural steroid injection (ESI)

Definitions

- Selective corticosteroid and long-acting anesthetic injection of lumbar nerve root at level of neural foramen

PREPROCEDURE

Indications

- Lumbar radiculopathy
  o Lumbar osteoarthritis
  o Posttraumatic osteoarthritis

Contraindications

- Coagulopathy
- Local or systemic infection
- Severe allergy to components of injectate
- Relative
  o Pregnancy, iodinated contrast allergy, recent live virus vaccination

Getting Started

- Things to check
  o Preprocedure imaging
    - Look for causative lesion and single or multilevel involvement
  o Laboratory data
    - Signs of infection or coagulopathy
  o Informed consent
- Medications
  o Corticosteroid
  o Long-acting anesthetic
  o Short-acting (local) anesthetic
  o Myelography-safe iodinated contrast

PROCEDURE

Patient Position/Location

- Best procedure approach
  o Prone
    - 2 approaches for lumbar SNRB
      □ Angle C-arm toward side to be injected and target foramen beneath pedicle/"eye" of "Scotty dog"
      □ Use anteroposterior projection and mark skin 6-8 cm lateral to neural foramen

Procedure Steps

- Procedural "time out"
  o Verify correct patient, side of injection, and procedure to be performed
- Carefully determine correct level(s) for injection
- Mark skin at appropriate level and perform sterile prep and drape
- Anchor 22-gauge spinal needle and check trajectory with AP and lateral fluoroscopy
- Carefully advance needle under intermittent frontal and lateral fluoroscopy until foramen or bone is reached

- Remove stylette, observe hub for blood, then attach contrast syringe/tubing
- Aspirate gently, then inject myelography-safe contrast
  o Watch for vascular enhancement and adjust needle tip if necessary
  o Should see contrast track along nerve root
- Remove contrast tubing then mix and attach injectate syringe
- Slowly inject, noting patient pain and whether characteristic pain is reproduced
- Remove needle and obtain hemostasis

Findings and Reporting

- Pain before, during, and after injection
  o Was pain reproduced by procedure?
- Level(s) injected including injectate volume and medications injected
  o SNRB ± transforaminal ESI

POST PROCEDURE

Expected Outcome

- Significant reduction in pain following injection
  o May experience worsening of pain between local anesthetic wearing off and corticosteroid taking effect (48-72 hours)

Things to Do

- Remind patient to keep pain diary until next clinic visit

Things to Avoid

- Bathing for 48-72 hours

OUTCOMES

Problems

- Failure of pain relief
  o Improper needle placement/extraforaminal injection
  o Improper level injected
- Vasovagal reaction

Complications

- Most feared complication(s)
  o Dural puncture (spinal cord injury, meningitis, CSF leak)
  o Vascular injury/intravascular injection (spinal cord ischemia)
- Other complications
  o Bleeding, nerve root injury, infection

SELECTED REFERENCES

1. Boezaart AP et al: Paravertebral block: cervical, thoracic, lumbar, and sacral. Curr Opin Anaesthesiol. 22(5):637-43, 2009
2. Eckel TS et al: Epidural steroid injections and selective nerve root blocks. Tech Vasc Interv Radiol. 12(1):11-21, 2009
3. Manchikanti L et al: Comprehensive review of neurophysiologic basis and diagnostic interventions in managing chronic spinal pain. Pain Physician. 12(4):E71-120, 2009
4. Roberts ST et al: Efficacy of lumbosacral transforaminal epidural steroid injections: a systematic review. PM R. 1(7):657-68, 2009

Epidural Steroid Injection, Lumbar Spine

TERMINOLOGY

- Corticosteroid/anesthetic injection into lumbar epidural space via interlaminar, transforaminal, or caudal approach

PREPROCEDURE

- Indications
  - Lumbar radiculopathy
  - Residual pain following vertebroplasty/kyphoplasty
- Things to check
  - Prior imaging: Adequate epidural space (especially important in postoperative back!)
- Avoid interlaminar approach in patient with severe canal stenosis without identifiable epidural space on preprocedure imaging
- Literature supports use of nonparticulate steroid (dexamethasone) to minimize possibility of small vessel vascular embolization

PROCEDURE

- Interlaminar epidural steroid injection (ESI)
  - Target superior lamina near midline
- Transforaminal ESI
  - Target superomedial neural foramen
- Caudal ESI
  - Target sacral hiatus at midline, and consider catheter placement in patients requiring higher lumbar level injections

POST PROCEDURE

- Expectations
  - Reproduction of pain with needle placement/injection
  - Significant improvement in pain after injection

OUTCOMES

- Most feared complications
  - Intravascular injection/spinal cord ischemia
  - Spinal cord puncture

Severe Central Canal Stenosis

(Left) Sagittal T1WI MR shows severe central canal stenosis ➡ at each disc level due to disc bulge/osteophyte and posterior ligamentous laxity. Note the epidural fat ➡ at levels above surgery. (Right) AP fluoroscopic image obtained during lumbar epidural steroid injection (ESI) shows anatomic landmarks and well-defined interlaminar space ➡. Note the spinous process ➡ and cortex of laminae above and below ➡.

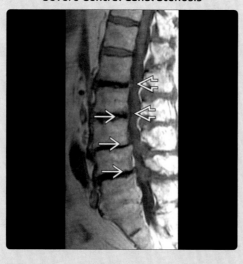

Needle Placement: Interlaminar ESI

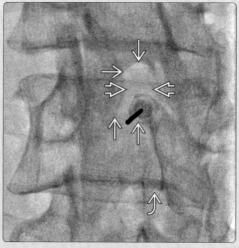

Transforaminal ESI

(Left) AP view obtained in this patient undergoing right L1/2 transforaminal ESI shows contrast ➡ spreading medial to the pedicle and cephalad within the lumbar epidural space. (Right) The lateral view provides additional confirmation that contrast is predominantly spreading within the dorsal epidural space ➡ and is noted to extend readily in a cephalad direction.

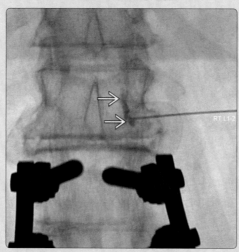

Contrast Spread in Dorsal Epidural Space

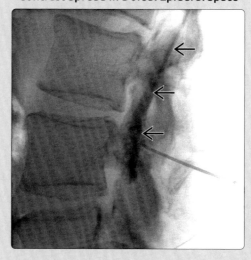

TERMINOLOGY

Abbreviations

- Epidural steroid injection (ESI)

Definitions

- Corticosteroid/anesthetic injection into lumbar epidural space via interlaminar or transforaminal approach

PREPROCEDURE

Indications

- Lumbar radiculopathy
  - Degenerative disc disease
  - Posttraumatic

Contraindications

- Coagulopathy
- Allergy to injectate
- Local or systemic infection
- Relative contraindications
  - Iodinated contrast allergy, pregnancy, active hepatitis

Getting Started

- Things to check
  - Laboratory data
    - Coagulation studies as indicated for patients undergoing anticoagulation therapy
      □ Prothrombin time, activated partial thromboplastin time, international normalized ratio, platelet count
- Equipment list
  - Interlaminar ESI
    - Glass syringe with preservative-free saline ("loss of resistance" technique)
    - 18- to 22-gauge Tuohy or Whitacre needle
  - Transforaminal ESI
    - 22-gauge spinal needle
  - Caudal ESI
    - 18- to 22-gauge Tuohy or Whitacre needle

PROCEDURE

Patient Position/Location

- Best procedure approach
  - Prone

Procedure Steps

- Steroid: Literature supports use of nonparticulate steroid (dexamethasone) to minimize possibility of small vessel vascular embolization
  - No strong literature support for better efficacy of particulate or Depo preparations
- **Interlaminar**
  - Target superior lamina near midline
  - Carefully "walk" off lamina superiorly, then attach glass syringe
  - Very carefully advance needle until loss of resistance occurs with glass syringe plunging
- **Transforaminal**
  - Target superomedial neural foramen
  - Slowly advance adjacent to exiting nerve root
- **Caudal**
  - Sacral hiatus/canal
  - Advance Tuohy needle through canal to epidural space using "loss of resistance" technique
    - If contrast does not opacify high enough into lumbar canal, consider use of catheter or vascular sheath
      □ Exchange needle over 0.035 wire, and navigate sheath or catheter over wire to desired level under fluoroscopic guidance
- Document needle placement with imaging
- Attach injectate, and slowly inject

Findings and Reporting

- Document level, amount of pain before and after procedure

POST PROCEDURE

Expected Outcome

- Reproduction of pain with needle placement/injection
- Improvement in pain after injection

Things to Avoid

- Interlaminar approach in patient with severe canal stenosis without identifiable epidural space on preprocedure imaging

OUTCOMES

Problems

- Incorrect level injected/failure of pain relief
- Vasovagal reaction

Complications

- Most feared complication(s)
  - Intravascular injection
    - Spinal cord ischemia
  - Spinal cord puncture

SELECTED REFERENCES

1. Dietrich TJ et al: Particulate versus non-particulate steroids for lumbar transforaminal or interlaminar epidural steroid injections: an update. Skeletal Radiol. 44(2):149-55, 2015
2. Fekete T et al: The effect of epidural steroid injection on postoperative outcome in patients from the lumbar spinal stenosis outcome study. Spine (Phila Pa 1976). 40(16):1303-10, 2015
3. Rathmell JP et al: Safeguards to prevent neurologic complications after epidural steroid injections: consensus opinions from a multidisciplinary working group and national organizations. Anesthesiology. 122(5):974-84, 2015
4. El-Yachouchi C et al: The noninferiority of the nonparticulate steroid dexamethasone vs the particulate steroids betamethasone and triamcinolone in lumbar transforaminal epidural steroid injections. Pain Med. 14(11):1650-7, 2013
5. Chang Chien GC et al: Digital subtraction angiography does not reliably prevent paraplegia associated with lumbar transforaminal epidural steroid injection. Pain Physician. 15(6):515-23, 2012
6. Peterson C et al: Evidence-based radiology (part 1): is there sufficient research to support the use of therapeutic injections for the spine and sacroiliac joints? Skeletal Radiol. 39(1):5-9, 2010
7. Wybier M et al: Paraplegia complicating selective steroid injections of the lumbar spine. Report of five cases and review of the literature. Eur Radiol. 20(1):181-9, 2010
8. Eckel TS et al: Epidural steroid injections and selective nerve root blocks. Tech Vasc Interv Radiol. 12(1):11-21, 2009

TERMINOLOGY

- Percutaneous cement augmentation of vertebral body

PREPROCEDURE

- STIR MR provides excellent depiction of bone marrow edema in acute fracture
- Clinical examination
  - Consistent with imaging findings
  - Point tenderness should be assessed prior to sedation

PROCEDURE

- Can be performed with unipedicular or bipedicular access
  - Ensure that medial pedicle cortex is not violated
  - Use of mallet may be advantageous with nonthreaded access needles
  - Once needle is clearly within vertebral body on lateral view, switch to frontal and lateral views for further needle advancement

- When needle is within anterior 1/3 of vertebral body, reassess position on direct AP and lateral fluoroscopy
- Inject polymethylmethacrylate (PMMA) cement under continuous fluoroscopy
  - Watch carefully for any signs of cement extravasation
  - Ensure that cement does not pass into posterior 1/4 of vertebral body on lateral view

POST PROCEDURE

- Significant improvement in pain following vertebroplasty
  - May require narcotic analgesics and muscle relaxants

OUTCOMES

- Problems: Incomplete pain relief, increased incidence of fractures at adjacent levels
- Most feared complications
  - Spinal cord injury by direct puncture or compression
  - PMMA-induced anaphylaxis
  - Pulmonary PMMA cement embolism

Compression Fractures

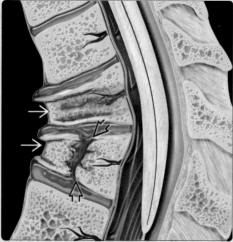

Needle Positioning

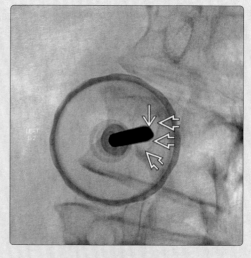

(Left) Sagittal graphic represents 2-level compression fractures ➡ of the lower thoracic spine. Note the vertical cleft ➡ predisposing to polymethylmethacrylate (PMMA) cement extravasation into intervertebral disc spaces. (Right) Oblique spot radiograph shows a needle ➡ positioned within the central/medial aspect of the pedicle. The needle should be within the posterior vertebral body on lateral view when this close to the medial pedicle cortex ➡.

Needle Position

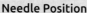
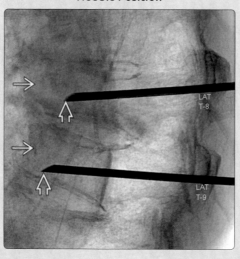

Inadequate vs. Adequate Cement Cross-Filling

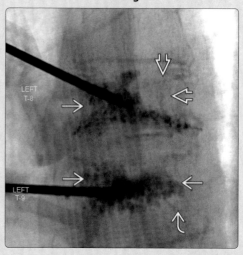

(Left) Lateral fluoroscopic spot radiograph in a patient with T8 and T9 osteoporotic compression fractures ➡ shows unipedicular access to each vertebral body, which was achieved with needle tip ➡ in anterior 1/3 of vertebrae. (Right) Anteroposterior fluoroscopic spot radiograph shows spread of PMMA cement within the T8 and T9 vertebrae ➡. Note failure to fill the right T8 hemivertebra ➡. Excellent cross-filling of T9 is seen extending to the contralateral pedicle ➡.

Vertebroplasty

TERMINOLOGY

Abbreviations
- Polymethylmethacrylate (PMMA)

Definitions
- Percutaneous cement augmentation of fractured vertebral body

PREPROCEDURE

Indications
- Symptomatic vertebral fracture refractory to medical management
  - Osteoporotic, posttraumatic, pathologic
- Impending vertebral fracture
  - Osteoporotic, pathologic

Contraindications
- Coagulopathy
- Inability to tolerate prolonged prone positioning
  - May require anesthesiology consultation

Preprocedure Imaging
- STIR MR provides excellent depiction of bone marrow edema in acute fracture

Getting Started
- Medications
  - Local anesthetic

PROCEDURE

Patient Position/Location
- Best procedure approach
  - Prone
    - C-arm angled obliquely toward pedicle to be accessed
    - Biplane affords advantage of continuous monitoring of needle depth on lateral fluoroscopy

Equipment Preparation
- Draw 10 of mL local anesthetic, and attach long 25-gauge needle
- Ensure all equipment for vertebroplasty is immediately available in desired quantity and sizes
- Angle C-arm for maximal visualization of pedicle to be accessed
- Will vertebral biopsy be performed prior to vertebroplasty?
  - Have biopsy system available
  - Procedure in place for proper specimen handling
- Will vertebral augmentation (cavity creation) be performed prior to vertebroplasty?
  - Ensure compatibility of pedicle access needle with augmentation device

Procedure Steps
- Procedure "time out"
- Initiate conscious sedation/general anesthetic
- Carefully reassess proper level for intervention
- Perform sterile prep and drape, anesthetic
- Anchor pedicle needle in subcutaneous tissue
- Carefully advance pedicle needle to central/lateral portion of vertebral pedicle under fluoroscopy
- Ensure favorable needle trajectory on both oblique and lateral views prior to gaining osseous purchase
- Carefully anchor needle in pedicle
- Incrementally advance needle through pedicle under intermittent oblique and lateral fluoroscopy
- Once needle is clearly within vertebral body on lateral view, switch to frontal and lateral views for further needle advancement
  - Depth best assessed on lateral view
- When needle is within anterior 1/3 of vertebral body, reassess position on direct AP and lateral fluoroscopy
- Repeat steps for contralateral pedicle as needed
- Obtain biplane fluoroscopic image to document needle placement
- Once ready to inject, mix PMMA bone cement per manufacturer's instructions
- Load injector, and check consistency of cement
- When consistency is adequate, per manufacturer's recommendation, attach injector extension stylette if desired, and preload
- Remove pedicle needle, and attach injecting system to pedicle access stylette
- Under constant fluoroscopy, slowly inject cement
- Watch for signs of cement extravasation
  - Ensure that cement does not pass into posterior 1/4 of vertebral body on lateral view
  - If incomplete filling is seen with resistance to antegrade injection
    - Stop injecting, and release forward pressure on injector
- If adequate vertebral filling is seen
  - Stop injection, and release forward pressure on injector
  - Switch to contralateral pedicle needle (if applicable)
- Rotate pedicle needle several times to break any cement adhering to tip
- Carefully remove needle

Alternative Procedures/Therapies
- Radiologic
  - Kyphoplasty
- Surgical
  - Stabilization/fusion

POST PROCEDURE

Expected Outcome
- Significant improvement in pain following vertebroplasty

OUTCOMES

Problems
- Incomplete pain relief
  - Pain may be multifactorial
- Fracture at adjacent levels

Complications
- Most feared complication(s)
  - Spinal cord injury
  - PMMA-induced anaphylaxis
  - Pneumothorax with thoracic vertebroplasty

KEY FACTS

TERMINOLOGY

- Vertebral fracture reduction via bipedicular balloon inflation followed by polymethylmethacrylate (PMMA) cement augmentation

PREPROCEDURE

- Carefully determine correct level
- STIR MR is most sensitive for vertebral edema
- Ensure level of pain is consistent with acutely fractured vertebra on imaging

PROCEDURE

- Angle C-arm toward side of pedicle to be accessed
  - Must have clear view of pedicle cortex
- Lateral fluoroscopy is essential in determining needle depth
- Needle tip in vertebra should allow inflated balloon to be centrally placed in hemivertebra
- Sudden decrease in pressure and heterogeneous contrast extravasation indicates balloon rupture

POST PROCEDURE

- Expectation: Significant decrease in pain following procedure
  - Some patients will develop periprocedural pain requiring narcotics ± muscle relaxants
- Problems: Fracture at additional/adjacent levels
  - Risk appears increased with PMMA cement extravasation into disc space

OUTCOMES

- Most feared complications
  - Spinal cord puncture during needle placement
  - Spinal cord compression by hematoma or cement extravasation

Compression Fracture

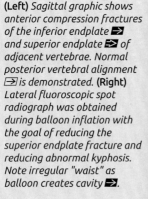
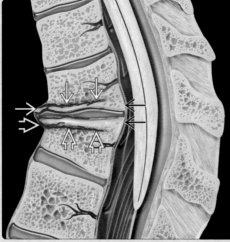

Balloon Inflation

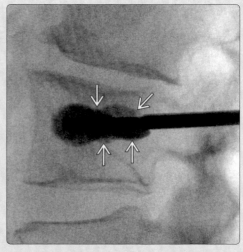

(Left) Sagittal graphic shows anterior compression fractures of the inferior endplate ➡ and superior endplate ➡ of adjacent vertebrae. Normal posterior vertebral alignment ➡ is demonstrated. (Right) Lateral fluoroscopic spot radiograph was obtained during balloon inflation with the goal of reducing the superior endplate fracture and reducing abnormal kyphosis. Note irregular "waist" as balloon creates cavity ➡.

Cement Injection: AP View

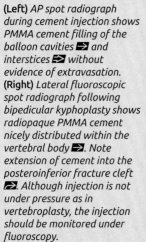
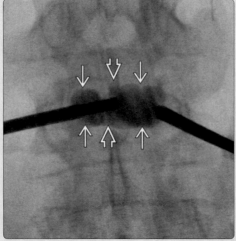

Post Kyphoplasty: Lateral View

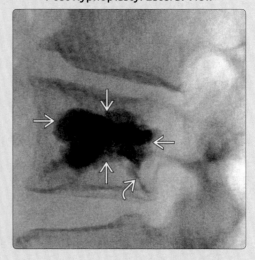

(Left) AP spot radiograph during cement injection shows PMMA cement filling of the balloon cavities ➡ and interstices ➡ without evidence of extravasation. (Right) Lateral fluoroscopic spot radiograph following bipedicular kyphoplasty shows radiopaque PMMA cement nicely distributed within the vertebral body ➡. Note extension of cement into the posteroinferior fracture cleft ➡. Although injection is not under pressure as in vertebroplasty, the injection should be monitored under fluoroscopy.

TERMINOLOGY

Abbreviations

- Polymethylmethacrylate (PMMA)

Definitions

- Vertebral fracture reduction via bipedicular balloon inflation followed by PMMA cement augmentation

PREPROCEDURE

Indications

- Painful vertebral fracture
  - Osteoporotic, posttraumatic
  - Pathologic fracture

Contraindications

- Coagulopathy, infection
- Unstable fracture
- Vertebra plana

Getting Started

- Things to check
  - Laboratory data
    - Evaluate coagulation parameters
  - Informed consent

PROCEDURE

Procedure Steps

- Procedure "time out"
  - Correct patient, level(s), procedure
- Initiate anesthesia or conscious sedation
- Carefully determine correct level(s) to be intervened upon
- Perform sterile prep and drape
- Angle fluoroscopy system to side of pedicle being accessed
- Create skin wheal, and apply local anesthetic to subcutaneous tissues
- If necessary, use 22-gauge spinal needle to reach pedicle under fluoroscopic guidance for deep anesthetic injection
- For thoracic levels, bilateral parapedicular access (outside lateral pedicle cortex) is suggested
- For lumbar levels, bilateral transpedicular approach vs. bilateral parapedicular approach
- Using anesthetic needle as guide, make dermatotomy to accommodate 13-gauge access needle
- Anchor 11- to 13-gauge needle in subcutaneous tissue, and check trajectory with fluoroscopy
- Under intermittent fluoroscopy, guide needle to pedicle cortex
- Prior to gaining purchase within bone, check tip placement on both oblique and lateral fluoroscopy
- Carefully advance access needle under intermittent fluoroscopy until safely within posterior vertebral body (~ 4 mm)
  - Should have "down the barrel" view of needle on oblique fluoroscopy
  - Ensure not to transgress medial pedicle cortex
- Mix PMMA cement
  - Most operators prefer consistency similar to toothpaste
- Remove stylette of 1 access needle

- Drill channel (under fluoroscopy) to accommodate balloon
  - Alternative is to perform core biopsy as indicated (also creates channel for balloon)
  - Place balloon through access needle
- Remove stylette of contralateral access needle, and repeat steps
- Under barometric control, inflate 1 balloon then other
  - For 15-mm balloon, usual injection volume is ≤ 4 mL
  - For 20-mm balloon, usual injection volume is ≤ 6 mL
- Assess degree of fracture reduction achieved with balloon inflation
- Watch carefully to avoid disruption of lateral cortex &/or endplates during inflation
- Sudden decrease in pressure and heterogeneous contrast extravasation indicate balloon rupture
- Deflate 1 balloon then other
  - Watch for signs of loss of fracture reduction
  - If fracture reduction is maintained, remove both balloons
- Inject PMMA cement through each needle
- After polymerization, twist needle several times to break connection between needle tip and cement
- Remove needles carefully to avoid injury to operator, equipment, and patient

Alternative Procedures/Therapies

- Radiologic
  - Vertebroplasty
  - Vertebral augmentation
  - Epidural steroid injection

POST PROCEDURE

Expected Outcome

- Significant decrease in pain following procedure
  - Some patients will develop periprocedural pain requiring narcotic pain medication ± muscle relaxants
  - Some may require pain injections (epidural or trigger point)

OUTCOMES

Problems

- Incomplete pain relief
- Balloon rupture
  - Generally not clinically significant
  - Likely related to aggressive inflation

Complications

- Most feared complication(s)
  - Spinal cord puncture during needle placement
  - Spinal cord compression by hematoma or cement extravasation
  - PMMA anaphylaxis
  - Pulmonary embolism
  - Endplate or lateral cortical fracture

SELECTED REFERENCES

1. Chen WJ et al: Impact of cement leakage into disks on the development of adjacent vertebral compression fractures. J Spinal Disord Tech. 23(1):35-9, 2010

KEY FACTS

TERMINOLOGY

- Percutaneous stabilization of sacral fracture via bone cement injection

PREPROCEDURE

- Indications
  - Insufficiency fracture
  - Pathologic fracture
  - Posttraumatic fracture
- Laboratory data
  - Coagulation parameters
  - Infection/inflammation markers
- Imaging
  - Consistent with acute/subacute fracture
  - Look for retropulsion of bone fragments into sacral canal or neural foramina
  - Look for cortical breakthrough and epidural extension associated with tumors

PROCEDURE

- Prone
  - AP fluoroscopy angled slightly to optimize visualization of entire sacrum
  - Direct lateral view is very important for optimal needle placement
  - Rotational flat-panel imaging may assist with confident needle placement prior to cement injection
- Advance needle through sacrum from dorsal S3 through upper S1 segment under intermittent fluoroscopic visualization
- Watch carefully for cement extravasation into sacroiliac joint, vasculature, &/or neural foramina

OUTCOMES

- Problems: Inability to diffuse polymethylmethacrylate throughout fracture/incomplete stabilization; cement extravasation into SI joints/sacral foramina/paraspinal veins

---

Sacral Insufficiency Fractures

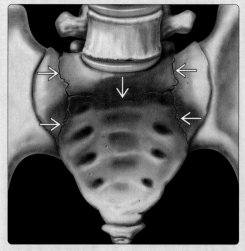

Sacral Insufficiency Fractures

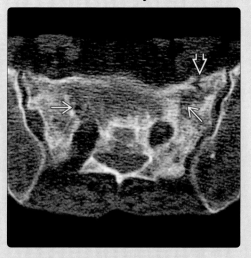

(Left) *Coronal graphic depicts the characteristic H-shaped sacral insufficiency fracture ➡ with bilateral vertical sacral alar and horizontal upper sacral fractures.* (Right) *Axial bone CT shows bilateral ill-defined sacral lucencies ➡ in keeping with sacral ala fractures. The left-sided fracture line extends to the anterior cortex ➡.*

Bilateral Needle Placement: AP View

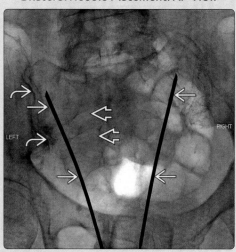

Cement Injection: Lateral View

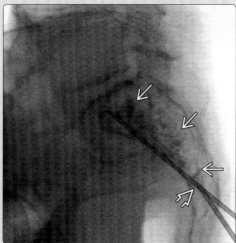

(Left) *An AP fluoroscopic spot radiograph was obtained following placement of bilateral 13-gauge vertebroplasty needles ➡ from the S3 through S1 segments. Note needle trajectory between the sacral foramina ➡ medially and the sacroiliac joint ➡ laterally.* (Right) *Lateral view obtained after injection of the right needle ➡ reinforces the need for cautious fluoroscopic observation in AP plane during injection, as the lateral view is obscured by preexisting cement ➡.*

TERMINOLOGY

Abbreviations

- Polymethylmethacrylate (PMMA)
- Rotational flat-panel imaging (RFPI)
- Sacroiliac (SI)
- Transient ischemic attacks (TIAs)

Synonyms

- Sacral augmentation

Definitions

- Percutaneous stabilization of sacral fracture via bone cement injection

PREPROCEDURE

Indications

- Sacral fracture
  - Insufficiency fracture
  - Pathologic fracture
  - Posttraumatic fracture

Contraindications

- Coagulopathy
  - Patients on anticoagulation
    - Hypercoagulable state, atrial dysrhythmias, TIAs, etc.
    - Patients with acute/chronic liver or renal disease
- Local or systemic infection

Getting Started

- Things to check
  - Coagulation parameters
    - Prothrombin time, activated partial thromboplastin time, international normalized ratio
    - Platelet count
  - Infection/inflammation markers
    - White blood cell count, fever
    - Cultures (if applicable)
    - C-reactive protein, erythrocyte sedimentation rate
  - Preprocedure imaging
    - Consistent with acute/subacute fracture
  - Informed consent
- Medications
  - Short-acting local anesthetic

PROCEDURE

Patient Position/Location

- Best procedure approach
  - Prone

Procedure Steps

- Procedure "time out"
  - Correct patient, procedure, side
- Provide conscious sedation/general anesthesia as indicated
- Perform sterile prep and drape, anesthetic
- Advance 13-gauge needle into S3 segment
  - Observe placement under lateral fluoroscopy
- Advance needle through sacrum from dorsal S3 to upper S1 segment under intermittent fluoroscopic visualization
  - Rotational flat-panel imaging may assist in confirmation of needle placement prior to cement injection
- Repeat steps for 2nd needle placement
- Confirm needle placement with RFPI if desired
- Mix PMMA bone cement
- Prepare injector per manufacturer's instructions
- Commercially available injection stylettes can be prefilled and passed through access needles
- Slowly inject 1 side of sacrum under continuous fluoroscopy
  - Watch carefully for cement extravasation into SI joint, vasculature, &/or neural foramina
- Withdraw needle as needed to allow cement to fill fracture lines of all 3 sacral segments
- Repeat injection through 2nd needle
  - Visualization will be impaired on lateral view due to previously placed bone cement
- Remove needles carefully after several twists
- Obtain hemostasis

Alternative Procedures/Therapies

- Radiologic
  - Adjunctive pain injections may be indicated in select patients
    - Caudal epidural steroid injection
    - Sacroiliac joint injection(s)
- Surgical
  - Open fracture fixation

POST PROCEDURE

Expected Outcome

- Successful percutaneous stabilization of sacral fracture
- Resolution or significant improvement in patient pain

OUTCOMES

Problems

- Inability to diffuse PMMA throughout fracture/incomplete stabilization
- Cement extravasation into SI joints/sacral foramina/paraspinal veins
- Residual pain after sacroplasty
  - May require anesthetic/steroid injection

Complications

- Most feared complication(s)
  - Compressive neuropathy secondary to PMMA extravasation into sacral foramina or caudal epidural space
  - Pulmonary PMMA embolization
  - PMMA anaphylaxis

SELECTED REFERENCES

1. Basile A et al: Sacroplasty for local or massive localization of multiple myeloma. Cardiovasc Intervent Radiol. 33(6):1270-7, 2010
2. Jayaraman MV et al: An easily identifiable anatomic landmark for fluoroscopically guided sacroplasty: anatomic description and validation with treatment in 13 patients. AJNR Am J Neuroradiol. 30(5):1070-3, 2009
3. Ortiz AO et al: Sacroplasty. Tech Vasc Interv Radiol. 12(1):51-63, 2009

TERMINOLOGY

- Image-guided percutaneous vertebral biopsy
- Cerebrospinal fluid

PREPROCEDURE

- Indications
  - Suspected tumor (biopsy ± vertebroplasty/kyphoplasty)
  - Osteomyelitis/discitis (identify responsible organism, determine antimicrobial sensitivity)

PROCEDURE

- Biopsy ± fine-needle aspiration (FNA)
  - ± vertebroplasty, kyphoplasty, vertebral augmentation
- Selection of biopsy system to use depends on
  - Lesion size, location
  - Operator experience/preference

POST PROCEDURE

- Ensure proper specimen handling, communication of results to clinician
- Follow-up on biopsy results
  - Operator quality assurance
  - Accountability to patient and referring clinician

OUTCOMES

- Problems
  - Nondiagnostic specimen
    - May be reduced by pathologist in attendance if FNA to be performed
      - FNA not practical to confirm specimen in cases of bone biopsy
- Complications
  - Most feared: Spinal cord or vascular injury, epidural/subdural hematoma, osteomyelitis, meningitis
  - Others: Local infection, bleeding, nerve injury

Fluoroscopy-Guided Biopsy

Transpedicular Approach

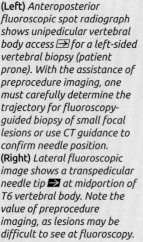
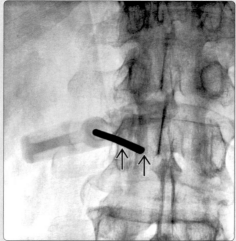
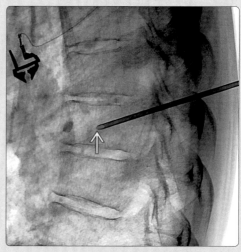

(Left) Anteroposterior fluoroscopic spot radiograph shows unipedicular vertebral body access ⇨ for a left-sided vertebral biopsy (patient prone). With the assistance of preprocedure imaging, one must carefully determine the trajectory for fluoroscopy-guided biopsy of small focal lesions or use CT guidance to confirm needle position. (Right) Lateral fluoroscopic image shows a transpedicular needle tip ⇨ at midportion of T6 vertebral body. Note the value of preprocedure imaging, as lesions may be difficult to see at fluoroscopy.

Pedicle Access

CT-Guided Biopsy

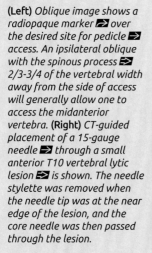
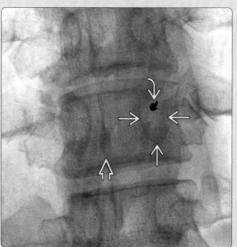
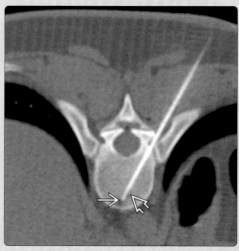

(Left) Oblique image shows a radiopaque marker ⇨ over the desired site for pedicle ⇨ access. An ipsilateral oblique with the spinous process ⇨ 2/3-3/4 of the vertebral width away from the side of access will generally allow one to access the midanterior vertebra. (Right) CT-guided placement of a 15-gauge needle ⇨ through a small anterior T10 vertebral lytic lesion ⇨ is shown. The needle stylette was removed when the needle tip was at the near edge of the lesion, and the core needle was then passed through the lesion.

Vertebral Biopsy

TERMINOLOGY

Abbreviations
- Fine-needle aspiration (FNA)

Definitions
- Image-guided percutaneous vertebral biopsy

PREPROCEDURE

Indications
- Suspected tumor
  - Biopsy for pathology
  - ± vertebroplasty/kyphoplasty
- Osteomyelitis
- Discitis

Contraindications
- Coagulopathy
- Anticoagulation
  - Patients with atrial fibrillation, TIA, etc.
- Contraindication to sedation/anesthesia
  - Unable to tolerate prolonged prone positioning

Getting Started
- Things to check
  - Check laboratory data
    - Coagulopathy/anticoagulation
      - Complete blood count, prothrombin time, activated partial thromboplastin time, international normalized ratio, bleeding time
    - Infection/inflammatory markers
      - White blood cell count, c-reactive protein, erythrocyte sedimentation rate, temperature
    - Cerebrospinal fluid studies if applicable
      - Cytology or increased white blood cell count
  - Obtain informed consent

PROCEDURE

Patient Position/Location
- Best procedure approach
  - Prone

Procedure Steps
- Procedure "time out"
  - Correct patient, level, procedure
- Under fluoroscopy or CT, localize optimal bone access point to reach lesion safely
  - Transpedicular: Angle fluoroscopy tube toward pedicle to be accessed
    - Ensure good visualization of pedicle margins
  - CT: Localize lesion in axial plane
    - Sagittal reformatted images may assist in determining correct level/needle trajectory
- Initiate conscious sedation
- Carefully localize target with imaging
- Perform sterile prep, drape, and anesthetic
- Transpedicular
  - Prior to anchoring needle in pedicle cortex
    - Carefully guide needle to pedicle

- Surgical clamps are helpful in holding needle without exposing hand in field of view
  - Ensure angle of entry is satisfactory
    - To reach biopsy target
    - To avoid medial pedicle cortex
  - Anchor transpedicular needle in pedicle
  - Advance carefully, checking frequently under fluoroscopy to ensure needle remains within pedicle
  - Advance to margin of vertebral lesion to be sampled
    - If FNA is desired, this may be performed through stylette
    - For biopsy without vertebroplasty/kyphoplasty/vertebral augmentation
      - Remove needle, and advance biopsy stylette (under gentle aspiration if applicable) through lesion under fluoroscopy
      - If desired, smaller coaxial biopsy can be obtained 1st with larger transpedicular biopsy needle used for 2nd specimen
      - Remove biopsy needle, and confirm adequate specimen
- Posterior element or cervical spine
  - Target specific lesion, and guide biopsy system under intermittent imaging to margin of lesion
    - CT guidance often preferred for posterior element and cervical spine lesions

Alternative Procedures/Therapies
- Surgical
  - Open biopsy
  - Corpectomy/fusion

OUTCOMES

Problems
- Nondiagnostic specimen
  - May be reduced by pathologist in attendance if FNA to be performed
    - Often not practical in cases of bone biopsy to confirm adequate specimen
      - Solid bone core often will not "touch off" onto slide for quick microscopic analysis

Complications
- Most feared complication(s)
  - Spinal cord injury
  - Vascular injury
  - Epidural/subdural hematoma
  - Osteomyelitis
  - Meningitis
- Other complications
  - Dural puncture
  - Nerve root injury
  - Infection
  - Bleeding

SELECTED REFERENCES

1. Powell MF et al: C-arm fluoroscopic cone beam CT for guidance of minimally invasive spine interventions. Pain Physician. 13(1):51-9, 2010
2. Bayley E et al: Percutaneous approach to the upper thoracic spine: optimal patient positioning. Eur Spine J. 18(12):1986-8, 2009
3. Dave BR et al: Transpedicular percutaneous biopsy of vertebral body lesions: a series of 71 cases. Spinal Cord. 47(5):384-9, 2009

Percutaneous Discectomy

TERMINOLOGY

- Percutaneous disc removal to reduce intradiscal pressure → protruded disc retracts back in place, reduced irritation on annulus nociceptive nerve receptors
  - Also decompresses nerve root from disc
  - Another proposed mechanism: Removing disc material may prevent release of chemical mediators that directly injure nerve root

PREPROCEDURE

- Radicular pain usually greater than back pain/neck pain
- Positive CT or MR scan for disc herniation
- Contained herniated disc of < 6 mm
  - Contained herniated discs have intact outer annulus with displaced disc material held within outer annulus of contained herniated disc
  - Noncontained herniated disc has localized displacement of disc material beyond intervertebral disc space & breach in outer annulus

- No improvement of symptoms after 6-8 weeks of conservative therapy
- Before percutaneous discectomy (PD), pain relief should be confirmed after selective nerve root block has been performed

POST PROCEDURE

- PD may provide appropriate relief in properly selected patients with contained lumbar disc prolapse
  - Reduced procedure time, lower costs, quick recovery, and low complication rates that can include discitis and possible nerve injury

OUTCOMES

- Complications: Nerve root or blood vessel injury
  - Infection, bleeding, discitis

Percutaneous Discectomy Approach

(Left) Percutaneous discectomy device reaches the disc via a posterolateral approach, passing just anterior to the superior articular facet, behind the nerve, in a trajectory toward the center of the disc. A contained foraminal protrusion is noted ➡. (Right) After local anesthesia, an incision of a few millimeters is performed, allowing the introduction of a coaxial trocar to the level of the disc. The decompression probe is then introduced, removing disc material.

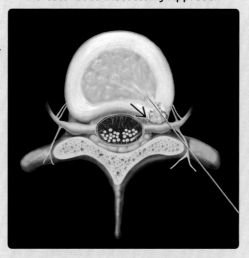

Sagittal Oblique Graphic of Percutaneous Discectomy

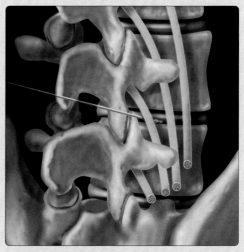

Lateral Oblique Radiograph of Percutaneous Discectomy

(Left) Oblique radiograph demonstrates the device tip in the target object ➡. Using only local anesthesia allows the patient to react to any nerve root impingement. If the patient experiences radicular pain during the procedure, the instruments are redirected, thus preventing a nerve root injury. (Right) Axial NECT shows an automated probe passing anterolaterally to the herniation and coming to rest in the center of the disc. Most of the disc removal occurs 1 cm anterior to the herniation.

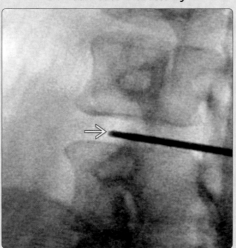

Axial CT of Percutaneous Discectomy

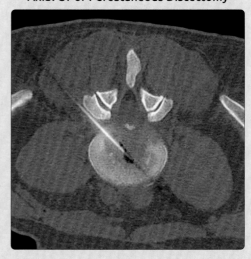

TERMINOLOGY

Abbreviations

- Percutaneous discectomy (PD)

Definitions

- Percutaneous disc removal reduces intradiscal pressure

PREPROCEDURE

Indications

- Radicular pain usually greater than back pain/neck pain
  - Symptoms include sensory loss, tingling, numbness, & muscle weakness
- Positive CT or MR scan for disc herniation
  - Contained herniated disc of < 6 mm
- No improvement of symptoms after 6-8 weeks of conservative therapy

Contraindications

- Evidence of acute or progressive degenerative spinal cord diseases
- Evidence of neurologic or vascular pathologies mimicking herniated disc
- Evidence of advanced spondylosis (significant bony spurs) with disc space narrowing, diffuse annular bulging, or spondylolisthesis
- Evidence of significant bony spurs blocking entry to disc space
- Evidence of cervical spinal canal or lateral recess narrowing
- Evidence of large extruded disc or sequestered disc fragment
- Existence of other pathologies or conditions, such as fractures, tumors, pregnancy, or active infections
- Previous surgery at site of herniated disc

Getting Started

- Things to check
  - Coagulation parameters, platelets, blood count
  - Allergies
- Equipment list
  - Stryker Dekompressor (Stryker Interventional Spine; Kalamazoo, Michigan)
    - Disposable, self-contained, battery-operated hand piece connected to helical probe
    - Outer cannula measures 1.5 mm with inner rotating probe
    - When activated, probe rotates creating suction to pull milled nucleus pulposus from disc up cannula to suction chamber at base of handheld unit
    - ~ 0.5-2.0 mL of nucleus pulposus is removed
    - Efficient removal of disc material decreases surgical procedure times to ~ 30 minutes with actual time of use for probe not exceeding 10 minutes
    - Procedure is done under fluoroscopic guidance

PROCEDURE

Patient Position/Location

- Best procedure approach
  - Lateral decubitus or prone position
  - Via posterolateral approach, instrument passes just anterior to superior articular facet, behind nerve, in trajectory toward center of disc

Procedure Steps

- Before PD, pain relief should be confirmed after selective nerve root block has been performed
- On AP view, align endplates and pedicles
  - Then rotate fluoroscope by ~ 30° to oblique position until superior articulating process bisects endplates
  - Object target is in site when disc is seen lateral to superior articulating process
- Stryker Dekompressor PD probe or MDS MicroDebrider System (Endius; Plainville, Massachusetts)
  - Terminal portion of probe is placed into herniated disc using fluoroscopic guidance
  - Device is used to suction out some or all degenerated central disc tissue
    - Dekompressor is activated and slightly pushed in and out ~ 1 cm
    - After running for 2 minutes, probe is removed, and distal portion is cut off and sent to pathology for quantitative and qualitative analysis

Alternative Procedures/Therapies

- Radiologic
  - CT-guided or performed under fluoroscopy
- Other
  - Laser discectomy, including YAG, KTP, holmium, argon, & carbon dioxide lasers
    - Procedure involves placing laser within nucleus under fluoroscopic guidance, after which laser is activated
      - Laser energy is transformed into heat to vaporize disc tissue
    - Due to differences in absorption, energy requirements & rate of application differ among lasers
  - Disc nucleoplasty procedure uses bipolar radiofrequency energy [Coblation (ArthroCare Spine: Sunnyvale, California)]
    - Small, multiple electrodes emit energy to ablate portion of nucleus tissue with low temperature

POST PROCEDURE

Expected Outcome

- PD may provide appropriate relief in properly selected patients with contained lumbar disc prolapse

OUTCOMES

Problems

- Dekompressor technique has yet to be studied in controlled clinical trial; results with this new automated technique are limited

Complications

- Most feared complication(s)
  - Nerve root or blood vessel injury

KEY FACTS

TERMINOLOGY

- Terminology
  - Heating of annulus to seal annular fissures
    - Denervate pain fibers along outer 1/3 of annulus
  - Relief of low back and referred leg pain may also be due to collagen modification
- Indications
  - Symptoms of degenerative lumbar disc disease at least 6-month duration
  - Failure to improve with minimum of 6 months of conservative therapy (pain medication and physical therapy)
  - Predominant low back pain ± radiculopathy
  - MR shows global disc degeneration or posterior/posterolateral annular fissure
  - "Positive" discography: Pain of "significant" intensity on disc injections and similar to patient's usual pain
- Contraindications

- Evidence of large contained or sequestered disc herniation
- Loss of > 50% of disc height at target level
- Neurogenic claudication due to spinal stenosis
- Previous back surgery at any level
- Spondylolisthesis at symptomatic disc level
- Coagulopathy
- Complications
  - Nerve/cord/vascular injury
  - Infection, epidural abscess

PROCEDURE

- Under fluoroscopy, navigable intradiscal catheter with thermal resistive coil is inserted into nucleus
- Heat conducted to annular wall
- Catheter tip should be within 5 mm of posterior vertebral margin

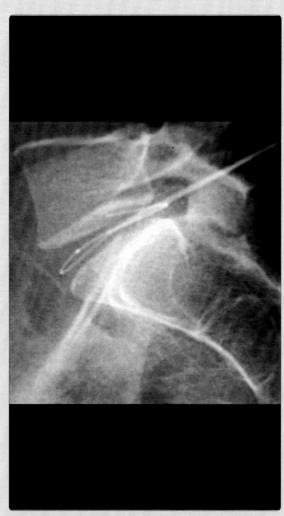

Navigable intradiscal catheter with thermal resistive coil is advanced anterolaterally inside nuclear tissue & directed circuitously to return posteriorly, providing an ideal position to heat the entire posterior annulus.

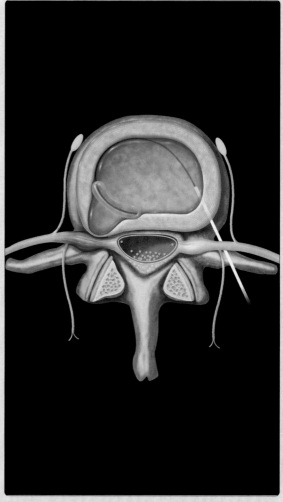

Axial graphic demonstrates a curved resistive heating wire threaded around the posterolateral annulus. The catheter tip should be within 5 mm of the posterior vertebral margin.

Nucleoplasty

TERMINOLOGY

- Method of percutaneous disc decompression using Coblation technology: Bipolar radiofrequency energy
- Radiofrequency energy dissolves portion of nucleus
- Advantage: Controlled and highly localized ablation resulting in minimal therapy damage to surrounding tissue

PREPROCEDURE

- Radicular/axial pain in lumbar/cervical spine
  - Leg pain > back pain
  - Unilateral radiculopathy or generalized cervical pain derived from contained herniated discs
  - MR evidence of contained herniated disc protrusion
  - Failure of 6 weeks of conservative therapy
- Axial back pain
  - MR evidence of contained disc protrusion
  - Discography positive for concordant pain
  - Failure of 6 weeks of conservative therapy

CONTRAINDICATIONS

- Large, noncontained disc herniation, sequestration, or extrusion
- Severe degenerative disc with > 33% loss of disc height
- Equivocal results of provocative and analgesic discogram
- Infection, tumor, fracture
- Cauda equina syndrome or newly developed signs of neurological deficit
- Uncontrolled coagulopathy and bleeding disorders

PROCEDURE

- Prone or decubitus position
- ~ 17-gauge needle introduced into posterolateral corner of disc through posterolateral extrapedicular approach

COMPLICATIONS

- Nerve or cord injury
- Vascular injury

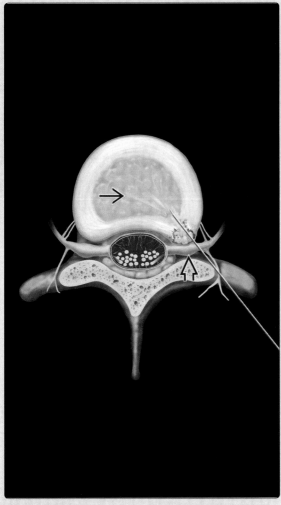

Axial graphic shows a probe removing a portion of the nucleus pulposus ➡. There is a focal contained left foraminal disc protrusion impinging upon the exiting nerve ➡.

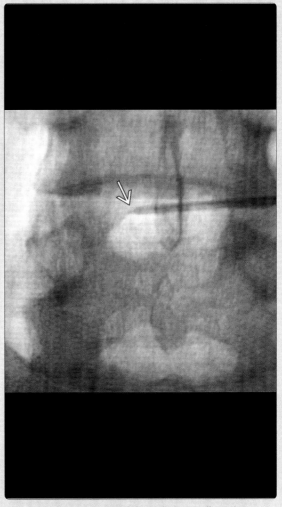

A wand-like device inserted through the needle and into the disc ➡ uses heat to remove disc material and seal the channel made by the needle. The needle should not transgress the transpedicular line.

TERMINOLOGY

- Fine-needle aspiration of intervertebral disc material ± core biopsy

PREPROCEDURE

- Coagulopathy/anticoagulation studies
  - Prothrombin time, activated partial thromboplastin time, international normalized ratio
  - Hemoglobin, hematocrit, and platelet count
- Suspected osteomyelitis/discitis
  - To confirm infectious organism

PROCEDURE

- For thoracic and lumbar levels use "Scotty dog" anatomy
  - Superimpose superior endplate of vertebra below disc to be intervened upon
  - Place "ear" of "Scotty dog" (superior articular process) at center of intervertebral disc by angling AP fluoroscopy plane toward desired side

- Needle entry should be at junction of middle 1/3 and outer 1/3 of disc (in front of Scotty dog "ear")
- CT guidance often preferred for cervical upper/mid thoracic disc aspiration/biopsies
  - Ensure patient can receive iodinated contrast if desired

POST PROCEDURE

- Careful evaluation for new neurologic symptoms following procedure

OUTCOMES

- Problem: Nondiagnostic specimen
- Most feared complications
  - Dural puncture with spinal cord injury, meningitis, or compressive epidural hematoma

---

"Scotty Dog" Anatomy

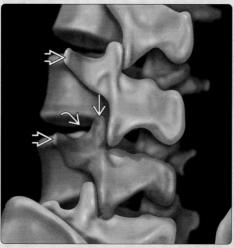

Needle Placement: CT Guidance

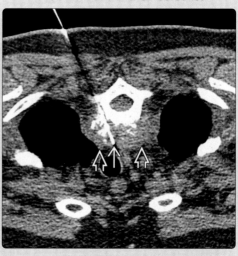

(Left) Oblique graphic shows "Scotty dog" anatomy at the L4 and L5 ➡ levels. Note the simulated needle placement ➡ with the needle entry just anterior to the superior articular process ("ear") ➡ at the midportion of the disc. (Right) This axial image is from the same patient after needle placement for L1/2 FNA/biopsy. Under intermittent CT guidance, the needle was advanced until the tip ➡ was within the anterior aspect of the soft tissue inflammatory changes ➡.

Preprocedure Imaging: Sagittal MR

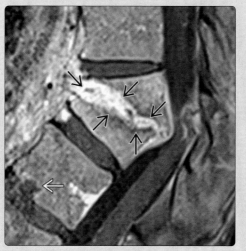

Needle Placement: Lateral View

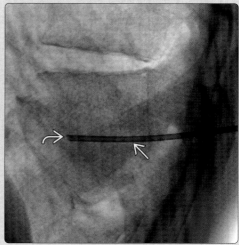

(Left) Sagittal contrast-enhanced, T1-weighted, fat-saturated MR in the same patient shows abnormal enhancement throughout the T10/11 disc and along the adjacent vertebral endplates ➡. Compare this appearance with that of a Schmorl node (intravertebral disc herniation) ➡. (Right) Lateral fluoroscopic spot radiograph in the same patient shows a 15-gauge biopsy cannula passing through the T10/11 disc space ➡ and into the superior endplate of T11 ➡.

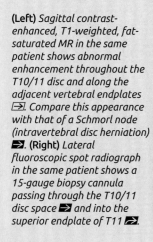

TERMINOLOGY

Definitions

- Fine-needle aspiration (FNA) or core biopsy of intervertebral disc material ± vertebral endplate

PREPROCEDURE

Indications

- Suspected osteomyelitis/discitis

Contraindications

- Coagulopathy
- Inability to tolerate prolonged prone positioning

Getting Started

- Things to check
  - Laboratory data
    - Coagulopathy/anticoagulation studies
      - Prothrombin time, activated partial thromboplastin time, international normalized ratio
      - Hemoglobin, hematocrit, and platelet count
    - Infection/inflammatory markers
      - White blood cell count, C-reactive protein, erythrocyte sedimentation rate
  - Imaging studies
    - Look for most accessible site if multiple sites of abnormality
  - Clinical presentation/history
    - Is patient taking antibiotics?
    - Anticoagulation/antiplatelet therapy?
- Equipment list
  - Needle for FNA/biopsy
    - May choose 22- to 25-gauge Chiba needle for FNA
      - Smaller gauge needle may be inadequate in setting of tenacious, purulent material
    - Larger gauge system preferred if doing biopsy (e.g., 13- to 16-gauge needle)
  - Specimen containers
    - Formalin vs. saline for tissue samples, depending on pathology suspected/institution protocol
      - Nonbacteriostatic saline for suspected infection

PROCEDURE

Equipment Preparation

- Imaging modality considerations
  - Fluoroscopy
    - Biplane allows easier triangulation compared with single plane/C-arm
      - Easier to frequently check AP and lateral fluoroscopy to ensure safe needle trajectory
  - CT
    - Preferred for cervical and thoracic discs by many interventionalists
    - Ensure renal function/contrast compatibility if intravenous contrast is contemplated
      - BUN/creatinine and glomerular filtration rate should be known
    - CT fluoroscopy generally offers shorter procedure times and lower radiation exposure to patient compared with conventional CT

Procedure Steps

- Insert FNA/biopsy needle
  - Utilize intermittent fluoroscopy to ensure safe trajectory
  - Check AP and lateral fluoroscopy to triangulate once needle anchored under skin
  - Obtain spot radiograph to document correct level and successful needle placement
- If bone encountered, usual culprit is facet
  - Check oblique/lateral fluoroscopy
  - If confirmed to be facet angle anteriorly
    - Often requires withdrawal (1-2 cm) 1st to allow redirection of needle tip
- Warn patient when passing near nerve root and prior to puncturing disc
  - May decrease sudden motion in response to pain
- Advance carefully under fluoroscopic guidance into disc
  - Where to start sampling depends on underlying pathology
    - Generally recommend sampling inflamed portion of disc/endplate such that sample includes nucleus, annulus, and endplate
    - FNA/biopsy of paraspinal inflammation may also increase diagnostic yield
- FNA
  - Apply small syringe (usually 3-5 mL) to 18- to 22-gauge Chiba needle, and gently aspirate
- Biopsy
  - e.g., Ostycut (Bard; Helsingborg, Sweden), Bonopty (AprioMed; Uppsala, Sweden): Remove needle, attach syringe, lock back, advance biopsy system slowly under fluoroscopy, release suction, withdraw specimen
- CT-guided FNA/biopsy
  - Cervical discs
    - Intravenous contrast helpful for improved visualization of vascular structures
    - Upper cervical spine
      - Positioning and skin entry depend on target lesion
    - Anterolateral approach
      - Preferred method for C4-T1 level
      - Can be used for CT- or fluoroscopy-guided procedure
      - Manually displace carotid artery and jugular vein posterolaterally
      - Atropine (0.6-1.0 mg) intravenously is recommended to avoid vasovagal response to manipulation of carotid body
      - Advance needle anterior to fingertips at ~ 30-40° angle between vessels and airway

POST PROCEDURE

Things to Avoid

- Dural puncture
- Intraspinal or extraspinal hematoma
- Meningitis
- Spinal cord injury

TERMINOLOGY

Definitions

- Sacrum is large triangular bone formed from 5 fused vertebrae at base of vertebral column

GROSS ANATOMY

Overview

- **Sacrum**
  - Consists of 5 fused vertebrae (S1-5)
  - Large, triangular-shaped; forms dorsal aspect of pelvis
  - 3 surfaces: Pelvic, dorsal, & lateral
  - Base: Articulates superiorly with L5
  - Apex: Articulates inferiorly with coccyx
- **Coccyx**
  - Consists of 3-5 rudimentary fused segments

Components of Sacrum

- **Bones**
  - Central body, lateral sacral ala, posterior triangular-shaped sacral canal
  - 4 paired ventral & dorsal sacral foramina extend laterally from sacral canal to pelvic & dorsal surfaces, respectively
  - **Pelvic surface**
    - Concave, forms dorsal aspect of pelvis
    - 4 paired anterior sacral foramina
    - 4 transverse ridges between anterior sacral foramina
  - **Dorsal surface**
    - Convex
    - **Median sacral crest** in midline ≈ fused spinous processes
    - Sacral groove on either side of crest
    - **Intermediate sacral crest** lateral to groove ≈ fused remnants of articular processes
    - 4 paired posterior sacral foramina are lateral to intermediate crest
    - **Lateral sacral crest** lateral to foramina ≈ remnants of transverse processes
    - **Sacral hiatus**: Dorsal bony opening below termination of median sacral crest
  - Lateral surface
    - Broad upper part, tapers inferiorly
    - Ventral articular surface for sacroiliac joint & dorsal roughened area for ligamentous attachment
- **Joints**
  - **Lumbosacral junction**
    - Joins with 5th lumbar vertebra by L5-S1 disc & facet joints
    - Superior base articulates with L5
    - Superior articular processes of S1 faces dorsally
  - **Sacrococcygeal joint**
    - Apex of sacrum & base of coccyx
    - Contains fibrocartilaginous disc
  - **Sacroiliac joints**
    - Ventral synovial joint: Between hyaline-covered articular surface of sacrum & fibrocartilage-covered surface of iliac bone
    - Dorsal syndesmosis: Interosseous sacroiliac ligament
- **Soft tissues**
  - **Thecal sac**
    - Thecal sac terminates at S2 level
    - Extradural component of filum terminale continues from S2 to attach at 1st coccygeal segment
  - **Nerves**
    - Sacral canal contains sacral & coccygeal nerve roots
    - Nerves emerge via ventral & dorsal sacral foramina
  - **Muscles**
    - **Piriformis**: Arises from ventral sacrum, passes laterally through greater sciatic foramen to insert on greater trochanter; nerves of sacral plexus pass along anterior surface of piriformis muscle
    - Gluteus maximus, erector spinae, & multifidus arise from dorsal sacrum
  - **Ligaments**
    - Anterior longitudinal ligament passes over sacral promontory
    - Posterior longitudinal ligament on dorsal surface of lumbosacral disc forming ventral margin of bony canal
    - Sacroiliac joint secured by broad anterior, interosseous, & posterior sacroiliac ligaments
    - Sacrospinous ligament bridges lateral sacrum to ischial spine
    - Sacrotuberous ligament bridges lateral sacrum to ischial tuberosity

IMAGING ANATOMY

Overview

- Lumbosacral junction
  - **Transitional vertebrae**
    - 25% of normal cases
    - **Sacralization** of lumbar body: Spectrum from expanded transverse processes of L5 articulating with top of sacrum to incorporation of L5 into sacrum
    - **Lumbarization** of sacrum: Elevation of S1 above sacral fusion mass assuming lumbar body shape
  - Sacrum lies at 40° incline from horizontal at lumbosacral junction
    - Axial load results in rotational forces at lumbosacral junction
    - Rotation forces checked by sacrotuberous, sacrospinous ligaments

ANATOMY IMAGING ISSUES

Imaging Pitfalls

- Lumbarization & sacralization may appear similar, require counting from C2 caudally to precisely define anatomy

SACRUM AND PUBIC SYMPHYSIS

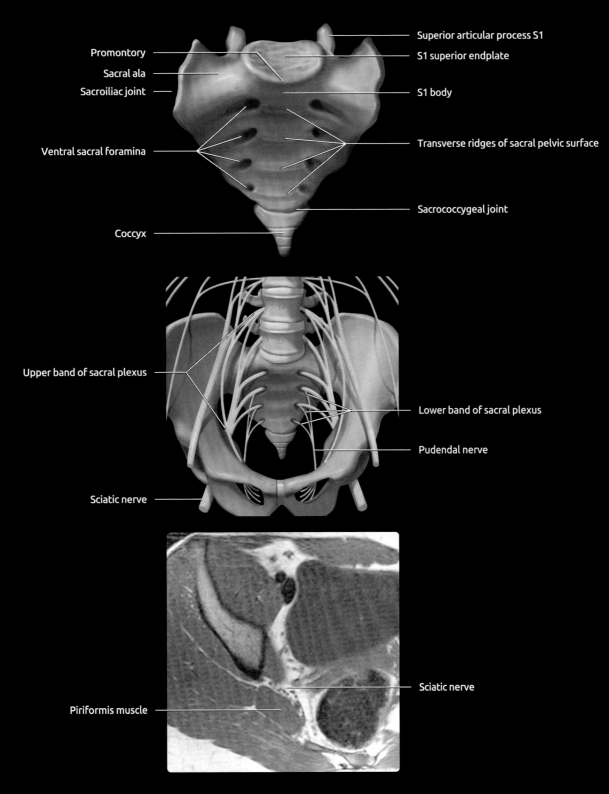

Promontory

Sacral ala

Sacroiliac joint

Ventral sacral foramina

Coccyx

Superior articular process S1

S1 superior endplate

S1 body

Transverse ridges of sacral pelvic surface

Sacrococcygeal joint

Upper band of sacral plexus

Sciatic nerve

Lower band of sacral plexus

Pudendal nerve

Piriformis muscle

Sciatic nerve

(Top) *Anterior graphic shows the sacrum, a large fused bony mass of 5 vertebra forming the posterior aspect of the pelvis. The superior articular facets arise off of the sacrum & articulate with the inferior articular processes of L5 to form the lumbosacral junction.* **(Middle)** *Coronal graphic depicts the upper and lower sacral bands of the sacral plexus. The primary terminal branch of the upper sacral band is the sciatic nerve, which supplies many thigh and all leg muscles (via the tibial and common peroneal nerves). The lower sacral band forms the pudendal nerve to the perineum.* **(Bottom)** *Oblique axial T1WI MR shows the sciatic nerve on the ventral piriformis muscle. Although the nerve (largest single nerve in the body) is enveloped by epineurium, the abundant fibrofatty epineurium gives the impression that the individual fascicles are free in pelvic fat.*

TERMINOLOGY

- Image-guided injection of corticosteroid and long-acting anesthetic into sacroiliac (SI) joint

PREPROCEDURE

- Indications
  - Diagnostic injection for hip/back/buttock pain
  - Sacroiliitis
  - Synovial cyst associated with SI joint

PROCEDURE

- Prone
  - Oblique tube angulation to "open" SI joint
- Advance needle under intermittent imaging until "pop" into joint space is felt or bone is reached
- Inject small amount of contrast under fluoroscopy to confirm intraarticular needle placement
  - Should see contrast track cephalad along SI joint

- Should **not** see pooling or "feathering" of contrast at needle tip
- Take note of pain before, during, and after injection
  - Whether or not concordant pain was elicited during procedure

OUTCOMES

- Expected
  - Improved pain score following injection
- Problems
  - Pain not relieved
  - Vasovagal reaction
  - Clinical failure: SI joint not pain generator
  - Technical failure: Extraarticular injection
- Most feared complications
  - Infection
  - Osteomyelitis
  - Septic joint

Sacral Anatomy

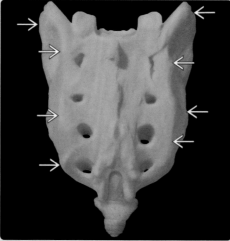

SI Joint Anatomy

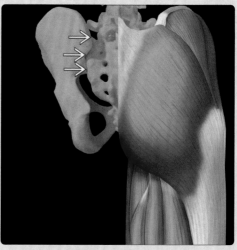

(Left) Graphic depicting a posterior view of the sacrum shows the angular configuration of the sacral ala ➡, which results in the complex oblique orientation of the sacroiliac (SI) joints. (Right) Graphic shows complex oblique articulation of the left SI joint ➡ and overlying gluteal and hamstring muscular groups as well as ligamentous supporting structures on the right.

Intraarticular Injection: Right Side

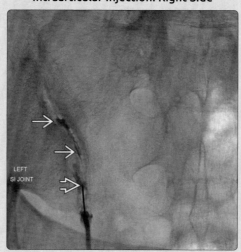

Extraarticular/Intramuscular Injection

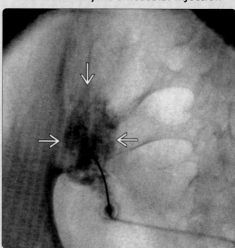

(Left) Anteroposterior fluoroscopic spot radiograph shows contrast injection within the left SI joint ➡. Note contrast extending cephalad within the synovial joint, away from the needle tip ➡. (Right) An overzealous contrast injection, as in this fluoroscopic spot radiograph, demonstrates a dilute, somewhat "feathery" appearance of contrast ➡ in keeping with an extraarticular, predominantly intramuscular injection.

TERMINOLOGY

Definitions

- Image-guided injection of corticosteroid and long-acting anesthetic into sacroiliac (SI) joint

PREPROCEDURE

Indications

- Diagnostic injection for hip/back/buttock pain
- Sacroiliitis
- Synovial cyst associated with SI joint

Contraindications

- Systemic or local infection
- Coagulopathy
- Allergy to injectate

Getting Started

- Things to check
  ○ Preprocedure imaging
    - Assess anatomy of SI joint
    - Look for osseous fusion
  ○ Coagulation parameters
  ○ Informed consent

PROCEDURE

Patient Position/Location

- Best procedure approach
  ○ Prone
    - Oblique tube angulation to "open" SI joint and establish needle trajectory
    - Target inferior 1/3 of SI joint

Procedure Steps

- Procedure "time out"
  ○ Correct patient, procedure, side
- Establish proper x-ray tube angulation to visualize joint space
- Mark skin overlying lower 1/3 of SI joint
- Perform sterile prep and drape
- Apply local anesthetic superficially and deep
- Spot fluoroscopy or CT imaging of numbing needle is helpful to confirm skin entry and needle trajectory
- Remove 25-gauge needle and anchor 22-gauge spinal needle in subcutaneous tissue
- Reconfirm skin entry and needle trajectory with fluoroscopy or CT imaging
- Advance needle under intermittent imaging until "pop" into joint space is felt or bone is reached
- If bone is encountered, confirm with imaging and "walk" needle tip into joint
- Remove stylette and observe hub of needle for blood
- Attach contrast tubing/syringe and gently aspirate to confirm extravascular needle tip position
- Inject small amount of contrast under fluoroscopy to confirm intraarticular needle placement
  ○ Watch for vascular opacification
  ○ Should see contrast track cephalad along SI joint
- Obtain spot radiograph to document intraarticular injection
- Attach injectate syringe and slowly inject

○ Take note of pain character and intensity before, during, and after injection

Alternative Procedures/Therapies

- Radiologic
  ○ Lumbar or sacral nerve root block
  ○ Caudal epidural steroid injection
- Surgical
  ○ Fusion
- Other
  ○ Cryoanalgesia

POST PROCEDURE

Expected Outcome

- Partial or complete cessation of pain related to SI joint

Things to Do

- Assist patient from procedure room
- Establish clinical follow-up
- Remind patient to keep a pain diary until next clinic visit

Things to Avoid

- Bathing for 48-72 hours

OUTCOMES

Problems

- Pain not relieved
  ○ Clinical failure
    - SI joint not pain generator
  ○ Technical failure
    - Extraarticular injection
- Vasovagal reaction

Complications

- Most feared complication(s)
  ○ Infection
    - Osteomyelitis
    - Septic joint
- Other complications
  ○ Bleeding
  ○ Nerve injury

SELECTED REFERENCES

1. Stone JA et al: Treatment of facet and sacroiliac joint arthropathy: steroid injections and radiofrequency ablation. Tech Vasc Interv Radiol. 12(1):22-32, 2009
2. Fritz J et al: Management of chronic low back pain: rationales, principles, and targets of imaging-guided spinal injections. Radiographics. 27(6):1751-71, 2007
3. Dussault RG et al: Fluoroscopy-guided sacroiliac joint injections. Radiology. 214(1):273-7, 2000

TERMINOLOGY

- Selective corticosteroid and long-acting anesthetic injection of sacral nerve root at level of neural foramen

PREPROCEDURE

- Malignant or benign neoplasm
- Imaging
  - Evaluate relevant anatomic landmarks
  - Search for other causes of patient pain

PROCEDURE

- Anchor 22-gauge spinal needle in subcutaneous tissue and confirm trajectory with fluoroscopy
  - Right side: Target foramen at 1-2 o'clock
  - Left side: Target foramen at 10-11 o'clock
- Pain score
  - Note patient pain before, during, and after injection
  - Whether pain was reproduced during procedure
- Alternatives
  - Caudal epidural steroid injection
  - Lumbar nerve root block
  - Sacroiliac injection

OUTCOMES

- Expected
  - Reproduction of pain during injection
  - Significant relief of pain following injection
- Problems
  - Extraforaminal injection failure of pain control/false-negative study
  - Diagnostic failure: Wrong level or selected root not sole pain generator
  - Nerve root injury, bleeding, infection
  - Vasovagal reaction

(Left) Anterior view of a 3D-VR NECT examination of the sacrum shows the location at which the sacral nerve roots exit via the 4 paired sacral foramina ⟶. The superior aspect of the sacrum articulates with the inferior endplate of L5. (Right) Sagittal T2WI MR shows multiple thin-walled cysts ⟶ within the sacral canal and enlarged neural foramina. Note displacement of the dorsal root ganglia peripherally ⟶.

Preprocedure Imaging: 3D CT

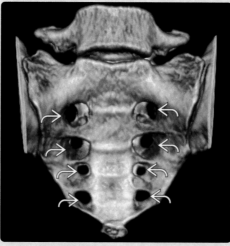

Perineural Cysts

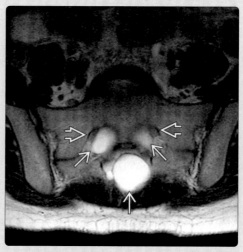

(Left) Fluoroscopic radiograph from a left S1 selective nerve root block shows that the needle appears centrally placed within the foramen on this view, and contrast is seen to fill a portion of the foramen ⟶ and track along the expected course of the exiting nerve root ⟶. (Right) Lateral fluoroscopic spot radiograph after contrast injection ⟶ shows that the needle tip ⟶ is in the superficial aspect of the neural foramen. Contrast outlines the neural foramen and extends slightly along the nerve root. This confirms satisfactory needle placement.

Foraminal Contrast Injection: AP View

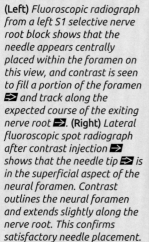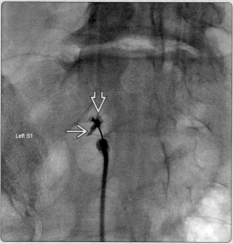

Needle Placement Confirmed: Lateral View

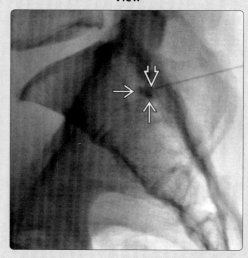

TERMINOLOGY

Abbreviations

- Nerve root block (NRB)

Synonyms

- Sacral selective nerve root injection

Definitions

- Selective corticosteroid and long-acting anesthetic injection of sacral nerve root at level of neural foramen

PREPROCEDURE

Indications

- Radiculopathy corresponding to sacral nerve root dermatome
- Acute or chronic sacral radiculopathy
- Osteoarthritis
- Compression of sacral nerve root

Contraindications

- Coagulopathy
- Allergy to components of injectate
- Local or systemic infection

Getting Started

- Things to check
  - Preprocedure imaging
    - Evaluate relevant anatomic landmarks
    - Search for other causes of patient's pain
  - Laboratory data
    - Evidence of infection or impaired coagulation
  - Informed consent

PROCEDURE

Patient Position/Location

- Best procedure approach
  - Prone
    - Angle of C-arm depends on lumbosacral lordosis

Equipment Preparation

- Draw 5 mL of local anesthetic, and attach 1.5-inch 25-gauge needle
- Draw 5 mL of myelography-safe contrast, and preload extension tubing
  - Tubing should be air-free
- Draw injectate
  - Generally 2 mL [e.g., 1 mL (80 mg) methylprednisolone + 1 mL 0.5% bupivacaine]

Procedure Steps

- Procedure "time out"
  - Correct patient, procedure, and side
- Angle C-arm to obtain optimal visualization of targeted sacral neural foramen
- Perform sterile prep and drape
- Create skin wheal with local anesthetic, and anesthetize subcutaneous tissues
- Anchor 22-gauge spinal needle in subcutaneous tissue, and confirm trajectory with fluoroscopy
  - Right side: Target foramen at 1-2 o'clock

- Left side: Target foramen at 10-11 o'clock
- Carefully advance spinal needle under intermittent fluoroscopy until intraforaminal or bone is reached
- If bone is reached, carefully "walk" needle into upper outer quadrant of foramen
- Remove stylette, and attach contrast tubing/syringe
- Inject contrast slowly
  - Communicate with patient prior to and during injection to
    - Avoid sudden movement secondary to pain
    - Learn whether or not pain is reproduced
  - Look for contrast flowing away
    - Intravascular injection
- Once needle tip position is confirmed in target foramen, attach injectate syringe
- Inject slowly
  - Note patient's pain before, during, and after injection
- Remove needle, and obtain hemostasis

Alternative Procedures/Therapies

- Radiologic
  - Caudal epidural steroid injection
  - Lumbar NRB
  - Sacroiliac injection
- Surgical
  - Decompression

POST PROCEDURE

Expected Outcome

- Significant reduction in pain related to nerve root injected

OUTCOMES

Problems

- Failure of pain control
  - Technical failure: Extraforaminal injection
  - Diagnostic failure: Sacral nerve root not sole pain generator
- Vasovagal reaction

Complications

- Most feared complication(s)
  - Nerve root injury
- Other complications
  - Bleeding, infection

SELECTED REFERENCES

1. Williams AP et al: The value of lumbar dorsal root ganglion blocks in predicting the response to decompressive surgery in patients with diagnostic doubt. Spine J. 15(3 Suppl):S44-9, 2015
2. Fritz J et al: Magnetic resonance neurography-guided nerve blocks for the diagnosis and treatment of chronic pelvic pain syndrome. Neuroimaging Clin N Am. 24(1):211-34, 2014
3. Boezaart AP et al: Paravertebral block: cervical, thoracic, lumbar, and sacral. Curr Opin Anaesthesiol. 22(5):637-43, 2009
4. Vranken JH et al: Continuous sacral nerve root block in the management of neuropathic cancer pain. Anesth Analg. 95(6):1724-5, table of contents, 2002

Image-Guided Procedures

TERMINOLOGY

- Selective image-guided injection of long-acting anesthetic and corticosteroid into piriformis muscle adjacent to sciatic nerve in treatment of piriformis syndrome
  - Some advocate intramuscular botulinum toxin A injection

PREPROCEDURE

- Injection is generally reserved for cases in which conservative measures/physical therapy have failed
- Preprocedure imaging
  - Look for signs of lumbosacral plexus compression
  - Evaluate sacroiliac joints
  - Rule out hip joint abnormality
  - Evaluate for pelvic musculature abnormality/asymmetry
- Nerve stimulator may further assist in confirming needle tip placement prior to injection

PROCEDURE

- Optimize patient positioning depending on imaging technique to be used
  - Can be guided by fluoroscopy, CT, or ultrasound
- Advance needle with intermittent imaging guidance until within fascial plane/muscle sheath at superficial margin of piriformis muscle
  - Intramuscular placement for botulinum toxin A injection
- Note patient's pain before, during, and after injection
- Complications:
  - Sciatic nerve injury
  - Bleeding, infection

POST PROCEDURE

- Maximal benefit may take 48-72 hours when corticosteroid takes full effect

Piriformis Syndrome

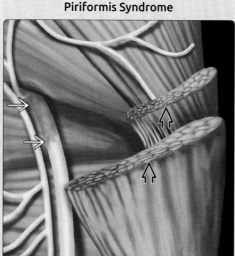

Anatomy

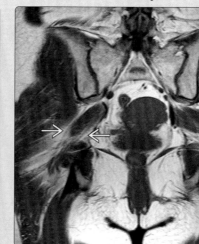

(Left) Red, swollen sciatic nerve ➡ passes through the sciatic notch in this patient with compressive neuropathy caused by an enlarged piriformis muscle. The gluteal musculature has been cut away ⊟. (Right) Coronal T1 MR shows sciatic nerve fibers ➡ on either side of the piriformis muscle. This is the most common anomalous course of the sciatic nerve, which may predispose patients to the piriformis syndrome.

Needle Placement: Final

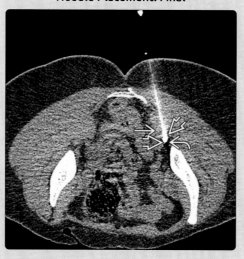

Contrast Tracking Adjacent to Sciatic Nerve

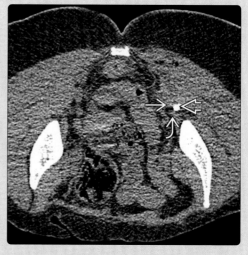

(Left) Axial CT image shows a dark artifact ➡ signifying the needle tip, which lies along the ventral margin of the piriformis ➡ muscle. The added hyperdensity ➡ at the tip is iodinated contrast. Always ensure that imaging includes the needle tip. (Right) Post contrast injection CT image confirms that the injection site ➡ is immediately lateral to the sciatic nerve ➡ along the ventral piriformis muscle ➡. With injection, the patient's symptoms immediately improved.

TERMINOLOGY

Definitions

- Selective image-guided injection of long-acting anesthetic and corticosteroid into piriformis muscle adjacent to sciatic nerve in treatment of piriformis syndrome
  - Some advocate intramuscular botulinum toxin A injection

PREPROCEDURE

Indications

- Piriformis syndrome
  - Buttock and leg pain (one of myriad causes of sciatica)
    - Hypertrophied piriformis muscle
    - Posttraumatic
      - Often sequelae of fall injury, fibrosis
- Sciatic notch pain
- Injection is generally reserved for cases in which conservative measures/physical therapy have failed

Contraindications

- Coagulopathy
- Systemic infection
- Known severe allergy to components of injectate

Getting Started

- Things to check
  - Preprocedure imaging
    - Look for signs of lumbosacral plexus compression
    - Evaluate sacroiliac (SI) joints
    - Rule out hip joint abnormality
    - Evaluate for pelvic musculature abnormality/asymmetry
      - Hypertrophic piriformis muscle
  - Laboratory data
    - Coagulation parameters
  - Informed consent

PROCEDURE

Patient Position/Location

- Best procedure approach
  - Fluoroscopy
    - Identify line connecting inferior aspect of sacroiliac joint and superolateral margin of acetabulum
    - Optimal target is 1/3 of distance from superolateral acetabulum along that line (2/3 of distance away from SI joint)
  - Computed tomography (CT)
    - Direct axial images with patient prone
    - Target is piriformis muscle adjacent to sciatic nerve

Procedure Steps

- Procedure "time out"
  - Identify correct patient, procedure, and correct side to be intervened upon
- Fluoroscopy
  - Place radiopaque marker over skin ~ 1/3 of distance medial to superolateral acetabulum along line from superolateral acetabulum to inferior SI joint
  - Perform sterile prep and drape, anesthetic
  - Assess trajectory under fluoroscopy
  - Advance needle until ilium is encountered
  - Withdraw needle ~ 2 mm
  - Remove needle stylette, and observe for blood return, aspirate
  - Inject 0.5-1.0 mL contrast under fluoroscopy
    - Observe feathery intramuscular appearance
      - Necessary for botulinum toxin injections
  - Needle tip confirmation can also be achieved via nerve stimulation
  - Slowly inject corticosteroid/anesthetic
- CT
  - Place radiopaque marker over affected side at level of sciatic notch
  - Identify piriformis muscle and overlying fascial plane containing sciatic nerve
  - Mark skin at appropriate site to allow perpendicular needle access to piriformis muscle near sciatic nerve
  - Perform sterile prep and drape, anesthetic
  - Obtain limited CT scan/CT fluoroscopy to determine trajectory
  - Advance needle with intermittent imaging guidance until within fascial plane/muscle sheath at superficial margin of piriformis muscle
  - Remove stylette and observe hub for blood, aspirate
  - Inject 0.5-1.0 mL contrast under CT fluoroscopy if available
  - Needle tip confirmation can also be achieved via nerve stimulation
  - Slowly inject corticosteroid/anesthetic

Alternative Procedures/Therapies

- Radiologic
  - SI joint injection
  - Lumbar/sacral nerve root block
  - Caudal epidural steroid injection

POST PROCEDURE

Expected Outcome

- Improvement in pain following injection
  - Maximal benefit may take 48-72 hours when steroid takes full effect

OUTCOMES

Problems

- Failure of pain control
  - Technical failure
    - Injection not properly localized
  - Clinical failure
    - Misdiagnosed as piriformis syndrome

Complications

- Most feared complication(s)
  - Sciatic nerve injury
  - Infection

SELECTED REFERENCES

1. Gonzalez P et al: Confirmation of needle placement within the piriformis muscle of a cadaveric specimen using anatomic landmarks and fluoroscopic guidance. Pain Physician. 11(3):327-31, 2008

INDEX

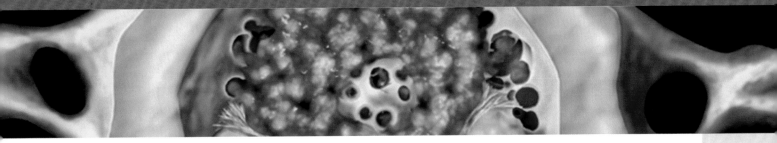

INDEX

INDEX

INDEX

INDEX

INDEX

INDEX

O

Q

R

S

INDEX